FREE Study Skills DVD Offer

Dear Customer,

Thank you for your purchase from Mometrix! We consider it an honor and a privilege that you have purchased our product and we want to ensure your satisfaction.

As a way of showing our appreciation and to help us better serve you, we have developed a Study Skills DVD that we would like to give you for FREE. This DVD covers our *best practices* for getting ready for your exam, from how to use our study materials to how to best prepare for the day of the test.

All that we ask is that you email us with feedback that would describe your experience so far with our product. Good, bad, or indifferent, we want to know what you think!

To get your FREE Study Skills DVD, email freedvd@mometrix.com with *FREE STUDY SKILLS DVD* in the subject line and the following information in the body of the email:

- The name of the product you purchased.
- Your product rating on a scale of 1-5, with 5 being the highest rating.
- Your feedback. It can be long, short, or anything in between. We just want to know your impressions and experience so far with our product. (Good feedback might include how our study material met your needs and ways we might be able to make it even better. You could highlight features that you found helpful or features that you think we should add.)
- Your full name and shipping address where you would like us to send your free DVD.

If you have any questions or concerns, please don't hesitate to contact me directly.

Thanks again!

Sincerely,

Jay Willis
Vice President
jay.willis@mometrix.com
1-800-673-8175

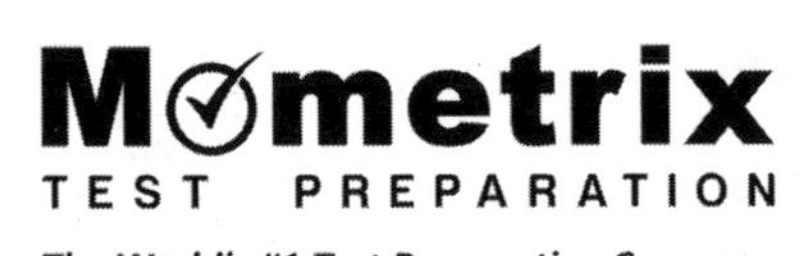

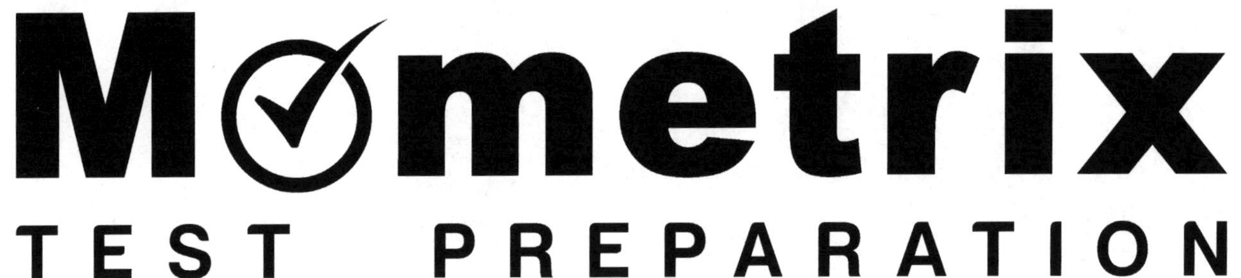

VTNE

Secrets Study Guide

Exam Review and VTNE Practice Test for the Veterinary Technician National Exam

Written and edited by Mometrix Test Prep

Printed in the United States of America

This paper meets the requirements of ANSI/NISO Z39.48-1992 (Permanence of Paper).

Paperback
ISBN 13: 978-1-5167-4801-3
ISBN 10: 1-5167-4801-8

DEAR FUTURE EXAM SUCCESS STORY

First of all, **THANK YOU** for purchasing Mometrix study materials!

Second, congratulations! You are one of the few determined test-takers who are committed to doing whatever it takes to excel on your exam. **You have come to the right place.** We developed these study materials with one goal in mind: to deliver you the information you need in a format that's concise and easy to use.

In addition to optimizing your guide for the content of the test, we've outlined our recommended steps for breaking down the preparation process into small, attainable goals so you can make sure you stay on track.

We've also analyzed the entire test-taking process, identifying the most common pitfalls and showing how you can overcome them and be ready for any curveball the test throws you.

Standardized testing is one of the biggest obstacles on your road to success, which only increases the importance of doing well in the high-pressure, high-stakes environment of test day. Your results on this test could have a significant impact on your future, and this guide provides the information and practical advice to help you achieve your full potential on test day.

Your success is our success

We would love to hear from you! If you would like to share the story of your exam success or if you have any questions or comments in regard to our products, please contact us at **800-673-8175** or **support@mometrix.com**.

Thanks again for your business and we wish you continued success!

Sincerely,
The Mometrix Test Preparation Team

TABLE OF CONTENTS

Introduction

Thank you for purchasing this resource! You have made the choice to prepare yourself for a test that could have a huge impact on your future, and this guide is designed to help you be fully ready for test day. Obviously, it's important to have a solid understanding of the test material, but you also need to be prepared for the unique environment and stressors of the test, so that you can perform to the best of your abilities.

For this purpose, the first section that appears in this guide is the **Secret Keys**. We've devoted countless hours to meticulously researching what works and what doesn't, and we've boiled down our findings to the five most impactful steps you can take to improve your performance on the test. We start at the beginning with study planning and move through the preparation process, all the way to the testing strategies that will help you get the most out of what you know when you're finally sitting in front of the test.

We recommend that you start preparing for your test as far in advance as possible. However, if you've bought this guide as a last-minute study resource and only have a few days before your test, we recommend that you skip over the first two Secret Keys since they address a long-term study plan.

If you struggle with **test anxiety**, we strongly encourage you to check out our recommendations for how you can overcome it. Test anxiety is a formidable foe, but it can be beaten, and we want to make sure you have the tools you need to defeat it.

Secret Key #1 – Plan Big, Study Small

There's a lot riding on your performance. If you want to ace this test, you're going to need to keep your skills sharp and the material fresh in your mind. You need a plan that lets you review everything you need to know while still fitting in your schedule. We'll break this strategy down into three categories.

Information Organization

Start with the information you already have: the official test outline. From this, you can make a complete list of all the concepts you need to cover before the test. Organize these concepts into groups that can be studied together, and create a list of any related vocabulary you need to learn so you can brush up on any difficult terms. You'll want to keep this vocabulary list handy once you actually start studying since you may need to add to it along the way.

Time Management

Once you have your set of study concepts, decide how to spread them out over the time you have left before the test. Break your study plan into small, clear goals so you have a manageable task for each day and know exactly what you're doing. Then just focus on one small step at a time. When you manage your time this way, you don't need to spend hours at a time studying. Studying a small block of content for a short period each day helps you retain information better and avoid stressing over how much you have left to do. You can relax knowing that you have a plan to cover everything in time. In order for this strategy to be effective though, you have to start studying early and stick to your schedule. Avoid the exhaustion and futility that comes from last-minute cramming!

Study Environment

The environment you study in has a big impact on your learning. Studying in a coffee shop, while probably more enjoyable, is not likely to be as fruitful as studying in a quiet room. It's important to keep distractions to a minimum. You're only planning to study for a short block of time, so make the most of it. Don't pause to check your phone or get up to find a snack. It's also important to **avoid multitasking**. Research has consistently shown that multitasking will make your studying dramatically less effective. Your study area should also be comfortable and well-lit so you don't have the distraction of straining your eyes or sitting on an uncomfortable chair.

The time of day you study is also important. You want to be rested and alert. Don't wait until just before bedtime. Study when you'll be most likely to comprehend and remember. Even better, if you know what time of day your test will be, set that time aside for study. That way your brain will be used to working on that subject at that specific time and you'll have a better chance of recalling information.

Finally, it can be helpful to team up with others who are studying for the same test. Your actual studying should be done in as isolated an environment as possible, but the work of organizing the information and setting up the study plan can be divided up. In between study sessions, you can discuss with your teammates the concepts that you're all studying and quiz each other on the details. Just be sure that your teammates are as serious about the test as you are. If you find that your study time is being replaced with social time, you might need to find a new team.

Secret Key #2 – Make Your Studying Count

You're devoting a lot of time and effort to preparing for this test, so you want to be absolutely certain it will pay off. This means doing more than just reading the content and hoping you can remember it on test day. It's important to make every minute of study count. There are two main areas you can focus on to make your studying count:

Retention

It doesn't matter how much time you study if you can't remember the material. You need to make sure you are retaining the concepts. To check your retention of the information you're learning, try recalling it at later times with minimal prompting. Try carrying around flashcards and glance at one or two from time to time or ask a friend who's also studying for the test to quiz you.

To enhance your retention, look for ways to put the information into practice so that you can apply it rather than simply recalling it. If you're using the information in practical ways, it will be much easier to remember. Similarly, it helps to solidify a concept in your mind if you're not only reading it to yourself but also explaining it to someone else. Ask a friend to let you teach them about a concept you're a little shaky on (or speak aloud to an imaginary audience if necessary). As you try to summarize, define, give examples, and answer your friend's questions, you'll understand the concepts better and they will stay with you longer. Finally, step back for a big picture view and ask yourself how each piece of information fits with the whole subject. When you link the different concepts together and see them working together as a whole, it's easier to remember the individual components.

Finally, practice showing your work on any multi-step problems, even if you're just studying. Writing out each step you take to solve a problem will help solidify the process in your mind, and you'll be more likely to remember it during the test.

Modality

Modality simply refers to the means or method by which you study. Choosing a study modality that fits your own individual learning style is crucial. No two people learn best in exactly the same way, so it's important to know your strengths and use them to your advantage.

For example, if you learn best by visualization, focus on visualizing a concept in your mind and draw an image or a diagram. Try color-coding your notes, illustrating them, or creating symbols that will trigger your mind to recall a learned concept. If you learn best by hearing or discussing information, find a study partner who learns the same way or read aloud to yourself. Think about how to put the information in your own words. Imagine that you are giving a lecture on the topic and record yourself so you can listen to it later.

For any learning style, flashcards can be helpful. Organize the information so you can take advantage of spare moments to review. Underline key words or phrases. Use different colors for different categories. Mnemonic devices (such as creating a short list in which every item starts with the same letter) can also help with retention. Find what works best for you and use it to store the information in your mind most effectively and easily.

Secret Key #3 – Practice the Right Way

Your success on test day depends not only on how many hours you put into preparing, but also on whether you prepared the right way. It's good to check along the way to see if your studying is paying off. One of the most effective ways to do this is by taking practice tests to evaluate your progress. Practice tests are useful because they show exactly where you need to improve. Every time you take a practice test, pay special attention to these three groups of questions:

- The questions you got wrong
- The questions you had to guess on, even if you guessed right
- The questions you found difficult or slow to work through

This will show you exactly what your weak areas are, and where you need to devote more study time. Ask yourself why each of these questions gave you trouble. Was it because you didn't understand the material? Was it because you didn't remember the vocabulary? Do you need more repetitions on this type of question to build speed and confidence? Dig into those questions and figure out how you can strengthen your weak areas as you go back to review the material.

Additionally, many practice tests have a section explaining the answer choices. It can be tempting to read the explanation and think that you now have a good understanding of the concept. However, an explanation likely only covers part of the question's broader context. Even if the explanation makes sense, **go back and investigate** every concept related to the question until you're positive you have a thorough understanding.

As you go along, keep in mind that the practice test is just that: practice. Memorizing these questions and answers will not be very helpful on the actual test because it is unlikely to have any of the same exact questions. If you only know the right answers to the sample questions, you won't be prepared for the real thing. **Study the concepts** until you understand them fully, and then you'll be able to answer any question that shows up on the test.

It's important to wait on the practice tests until you're ready. If you take a test on your first day of study, you may be overwhelmed by the amount of material covered and how much you need to learn. Work up to it gradually.

On test day, you'll need to be prepared for answering questions, managing your time, and using the test-taking strategies you've learned. It's a lot to balance, like a mental marathon that will have a big impact on your future. Like training for a marathon, you'll need to start slowly and work your way up. When test day arrives, you'll be ready.

Start with the strategies you've read in the first two Secret Keys—plan your course and study in the way that works best for you. If you have time, consider using multiple study resources to get different approaches to the same concepts. It can be helpful to see difficult concepts from more than one angle. Then find a good source for practice tests. Many times, the test website will suggest potential study resources or provide sample tests.

Practice Test Strategy

When you're ready to start taking practice tests, follow this strategy:

1. Take the first test with no time constraints and with your notes and study guide handy. Take your time and focus on applying the strategies you've learned.
2. Take the second practice test open-book as well, but set a timer and practice pacing yourself to finish in time.
3. Take any other practice tests as if it were test day. Set a timer and put away your study materials. Sit at a table or desk in a quiet room, imagine yourself at the testing center, and answer questions as quickly and accurately as possible.
4. Keep repeating step 3 on a regular basis until you run out of practice tests or it's time for the actual test. Your mind will be ready for the schedule and stress of test day, and you'll be able to focus on recalling the material you've learned.

Secret Key #4 – Pace Yourself

Once you're fully prepared for the material on the test, your biggest challenge on test day will be managing your time. Just knowing that the clock is ticking can make you panic even if you have plenty of time left. Work on pacing yourself so you can build confidence against the time constraints of the exam. Pacing is a difficult skill to master, especially in a high-pressure environment, so **practice is vital**.

Set time expectations for your pace based on how much time is available. For example, if a section has 60 questions and the time limit is 30 minutes, you know you have to average 30 seconds or less per question in order to answer them all. Although 30 seconds is the hard limit, set 25 seconds per question as your goal, so you reserve extra time to spend on harder questions. When you budget extra time for the harder questions, you no longer have any reason to stress when those questions take longer to answer.

Don't let this time expectation distract you from working through the test at a calm, steady pace, but keep it in mind so you don't spend too much time on any one question. Recognize that taking extra time on one question you don't understand may keep you from answering two that you do understand later in the test. If your time limit for a question is up and you're still not sure of the answer, mark it and move on, and come back to it later if the time and the test format allow. If the testing format doesn't allow you to return to earlier questions, just make an educated guess; then put it out of your mind and move on.

On the easier questions, be careful not to rush. It may seem wise to hurry through them so you have more time for the challenging ones, but it's not worth missing one if you know the concept and just didn't take the time to read the question fully. Work efficiently but make sure you understand the question and have looked at all of the answer choices, since more than one may seem right at first.

Even if you're paying attention to the time, you may find yourself a little behind at some point. You should speed up to get back on track, but do so wisely. Don't panic; just take a few seconds less on each question until you're caught up. Don't guess without thinking, but do look through the answer choices and eliminate any you know are wrong. If you can get down to two choices, it is often worthwhile to guess from those. Once you've chosen an answer, move on and don't dwell on any that you skipped or had to hurry through. If a question was taking too long, chances are it was one of the harder ones, so you weren't as likely to get it right anyway.

On the other hand, if you find yourself getting ahead of schedule, it may be beneficial to slow down a little. The more quickly you work, the more likely you are to make a careless mistake that will affect your score. You've budgeted time for each question, so don't be afraid to spend that time. Practice an efficient but careful pace to get the most out of the time you have.

Secret Key #5 – Have a Plan for Guessing

When you're taking the test, you may find yourself stuck on a question. Some of the answer choices seem better than others, but you don't see the one answer choice that is obviously correct. What do you do?

The scenario described above is very common, yet most test takers have not effectively prepared for it. Developing and practicing a plan for guessing may be one of the single most effective uses of your time as you get ready for the exam.

In developing your plan for guessing, there are three questions to address:

- When should you start the guessing process?
- How should you narrow down the choices?
- Which answer should you choose?

When to Start the Guessing Process

Unless your plan for guessing is to select C every time (which, despite its merits, is not what we recommend), you need to leave yourself enough time to apply your answer elimination strategies. Since you have a limited amount of time for each question, that means that if you're going to give yourself the best shot at guessing correctly, you have to decide quickly whether or not you will guess.

Of course, the best-case scenario is that you don't have to guess at all, so first, see if you can answer the question based on your knowledge of the subject and basic reasoning skills. Focus on the key words in the question and try to jog your memory of related topics. Give yourself a chance to bring the knowledge to mind, but once you realize that you don't have (or you can't access) the knowledge you need to answer the question, it's time to start the guessing process.

It's almost always better to start the guessing process too early than too late. It only takes a few seconds to remember something and answer the question from knowledge. Carefully eliminating wrong answer choices takes longer. Plus, going through the process of eliminating answer choices can actually help jog your memory.

Summary: Start the guessing process as soon as you decide that you can't answer the question based on your knowledge.

How to Narrow Down the Choices

The next chapter in this book (**Test-Taking Strategies**) includes a wide range of strategies for how to approach questions and how to look for answer choices to eliminate. You will definitely want to read those carefully, practice them, and figure out which ones work best for you. Here though, we're going to address a mindset rather than a particular strategy.

Your chances of guessing an answer correctly depend on how many options you are choosing from.

How many choices you have	How likely you are to guess correctly
5	20%
4	25%
3	33%
2	50%
1	100%

You can see from this chart just how valuable it is to be able to eliminate incorrect answers and make an educated guess, but there are two things that many test takers do that cause them to miss out on the benefits of guessing:

- Accidentally eliminating the correct answer
- Selecting an answer based on an impression

We'll look at the first one here, and the second one in the next section.

To avoid accidentally eliminating the correct answer, we recommend a thought exercise called **the $5 challenge**. In this challenge, you only eliminate an answer choice from contention if you are willing to bet $5 on it being wrong. Why $5? Five dollars is a small but not insignificant amount of money. It's an amount you could afford to lose but wouldn't want to throw away. And while losing $5 once might not hurt too much, doing it twenty times will set you back $100. In the same way, each small decision you make—eliminating a choice here, guessing on a question there—won't by itself impact your score very much, but when you put them all together, they can make a big difference. By holding each answer choice elimination decision to a higher standard, you can reduce the risk of accidentally eliminating the correct answer.

The $5 challenge can also be applied in a positive sense: If you are willing to bet $5 that an answer choice *is* correct, go ahead and mark it as correct.

Summary: Only eliminate an answer choice if you are willing to bet $5 that it is wrong.

Which Answer to Choose

You're taking the test. You've run into a hard question and decided you'll have to guess. You've eliminated all the answer choices you're willing to bet $5 on. Now you have to pick an answer. Why do we even need to talk about this? Why can't you just pick whichever one you feel like when the time comes?

The answer to these questions is that if you don't come into the test with a plan, you'll rely on your impression to select an answer choice, and if you do that, you risk falling into a trap. The test writers know that everyone who takes their test will be guessing on some of the questions, so they intentionally write wrong answer choices to seem plausible. You still have to pick an answer though, and if the wrong answer choices are designed to look right, how can you ever be sure that you're not falling for their trap? The best solution we've found to this dilemma is to take the decision out of your hands entirely. Here is the process we recommend:

Once you've eliminated any choices that you are confident (willing to bet $5) are wrong, select the first remaining choice as your answer.

Whether you choose to select the first remaining choice, the second, or the last, the important thing is that you use some preselected standard. Using this approach guarantees that you will not be enticed into selecting an answer choice that looks right, because you are not basing your decision on how the answer choices look.

This is not meant to make you question your knowledge. Instead, it is to help you recognize the difference between your knowledge and your impressions. There's a huge difference between thinking an answer is right because of what you know, and thinking an answer is right because it looks or sounds like it should be right.

Summary: To ensure that your selection is appropriately random, make a predetermined selection from among all answer choices you have not eliminated.

Test-Taking Strategies

This section contains a list of test-taking strategies that you may find helpful as you work through the test. By taking what you know and applying logical thought, you can maximize your chances of answering any question correctly!

It is very important to realize that every question is different and every person is different: no single strategy will work on every question, and no single strategy will work for every person. That's why we've included all of them here, so you can try them out and determine which ones work best for different types of questions and which ones work best for you.

Question Strategies

Read Carefully

Read the question and answer choices carefully. Don't miss the question because you misread the terms. You have plenty of time to read each question thoroughly and make sure you understand what is being asked. Yet a happy medium must be attained, so don't waste too much time. You must read carefully, but efficiently.

Contextual Clues

Look for contextual clues. If the question includes a word you are not familiar with, look at the immediate context for some indication of what the word might mean. Contextual clues can often give you all the information you need to decipher the meaning of an unfamiliar word. Even if you can't determine the meaning, you may be able to narrow down the possibilities enough to make a solid guess at the answer to the question.

Prefixes

If you're having trouble with a word in the question or answer choices, try dissecting it. Take advantage of every clue that the word might include. Prefixes and suffixes can be a huge help. Usually they allow you to determine a basic meaning. Pre- means before, post- means after, pro - is positive, de- is negative. From prefixes and suffixes, you can get an idea of the general meaning of the word and try to put it into context.

Hedge Words

Watch out for critical hedge words, such as *likely*, *may*, *can*, *sometimes*, *often*, *almost*, *mostly*, *usually*, *generally*, *rarely*, and *sometimes*. Question writers insert these hedge phrases to cover every possibility. Often an answer choice will be wrong simply because it leaves no room for exception. Be on guard for answer choices that have definitive words such as *exactly* and *always*.

Switchback Words

Stay alert for *switchbacks*. These are the words and phrases frequently used to alert you to shifts in thought. The most common switchback words are *but*, *although*, and *however*. Others include *nevertheless*, *on the other hand*, *even though*, *while*, *in spite of*, *despite*, *regardless of*. Switchback words are important to catch because they can change the direction of the question or an answer choice.

Face Value

When in doubt, use common sense. Accept the situation in the problem at face value. Don't read too much into it. These problems will not require you to make wild assumptions. If you have to go beyond creativity and warp time or space in order to have an answer choice fit the question, then you should move on and consider the other answer choices. These are normal problems rooted in reality. The applicable relationship or explanation may not be readily apparent, but it is there for you to figure out. Use your common sense to interpret anything that isn't clear.

Answer Choice Strategies

Answer Selection

The most thorough way to pick an answer choice is to identify and eliminate wrong answers until only one is left, then confirm it is the correct answer. Sometimes an answer choice may immediately seem right, but be careful. The test writers will usually put more than one reasonable answer choice on each question, so take a second to read all of them and make sure that the other choices are not equally obvious. As long as you have time left, it is better to read every answer choice than to pick the first one that looks right without checking the others.

Answer Choice Families

An answer choice family consists of two (in rare cases, three) answer choices that are very similar in construction and cannot all be true at the same time. If you see two answer choices that are direct opposites or parallels, one of them is usually the correct answer. For instance, if one answer choice says that quantity *x* increases and another either says that quantity *x* decreases (opposite) or says that quantity *y* increases (parallel), then those answer choices would fall into the same family. An answer choice that doesn't match the construction of the answer choice family is more likely to be incorrect. Most questions will not have answer choice families, but when they do appear, you should be prepared to recognize them.

Eliminate Answers

Eliminate answer choices as soon as you realize they are wrong, but make sure you consider all possibilities. If you are eliminating answer choices and realize that the last one you are left with is also wrong, don't panic. Start over and consider each choice again. There may be something you missed the first time that you will realize on the second pass.

Avoid Fact Traps

Don't be distracted by an answer choice that is factually true but doesn't answer the question. You are looking for the choice that answers the question. Stay focused on what the question is asking for so you don't accidentally pick an answer that is true but incorrect. Always go back to the question and make sure the answer choice you've selected actually answers the question and is not merely a true statement.

Extreme Statements

In general, you should avoid answers that put forth extreme actions as standard practice or proclaim controversial ideas as established fact. An answer choice that states the "process should be used in certain situations, if..." is much more likely to be correct than one that states the "process should be discontinued completely." The first is a calm rational statement and doesn't even make a definitive, uncompromising stance, using a hedge word *if* to provide wiggle room, whereas the second choice is a radical idea and far more extreme.

Benchmark

As you read through the answer choices and you come across one that seems to answer the question well, mentally select that answer choice. This is not your final answer, but it's the one that will help you evaluate the other answer choices. The one that you selected is your benchmark or standard for judging each of the other answer choices. Every other answer choice must be compared to your benchmark. That choice is correct until proven otherwise by another answer choice beating it. If you find a better answer, then that one becomes your new benchmark. Once you've decided that no other choice answers the question as well as your benchmark, you have your final answer.

Predict the Answer

Before you even start looking at the answer choices, it is often best to try to predict the answer. When you come up with the answer on your own, it is easier to avoid distractions and traps because you will know exactly what to look for. The right answer choice is unlikely to be word-for-word what you came up with, but it should be a close match. Even if you are confident that you have the right answer, you should still take the time to read each option before moving on.

General Strategies

Tough Questions

If you are stumped on a problem or it appears too hard or too difficult, don't waste time. Move on! Remember though, if you can quickly check for obviously incorrect answer choices, your chances of guessing correctly are greatly improved. Before you completely give up, at least try to knock out a couple of possible answers. Eliminate what you can and then guess at the remaining answer choices before moving on.

Check Your Work

Since you will probably not know every term listed and the answer to every question, it is important that you get credit for the ones that you do know. Don't miss any questions through careless mistakes. If at all possible, try to take a second to look back over your answer selection and make sure you've selected the correct answer choice and haven't made a costly careless mistake (such as marking an answer choice that you didn't mean to mark). This quick double check should more than pay for itself in caught mistakes for the time it costs.

Pace Yourself

It's easy to be overwhelmed when you're looking at a page full of questions; your mind is confused and full of random thoughts, and the clock is ticking down faster than you would like. Calm down and maintain the pace that you have set for yourself. Especially as you get down to the last few minutes of the test, don't let the small numbers on the clock make you panic. As long as you are on track by monitoring your pace, you are guaranteed to have time for each question.

Don't Rush

It is very easy to make errors when you are in a hurry. Maintaining a fast pace in answering questions is pointless if it makes you miss questions that you would have gotten right otherwise. Test writers like to include distracting information and wrong answers that seem right. Taking a little extra time to avoid careless mistakes can make all the difference in your test score. Find a pace that allows you to be confident in the answers that you select.

KEEP MOVING

Panicking will not help you pass the test, so do your best to stay calm and keep moving. Taking deep breaths and going through the answer elimination steps you practiced can help to break through a stress barrier and keep your pace.

Final Notes

The combination of a solid foundation of content knowledge and the confidence that comes from practicing your plan for applying that knowledge is the key to maximizing your performance on test day. As your foundation of content knowledge is built up and strengthened, you'll find that the strategies included in this chapter become more and more effective in helping you quickly sift through the distractions and traps of the test to isolate the correct answer.

Now it's time to move on to the test content chapters of this book, but be sure to keep your goal in mind. As you read, think about how you will be able to apply this information on the test. If you've already seen sample questions for the test and you have an idea of the question format and style, try to come up with questions of your own that you can answer based on what you're reading. This will give you valuable practice applying your knowledge in the same ways you can expect to on test day.

Good luck and good studying!

Pharmacy and Pharmacology

Preparing Medications and Educating the Client

Preparation of Eye Medication and Information on Prescription Label

Eye medications come in suspensions, ointments, and serum drops. If the veterinarian asks to have a certain eye medication filled for the patient, the veterinary technician must create a label for the medication. You must be sure you have the patient's name, client's first and last names, and date on the label. The name of the medication as well as the strength of the medication must be on the label also. For instructions, you must include how many drops or how much ointment to apply to which eye or both eyes, how many times per day, and for how long. All instructions must be gone over with the client to ensure compliance.

Instruments to Cut and Count Tablets of Medication

A **pill cutter** is commonly used to cut pills in half or in quarters in order to get the correct strength of medication that the patient will need. A **pill counter tray** is a smooth-surfaced, plastic tray used to sort and count pills or capsules with a small plastic spatula. Using the spatula to sort and count the pills limits handling by the veterinary technician and allows for a more convenient and accurate count. Depending on what the veterinarian's instructions will be, the veterinary technician must be able to calculate the appropriate amount and strength of medication to go home with the patient. For example, the veterinarian asks for 30 days' worth of cefpodoxime 100 mg tablets to be given at half a tablet twice daily. Using the pill counter tray and spatula, by increments of 5, count out 30 tablets. Then using the pill cutter, cut all of the tablets in half.

Anaphylactic Reaction to Vaccines

Anaphylactic reactions are severe allergic reactions sometimes seen after a vaccination. Anaphylactic reactions can occur after the first vaccine the patient gets or the third — it is impossible to predict — but if the patient has had a previous reaction, they can be given an antihistamine injection prior to the vaccine to prevent a reaction in the future. Anaphylactic reactions normally happen less than 24 hours from vaccination and cause itching, weakness, apnea, sudden onset of diarrhea and vomiting, facial swelling, pale gums, and seizures. If this type of reaction is not treated immediately, it can lead to respiratory failure, heart failure, and shock. Treatment for anaphylaxis includes administration of epinephrine (adrenaline), antihistamines, oxygen therapy, and intravenous (IV) fluids if necessary.

Administering Ear Medications for Yeast, Bacterial, or Ear Mite Infections

In order to effectively **administer ear medications** to the patient, the medication must get into the ear canal where the infection is. For bacterial or yeast infections, the ears can be treated with regular ear cleanings, topical or oral antibiotics, or antifungals. Antibiotics and antifungal medications are normally administered by putting a quarter-sized amount of medication down into the ear canals and then massaging underneath the ear to move the medication further down. The ears can be cleaned with a cleansing and drying cleaner as well, which works by drying once it is inside the ear so when the pet shakes its head, the debris is expelled. Ear mites are treated by using a one-time-use medication in each ear that kills the ear mites. The veterinarian should remind the client to come back to recheck the ears once done medicating to make sure the infection has cleared up.

Educating Client with Newly Diagnosed Diabetic Pet

To properly store **insulin**, it must be kept in the refrigerator. Prior to administering insulin, the pet must eat because if they receive an insulin dose without eating, this can lead to dangerously low blood sugar (hypoglycemia). The veterinary technician must educate the client on what signs to watch for that can indicate hypoglycemia, such as shaking, seizures, weakness, and lethargy. If any of these signs occur, the owner should always have some light corn syrup available and can give a little amount by mouth as long as the pet can swallow. The veterinary technician needs to make sure that the owner knows to always double-check the amount of insulin they drew up and the syringe type before administering. Human insulins are made in different concentrations than veterinary insulins; therefore, they each require their own dosing syringes. Veterinary insulin (Vetsulin for dogs) is made at 40 units per ml and requires U-40 syringes, whereas human insulin (Humulin N) is made in 100 units of insulin per ml and requires U-100 syringes.

Demonstrating How to Administer Insulin

To demonstrate to the owner how to **administer insulin** at home, use an insulin syringe and sterile saline instead of insulin for the demonstration. Demonstrate with the sterile saline vial how to roll the vial between the palms of your hands to mix (instead of shaking). Show the owner on the insulin syringe how the units are marked and how many units their pet is going to be receiving. Draw up sterile saline to the amount they are directed to give, and have the owner watch you draw it up. Also, show the owner how to hold the patient and to lift up on the skin behind the neck to form a tent. Insert the needle into the subcutaneous (SQ) tissue up to the hub and push the plunger of the syringe to inject the insulin. Pull the needle straight out, and place it in a sharps container that the owner should have as well. Let the owner practice with saline with you until they are comfortable.

Giving Tablets or Liquid to Pets Orally

Often, pet owners will have to **administer medications orally** to their pet whether it be for a couple of weeks or a lifelong medication. Giving a pet an oral medication that is tablet or capsule form can be done for a dog by holding open its mouth wide and placing the pill as far back in the throat as possible and then closing its mouth. Hold the dog's head up, and rub its neck while holding the mouth shut with one hand to be sure the pill is swallowed. Sometimes it is not possible for the owner to put the medication into the dog's mouth, especially if it is trying to bite. The pill can be hidden inside of a soft treat or some canned food in the form of a small ball and then is fed to the dog. As for cats, to administer a tablet or capsule form of medication, the easiest way is to open its mouth and place it quickly on the back of the tongue. Because the cat's tongue is rough and the pill will stick to it, swallowing it is easy. Liquid medications are usually administered through a dropper or syringe, and by putting the end of the dispenser in the corner of the pet's mouth, the medication can be administered slowly to ensure they swallow it all.

Determining Fluid Rate

The **fluid rate** will be determined based on the percent of dehydration, ongoing losses such as diarrhea, and the maintenance requirement. The percent of dehydration is determined by taking the animal's weight in kilograms multiplied by the percent dehydration in decimal form. Ongoing losses may be estimated or measured accurately; for example, urine can be measured if a catheter is placed and a collection system is attached. Maintenance fluids are the required amount of fluid needed per day, and this is calculated at 40–60 ml multiplied by weight in kilograms. In order to calculate for the patient's fluid deficit, the patient's body weight in pounds is multiplied by the percent dehydration (in decimal form) and then multiplied by 500. This will be the amount that the patient will require to become rehydrated if there are no ongoing losses (e.g., urine, vomiting, diarrhea). If there are ongoing losses, they are added to the fluid deficit.

SENSIBLE AND INSENSIBLE FLUID LOSSES

Sensible losses are losses that can be measured, such as urine. Urine can be measured if a urinary catheter is placed and a collection system is attached. The collection system can be emptied and measured throughout a hospitalization. Insensible losses cannot be measured and can only be estimated by the veterinarian. **Insensible losses** include losses due to fevers, excessive panting respiratory loss, and fluid lost in feces. Both categories of loss must be included in the calculation for the total fluid deficit. Crystalloids are used to maintain the fluid level of the patient to keep up with the sensible and insensible losses in patients that are not eating or drinking as they should under hospitalization.

Calculating Dosage

INTERPRETING AND CALCULATING DOSAGE

Dosage is the term given to describe how much of a medicinal substance should be administered in the treatment of a given condition. Most medications are produced as pills, capsules, or liquids, with the relative strength measured in units known as milligrams or milliliters. The dosage should also indicate how much of the drug (described in the units of measurement) is to be given to the patient at any **one time interval**, along with the recommended **interval of time between administrations** of the recommended amount of medication. The animal's weight must be included in the calculation. Thus, the dosage will be determined with this weight in mind. For instance, short-hand phrases such as 100 mg/kg, mL/kg, or tablets/kg each relate to the amount of the dosage to be delivered based on the animal's weight expressed as kg or kilograms. A kilogram is the basic metric unit of mass, with 1 pound equivalent to 0.45 kilograms. Therefore, a 10-pound animal weighs 4.5 kilograms. The drug is administered to the patient based on its weight in order to achieve a certain concentration, as identified by the manufacturer.

DOSAGE AND BODY WEIGHT

Most veterinary medications **intended for ingestion or injection** have dosages calculated in terms of an **animal's body weight**. In this way, therapeutic medication concentrations can be achieved. In administering a dosage that is denoted by a milligram, the veterinarian should multiply the unit strength by the weight of the animal in kilograms to arrive at the proper dose. For instance, a medication produced in 10 milligram units would indicate a proper dosage to be 10 mg/kg. Thus, an animal that weighed 30 kg would receive 300 mg (milligrams) of medication. Medications administered in milliliters would be figured by dividing the dose in milligrams by the concentration of the drug in mg/mL.

Further, consider the administration of a liquid drug with a concentration of 40 mg/mL, from which a dose of 150 mg is to be given. The patient would be given a dosage calculated in milliliters as a 3.75 mL dose.

DOSAGE CALCULATION EXAMPLE

First, to **determine the dosage**, which is the amount of medication based on the **weight of the patient**, you will use the following formula: weight (kg) × dosage (mg/kg) = dose (mg). To calculate the dose in milliliters, you will take the dose divided by the concentration, which is decided by the manufacturer and found on the bottle of medication in terms of mg/ml. Use the following formula: dose (mg) ÷ concentration (mg/ml) = dose (ml). Therefore, first calculate pounds of body weight to kilograms by dividing 80 lb by 2.2 = 36.4 kg. Next, following the dose formula, take 36.4 kg × 20 mg/kg (dosage) = 728 mg. Then, to calculate the dose in milliliters, follow the formula taking 728 mg ÷ 100 mg/ml (concentration) = 7.3 ml of cefazolin.

Solution Terminology

The veterinarian who uses a concentrated form of the medication may need to dilute or reduce the strength of the medication. **Dilution** occurs when the **strength of a substance is lowered** by mixing a dilutant into the concentration. The added dilutant can consist of one or more substances that have a compatible composition. The solute must be able to be dissolved and absorbed by the diluting substance. This other substance is the called the **solvent**. The final mixture is known as the **solution**. The **concentration** of this solution reflects the amount of solute that was combined with the solvent. This concentration may reflect a strong or a weak solution. The concentration can be measured according to its percentage: volume solute per volume solvent, which is written as (v/v). This is typically expressed as a percentage — for liquids, the volume of solute in milliliters per 100 mL of total solution. The concentration can also be measured as weight per volume, written as (w/v). This indicates the percentage mass of the solute in units such as grams or milligrams in relation to 100 mL of total solution. Finally, the concentration may be reflected as percentage weight per weight, which is written as (w/w). This indicates the weight of the solute in a unit such as grams in relation to 100 g of the total solution.

Solution Strength

The veterinarian must use a computation to determine the **concentration or strength of solution**. The **mass of the solute** is measured in grams. This number is then divided by the **volume of liquid** as measured in milliliters (i.e., weight/volume — typically written as w/v). The calculation formula is g/mL. For instance, the strength of a solution with a mass of 50 g of solute that is divided by 200 mL of solvent yields a final solution concentration of 0.25 g/mL. Another computation is needed to determine the percentage of strength of the solution. This computation takes the solvent's concentration measurement and multiplies that by 100. In this case, 0.25 is multiplied by 100 to arrive at a percentage indicating a 25% solution. The equation may need to be figured in a different order to arrive at the other values available through the computation. The rearrangement of the formula will bring about these values. This rearrangement may begin with the calculation of the mass in a gram of measurement. Computation (g/mL) means that the mass of the solute measured in grams is divided by the volume measured in milliliters to obtain the concentration of the solution. Computation (mL/mL) means that the solute volume as measured in milliliters is divided by the solvent measured in milliliters to determine the concentration of the solution. Computations are easiest when an "aliquot" of a given solution is used – i.e., a known fraction of a whole; an exact divisor of some quantity (for example, 4 is a one-third aliquot of 12).

Stock and Working Solutions

Pure solutions that are free from contamination or foreign substances are written as a 100% solution — or, 100 g of solute in 100 mL of solution. A **"stock" solution** is a 100% concentrated solution that must be diluted to produce a **"working" solution**. Dilution denotes the mixing of this 100% pure solution with a given amount of solvent. The solvent is mixed into the pure solution in an effort to weaken or reduce the strength of the solute in the solution. If you need to reduce this solution further, then you will need to mix or dilute the solution with more solvent. If you need to increase the potency or strengthen a solution, then you will need to mix a new solution that has not been diluted as much — or add more solute (i.e., the active ingredient). Alternately, you may wish to add more of the pure solution to the stock solvent to obtain a stronger concentration. To determine any change in concentration between an initial and final solution, use the equation M1V1 = M2V2. M1 is the solute concentration in the initial (stock) solution, M2 is the solute concentration in the final solution, V1 is the volume of initial (stock) solution used, and V2 is the total volume of the final solution. To create a specific dilution, determine the volume of solvent (Vs) to mix with the selected volume (i.e., aliquot) of stock solution (V1). This can easily be computed using Vs = V2 - V1.

Drip Rates

Medications may be administered through IV tubes over time. To determine how much medication is being given, IV tubing is rated as delivering a certain **number of drips per milliliter** (also called "cc"—for cubic centimeter). The number of drops per cc or mL of fluid is known as the "drop factor," arising from the diameter of the IV tubing. Three common IV tube drop factors are 15 gtt/cc, 10 gtt/cc, and 60 gtt/cc (also known as "micro drip tubing"). The **drop factor** is printed on the IV packaging. Facilities use 60 for situations needing close monitoring (i.e., very small animals, vasoactive medications, etc.).

The computation required for the drip rate is the **number of drops** delivered during each **1-minute interval** — often written gtt/min, meaning "guttae" (drips) per minute. The symbol mL is used to indicate milliliters. The medication package gives clear directions regarding optimum delivery time in minutes or hours. A prescribed delivery rate may be given as follows: a 0.5 L solution with 15 drops/mL and an administration time of 3 hours. To determine the proper drip rate, take the time in hours and compute: 3 hours multiplied by 60 minutes equals 180 minutes total. The second step is to take the 0.5 L (500 mL) and multiply by 15 drops/mL, totaling 7500 drops. 7500 divided by 180 minutes equals a drip rate of 41.67 gtt/min. Note: drip rate must never be confused with "flow rate" — which is the rate of delivery provided by an IV infusion pump, independent of drips per minute.

Therapeutic Index (TI)

The **Therapeutic Index** or TI (also known as the Therapeutic Ratio) is used to address the **relative safety of a drug**. The Therapeutic Index is expressed by the following formula: TI = LD50/EC50.

LD50 refers to the lethal dosage for 50% of a designated population, while EC50 refers to the minimum effective dosage for 50% of that same population.

Drugs that are deemed to be safer will have a higher TI than drugs deemed to be less safe. Drugs with a lower TI provide a **narrower available dosage range** between a desired therapeutic effect and toxic or poisonous results. Thus, drugs with a lower TI offer fewer dosage options in treating a given condition before adverse effects may begin to arise. They can also be very hazardous to handle, and much more difficult to prescribe and manage. Typically, more frequent provider contacts are required, more detailed status reports are needed, and laboratory testing for both therapeutic levels and signs of deleterious secondary effects are more critical.

Microbes, Antimicrobials, and Antibiotics

Pathogenic microbes are microscopic organisms with the capacity to infect and induce diseases in other life forms. Some examples of microbes include bacteria, fungi, viruses, and parasites. **Antimicrobials** are medications that are able to kill off or slow the growth of disease-causing microbes. **Antibiotics** are medications that have been isolated from natural sources, or synthetically produced, to kill or inactivate certain kinds of bacteria. Antibiotics are most effective when given clear passage to the site of infection. Antibiotics given in the proper dosage and concentration, and over a sufficient duration of time, can kill or impede the growth of many disease-causing microbes. However, when antibiotics are not given as prescribed, the bacteria may survive to develop a resistance to the drug.

Antibiotics themselves can have **adverse effects** on some patients. In addition, not all antibiotics are effective in the treatment of certain microbes. With the passage of time, more and more bacteria are becoming resistant to antibiotics commonly given to both humans and animals. Once this resistance has developed, the bacteria are able to survive despite the presence of the antibiotic within the body. Further, the bacteria's offspring will inherit this same resistance. Consequently, animal caregivers should be aware of the **need for proper antibiotic administration** and complete treatment of all disease-causing microbes.

Inhibition of Microbial Protein Synthesis

Antimicrobials can be effective in **obstructing microbial protein synthesis**. This interference is accomplished as the antimicrobial substance is introduced into the microbe and fastens itself to the microbial ribosomes. Ribosomes are submicroscopic clusters of proteins and RNA found within the cytoplasm of cells which are necessary for protein synthesis.

Many **aminoglycosides**, some of which also **prevent microbial protein synthesis**, are bactericidal in nature. By contrast, other antibiotics such as Tetracycline, lincosamide, chloramphenicol, and macrolides, which also use this mechanism, are bacteriostatic agents — they do not kill the bacteria outright (except in high concentrations) but rather inhibit growth and reproduction.

Still other **antimicrobial drugs slow down nucleic acid production** in an invading organism. **Nucleic acid** is a complex acid which found in all living cells, and includes both DNA and RNA. The purpose of nucleic acid is to transmit genetic information during cell division and reproduction, and to create enzymes and proteins for use within and around cells. When antimicrobial drugs slow down the production of nucleic acid in the microbial organism, genetic information transmissions and protein and enzymatic processes and syntheses are also reduced. Thus, bacteriostatic drugs may also be responsible for microbial inability to divide, as they interrupt microbial metabolic activity.

Eliminating Drugs from the Body

Medications are identified by the body as **foreign substances** to be eliminated as expeditiously as possible. Elimination occurs by a metabolic process of breaking down and reconfiguring the original substance until it can be successfully excreted. The liver is the primary organ in this metabolic process, although other organs may be involved, as well. The liver uses enzymatic systems to change or break down the drug, which is then referred to as a metabolite. Some common examples of enzymes involved in these metabolic processes include cytochrome P450 oxidase and flavin-containing monooxygenase.

Some metabolites can be more potent or toxic to the animal than the original drug. Once a water-soluble metabolite is formed, the kidneys remove it from the body via the **urine**. Metabolites may also be excreted in **sweat** and **feces**. However, a patient that has poorly functioning kidneys or a damaged liver may not be able to metabolize and discharge drugs at a sufficient rate to avoid a systemic build-up and consequent toxic effects.

Hydration Status

A patient's **hydration status** can be evaluated a few different ways; the first is to perform a **skin tent test**. The skin tent test will check the amount of moisture in the skin by pulling the skin over the thorax or lumbar region away from the back. If the patient is well hydrated, the skin will return immediately to its normal position, but if the skin stays standing, that means the patient is dehydrated. If there is a slight loss of the **skin's elasticity** from the skin tent test, that indicates a 5%–6% dehydration. If the patient has an increased capillary refill time, sunken eyes, and a more obvious delay in the skin returning to its normal position during the skin tent test this indicates a

7%–10% dehydration level. Dry mucous membranes, sunken and dull eyes, tachycardia, rapid and weak pulses, along with no return of the skin to its natural position during the skin tent test is a 10%–12% dehydration level. A 12%–15% dehydration level can lead to death.

Measurement of Solids and Liquids

When instructing the owner of an animal on measuring dosage, be sure to stress the need for accurate measurement tools. **Measurements** in teaspoons and tablespoons are not accurate, especially when using common kitchen silverware. A household teaspoon can range from 2–7 ml, resulting in either an **overdose** of the medication or an **underdosing**. A syringe or measured dropper is commonly used to measure and administer liquid medication to a patient. Common quantities are converted such as 1 tsp = 5 ml and 1 T = 15 ml, 1 liter converts to 1,000 ml, 1 fl oz = 30 ml, and 1 gal = 3,785 ml. Solid measurements are often used in veterinary medicine. For example, the veterinarian may need the technician to convert an animal's weight in pounds to kilograms to calculate a dosage. Conversions of solids include 1,000 g = 1 kg, 1 kg = 2.2 pounds, 1 lb = 16 oz, 1,000 mg = 1 g, and 1,000 μg = 1 mg.

Drug Inventory and Dispensing

Medication Labels

When a licensed veterinarian provides a prescription, the label of the drug should include certain specific information:

1. the name and address of the **prescribing veterinarian**;
2. the name of the drug or **active ingredient** that is used to make the drug;
3. the identification of the **animal or herd to be treated**;
4. the date of **expiration**;
5. any specific management and administration directions pertinent to the drug;
6. directions regarding **how often the drug should be given** and how long the drug can be taken, spelled out in detail;
7. directions about whether the drug should be given by mouth, rectum, injection, or other method;
8. any **warnings** that should be followed; and,
9. directions regarding the **proper management and storage** of the medication to ensure patient safety.

Prescription Labels and Dispensing Drugs

Prescription drugs are intended for the animal that has received the prescription. No other animal should be given another's prescription medications. If the state of residence requires it, then a childproof container must also be used. It is important to follow dosage amounts as provided on a typed package label. The use of abbreviations is not allowed on this typed label. The veterinarian will have specified all requisite dosing and handling information in detail on the label of the prescription. At a minimum the label will state the date, name, address, veterinarian's telephone number, patient's name, and client's last name. There may be information about the species of the animal as required by individual state law. The label will also include: the drug's name, concentration, dosage amount, any state-required drug identification number (or DIN), and the number of available refills. The label will have directions concerning whether the drug should be given with food, on an empty stomach, or with liquids. The same management should be applied to prescription drugs for extra-label use. If the medication is sensitive to light, then an amber vial is used to obstruct the ultraviolet rays. Other instructions may include special storage requirements, administration needs, toxicity criteria, or withdrawal period.

Guidelines for Dispensing Drugs

Very specific laws govern the issuance of veterinary prescription drugs. These drugs may only be given out by a licensed veterinarian using proper documents. In addition, the drugs must be administered through a valid **veterinarian-client-patient relationship** (abbreviated as VCPR). Three conditions must be met for a VCPR to be considered valid. The first condition requires that the clinical judgments regarding the patient's health are **decided by the treating veterinarian**. Second, this veterinarian must agree to be **accountable for the treatments prescribed**. Finally, the client or animal owner must **agree to abide by the veterinarian's instructions for care**. The barest amount of care should include a general or preliminary exam of the patient. The veterinarian must also stay available should the patient have need of follow-up or emergency care due to an adverse reaction. If the veterinarian is unavailable, then an alternative doctor should be available to act in the veterinarian's place.

Veterinarian-Client-Patient Relationship

In order for the veterinarian to prescribe medications to a patient, a relationship between the client and veterinarian must be established, as well as between the patient and veterinarian (**veterinarian–client–patient relationship**). This is required by law in most states, but overall it is in the best interest of the patient. In order to prescribe the appropriate medication, the veterinarian must have the patient's history, which is provided by the owner, as well as a thorough exam of the patient to assess its overall health. With a proper medical history of the patient, the veterinarian will know if they are on any current medications, have any underlying health issues, and any lab results. This can all be beneficial when trying to prescribe medication for the current issue to be sure it can be given in conjunction with certain medications the pet may be taking or if the pet may need comprehensive blood work done if there is an underlying health issue. Without thoroughly examining a patient and having knowledge of its previous medical history and vaccination status, then no medical advice should be given and no medications should be prescribed.

Accounting for Controlled Drugs Used in the Hospital

There needs to be a system in each hospital that shows the balance on hand of each **controlled substance**. Frequently updated written logs or computerized logs work well. The patient's name, client's name, the date, drug name, and drug amount used must be recorded. If an injectable drug is prescribed, then the amount drawn up and the amount actually administered to the patient must be recorded. Regular inventory counts should be done to ensure that the amounts correspond to the actual log books. Having one person, whether it is a veterinarian or a veterinary technician, responsible for keeping track of the controlled drug logs is ideal; that way, that person will be able to notice and keep track of trends.

Handling Shortages Within the Controlled Drugs Log

If a **shortage** is noticed in the **controlled drug log**, usually it is due to a miscalculation or record-keeping error, so the record book must be calculated through to catch any adding or subtracting errors, and drug doses and strengths must be checked for accuracy. Also, checking the computer and comparing it to the log book to determine if any controlled drug prescriptions were filled and not logged will catch errors as well. If the problem is identified, then an entry can be made to correct the balance appropriately. If **theft** is the cause, then a report will have to be filled out for the **Drug Enforcement Agency** of what is missing, and an explanation but no evidence is required.

Schedules of Controlled Drugs

Controlled drugs are labeled in specified **schedules** ranging from I–V. Schedule I substances, such as heroin, LSD, and cannabis, have **no medical use** and are not safe even with medical supervision with the risk of high abuse. Schedule II drugs, such as opium, morphine, ketamine, fentanyl, and hydromorphone, have a **high risk of abuse** and severe physical and psychological dependence. Schedule III drugs, including buprenorphine, tramadol, and midazolam, have a **lower abuse potential** than Schedules I and II drugs. Schedules II and III drugs require strict record keeping for tracking the use or dispensation of these drugs. Schedule IV drugs, including phenobarbital and diazepam, have a **low potential for abuse**. Schedule V substances include medications that are **available without a prescription** such as antitussives that may contain small quantities of a narcotic drug such as codeine. Schedules II–V drugs are all accepted for medical use in the United States.

Classifications of Drugs

Drugs, Poisons, and Generics

The terms **drug, poison**, and **generic** may be defined as a chemical compound that can be beneficial when used correctly in the prescribed amounts. Drugs can cause significant physiological changes within the body and can work to improve the body's ability to function properly. Drugs can also be applied in preventive care. A drug can be given in response to a specific diagnosis, as a prescribed treatment. Some drugs are given to bring relief for specific symptoms involving pain or other distress, as opposed to restoration of the body.

Poison is defined as **a toxic substance** which can produce injury, sickness, or death. Drugs that are not applied in the correct dosage may produce poisonous results. Toxic substances may be given through ingestion, injection, inhalation, or absorption through the skin, or they may be created by chemical processes within the body. Many common substances like water or vitamins can be harmful or poisonous when **taken in excess.**

Generic is a term given to designate the name of a **drug in its basic chemical form**. It may or may not hold the same chemical formula as brand-name medications (often depending upon whether or not the patent has expired). The chemical name or generic name of a drug can be used in place of other proprietary or trademark names for the same drug substance.

Drug Reference Materials

A review of the packet insert or other drug reference material is required to gain specific knowledge about a **drug's potential for harm**, as well as its **intended beneficial effects**. In reading the indications for a drug, one should note the explanation concerning the expected therapeutic benefits. One should also note the appropriate use and application of the drug. Further, the literature should indicate if there are any known **precautions** or special considerations necessary to safely take the drug. Likewise, the literature should also note any explicit contraindications.

Contraindications are specific actions that are inadvisable to take while using a certain drug (i.e., concurrently taking certain other prescriptions, over-the-counter medications, or vitamins; eating certain foods; or engaging in certain activities; etc). These actions could lead to adverse consequences. The literature should state any mild or significant side effects that could arise with typical usage of the drug. The literature may also provide directions to follow should accidental overdose occur, or steps to take in the event that serious but unintended effects of the drug arise.

Dosage Schedule and Tolerance

The packet inserts or **drug reference material** includes information on when and where the drug should and should not be taken. For example, there may be a warning that the drug should be taken only on an empty stomach, or only with meals. Further, warnings may advise against certain activities or going out for prolonged periods in the sun. The literature should include information concerning appropriate dosages along with the required administration method (oral, suppository, patch, etc.) and amount of the drug to be administered at requisite intervals.

There are times that the body can build up a **tolerance for a drug**, and warnings to this effect may also appear in any explanatory literature. Tolerance indicates that the response to the drug has lessened due to continued exposure over a long period of time. Tolerance may sometimes lead to higher amounts of medication usage than at prescribed intervals, to the point that the drug may become toxic to the body. In these cases, a drug overdose can occur. The literature should also explain what to do in cases of overdose. Both intentional and unintentional overdoses can be dangerous or even fatal, and thus will likely require prompt medical attention.

Extra-Label Drug Use (ELDU)

FDA is an acronym for the **Federal Drug Administration**, which is an agency of the government of the United States. This federal agency is responsible for the approval of all drugs to be used in the United States. Drugs that are approved by the FDA are approved for use under the specific conditions and diseases against which they were tested. However, not all drugs are used solely for the purposes approved by the FDA. In certain circumstances the known pharmacological properties of a drug may suit it well for treating other diseases and conditions.

Therefore, a veterinarian may sometimes apply a drug in a manner other than for its approved purpose. In recognition that it is not possible to test every drug for every possible use, the FDA has made provisions for certain "off label" drug use — or "**extra-label drug use**" (ELDU) as it is formally called. However, ELDU practices in veterinary medicine are still regulated by the Animal Medicinal Drug Use Clarification Act (AMDUCA) of 1994. This act specifies that ELDU medications can only be prescribed: a) by a licensed veterinarian, b) when the veterinarian has a legitimate veterinarian-client-patient relationship, and c) when no contaminants will result when the medication is provided to food-producing animals.

Animal Medicinal Drug Use Clarification Act of 1994 (AMDUCA).

Further ELDU criteria as clarified by the **Animal Medicinal Drug Use Clarification Act of 1994** includes the following: Medications considered for ELDU must still be listed for at least one approved purpose under FDA regulatory criteria before being administered to an animal or to a human being. The ELDU was not created to facilitate the mass production of drugs targeted for ELDU applications; instead, ELDU applications must be solely for therapeutic reasons in individually determined cases. The ELDU is applicable to those drugs that are given in the manufactured form of the drug or dispensed in a water solution.

ELDU drugs cannot be given as a supplement to the food supply of an animal. ELDU strictly forbids the use of any drug that can become a contaminant to the food supply or the environment. Specifically, any remaining residue that can have a negative impact or risk on the well-being of individual consumers or the community is strictly prohibited from use by the ELDU. Once the FDA has issued a ban against a specific ELDU drug application, then that ELDU option is no longer permitted.

Drugs with High Potential for Abuse

Drugs that have a medical purpose, but that also have a **high potential for physiological and psychological dependence and abuse** are classified as Schedule II drugs. Pharmaceutical medications under the Schedule II label can be used in veterinary practice. However, Schedule II

drugs require strict record keeping and storage arrangements, and many
carefully restricted ways. Thus, the veterinarian must adhere to strict me
or her prescription and distribution of these drugs.

Schedule III drugs and substances have moderate to low physiological depen
psychological dependence features. Schedule IV drugs and substances may le
physiological or psychological dependence, as compared with Schedule III dru
V drugs and substances are those with the lowest abuse potential, as compared
drugs. Even so, drugs under the label of Schedule III, IV, and V require strict rec
storage arrangements. The Controlled Substance Act of 1970 mandates these cri ... United
States.

Controlled Drugs

The United States Congress has passed laws regarding controlled substances (i.e., drugs, both licit and illicit). These laws have been in effect since 1970. The codified law is called the **Controlled Substance Act** or the CSA. The law consists of regulations governing the manufacture, importation, possession, and distribution of certain drugs within the boundaries of the United States. Subject to this Act, the FDA, or Food and Drug Administration, is also in charge of regulating any pharmaceutical drug that has the potential for abusive use. Finally, the Drug Enforcement Agency, or DEA, is responsible for enforcing these drug laws and regulations.

Those drugs which fall under these 2 agencies' jurisdiction are known as **controlled drugs**. The DEA has classified the controlled drugs in accordance to their abuse potential. Drugs that have the most likelihood for abuse are classified as C-I. Drugs that have the least likelihood for abuse are classified a C-V. Schedule I (C-I) drugs are those that have a high risk for being abused. Drugs labeled under the Schedule I designation do not have an acceptable medical purpose, nor do these drugs have approved safety data. The licensed veterinarian will not be using these drugs in his or her veterinary practice.

Antimicrobial Mechanisms

Antimicrobials are classified by their microbial eradicating and/or inhibiting capabilities. Antimicrobials with the suffix "-cidal" are able to **directly eradicate bacteria**. Antimicrobials with the suffix "-static" primarily **impede bacterial growth**. Antimicrobial drugs work in many ways. These include: 1) hindering cell wall growth, 2) preventing the organism from synthesizing proteins, 3) inhibiting nucleic acid synthesis, 4) inhibiting metabolic pathways in the bacteria that do not exist in the host, and 5) damaging cytoplasmic membranes.

When bacterial cytoplasmic membranes are damaged, the cell wall membrane may become permeable or porous. The permeable membrane allows the antimicrobial drug to diffuse into the cell. The bacteria may then break open through a process known as "lysis." Antibiotics that work in these ways are generally efficient in preventing or reducing bacterial growth.

General Anesthesia

General anesthesia serves to bring a patient into a coma-like state of deep unconsciousness, sufficient to produce a loss of all sensation. General anesthetics are administered to the patient as inhalants or injectables. Death can occur if an overdose of some general anesthetics occurs.

Nearly all animal euthanizing agents utilize sodium pentobarbital as the primary active agent. **Pentobarbital**, without any other additives, is rated as a Schedule II (C-II) drug by the DEA. However, some pentobarbital-based euthanizing agents have additives that work as cardiac depressives. These combined drugs are then reclassified as C-III. Pentobarbital-based animal [illegible] drugs with cardiac depressive additives include Euthanasia-D with phenytoin, and FP-3 [illegible]h) with lidocaine.

Sodium pentobarbital injected perivascularly has the ability to induce necrosis. Necrosis is described as the death and decay of tissues or organs within the body. Conversely, lower-dose sodium pentobarbital also has the ability to postpone or prevent death in some cases. Animals that will be consumed as food must not receive any general anesthetics due to the danger that residual medications can be passed on to the human consumer.

Analgesics and Anti-Inflammatory Drugs

Opioid or **narcotic analgesics**, **corticosteroids**, and **nonsteroidal anti-inflammatory drugs** are defined as analgesic and/or anti-inflammatory drugs. The function of these drugs is to provide immediate pain relief and ongoing control.

Nonsteroidal anti-inflammatory drugs may also be referred to by their acronym "**NSAIDs**." Common NSAIDs include phenylbutazone, aspirin, ibuprofen, etodolac, and carprofen. Nearly all NSAIDs work to block the prostaglandin production that results from the inflammatory process. However, NSAIDs are not useful in counteracting visceral (organ) pain nor the pain associated with broken bones, as they do not produce sufficient analgesic effects.

By contrast, **opioid analgesics** can entirely **block all awareness of neural pain impulses**. Thus, opioids can control more intense pain symptoms, such as those related to visceral pain and the pain of broken bones. Morphine, meperidine, oxymorphone, butorphanol, and codeine are all types of opioid pain control medications.

Many of the perianesthetic medications are also **opioids**. These medications work as both analgesics and sedatives. Many sedatives can also be effective as tranquilizers.

Corticosteroids are anti-inflammatory drugs which can also relieve pain. However, it is important to use caution with these drugs, as they can have negative effects on the endocrine and immune systems. The most widely used corticosteroids are dexamethasone and prednisone.

Drugs that Affect the Central Nervous System

The breathing center of the brain is stimulated via neural, chemical, and hormonal signals that control the respiratory rate, tidal volume, etc. This center can also be **stimulated** by intravenous administration of the drug doxapram hydrochloride. Some patients may require this treatment for **respiratory problems**, particularly those that have been brought about by medication overdoses, lung diseases, or from the postoperative effects of general anesthesia.

Toxicity may be defined as the threshold at which a drug begins to cause untoward effects or outright physiological damage, coupled with how quickly that damage escalates with increasing levels of the drug. Virtually **all stimulants can become toxic** in animals as dosages are increased. Examples of stimulants that may readily cause this effect include caffeine, amphetamines, and theobromine.

Antidepressants are used to reduce symptoms of depression. Antidepressants may also be applied in the treatment of separation anxiety or canine cognitive dysfunction. Clomipramine, also known as Clomicalm, is an antidepressant often used for separation anxiety. This is a condition in which the patient experiences a high degree of anxiety or stress when separated from a primary caregiver or companion. Selegiline, also known as Anipryl, is an antidepressant used for canine cognitive dysfunction.

Controlled Drugs that Affect the Central Nervous System

Drugs that impact the central nervous system include the so-called "**controlled drugs**." Examples of controlled drugs include anesthetics, analgesics, tranquilizers and sedatives, anticonvulsants, stimulants, and other psychoactive medications.

Tranquilizers and **sedatives** are usually applied when patients are overwhelmed with agitation, need assistance in easing some anxiety, or need an aid to induce sleep. These drugs can produce a mental state of tranquility and/or sleepiness in the patient. Benzodiazepines and phenothiazines are examples of tranquilizers and sedatives (phenothiazines are commonly used as antipsychotics, as well).

Anticonvulsants are used for controlling seizures, both preventatively and when in progress. Two examples of anticonvulsants are diazepam and pentobarbital. These drugs produce a pronounced antiseizure effect in a short period of time. The drugs are often given to patients in the hospital setting, with other medications being prescribed for more long-term seizure management. Two types of oral medications commonly given to seizure-prone animals in the home or field setting are phenobarbital and potassium bromide.

Cardiovascular Drugs

There are a multitude of drugs which can be used to effectively treat various symptoms and conditions involving the heart. These drugs include cardiovascular drugs, antiarrhythmics, diuretics, positive inotropics, catecholamines, and vasodilators.

Antiarrhythmic drugs can be useful in the restoration of normal electrical activity in the heart. Lidocaine and procainamide are known as sodium channel blockers, as they restrain or limit the flow of the electrolyte sodium (Na^+). Propranolol hydrochloride is a negative inotrope. It can obstruct beta-adrenergic receptors, which might otherwise reduce myocardial contractility.

Myocardial contractility refers to the "pumping" movement of the thick muscular wall of the heart. Calcium channel blockers are antiarrhythmics and include verapamil and diltiazem. Antiarrhythmics such as these slow the conduction or transmission of electrical activity in the heart, thereby allowing cardiac functions to more readily normalize.

Finally, positive **inotropes and catecholamines** are drugs which are used to make the cont**ractions of the heart stronger**. One example of a positive inotrope is digoxin. Digoxin can increase the quantity of calcium accessible to the heart.

Drugs that Affect the Autonomic Nervous System

The **autonomic (i.e., unconscious, self-regulating) nervous system** has 3 divisions: **sympathetic**, **parasympathetic**, and **enteric**. The sympathetic division manages rapid-demand changes (i.e., flight-fight responses, etc.), while the parasympathetic system modulates and complements those responses, seeking balance over time. The enteric system regulates autonomic digestive system processes.

Parasympathetic changes can be caused by cholinergic and adrenergic agents. In general, adrenergic agents act on sympathetic processes (principally by releasing epinephrine and norepinephrine), while cholinergic agents act upon parasympathetic processes (principally by producing, altering, releasing, or mimicking acetylcholine). Both of these agents can be circumvented by anticholinergics and adrenergic blockers. The cholinergic drug pilocarpine reduces intraocular pressure, while Metoclopramide stimulates the gastrointestinal system, and Urecholine quickens the urinary system.

The **parasympathetic nervous system** may be overstimulated by the introduction of cholinergics. These effects can be moderated by anticholinergics such as aminopentamide, atropine sulfate, and glycopyrrolate. Aminopentamide has the ability to slow down gastrointestinal motility (movement). Atropine sulfate and glycopyrrolate can cause the pupils to dilate and the heart rate to increase, as well as secretions to dry up. Anticholinergics normally produce adverse effects if administered in the wrong dosage.

Antifungal Agents

Antifungal drugs work by attempting to **exploit distinguishing features** between mammalian and fungi cells. This has been challenging as both are eukaryotic, both have DNA organized into chromosomes in a nucleus, and both have similar intracellular organelles. They even have similar biosynthetic processes for DNA replication and protein synthesis.

However, one important difference has been noted. While mammalian cell walls contain significant amounts of cholesterol (about 25% of the cell membrane, by weight), fungi cell walls contain primarily "ergosterol".

Several antifungal agents have been designed to exploit this difference in **sterol content**, including the polyenes, azoles, and allylamines. Polyene antifungals bind with the sterols in the fungal cell wall, producing a **permeable condition**. This allows the cellular contents to spill out and ultimately results in the elimination of the cell. The cholesterol found in animal cells is less susceptible to this process, leaving these cells structurally undisturbed. Two kinds of polyene antifungals are nystatin and amphotericin B.

Azole Antifungal Agents

Imidazole and triazole are 2 antifungal drugs of the azole family that work by **blocking or obstructing an enzyme essential to ergosterol synthesis** in the fungal cell wall. Enzymes are complex proteins that act as catalysts to encourage biochemical reactions. The enzyme is not changed chemically through this process, and thus it remains effective throughout the biochemical intervention and available for continued bioactivity. The azole antifungal agents target a lanosterol demethylase enzyme necessary to convert or change lanosterol to ergosterol. In this way fungi are unable to obtain and maintain sufficient ergosterol to sustain cell wall integrity.

By blocking certain kinds of sterol syntheses in the cell, imidazole and triazole cause a **depletion of normal sterols and an abnormal accumulation of sterol precursors**, resulting in fungal cell toxicity and subsequent demise. Triazole antifungal drugs are not as toxic or as poisonous as many other drugs used for a similar purpose. Further, the triazoles often produce a more positive result than the imidazoles, thus they may be among the more preferred antifungal drugs available. Two examples of triazoles are fluconazole and itraconazole. Two examples of imidazoles are miconazole and ketoconazole.

Cephalosporin Antibiotics

Cephalosporins are of the beta-lactam antibiotic family (along with the penicillins, carbapenems, and monobactams). Cephalosporins can be effective against both gram-positive and gram-negative bacteria. Cephalosporins function to interrupt mucopeptide synthesis in the bacterial cell wall. This formation is needed to secure and maintain the structural integrity of the cell wall, without which the **bacterial cell cannot survive**.

In contrast to penicillin, the cephalosporins are resistant to the process of enzymatic hydrolysis of the beta-lactam ring. Enzymatic hydrolysis renders an antibiotic ineffective, and occurs when bacteria produce the enzymes beta-lactamase or penicillinase. These enzymes are secreted by significant numbers of bacteria, thus this resistance is important.

There are 4 generations of cephalosporins. The first generation usually had a positive effect only against gram-positive bacteria. However, the generations of cephalosporins which followed have been increasingly effective against gram-negative bacteria. Thus, the fourth generation has been classified as a true broad-spectrum antibiotic, effective against both gram-negative and gram-positive bacterial infections. Patients with a known allergy to penicillin should not be administered first-generation cephalosporins, which include: cefadroxil, cefazolin, and cephalexin. An example of a second-generation cephalosporin is cefoxitin, while ceftiofur is a third-generation cephalosporin.

Use of Sedatives in Veterinary Medicine

Sedatives and **tranquilizers** are commonly used medications. Some examples of sedatives and tranquilizers include acepromazine, diazepam, medetomidine, midazolam, and xylazine.

The sedative acepromazine is manufactured under the trade name Atarvet. It should be noted that acepromazine is not advisable for use with animals that have recently been treated for fleas using any organophosphate-based pesticide. While organophosphates are useful to kill fleas, any residual phosphate compounds coupled with acepromazine can cause negative side effects, including hypotension (low blood pressure).

Diazepam (Valium) is considered one of the "classical" benzodiazepines, having been only the second benzodiazepine derivative developed. Others include clonazepam, lorazepam, oxazepam, alprazolam, nitrazepam, flurazepam, bromazepam, and clorazepate. Diazepam is both an anxiolytic and a sedative. An anxiolytic is a drug that relieves anxiety, while a sedative induces rest and sleep. However, diazepam can also be used as a muscle relaxant, appetite stimulant, and anticonvulsant. Other uses include treating insomnia and muscle spasms. Because it can be used to address such a broad array of conditions, it has become one of the most widely used medications in the world.

Medetomidine, Midazolam, and Xylazine

Medetomidine is an alpha-2 agonist. It is manufactured under the trade name Domitor. This drug has a **short elimination half-life**. Medetomidine is a highly potent anxiolytic, hypnotic, anticonvulsant, muscle relaxant, sedative, and analgesic. However, medetomidine can also produce serious side effects under certain conditions, including bradycardia, hypothermia, decreased respiration, urination, occasional AV blocks, and vomiting with the accompanying potential for aspiration pneumonia. Thus, this medication should be administered cautiously, particularly to very young or very old dogs. The more significant side effects to medetomidine should be treated through pharmacological reversal of the drug.

The drug **midazolam** is manufactured under the trade names Dormicum, Flormidal, Versed, Hypnovel, and Dormonid. Midazolam can be substituted for diazepam when it is otherwise advantageous.

The drug xylazine is manufactured under the trade names Rompun and Anased.

Xylazine can be used as an **analgesic** to treat pain. It is also useful for muscle relaxation, anesthesia, and sedation. The more serious side effects of xylazine include: bradycardia, cardiac conduction disturbances, myocardial depression, and vomiting. The reversal drug for xylazine, yohimbine, may be used when severe side effects persist.

Antitussives, Expectorants, Mucolytic, and Bronchodilating Medications

Cough medicine is used to suppress or reduce the cough reflex. Typically, cough medicines have an **antitussive additive** such as codeine (i.e., dihydrocodeine phosphate) to achieve this end. Antitussives can be administered to a patient with a **dry, hacking cough**. However, antitussives may be **contraindicated** or **inadvisable** for productive coughs, which may respond better to expectorant medication to aid in clearing congestion. A productive cough is beneficial because it decreases mucus and other organic debris that may otherwise accumulate in the airways. Antitussives can also be used to treat **tracheobronchitis**, which is commonly referred to as **kennel cough.**

Expectorants are used to increase the fluidity or the liquid consistency of the mucus in the airways. Mucus that has greater fluidity is easier to expel or to cough up. Human expectorants sold over the counter have not been found beneficial to animals. Instead, mucus in animals can best be thinned by **moistening the air they breathe** through a process of **humidification**.

Mucolytic agents are beneficial in the improvement of **bronchial airflow**. Mucolytic agents are able to reduce the viscosity or the thickness of the mucus. Thus, mucolytic agents help to more readily break up the mucus.

Bronchodilators expand breathing passages and reduce respiratory burdens. Some common bronchodilators include albuterol, terbutaline, aminophylline, and theophylline. Bronchodilators help the **smooth muscles in the lungs to relax.** This allows an expansion of the air passages, which produces a more comfortable state of breathing. The general side effects associated with the use of albuterol are related to the amount of medication that has been administered. These side effects are not usually long lasting. However, caution should be used to reduce the likelihood of exhaled air entering the injection vials, as carbon dioxide can substantially accelerate the effects of aminophylline.

Examples of Antitussives

Three examples of **antitussive medications** are butorphanol, dextromethorphan, and hydrocodone. These antitussives are effective in controlling the desire or impulse to cough, which often accompanies some illnesses.

Acetylcysteine is a mucolytic drug. This drug can reduce the thickness and viscosity of the mucus in the lungs. Acetylcysteine can be given by inhalation, orally, or intravenously.

Treating Respiratory Ailments

Bronchodilators are given to the patient to improve bronchial airflow. This improvement is produced when the bronchioles in the lungs are expanded and widened in response to an application of **dilating medication**. Bronchodilation can be accomplished by stimulating the Beta2-receptors in the lung. This produces a state of relaxation in the lungs as the smooth muscles become less tense.

Antihistamines, **corticosteroids**, **diuretics**, and **oxygen** are able to improve breathing conditions in animals that have respiratory ailments. Antihistamines can keep the body's histamine response from further affecting the respiratory tract. The antihistamine medications prophylactically work to help reduce infection and disease, to which the lungs may be predisposed when bronchial restriction accompanies a marked histamine response.

When inflammation in the lungs is severe, the application of corticosteroids is also recommended. In addition, excess fluids can be eliminated from the lungs when a patient is given diuretics. Finally, when a condition is present that seriously compromises breathing or airway perfusion, the recommended procedure is to give the patient supplemental oxygen.

Antihistamines and Allergy Treatment

Histamines are an important part of the body's immune system. However, if overstimulated by omnipresent allergens or an allergen which causes **anaphylaxis** (an exaggerated allergic reaction), then untoward side effects can ensue. These may include respiratory difficulties, itching, rashes, and other inflammatory responses.

Antihistamines are drugs which are able to **block histamine release** or their uptake by specific cell receptors. These drugs can be used to prevent or reduce severe allergic reactions. Common antihistamines include chlorpheniramine, cyproheptadine, diphenhydramine, hydroxyzine, and clemastine. These drugs often produce somnolence as an undesirable side effect, and patients may also exhibit symptoms of dry mouth or marked thirst.

Some antihistamines have additional treatment purposes, as well. For example, cyproheptadine can enhance feline appetite for food.

Treating Anaphylactic Shock

Diphenhydramine (trade name Benadryl) is given to patients in anaphylactic shock. **Anaphylactic shock** is an allergic reaction severe enough to cause the death of the patient. Patients in anaphylactic shock may have symptoms of low blood pressure, itching, swelling, and extreme respiratory problems. In such situations diphenhydramine should be given **intravenously** to offer maximal support.

Decongestants are normally used to **reduce sinus and nasal congestion** accompanying a cold. Patients will often have copious amounts of fluid or mucus built up in the nasal and sinus cavities, and decongestants can help them breathe easier. They typically work to constrict blood vessels in the nasal passages, thereby reducing nasal swelling and allowing air to pass more easily. However, decongestants can also serve other purposes. For example, the decongestant phenylpropanolamine can be used to treat urinary incontinence in animals. Urinary incontinence (where the animal is unable to adequately control the bladder) can become a significant problem for animals as they age.

Stimulant drugs are sometimes given to patients to temporarily increase their ability to function properly. Doxapram is a known stimulant that has the ability to transiently boost the respiratory rate in animals being treated for respiratory related problems.

Antidiarrheals

Antiemetics are beneficial in the treatment of **burdensome nausea symptoms**. Antiemetics are employed to stop or reduce patient vomiting. The selection of the antiemetic will be made after due consideration of the causes contributing to the vomiting. Some patients vomit as a result of motion sickness (often induced by automobile or boat travel). Patients with motion sickness have been known to respond favorably to chlorpromazine, diphenhydramine, and dimenhydrinate. Patients who suffer from gastrointestinal spasms may respond well to metoclopramide or aminopentamide. These medications may also help improve peristaltic movement in the gastrointestinal system.

The patient with watery, diarrheal bowel movements may benefit from antidiarrheal drugs. However, the veterinarian should investigate the underlying cause of the diarrhea before administering an antidiarrheal drug. For example, hypersecretions (diarrhea) may be caused when bacteria emit poisons that induce fluid retention in the bowel and accelerate the excretory process. Common treatments for diarrhea include loperamide and diphenoxylate. Other diarrhea medications include aminopentamide and various antispasmodics. Some diarrhea treatments like bismuth, kaolin, pectin, and activated charcoal do not require a prescription.

Emetics

Emetics are drugs which are used to **induce vomiting**. Typical applications include emptying stomach contents of contaminated foods or poisonous substances. Upon ingestion of the drug, the animal vomits up the contents of its stomach. These drugs should not be used in situations where regurgitation can cause further damage (i.e., where the substance may be better neutralized by other treatments). Generally, the contents of the stomach can be safely regurgitated when a noncorrosive toxin has been swallowed by the patient. The noncorrosive toxin must be eliminated from the patient's stomach as soon as possible. The administered emetic will produce the desired results quickly.

Emetics are also **beneficial prior to anesthesia** in cases where the patient has ingested food shortly before surgery, creating a risk of anesthesia-induced emesis and pulmonary aspiration. Emetics work by irritating the gastric mucosa, which then stimulates the central nervous system and causes vomiting to occur. Examples of emetic drugs are syrup of ipecac and hydrogen peroxide.

Saline and Bulk Laxatives

Magnesium salts are a form of **saline laxative**. Saline laxatives are able to osmotically induce the movement of water into and out of the small intestines, and thereby swiftly drain the lower intestines of its contents.

Other laxatives use combinations of **fibers and water**. These laxatives are referred to as bulk-producing laxatives. Insoluble, water-absorbing fiber can often relieve constipation. Undigested fiber is transported via the GI tract where peristalsis (fecal-moving muscle contractions) pushes along the swollen, fibrous bulk that has taken on water.

However, bulk-producing laxatives are unable to work without the addition of water and other liquids into the body. Thus, the patient must be encouraged to take adequate fluids to ensure the laxative works correctly and to avoid otherwise dehydrating the bowel and its contents further.

Hyperosmotic and Disaccharide Laxatives

Constipation is a condition in which the intestinal tract is blocked or obstructed with an accumulation of hardened and somewhat dehydrated fecal matter. This condition can often be alleviated with the administration of a laxative. The laxative draws fluids into the bowel, and thereby eases the constipating symptoms. Hyperosmotic laxatives such as lactulose and magnesium salts are able to draw water from the surrounding tissues, thereby softening the feces.

Certain kinds of **disaccharides (sugars) may also aid in resolving constipation**. Some disaccharides are irregular sugars which cannot be digested by mammals. One example is lactulose, which remains undigested throughout the gastrointestinal tract. Inside the large intestine, lactulose attracts bacteria which produce acids and thereby bring water into the bowel. The resulting hydration can relieve the dry hardness of the feces and aid in their expulsion.

Antacids

Effective antacids work by **reducing levels of acids** that cause discomfort (i.e., "heartburn" or pyrosis) within the stomach. Most antacids are designed to produce a chemical buffer which results in a rise in overall gastric pH measurements. The rise in pH occurs as the antacid neutralizes the gastric acids. Following treatment with a buffering antacid, any stomach contents that reflux up into the esophagus will no longer cause the painful, burning symptoms characteristic of acidic fluid exposure.

Histamine H_2-receptor antagonist antacids work by **reducing the amount of gastric acids produced**. As histamine is the most important positive regulator of gastric acid production, blocking histamine receptors interrupts the production cycle. The H_2-receptor is a cell that can be motivated to create histamines in the stomach responsible for gastric secretions. Drugs which block the H_2-receptor thus stop some of the production of gastric acids.

Common H_2-receptor antagonists include cimetidine, ranitidine, and famotidine (with trade names of Tagamet, Zantac, and Pepcid, respectively). However, there are other receptors which can also produce acid in the stomach which are not effectively held in check by the H_2-receptor–blocking drugs. Thus, other adjunctive treatments and management approaches may be necessary.

Types of Laxatives

Other **beneficial laxatives** work by **lubricating the intestinal tract** and the **waste material** contained therein. Examples of **lubricant laxatives** are mineral oils and petroleum-based products. These lubricants work to ease the friction between the stool and the intestinal tract. The involved surfaces become coated in a waterproof covering of indigestible grease or oil. This coating not only fills the entire GI tract, but covers and mixes with the feces as well. Water consumption is maintained to keep the stool soft. The lubricant and water are beneficial in producing fecal matter that is softer and more easily expelled.

Emollient laxatives (stool softeners), such as Colace, are used to help alleviate uncomfortable symptoms in the patient experiencing constipation. These laxatives contain a surfactant such as docusate that helps to "wet" and soften the stool. Emollient laxatives may take a week or longer to be effective. Even so, they are used frequently by postoperative patients, postpartum women, and individuals suffering from hemorrhoids.

Ulcers

Ulcers are **sores which are found on the membranous lining of the digestive system**. There are drugs which can reduce the formation of these sores. These drugs are known as antiulcer drugs. Antiulcer drugs are listed under 4 classifications: antacids, H_2-receptor blockers, proton pump inhibitors, and cytoprotective agents.

Antacids are beneficial in reducing the stomach acids which can cause discomfort to the patient. The acids are neutralized by drugs like Amphojel, Maalox, Basaljel, and Tums. It should be noted that some drugs are not absorbed into the bloodstream as readily when antacids are given to the patient. Therefore, the absorption of other drugs should be more carefully considered when antacids are being prescribed, or over-the-counter preparations are being used.

The stomach contains gastric parietal cells which produce stomach acid. Parietal cells interact with the proton pump or the ATPase pump, which is responsible for the release of histamine. Histamine is the most important positive regulator of the secretion of gastric acid in the stomach. If histamine is not released, then the proton pump cannot produce acid as readily. When stomach acid levels fall, ulcer healing can more readily take place.

Proton Pump Inhibitors (PPI)

Animals who don't respond to traditional antacids and acid blockers may require acid control treatment with a **proton pump inhibitor (PPI).** The gastric hydrogen/potassium ATPase enzyme is often called the "proton pumps" (acidification) system of the stomach. PPIs denature the ATPase enzyme and allow it to be digested, stopping acid production by up to 99%.

The quantity of acid can be measured in proportion to the number of protons found in the stomach. The acid is reduced as the relative amount of proton pumps are prevented from secreting acids in the stomach. The proton pump inhibition systems are considered to be powerful antacids.

One common type of proton pump inhibitor medication is omeprazole, marketed under the trade name Prilosec. Another kind of effective antacid is misoprostol, marketed as Cytotec. It works to trigger an increase in secretions found in the lining of the gastrointestinal tract. These increased secretions more fully protect and lubricate the gastrointestinal tract from the effects of gastric acids.

Antiulcer Drugs

Some drugs block histamine H_2-receptors in the stomach, and thereby reduce the amount of gastric acid. Effective H_2-receptor– blocking drugs include famotidine, ranitidine, and cimetidine (marketed under trade names Pepcid, Zantac, and Tagamet, respectively).

Other antiulcer drugs work to stop enzyme-based proton pumps from producing acid in the stomach. Proton pump inhibitors are effective in denaturing the ATPase enzyme. If this enzyme is blocked then acid is not produced. One type of proton pump inhibitor medication is omeprazole. The trade name for omeprazole is Prilosec.

Another type of antiulcer drug is sucralfate or Carafate. This drug creates a protective lining along the surface where the ulcer has formed. Similarly, misoprostol (Cylotec) also forms a protective coating by increasing the production of mucus in the lining of the gastrointestinal tract.

However, the absorption of some medications may be impaired by antacids. Thus, absorption factors as related to gastric acidity should be considered when treating a patient — particularly one who has been given proton pump inhibitors — as the reason for impaired absorption may be the stomach's low gastric pH levels.

Reproductive Drugs

Two categories of reproductive drugs are **estrogen** and **progestins**. One type of estrogen, Diethylstilbestrol or DES, is formed synthetically through means of a chemical process. This drug is used to prevent a successful pregnancy when breeding of the animal was not planned. The function of this drug is to cause the fertilized egg to be reabsorbed, so that the reproductive cell or the ova cannot make its way to the uterus. Potential negative side effects from this drug include bone marrow suppression, aplastic anemia, pyometra, or death. Aplastic anemia is a particularly serious condition in which the bone marrow cannot produce enough red blood cells.

A semi-synthetically produced estrogen is known as estradiol cypionate or ECP. This drug is used for hormone replacement therapy, to prevent embryo implantation within 72 hours of mating, and to treat animals that are experiencing urinary incontinence. Some horses respond favorably to this drug and become more responsive to the sexual advances of other horses. However, this drug should not be given to animals that are pregnant with unborn offspring. To date, the drug ECP has not been reported as having serious side effects.

Prostaglandin Reproductive Drugs

The synthetic prostaglandins constitute another category of reproductive drugs. **Dinoprost** is one example of a synthetic analog of prostaglandin. This drug is effective in bringing about a faster birth at the end of a pregnancy. Dinoprost can also be used to bring about a premature end to a pregnancy by miscarriage.

Prostaglandin is a naturally occurring hormone in female mammals. Secreted by the uterus, this substance is beneficial in adjusting and controlling the length of time that the corpus luteum exists. The corpus luteum can be defined as a yellow mass of tissue that manifests itself after ovulation has occurred in the mammal, and is necessary to establish and maintain a pregnancy. Ovulation is the condition in which an egg reaches the right stage to be released from the ovary, and the corpus luteum develops from an ovarian follicle following this release.

This process produces **optimum conditions for fertilization** of the egg. Gloves and other protective covering should be worn whenever administering this drug to an animal, as the drug can be absorbed through the skin.

Progestins

A second category of reproductive drugs is known as **progestins**. Progestins are beneficial to animals that are having difficulty adjusting or controlling periods of sexual excitement during their estrous cycle.

Animals typically experience a stage of **sexual inactivity just after a breeding period**, which is known as the transitional anestrus stage. Progestins can be administered to animals in the anestrus stage to keep them from entering the proestrus period in preparation for sexual activity. The proestrus period is the stage immediately preceding estrus, which is the period of heightened sexual responsiveness and fertility.

One example of this medication is megestrol acetate. Similar to naturally occurring progesterone, megestrol acetate has anti-estrogen properties that produce the necessary effects. However, gloves and other protective covering should be worn when administering progestin drugs, as the liquid form can readily be absorbed through the skin.

Oxytocin, Fluprostenol, and Eleprostenol

Oxytocin is another type of **reproductive drug**. This drug is beneficial in facilitating the birth process. This drug may also be used to increase milk production in the female, providing the offspring with the enhanced benefit of natural mother's milk. Maternal milk is rich in nutrients such as protein, fats, lactose, and vitamins.

The veterinarian should administer oxytocin when the cervix is dilated. The cervix is the lower portion of the uterus with an opening, called the os, which connects the uterus to the vagina or birth canal. Oxytocin is a drug which benefits the uterus, causing the smooth muscles to contract, helping the uterus to discharge its contents.

Other drugs used for reproductive purposes are fluprostenol and eleprostenol. These drugs are used in the reproductive treatment of large-sized animals. The preferred method of use is through subcutaneous (i.e., under the skin) injection.

Diabetes

Diabetes is a serious medical condition. Patients that suffer with diabetes experience hyperglycemia, a condition in which blood sugar reaches unsafe levels. Patients with diabetes may also experience blood sugars that are too low. These fluctuations are caused by the body's failure to control and adjust blood sugar levels by means of the hormone insulin. Insulin is described as a polypeptide hormone which is secreted by beta cells found in the islet of Langerhans, in the pancreas. This hormone is responsible for moving glucose out of the blood and into the cells, where it is burned for energy or stored for later use. If this hormone is not produced in sufficient supply, the patient will become diabetic.

Animals are prone to contracting 2 kinds of diabetes: 1) uncomplicated diabetes, and 2) diabetes with ketoacidosis. Uncomplicated diabetes primarily involves reduced insulin production. If the animal cannot manufacture enough insulin, then the animal becomes dependent on artificial sources of insulin. Diabetic ketoacidosis (DKA) occurs when fatty acid–derived ketone bodies become the primary cellular energy source instead of glucose. The metabolism of fats produces an acidic state in the blood that often further complicates the diabetes, and rising levels of ketones may become toxic. Thus, animals with DKA may be very ill, vomiting, and depressed.

Insulin and Insulin Facilitators

There are two medications which a veterinarian might prescribe for treatment of diabetes. These medications are **insulin** and **insulin facilitators** such as sulfonylurea-based medications.

Insulin is available as a hormone in 3 classifications. The first type of insulin is given to patients who require their blood sugars to be decreased rapidly. An example of this kind of insulin medication for animals is Vetsulin. Patients who require a daily control method should be given NPH. NPH is insulin which is classified as an intermediate acting hormone.

Finally, insulin can be blended with protamine to produce a product that can last for an extended period of time. This mixture can also be given to the patient through injections. Animal patients with diabetes will benefit from the administration of protamine zinc insulin. The extended release nature of this medication gradually releases insulin over a 24 hour period.

The veterinarian may also administer insulin in concentrated forms. The concentrations have been measured in accordance with international unit (IU) per milliliter (mL) standards. In determining the kinds of insulin to use and the dosages and concentrations, the veterinarian must apply proper evaluative standards based on the individual patient and the presenting circumstances.

Insulin Resistant Diabetes and Ketoacidosis

Another form of diabetes is called **insulin resistant** or **IR diabetes**. In this condition, the patient is not utilizing or processing the insulin that is available. This form of diabetes is more common in canines, but can also occur in horses, cats, and cattle. The patient may exhibit symptoms of extreme thirst and/or an excessive need for urination. The patient may initially gain weight, although the extended progression of this disease is characterized by weight loss. The patient may also become lethargic and exhibit sluggishness or exhaustion. Further, the patient may experience vision problems due to cataracts (as they are 40 to 60% more likely to develop this problem as a complication of the disease). The patient's coat or fur may also show signs of distress.

In addition, the animal will likely have **ketoacidosis**. Ketoacidosis is categorized by the body's breakdown of fats as a primary energy source, as opposed to glucose and carbohydrates. The level of ketone bodies in the blood may become toxic in the diabetic patient. The condition may cause the patient to present with "fruity" smelling acetone breath as the ketone concentration rises. Blood or urine testing will definitively reveal the level of ketones. Treatment typically involves intravenous fluid replacement (to correct dehydration and dilute acids and ketones) and the administration of insulin until the situation becomes more stable.

Insulin-Specific Syringes

Insulin is always taken by injection, as it cannot tolerate the digestive process. A veterinarian must use insulin syringes that have been appropriately marked for this purpose. Insulin syringes that have not been marked in "IU's" or international units of measurement should not be used by the veterinarian. Insulin syringes have been specifically designed for the administration of a given solution strength of insulin. For instance, the syringe marked with U-40 is for patients in need of 40 units of insulin hormone, while the syringe marked with U-100 is for patients in need of 100 units of insulin hormone. Therefore, use of the wrong syringe can result in the wrong dosage of insulin. This can potentially result in the death of the animal.

Certain other medications can be used to treat some diabetic patients, particularly those who still produce some natural insulin. One classification of these medications is the sulfonylureas. A common sulfonylurea-based antidiabetic drug is glipizide. Glipizide (Glucotrol) is given to animals which still possess the ability to produce some insulin by natural means, but with a diagnosis of insulin-independent diabetes. This medication is best if given twice a day during the mealtimes.

Hyperthyroidism

The thyroid is part of the endocrine (glandular) system. The **endocrine system** regulates, controls, and adjusts the provision of chemical energy, enzymatic catalysts, and nutrients as needed for a healthy metabolism. Thus, endocrine disorders can be quite complex and damaging. In the case of an overactive thyroid, the thyroid gland produces an overabundance of certain hormones. This condition is diagnosed as hyperthyroidism. The thyroid secretes the hormones thyroxin (T4) and triiodothyronine (T3). This condition is rarely diagnosed in canines and is more commonly found in felines.

Upon further inspection, the cat will usually be secondarily diagnosed with a thyroid tumor. The tumor is typically comprised of thyroid cells, thus accounting for the increased production of thyroid hormones. Felines diagnosed with hyperthyroidism can range from 4 to 22 years of age. Some cats suffering from hyperthyroidism may experience weight loss, while others may have an increased appetite. The condition can be exacerbated by a heart murmur or elevated heart rate. The cat may also exhibit marked thirst and an excessive need to urinate.

Treating Hyperthyroidism

Hyperthyroidism is evident in the overproduction of thyroxin (T4) and triiodothyronine (T3). Hyperthyroidism can be detected through a simple blood test. In most cases the veterinarian will surgically remove the diseased thyroid — often referred to as **surgical ablation** (i.e., removal or reduction) of the thyroid. However, this surgery does come with significant risks to the parathyroid gland. The parathyroid gland is responsible for producing hormones that regulate calcium and phosphorus in the body's skeletal system. The removal of the entire thyroid will precipitously cause hypothyroidism, and even partial ablation often produces a change from hyperthyroidism to hypothyroidism. In cases of hypothyroidism the animal will require thyroid supplements to regulate the body's metabolism. Periodic blood tests will be necessary to determine how much of the supplement drug needs to be administered to the animal. Options to surgical ablation include radioactive and chemical ablation.

Antithyroid Agents and Radioactive Iodine Treatment

There are **alternative treatments for hyperthyroidism** that are not surgical in nature. Alternatives include radioactive iodine treatment and antithyroid agents such as methimazole, marketed as Tapazole.

Tapazole is beneficial in obstructing enzymatic processes in the thyroid necessary for the production of triiodothyronine (T3) and thyroxin (T4). The animal should be monitored for side effects following this treatment, as it may induce vomiting, malaise, and fatigue.

Radioactive iodine treatments make use of the thyroid's natural demand for iodine. The thyroid is the only organ in the body that requires iodine to work properly. The thyroid absorbs radioactive iodine the same way that it absorbs normal iodine. The radioactive iodine focuses its strength on any hyperplastic tissue or tumor found inside the thyroid.

Hyperplastic tissue has formed from an increase in the number of cells, and tends to utilize greater quantities of iodine than normal thyroid tissue. Thus, this abnormal tissue is exposed to greater levels of radiation from the radioactive iodine. The radiation works to destroy the tumor and/or reduce the numbers of hormone- producing cells. This treatment usually does not harm the majority of normal cells found in the thyroid.

Hypothyroidism

Hypothyroidism may cause a myriad of other conditions and symptoms. For example, excessive weight gain may create secondary problems. Not only can the animal's joints and cardiac and respiratory status be compromised, but when muscle and other tissues atrophy and waste away, accumulating fat may infiltrate where the tissues have become structurally diminished. Further, because normal thyroid hormone levels are necessary for healthy hair and nails, an animal's fur may thin and appear dull and lackluster, and the nails and the skin may become cracked and flakey. The animal may also exhibit marked alopecia — a condition in which its hair falls out.

The animal may also suffer from anemia and/or high blood cholesterol. Anemia is a blood disorder characterized by hemoglobin deficiency and reduced numbers of red blood cells. This causes the animal to become weak. High blood cholesterol can also be linked to the development of atherosclerotic heart disease. The animal's skin may exhibit hyperpigmentation, which discolors the skin.

The animals most commonly affected by hypothyroidism are dogs ranging in age from 4 to 10 years. The dogs are more typically medium or large in size. Smaller dogs do not develop hypothyroidism as often as larger-sized dogs.

Treating Hypothyroidism

Hypothyroidism can sometimes be the result of a hypothalamus or a pituitary gland dysfunction. The hypothalamus releases a hormone called **Thyrotropin Releasing Hormone** (TRH), which stimulates the pituitary to release a hormone called **Thyroid Stimulating Hormone** (TSH). TSH in turn stimulates the thyroid to produce its metabolic regulatory hormones, triiodothyronine (T3) and thyroxin (T4). A breakdown at any point in this system of endocrine relays will result in hypothyroidism. Thus, the production and release of TRH and TSH is critical in the regulation of thyroid hormones required for a healthy metabolism.

In the event that the thyroid's production levels of T3 and T4 are diminished — whether due to hypothalamus or pituitary dysfunction, or due to dysfunction of the thyroid gland itself — the patient's condition will be diagnosed as hypothyroidism. Hypothyroidism can be detected through simple blood tests. The blood tests are analyzed based on measurements of T3, T4, and TSH. The veterinarian will use this data to determine the amount of medications that the patient needs. The patient may be given supplemental thyroid hormones, as T3 and T4 can be produced synthetically.

Supplemental Medications for Hypothyroidism

Hypothyroidism causes a slowing of the animal's metabolic rate due to a **decrease in thyroid hormone production**. Resolution of persistent hypothyroidism requires the administration of supplemental thyroid hormones. Natural thyroid hormones are available from desiccated porcine (pig) thyroids. However, obtaining accurate standardized dosages may be problematic. Synthetic T3 and T4 are both available, but the veterinarian will normally select T4 to be administered due to the complications involving T3 supplementation. T3's dosage is often difficult to regulate, and overmedicating the patient is an ongoing challenge.

T4 supplementation alone may be sufficient, as the thyroid is able to transform some T4 into T3. However, this is not always the case with a malfunctioning thyroid, and thus combined synthetic T3/T4 supplementation may sometimes be required. The animal's hormone levels and reaction to the drugs should be monitored to ensure proper dosage and medication management over time. Periodic blood tests will be beneficial in determining how much of the drug needs to be administered at optimum intervals. Careful ongoing monitoring of the patient's blood levels should produce the data needed to successfully regulate the animal's metabolic functioning.

Common Symptoms of Hypothyroidism

Hypothyroidism is a condition in which the thyroid finds itself unable to secrete enough hormones to promote healthy metabolic functioning. This condition affects both felines and canines, although it is more commonly found in dogs. Indeed, it is the most common endocrine disorder occurring in canines.

Upon closer inspection, the veterinarian usually discovers that the thyroid gland has been destroyed by the animal's immune system — with elements of the animal's own immune system attacking the previously healthy thyroid cells. This condition is known as **autoimmune thyroiditis**.

Animals with hypothyroidism frequently gain weight, even with only modest nutritional intake. Additional symptoms include increased fatigue, anemia, constipation, poor blood clotting, increased susceptibility to infections and illnesses, depression, mental dullness, cold intolerance, and mild bradycardia.

Vaccines

Vaccines are given to patients to **reduce the likelihood of a particular virulent or damaging disease**. Successful vaccination requires the administration of a subclinical (small, insufficient to infect) amount of the target germs or viral matter to the animal. The germs or viral matter administered (referred to as the inoculant or inoculum) may be either live (active), modified (attenuated or denatured), or killed (dead). The administration of an inoculant is referred to as an inoculation. The inoculation can take the form of an oral dose, an injection, or an inhalation. Regardless, the inoculant is introduced into the animal's immune system.

The animal's immune system then works to fight off the small amount of infection which has been introduced. Dead inoculant offers the least amount of immunization from a disease. However, the dead inoculant is also the safest one to be introduced into the body. Both living and modified inoculants are more dangerous to the patient. Even so, they do offer more protection from the disease. This is because live or attenuated inoculants produce a stronger immune response, as measured in greater numbers of antibodies produced and their longer persistence in the body. These antibodies will attack any inoculant-specific infection that the patient may later acquire, as long as they continue to be produced by the body.

Vaccine Efficacy

If a **vaccination is effective**, it will cause **antigens** to be produced by the body. Antigens are large protein molecules found on the outer surface of the microorganisms which cause disease. The antigens are responsible for the body's creation of antibodies to fight off the disease. The body's immune system identifies the foreign antigens when an exposure has occurred. With a vaccine, the first exposure occurred at the time of inoculation. The body then learns to synthesize proper antibodies to fight the specific antigens encountered.

Later, subsequent contacts with the disease allow the body to fight off the microorganisms with a larger, existing collection of antigen-specific antibodies. The degree of vaccination success and duration of antibody persistence will depend upon certain conditions, including the animal's age, breed, and health; the strength of the animal's immune system; the method of storage of the vaccine; and the inoculation method and type chosen by the veterinarian.

Efficacy and Passive Immunity

Vaccines should be stored in such a way as not to reduce their potency. The vaccine usually does not become effective in fighting the disease for up to 3 weeks following the first injection. Vaccines given nasally may take only a few days to become effective, but nasally administered vaccines tend to produce fewer antibodies, even when weakened live inoculants are used (versus the dead inoculants provided by injection).

Some **natural immunizations** may occur between mothers and their offspring. Mothers are able to pass some antibodies on to their unborn babies through the placenta. This form of immunization is known as maternal passive immunity. However, some difficulty exists in determining how long passive immunity lasts. Therefore, the baby should be given additional dosages of vaccine over a period of time to ensure protection. Antitoxins are described as antibodies taken from plants, animals, and certain bacteria that are able to fight off specific toxins or poisons. Antiserums are obtained from animals or humans that have been able to produce antibodies to a particular disease. The blood serum of an antibody-bearing host is used to transfer antibodies to an otherwise susceptible host. One common type of antiserum is antivenin, obtained from animals which have been inoculated with increasing doses of snake venom until they have developed high antibody concentrations. Both antitoxin and antiserum administrations confer passive immunity to the recipient.

Immunosuppressives

Some diseases trigger the immune system to such a degree that the animal is harmed. Harmful effects arising from an **overactive immune system** can be relieved with the administration of certain kinds of drugs. These various drugs are referred to as immunosuppressants. These same drugs have also been used in the treatment of patients that have received organs or tissues from donors. The body's natural immune system will try to attack and destroy donated organs, as they are seen as foreign invaders. However, immunosuppressant drugs can help the body to accept the organs or tissues more gradually, while holding an aggressive immune system at bay.

Patients that have a disease that is autoimmune in origin may also benefit from the administration of these drugs. Diseases that fall in this category include rheumatoid arthritis, lupus erythematosus, inflammatory bowel disease, and ulcerative colitis. Drugs that are classified as immunosuppressants (and their trade names) include azathioprine (Imuran), cyclosporine (Sandimmune), cyclophosphamide (Cytoxan), corticosteroids, and metronidazole (Flagyl).

Antimetabolites

An **antimetabolite** is a drug which has the ability to interrupt normal metabolic processes, such as cell growth. The composition of antimetabolites targeting cell growth is similar to the metabolites that promote cell growth. The essential difference is that the antimetabolite uses altered cell replication nucleotides in place of the nucleotides necessary to sustain cell division. Purines and pyrimidines are organic nucleotides needed for cell DNA replication. One form of cell antimetabolite uses similar-looking purine and pyrimidine analogs, but ones that are unable to complete the replication process. The tumor cell introduces these nucleotide analogs in an effort to replicate the tumor cell's DNA. However, this similar-looking compound does not produce the same results. Further, because they are made abundantly available, the antimetabolites are largely able to prevent the true purines and pyrimidines from being introduced into the tumor cell. In this way, cancerous tumor growth is substantially inhibited by the antimetabolite.

Common Antimetabolite Drugs

Although originally designed for use in human hosts, veterinarians can also utilize **antimetabolite drugs** to stop or **interrupt the growth of cancerous cells** in animals. Hydroxyurea, cytarabine, methotrexate, and 5-fluorouracil are all cell-cycle–specific drugs (i.e., drugs that inhibit the process of cell division) and are thus classified as antimetabolites. When used, the veterinarian should carefully monitor the patient for any untoward side effects, as these drugs may cause bone marrow suppression. The drug hydroxyurea is typically given to patients with blood, bone marrow, and lymph node cancers. The drug cytarabine is given to patients with leukemia. Methotrexate is given to patients with cancer of the breast, head and neck, lung, blood, and bone, and has recently also come to be used in the treatment of certain autoimmune diseases. The drug 5-fluorouracil is given to patients with bowel, breast, stomach, and esophageal cancers. However, 5-fluorouracil is not safe for use with felines.

These drugs have all been effective in the treatment of patients previously diagnosed with cancer.

Immunostimulants

The immune system can be medically assisted with drugs known as **immunostimulants**. Immunostimulants work to increase the body's immunological response against unwanted viruses and cancer cells. The animal diseases that are most commonly treated with immunostimulants include FLV or feline leukemia virus, FIV or feline immunodeficiency virus, and canine lymphoma. Dogs that develop canine lymphoma can receive a boost to their immune system through the administration of canine lymphoma monoclonal antibodies. The abbreviated term for canine lymphoma monoclonal antibodies medication is CL/MAb 321. These antibodies are produced in a laboratory. The animal will benefit greatly when the stimulated immune system begins to inflict damage on cancer cells.

Acemannan is an immunostimulant that is beneficial in the treatment of patients with FLV, FIV, and specific cancers. Acemannan is produced by synthesizing aloe vera and propionibacterium acnes. The trade name for acemannan is Immunoregulin.

Alkylating Agents

Alkylating agents are formed out of an alkyl group and small carbon-hydrogen compounds. These agents can hinder cancerous growths in 3 ways, all involving cellular DNA. First, they may stop tumor cell growth by cross-linking nucleobases found in the cell's DNA strands. This action renders the DNA incapable of uncoiling and separating itself for transcription, which is necessary for replication. Second, alkylating agents can attach alkyl groups to DNA bases. Sensing alteration, DNA repair enzymes will inadvertently separate and fragment the DNA in unsuccessful efforts to replace the altered DNA bases. Third, alkylating agents can also induce the mispairing of DNA nucleotides. The double-strands of DNA must pair specific nucleotides in each strand with each other in order to form and maintain the coiled, double-helix formation necessary for proper DNA function. If the nucleotides mispair with alternate nucleotides then DNA mutations result, preventing DNA replication and subsequent cell division.

Mitotic Inhibitors

Some cancers can also be treated with medications known as **mitotic inhibitors**. These drugs are derived from plant alkaloids, and are able to stop the cellular process of mitosis — i.e., nucleus (chromosomal) replication in preparation for cell division, followed by cytokinesis, in which all other cell contents replicate/separate and divide. Mitosis is stopped by disrupting a process known as microtubular polymerization. This process involves the joining of protein pairs, called dimers, into protofilaments and then into microtubules. A polarization process is also involved, causing the protofilaments to join only end-to-end, thereby producing long filaments capable of creating extended microtubules. Cells use microtubules to construct the cytoskeleton, mitotic spindle, and other intracellular components. These microtubules are derived from structural proteins known as tubulin. Mitotic inhibitors work to inhibit or suppress the tubulin dimers. This stops mitosis from being carried out in the cell and thus cell replication does not take place.

Alkylating Agents

Alkylating agents produce an altered DNA which is unable to replicate or copy its genetic material. Cisplatin, carboplatin, chlorambucil, and cyclosphamide are drugs which work with the use of alkylating agents. All can be used in animal populations, although the drug cisplatin is contraindicated for use with felines.

Some alkylating agents (and other drugs) fall into the category of "**prodrugs**." A prodrug is one that is largely or entirely inactive in its administered form. These drugs must be changed or altered by a predetermined mechanism in the body to become active. The purposes behind prodrugs are twofold: 1) to increase bioavailability (often to improve gastrointestinal absorption), and 2) to target certain cells such as cancer cells (allowing, for example, properties unique to those cells to activate the drug).

The drug known as cyclophosphamide is considered a prodrug. This drug must first be changed by the liver in order to activate the drug's alkylating agents. The patient given these drugs should be monitored for side effects such as bone marrow suppression, gastrointestinal disturbances, and hemorrhagic cystitis (severe bleeding in the bladder due to the chemotherapy).

Antineoplastic Agents

Antineoplastic agents (cytotoxic chemotherapy drugs) are beneficial in treating patients with cancer. These drugs work by traveling throughout the body and killing off cancerous cells that can develop into tumors. A tumor (neoplasm) is an uncontrolled growth of malignant or benign cells. Left unchecked, benign tumors can encroach on normal tissues and functions, and cancerous tumors can spread and overwhelm the body.

The veterinarian who uses this drug should wear safety equipment. The recommended safety gear includes gloves and protective clothing. The person administering this drug is at risk because the antineoplastic agent in the drug is not end-cell selective, and thus will kill off both cancer and non-cancer cells in life-forms. Thus, healthy human and healthy animal cells can be accidentally destroyed by this drug when contact precautions are not followed. The antineoplastic drug works by seeking out any cell that can multiply rapidly. Typically, the gastrointestinal cells, tumor cells, bone marrow cells, and reproductive tract cells are the ones targeted. However, the drug can also result in lasting harm to the DNA, which cannot be repaired.

Classifications of Antineoplastic Drugs

There are **5 classifications of antineoplastic drugs**: alkylating agents, antimetabolites, plant alkaloids, antibiotics, and hormonal agents.

The veterinarian should prepare the starting dosage based on body surface in square meters rather than on the animal's body weight, as this figure closely approximates total blood volume. Adjustments to avoid toxicity (based on individual metabolism, liver and kidney function, etc.) may later be needed.

The veterinarian must also consider the type of cancer and its stage of progression when selecting an antineoplastic drug and in determining a specified regimen of chemotherapy. It is not uncommon for a veterinarian to select a combination of these drugs in treating a patient with cancer. However, the veterinarian should remember to always use safety equipment when handling and administering antineoplastic drugs.

Monitoring Mitotic Inhibitors

Mitotic inhibitors are known as Vinca alkaloids, because the alkaloid components, Vincristine and Vinblastine, are derived from the Madagascar Periwinkle, once botanically classified as Vinca rosea (now classified as Catharanthus roseus). Vinca alkaloid drugs are beneficial in the treatments of patients who have cancer, as these alkaloids prevent cancer from completing mitosis and subsequent cell replication.

However, the veterinarian should be careful in administering these drugs because Vinca alkaloids are not target-cell specific. This means that these drugs can produce adverse conditions by stopping all replicating cells. Thus, the intestinal epithelium and bone marrow cells, for example, can also be prevented from replicating (albeit the cancer cells are stopped from replicating, along with these essential cells). Therefore, the patient's drug levels as relevant to toxicity must be carefully and regularly monitored. Toxicity may manifest as gastrointestinal disturbances, bone marrow suppression, and alopecia. The drug is a vesicating (blister-producing) agent and does cause skin irritation when it has been exposed. The drug Vincristine is given to patients who have lymphoma. The drug Vinblastine is given to patients who have mast cell tumors.

Erythropoietin for Treating Anemia

Cancer chemotherapeutic treatments can induce bone marrow suppression, reducing red blood cell production and creating an anemic condition. **Anemia** (low hemoglobin) can also be caused by other conditions. To remedy anemia, patients may be given "**blood building**" products called **hematics** (or hematinics). Three types of hematics include erythropoietin, androgens, and blood substitutes. Patients that take hematics will experience an increase in the oxygen carrying capacity of the blood, as available hemoglobin increases. Hemoglobin is described as a protein-containing iron that is capable of carrying oxygen from the lungs to the other parts of the body. Red blood cells need hemoglobin to function properly. The patient that exhibits symptoms of anemia should be given a blood test. The test will determine the volume of hemoglobin that is present (typically measured in grams per deciliter of blood). Patients with anemia will have lower volumes of hemoglobin. Erythropoietin (also called hematopoietin or hemopoietin) is a hormone that regulates the production of red blood cells. Both the kidney and the liver, to a lesser degree, produce this hormone in response to low blood levels. Where hemoglobin levels have fallen precipitously, the patient can be given a synthetic version in the form of an injection to boost red blood cell production and related hemoglobin availability.

Anticoagulants and Thrombolytics

The patient afflicted with **blood clots** (thrombi) can typically benefit from the administration of **anticoagulants** and **thrombolytics**. Anticoagulants are given to **stop the formation of blood clots** in the circulatory system of the patient. Thrombolytics can **break up and dissolve blood clots** in the body. Blood clots are formed from the process of coagulation by a protein known as thrombin. Thrombin is a blood enzyme which is responsible for increasing the conversion rate of fibrinogen to fibrin. Fibrin is a protein which induces the blood to clot. Antithrombin is a protein molecule that inactivates several enzymes in the body's coagulation system, including the enzyme thrombin. Thrombin is also stopped by the use of a medication called heparin and its various derivatives. However, while heparin inhibits clot formation, it does not actively break up existing clots. Thrombolytics such as t-PA (alteplase Activase), streptokinase (Kabikinase, Streptase), and urokinase (Abbokinase) serve this purpose. Thrombolytics work to activate the production of plasmin. Plasmin is an enzyme which works to separate and disintegrate the strands of fibrin within a blood clot.

Androgens and Blood Substitutes for Treating Anemia

The hormone erythropoietin stimulates the **production of red blood cells in the bone marrow**. However, if the body does not produce sufficient erythropoietin, red blood cell production will also fall and cause anemia. While the liver does produce erythropoietin, about four-fifths of all erythropoietin is produced by the kidneys. Patients suffering from chronic anemia can be given androgens or anabolic steroids to stimulate the kidney's production of erythropoietin. However, the administration and secondary effects of androgens can be problematic. Therefore, this is not the drug of choice in the care of most patients with anemia.

A useful **blood substitute** that may be given to patients suffering from anemia is known as **Oxyglobin**. Oxyglobin is derived from chemically stabilized bovine hemoglobin. This substance gives short-term relief to the patient. Oxyglobin is able to raise and sustain higher oxygen levels in the blood. However, Oxyglobin is only intended for use with animals. Hemopure is a similar product designed for human use.

Topical Medications

Topical medications are drugs which are applied to the skin's surface and to the mucous membranes of the body. The mucous membranes line the surface of all moist body passages and features including the eyes, inner ears, nostrils, tongue, rectum, urethra, and vagina. Applying topical medications to the skin is normally easily accomplished. However, the mucous membranes can be very sensitive, and thus application of topical medications to these tissues requires special preparation. Topical medications can be applied otically in the form of ear drops; ophthalmically in the form of eye drops or ointments; intranasally as drops, creams, or ointments; and sublingually by placing the medication under the tongue. Cream and ointment topical medications can be applied directly to rectal and vaginal areas. The veterinarian should follow the instructions packaged with a medication explicitly. Particular caution is also required to compensate for animal biology and behaviors. For example, animals are known to pass their tongue over injured regions of the body in a cleansing and mollifying action. However, some human topical products can be poisonous to the animal. Topical treatments have a tendency to be poorly absorbed by the animal's system as a whole. Other topical drugs like nitroglycerin and certain pour-on preparations will produce a systematic effect.

THROMBOEMBOLISM

Patients suffering with **thromboembolism** may have one or more blood clots in the **pulmonary vasculature** — the blood vessels involving the lungs. The situation becomes life-threatening if the blood clots totally obstruct the flow of blood in the pulmonary vessels.

The drugs used in the treatment of this disease are **anticoagulants** and **thrombolytics**. However, research indicates that thrombolytics are not fully effective in treating this disease in veterinary patients. Anticoagulants, rather than thrombolytics, are more effective in veterinary patients with thromboembolism. Anticoagulants can be administered to the patient by injection with a syringe. They also work to stop the formation of clots in the blood samples drawn for use in medical tests. Uncoagulated whole blood is often necessary to obtain accurate results in laboratory tests.

ANESTHETIZING AND LUBRICATING OPHTHALMIC AGENTS

There are **ophthalmic anesthetics** that can be applied to the eye to numb and reduce the sensation of feeling in exposed eye membranes. Topical anesthetics appropriate for use in the eye which can produce this result include proparacaine and tetracaine.

Individuals may have environmental or health situations arise which **reduce the natural lubricants** of the eye (tears). For transient relief, drops of "**artificial tears**" are available. Conditions which cause enduring dryness of the eyes require more aggressive intervention. The disease keratoconjunctivitis sicca causes a patient to become incapable of producing adequate tears. Patients suffering from keratoconjunctivitis sicca can be given a medication called cyclosporine.

Cyclosporine seems to both reduce inflammatory cells and increase the number of mucin-secreting goblet cells, thus gaining the patient the ability to make tears in greater amounts.

Other anti-infective and anti-inflammatory agents can be applied in the treatment of the eyes. These drugs can reduce infection and irritation. However, the veterinarian should not use any medications with a steroid base for patients afflicted with a corneal ulcer.

COMMON OPHTHALMIC AGENTS

Patients are given ophthalmic agents to treat various conditions of the eyes. The medication can be produced as eye drops or eye ointments. Typically, ophthalmic agents require several applications before full relief is experienced by the patient.

Mydriatics are medical agents which produce a dilation of the pupils in the eyes. Tropicamide is a mydriatic agent which consistently produces a rapid result. This drug is beneficial when the patient requires an examination of the interior of the eye (i.e., the ocular fundus, etc.).

In some situations it becomes necessary to constrict the pupil. At such times the patient is given a miotic agent to produce a constriction of the pupil. The patient with glaucoma may be given a miotic agent called pilocarpine to constrict the pupil. This constriction is necessary to transiently increase the intraocular pressure. Glaucoma is a disease with abnormally high intraocular pressure. However, a temporary increase in pressure, such as that caused by constriction induced via a miotic agent, allows the excess aqueous humor (i.e., the transparent fluid in the eye) to drain away. This ultimately reduces the intraocular pressure that so often damages the sensitive interior structures of the eye.

Acetylcysteine

The medication acetylcysteine has multiple uses, one of which is as an antidote. This drug can be given in situations of **acetaminophen overdose**. Acetylcysteine is also used to reduce and dissolve mucus in conditions with excessive or thick mucus production such as emphysema, bronchitis, tuberculosis, and pneumonia.

As an antidote, **acetylcysteine** provides important protective effects. When metabolized in the liver, acetaminophen produces a toxic byproduct known by its acronym, NAPQI. This metabolite is typically removed from the body by glutathione, found in the liver. In situations of overdose, however, there are insufficient reserves. Acetylcysteine is able to stimulate the production of glutathione and bind with NAPQI, reducing its liver-toxic effects.

Unopened vials of acetylcysteine solutions should be kept at room temperature to ensure optimal results. However, upon opening the vial, it may only be refrigerated for a period of 96 hours or less. After 96 hours any previously opened medication should not be used. The medication is typically given intravenously due to low oral bioavailability and its very unpleasant taste and odor. The patient should be observed for possible side effects, including nausea, vomiting, and urticaria (hives).

Mucolytic Uses of Acetylcysteine

One of the side effects of acetylcysteine includes urticaria. **Urticaria** is a skin rash (i.e., hives) that indicates the patient is having an **allergic reaction** to the medication. With continued administration, the reaction will only get worse, and thus alternative treatment options will be necessary.

Acetylcysteine is also given to patients that are afflicted with lung disease, corneal ulcers, and keratoconjunctivitis.

When given in situations of mucus-producing pulmonary disease, the patient benefits from a reduction in the quantity and viscosity of the mucus produced. Treatments are given to the patient with a nebulizer. The nebulizer can be attached to the animal's face by way of a mask. The mask allows the animal to inhale the medication through either its nose or mouth. The nebulizer works to dissolve the mucus found in the animal's respiratory tract. The patient should be monitored for possible side effects, including heaviness or tightness in the chest area and urticaria. The patient may also experience a feeling of squeezing or constriction in the bronchi (or air passages) leading to the lungs, as well as irritation or a painful reaction to the medication in the respiratory tract.

Dormitor and Atipamezole

Domitor is a sedative medication often used to facilitate the handling of animals during clinical examinations, or when undergoing difficult or uncomfortable medical procedures. Domitor is also called medetomidine hydrochloride. For example, an animal that has come into contact with a porcupine may need to have the quills removed and can be given domitor as a calming sedative. However, the animal must not need a drug that produces muscle relaxation such as that required for respiratory intubation. At the conclusion of the procedure, the animal can be given atipamezole to reverse the effects of the Domitor. Atipamezole is given to the patient by intramuscular injection. **Atipamezole** is fast-acting, so the patient should recover from the effects of the sedative within 5 to 10 minutes. Some animals may experience transient behavioral problems, such as a readiness to attack or extreme nervousness. Thus, due caution should be exercised.

Side Effects Associated with Atipamezole.

Animals receiving **atipamezole** may temporarily become **inordinately anxious** or **nervous**, and may even exhibit a readiness to attack that is not normally part of their behavior. Therefore, the veterinarian should place the animal in a quiet and darkened recovery area that is not otherwise utilized while the animal is regaining consciousness and the effects of the sedative are wearing off.

In addition, the animal should be monitored for other side effects. In particular, the animal's blood pressure should be checked as the drug tends to induce hypotension. In some cases, the animal's heart and respiratory rates may rise. The patient should also be monitored for nausea and vomiting. Finally, the patient may also experience symptoms of diarrhea, hypersalivation, shivering or tremors, overstimulation, and nervousness.

Pregnant or nursing animals should not be given the drug, as the fetal and developmental effects are unknown.

Primary Symptoms of Organophosphate Poisoning

Organophosphate poisoning can easily lead to an animal's death. Typically, the animal that dies has experienced extreme respiratory distress produced from the toxic substance. The patient may exhibit the following: drooling, vomiting, stress defecation, diarrhea, constricted pupils, difficulty breathing (often due to laryngospasm, bronchospasm, bronchorrhea, or seizures), tremors, and muscle twitching. The antidote, atropine, lowers the secretions or the discharges caused by the poison and relaxes and expands the air passageways that were constricted from the spasmodic effects of the poison. The patient should be closely monitored for possible side effects. In particular, the patient may experience seizures, dilated pupils, and tachycardia. Patients experiencing a seizure may experience a very sudden onset and attack. The patient's pupils may dilate, becoming much wider or larger. The patient may even show signs of a rapid heart rate. Early administration of the antidote, atropine, should substantially reduce the toxic effects of organophosphate poisoning. Therefore, the veterinarian should administer the antidote as quickly as possible.

Common Organophosphates and Treatment

Organophosphates can be found in various insecticides and herbicides that animals (and humans) may sometimes ingest. The patient that has symptoms of organophosphate poisoning can be given atropine. **Atropine** serves as an antidote due to its **anti-cholinergic properties**. Atropine is produced from a substance found in a plant known as Atropa belladonna. A patient in need of medication with antispasmodic capabilities can be given atropine, as it has properties that will reduce the spasms the patient is experiencing. Atropine is also a form of a mydriatic (pupil dilatant).

Some **common insecticides** that contain organophosphates are Malathion, Parathion, Diazinon, Chlorpyrifos, and Chlorfenvinphos. **Organophosphates** are readily absorbed through the skin and can also enter through the gastrointestinal and respiratory tracts of the animal. An animal that has had contact with the poison may begin to show symptoms in just a few minutes. However, some of these poisons may only show up days later. The feline species is particularly susceptible to organophosphate poisoning.

Step Method for Conversion of Measurements

The **metric system** is a method used to measure the quantity of something. The method utilizes a set of procedures which allows the **conversion of measurements between varying related unit terms**. The units which can be assigned include meter (for spatial dimension), gram (for weight), or liter (for volume) measurements, depending upon the qualitative nature of the material being measured. The initial method of conversion between like-kinds of materials applies the "step method" to the problem. The step method is carried out by moving the decimal to the right to utilize a smaller unit of measurement. If the step method is carried out by moving the decimal to the left, then the unit of measurement utilized will be one larger. For example, suppose 300 milligrams (where "milli" refers to 1000) needs to be converted to a gram unit of measurement. Then the decimal should be carried over 3 decimal places to the left side (i.e., 0.3 grams), as the problem is asking for a larger unit term to be used — with "larger" indicating that the move must be to the left..

Example Conversion of Measurement

The **step method** is carried out by moving the decimal to the right to obtain a smaller unit of measurement. Thus, if the problem were asking for a smaller measurement unit, then the move would be to the right. Milligrams are smaller than grams by a factor of 1000. Thus, milligrams are 1/1000 of a gram. This dictates that the move should be 3 decimal places. Thus, if the above example of 300 milligrams is converted to grams, the answer would be 0.3 g. However, if the example asked that 0.2 grams be converted into milligrams, then the correct answer would be obtained by moving 3 decimal places to the right, which would produce 200 mg or milligrams. The step method allows a smaller unit or a larger unit of measurement to be utilized based upon simple movements of the decimal point. Grams are abbreviated as (g) and milligrams are abbreviated as (mg).

Metric Time and Date

The proper configuration used to write the **metric date** is the **year/month/day/time**. The time entered is based on a **24 hour block**. This 24 hour block of time is counted from midnight to midnight. For example, the date of April 1, 2005, 7:15 PM would be given in the following format: 2005/04/01/19:15. Notice that the time is written with 4 digits and without the use of the afternoon or morning designations of PM or AM. The first 2 digits denote the hours elapsed from midnight. The 2 digits following the semicolon denote the elapsed minutes in the ensuing hour. The general population in the United States does not yet make use of the use of the metric time and date, and instead uses the following configuration to write the month/day/year: 04/01/05, 04-01-05, or 04,01,2005. This format allows the use of a backslash, a dot, or a space to separate the time reference values.

ChelationTreatment

The metal substances lead, mercury, and arsenic can present a **threat of poisoning** to humans and animals alike. This type of poisoning can sometimes be adequately treated via **chelation therapy**. Chelation therapy incorporates chelating (binding) agents that are able to produce a chemical bond with these metal substances. A **chelated chemical bond** gives the animal a **safe way to discharge the poison from its system**. Succimer, dimercaprol, calcium EDTA, and penicillamine are all chelating agents applied in the treatment of heavy metal poisoning in animals. The common abbreviation for Succimer is DMSA. Succimer is a powder that has the ability to combine its white crystalline base with mercury or other heavy metals through a chemical binding process. Succimer can bind itself to the poisons in the brain by breaking through the blood-brain barrier which normally limits what can diffuse from the blood into the brain. Once chelated, the animal urinates to rid itself of the poisonous metal, bound with the chelating agent.

Chelating Agents

One **chelating agent** is known as dimercaprol or British anti-Lewisite (abbreviated BAL), as it was developed by British biochemists at Oxford University. It is produced in a peanut oil base, and works by joining the target heavy metals with its 2 nonmetallic thiol groups. Thiol is a sulphur-based compound that effectively chelates arsenic. Dimercaprol is a potentially poisonous substance which is transparent and thick. It has a narrow therapeutic index which means that it is not recommended for long-standing use in treatment.

Another chelating agent is penicillamine, also known by the name Cuprimine. This substance is a penicillin derivative, although it has no antibiotic properties. Penicillamine is incorporated as a chelating agent to rid the body of numerous heavy metals including lead, mercury, and arsenic.

Treating Ethylene Glycol Poisoning

Pets and other animals are attracted to the **sweet taste of antifreeze**. One of the key ingredients of antifreeze is the poison known as **ethylene glycol**. Animals that have ingested ethylene glycol will initially show signs of illness such as staggering, rapid pulse, and various abnormal behaviors. These initial signs are followed by other symptoms such as vomiting, respiratory distress, agitation, increased unsteadiness, seizures, and coma. The patient will eventually experience acute renal failure. These are life-threatening conditions that will only worsen without treatment.

The veterinarian should treat the animal with an appropriate antidote. The antidotes chiefly used are **ethanol** (drinking alcohol) and **4-methylpyrazole**. The trade name for the antidote 4-methylpyrazole is called Antizol-Vet. Time is of the essence. The veterinarian should administer the antidote within 8 hours of the animal's poisoning. A timely intervention will provide the animal with the best chance for survival.

Glucosamine for Joint Health in Dogs

Glucosamine naturally occurs in the dog's body and produces glycosaminoglycan, which is used to form and repair cartilage. As the dog gets older, this natural glucosamine production decreases, so the natural formation and repairing of cartilage slows, and the dog will experience joint pain. The dog's activities will continue to wear on the joints with everyday activity, and this combined with the slowed production of glucosamine lead to arthritis. Glucosamine supplements can be given to the dog to help rebuild the cartilage and provide lubrication to the joints, improving the dog's overall activity level and joint health. To help combat the pain associated with arthritis, glucosamine also has an anti-inflammatory effect.

Antihistamines

Antihistamines work in one of two ways: by blocking either H_1 receptors or H_2 receptors in the body. The H_1 receptors in the body are responsible for pruritus (itching) and also cause inflammatory cells to be drawn to the site. Antihistamines that are H_1 blockers try to beat the histamine to the H_1 receptor sites by antagonizing the histamine instead of blocking histamine release. The H_1-blocking antihistamines are effective for treatment of anaphylaxis because they stop bronchoconstriction and vasodilation, but they are less effective as anti-inflammatories or for allergy treatment because histamine is not the only factor for the body's entire inflammatory response and most allergy cases require a multimodal approach for treatment. The other form of antihistamines is H_2 antagonists, which are used to suppress gastric secretory effects caused by histamine and also have low anti-inflammatory effects. Benadryl and Claritin are H_1-blocking antihistamines; famotidine is an H_2-blocking antihistamine.

Benzodiazepines

Benzodiazepines act as sedatives through depression of the limbic system (the system of nerves and networks in the brain), the thalamus, and the hypothalamus. Benzodiazepines also have muscle-relaxing effects caused by the inhibition of the neurons on the spinal cord. Benzodiazepines such as diazepam are anticonvulsants as well as anxiolytic (antianxiety) drugs (alprazolam) that are primarily metabolized through the liver and excreted through urine and should be used with caution in patients with kidney or liver disease. Benzodiazepines are absorbed quickly and completely. Some patients may experience central nervous system (CNS) depression, ataxia, weakness, disorientation, nausea, and vomiting; other patients may exhibit CNS excitation followed shortly by CNS depression.

Dissociative Anesthetics

Dissociative anesthetics are *N*-methyl-D-aspartate (NMDA) antagonists. They work by dissociating the thalamocortical and limbic systems, which produces altered consciousness. They also produce amnesia and provide analgesia. By working as NMDA antagonists, this blocks the excitatory pathway but doesn't produce sleepiness, so patients that are anesthetized with dissociative agents (ketamine) don't appear sleepy and often have their eyes open and have increased muscle tone. However, that does not mean that they are not adequately anesthetized. Ketamine provides analgesia by preventing wind-up pain in the dorsal horn of the spinal cord. Ketamine causes increased cranial pressure as well as cerebral oxygen demands, increases cerebral blood flow, lowers the seizure threshold, and increases intraocular pressures. Along with this, ketamine increases sympathetic (fight-or-flight) tone resulting in an increased heart rate and high blood pressure. Ketamine could also cause respiratory depression and cause apneustic breathing (fast breaths followed by holding breaths on inspiration).

Vaccines

Vaccines protect pets from contagious and deadly diseases. Vaccinations also prevent diseases that can be transmitted from animals to animals, as well as animals to humans (zoonotic), such as rabies. Modified live forms of vaccines are composed of a weak form of the pathogen, and when this vaccine is administered, the pathogen replicates but will not cause disease. Killed vaccines are composed of the killed pathogen, and once they are administered to the animal, they cannot cause disease. More booster vaccines may be required with killed vaccines to adequately stimulate the immune system because they have a shorter duration of immunity than modified live vaccines. Recombinant subunit vaccines consist of certain non-disease-causing proteins normally produced by the pathogen. The protein gene is removed from the pathogen and transmitted to a different organism and grown in a laboratory; then these proteins are concentrated into a vaccine. Antibodies created to recognize the proteins by the immune system will also recognize them as a part of the pathogen if it invaded the animal. Recombinant vector vaccines are obtained by administering genetically altered organisms from a laboratory through the vaccine to the animal.

Antimicrobials

Antimicrobials kill microorganisms or prevent them from multiplying, and they are used to treat infection caused by bacteria, fungi, viruses, and protozoa. Antimicrobials are effective in the treatment of urinary tract infections. Certain antimicrobials used for urinary tract infection therapy include amoxicillin, amoxicillin-clavulanic acid, cephalexin, cefpodoxime, and enrofloxacin. Many antimicrobials are secreted and reabsorbed through the kidneys. A high antimicrobial concentration in the urine helps to eliminate bacteria present in the urine; however, an antimicrobial will have to have concentrations within the tissues in order to treat bladder wall or kidney infections.

Chondroitin

Chondroitin is a naturally occurring main glycosaminoglycan in the dog's body found in the cartilage that is responsible for maintaining appropriate shock absorption and joint tissue health by providing elasticity and water retention in the cartilage. Chondroitin stops the production of inflammatory mediators that destroy the joints as well as provides increased mobility and improves the dog's strength. Chondroitin is normally used in conjunction with glucosamine. Whereas chondroitin blocks the enzymes that try and destroy cartilage in the joints, glucosamine works to repair them.

Crystalloid Solutions

Crystalloid solutions are fluids that hold electrolyte and nonelectrolyte solutes that move freely around the body's fluid compartments. Crystalloid solutions come in three forms: isotonic, hypertonic, and hypotonic. Isotonic solutions are balanced electrolyte solutions that are equal to the osmolality of the red blood cells (RBCs) and plasma of the patient. Isotonic solutions such as lactated Ringer's, Normosol-R, and Plasma-Lyte are used to support perfusion and volume replacement. Hypertonic solutions have a higher osmolality than the RBCs and plasma, causing fluids to be drawn from the intracellular space into the intravascular space making these solutions useful for those patients who need large amounts of fluids quickly. Hypotonic solutions such as 5% dextrose in water and 0.45% sodium chloride have lower osmolality than the intravascular fluid and draw the fluids into the cells; they are primarily used to correct electrolyte imbalances.

Colloid Solutions

Colloid solutions have large molecules and only compose the plasma compartment of the body. Natural colloids include whole blood and plasma that can be used in patients who are anemic. Synthetic colloids include hetastarch, pentastarch, and dextran. Hetastarch aids in retaining fluids in the intravascular compartment. Patients in shock experience a metabolic disturbance caused by the circulatory system failing to provide adequate perfusion to the body's vital organs. Colloids are used to restore the body's organ perfusion, and colloid solutions are also used in patients with pulmonary contusions and head trauma. A major benefit of colloid use is that resuscitation is achieved at a lower rate than that of crystalloids because colloids stay in the vascular space for a longer time frame than do crystalloids.

Non-Steroidal Anti-Inflammatory Drugs (NSAIDs)

NSAID stands for nonsteroidal anti-inflammatory drug. NSAIDs are used to control pain and inflammation as well as reduce swelling. They do this by blocking the production of prostaglandin molecules that promote pain. They also provide analgesia by reducing inflammation that triggers the pain sensation. They also provide antipyretic (fever-reducing) effects. NSAIDs are commonly used for postoperative pain control in small-animal practice. They are also used long term in certain patients with osteoarthritis. If used long term, baseline and annual blood work are ideal to use for checking kidney and liver function. Side effects of NSAID use include kidney and liver toxicity, gastrointestinal (GI) ulcers, and possible stomach bleeding. More common side effects include vomiting, diarrhea, loss of appetite, and lethargy.

Opioids

Opioids are analgesics (painkillers). Opioids act on the CNS to relieve pain and may produce side effects including mood changes, excitement, and sedation. There are two classes of opioids: pure mu agonists such as morphine, hydromorphone, fentanyl, and meperidine and partial mu agonists such as buprenorphine. Pure mu agonists will provide a more effective analgesia, but they can also cause side effects such as vomiting, respiratory depression, and sedation. Partial mu agonists, however, bind with the less effective analgesic receptor (k receptor). Butorphanol is neither a pure mu or partial mu agonist, but rather a mu antagonist that reverses the effects of the pure mu opioids, leaving the patient with weaker analgesic effects. Butorphanol has a short duration of action and does not provide adequate analgesia for more painful procedures.

Alpha 2 Agonists

Alpha 2 agonists, such as dexmedetomidine, xylazine, and medetomidine are sedatives that also provide analgesia and muscle relaxation. The α_2-agonists should be used with caution because they can have cardiovascular side effects such as bradycardia (slow heart rate), hypertension (high blood pressure), and a reduced cardiac output. The α_2-agonists should not be used in patients with cardiovascular disease, liver disease, or kidney disease. The α_2-agonists such as dexmedetomidine can be used as a premedication for general anesthesia, greatly decreasing the amount of induction agent and inhalant needed to maintain the patient. Fortunately, dexmedetomidine can be reversed with atipamezole, which is the appropriate way to treat for bradycardia rather than using an anticholinergic such as atropine because this can cause the heart to work harder than it already is.

Propofol

Propofol is an anesthetic that provides smooth, rapid induction and recovery from anesthesia. Propofol is given intravenously as a hypnotic agent used for sedation in ventilated patients, as well as induction and maintenance of anesthesia (up to 20 minutes). Propofol should be titrated (given to effect) for up to 1 minute or until the patient exhibits signs of onset of anesthesia. Rapid IV injection of propofol can cause apnea, hypotension, and oxygen desaturation. Maintenance of anesthesia with propofol may be used for shorter procedures (20 minutes) or as a transition to inhalant anesthetic. Propofol decreases cardiac output and causes vasodilation and should be used with caution in patients with hypotension (low blood pressure), hypovolemia (a condition in which the blood plasma is too low), or cardiovascular insufficiencies. Propofol is metabolized in the liver and excreted through the urine. Propofol provides a rapid recovery in which the patient is standing in fewer than 20 minutes; however, certain drugs in the premedications may prolong this recovery.

Antibiotics

Antibiotics are used to stop bacterial infections by either preventing them from growing (bacteriostatic) or by killing the organisms (bactericidal). Antibiotics do NOT kill off viruses, but they can be effective in treating secondary bacterial infections that can occur while patient is ill from a virus. There are various classes of antibiotics, including quinolones, penicillins, tetracyclines, and macrolides. Some antibiotics are effective against a wide range of bacteria (broad spectrum) and some antibiotics may be more effective against certain bacteria and less effective against others (narrow spectrum).

Drug Administration

Five Rights of Drug Administration

Medicines should be given in accordance with the "**Five Rights of Drug Administration**." These Five Rights, which are designed to produce a **standard for dispensing drugs** properly, are as follows:

1. The patient has the right to be the **proper recipient** (i.e., drugs must not be administered to the wrong patient).
2. The patient has the right to receive the **proper medication** (i.e., the wrong drugs must not be given to the properly identified recipient).
3. The patient has the right to receive the **proper dosage**.
4. The patient has the right to be given the drug by the **proper route** (oral, injection, etc.).
5. The patient has the right to receive the medication **on time**.

To facilitate these rights, the attending veterinarian is responsible for ensuring that the medication orders are clear and easily understood. The drug's label should be checked carefully, ideally 3 times, before being given to the patient: 1) when it is taken off the shelf, 2) when the dosage is being prepared (pills counted, injectables drawn up, etc.), and 3) when the dosage is being administered to the patient.

Medication Adjustments

In addition to the Five Rights, there are other considerations of particular concern in veterinary medicine. For example, **animal size** can be a significant concern as related to standard dosage. While human medications are produced in prepackaged dosages for infants, children, and adults, veterinary medications may require additional calculation. The concentration or strength of a drug should be checked to make sure that the amount administered is appropriate for the size of the animal. Larger animals require larger doses of medication than smaller animals, and dosages may need to be adjusted accordingly.

Adherence to the prescribed **route of medication delivery** is also important. The efficacy of a medication can vary widely according to the route of administration into the body. Thus, the approved route of administration should always be utilized to ensure that the drug is administered properly. Alternate routes may not produce the desired results, as they may cause the drug to be absorbed incorrectly or not at all. Consequently, alternate routes can harm the patient. By careful adherence to medication management protocols, drug efficacy and patient safety can be optimally secured.

Factors Affecting Absorption of Drugs

Drugs that are effective are **absorbed into the animal's bloodstream** and distributed to the tissues through a variety of mechanisms. Absorption frequently occurs directly through the mucous membranes and the digestive tract, as the body seeks to equilibrate by taking in the substances found in the drug. Some drugs are less soluble and may not be absorbed and distributed as rapidly as other more soluble drugs. Further, a variety of additional factors unique to the body can impact drug absorption and distribution rates, including the drug's pKa (or ionization tendency), the pH (acidity or alkalinity) of the tissues, the perfusion of the tissues, and the overall volume of distribution (or Vd).

These factors can make the drug more unstable in the stomach and/or less able to penetrate the blood-brain barrier. Further, drugs given by mouth are absorbed into the intestines and then enter the hepatic portal circulation, which transports them directly to the liver. In the first-pass effect, the liver metabolizes many drugs using a biochemical process which prevents much of the original drug from entering the systemic circulation. Alternate routes of administration include intravenous, sublingual, and intramuscular injection methods. These methods can be used to avoid the first-pass effect.

Common Abbreviations in Drug Administration

There are many **abbreviations** that the veterinarian may use to relay a prescription refill to the technician, e.g., SID, once a day; BID, twice a day; and TID, three times a day. Abbreviations referring to the route of administration will be used also, including PO, by mouth; IM, intramuscular; and SQ, subcutaneous. Many times, the veterinarian will write instructions using this terminology; for example, give 1 tablet PO BID means to give one tablet by mouth twice a day. Other abbreviations will use the letter q, which stands for every; therefore, qh stands for every hour, and q4h stands for every 4 hours. When referring to the patient's eyes or ears, abbreviations including OD (right eye), OS (left eye), and OU (both eyes) are used as well as AD (right ear), AS (left ear), and AU (both ears).

Safe Storage and Handling

Storing Prescription Medications

There are specific **regulations** governing the **safe storage of medications** in veterinary medical settings. Prescription medications must be kept in a **secure, locked setting** within a veterinary hospital. The hospital must adequately **monitor environmental conditions** like the **temperature**, **humidity**, and **light** exposure that could affect stored medications. The medication's **expiration** date must be noted, and a review system must be in place to ensure expired medications are properly discarded. The expiration date is the date that the drug is deemed no longer safe for continued use.

The **reconstitution**, **storage**, and **handling** instructions must also be written on the label or packet insert. This literature is useful for describing the care that should be taken with each stored drug. The **Safety Data Sheet** or the SDS specific to each drug is a necessary document that presents complete safety, handling, clean-up, and disposal criteria for every drug stored in the hospital. Those drugs which are labeled as hazardous must also be handled in accordance with the guidelines published by the Occupational Safety and Health Administration or OSHA, as specific to the state in which the drugs are maintained. Drugs require a written prescription before they can be given to a patient.

Storing Controlled Drugs

Controlled drugs should be stored in a locked cabinet with hidden hinges or in a safe that is secured to a cabinet or wall that cannot be easily moved. The attending veterinarian should be the only one with access to the controlled drug unit to ensure tight security. If using a mobile unit for controlled drug storage, there should only be drugs in the unit for that specific procedure and the rest should be kept in a secure location in the hospital. The controlled drugs should be kept in a secure, hidden, locked unit if being transported by vehicle and unsupervised.

Storing Vaccinations

Vaccines need to be stored in the dark and at a temperature of 35-45 °F (refrigerated). Vaccines should be stored in a dedicated refrigerator, meaning they should not be stored in the same refrigerator as employees' food and drinks as well as opened pet food that is used for patients. The vaccines should be stored in the center of the refrigerator because temperatures in the fridge can vary. The temperature of the refrigerator should be monitored daily to ensure that the vaccines are kept at a regulated temperature because being exposed to temperatures outside of the recommended range can reduce the effectiveness of the vaccines. A thermometer can be kept in the middle of the refrigerator and compared to the temperature on the refrigerator itself daily to ensure that it is at the correct temperature.

Handling Vaccines

Vaccines should always be drawn up with a new and sterile needle and syringe, and they should not be drawn up until they are going to be administered. Once reconstituted, the vaccine could be more temperature sensitive; plus, the risk of bacterial contamination increases the longer that the vaccine is reconstituted and sitting in the syringe. Vaccines should be administered within 30 minutes after being reconstituted. Certain vaccines look similar once they are reconstituted; one way to prevent vaccines from being mistaken for the other is to peel off the sticker from the vaccine vial and place it around the syringe used to draw up that vaccine. Vaccines should be mixed thoroughly before drawing them up into the syringe.

Transporting Vaccines

The priority for **transport of vaccines** is to maintain a temperature of 35-45 °F. While being transported from the manufacturer to the clinic, they must be kept inside of an insulated cooler with ice packs if needed. Ice packs should be wrapped in paper or some sort of layer to prevent them from contacting the vaccines, which could make them too cold. A cooler with vaccines should not be kept in a trunk or the bed of a truck because these areas are more susceptible to the weather outside and could get too cold in the winter and too hot in the summer, so vaccines need to be kept in the center of the transport vehicle where it is temperature controlled. Modified live vaccines are heat sensitive, whereas adjuvanted vaccines are more sensitive to freezing temperatures, causing the adjuvant to separate from the antigen to form a precipitate that can cause local inflammation at the administration site, so maintaining the proper temperature for vaccines is crucial.

Drug Withdrawal Times

A drug introduced into an animal that is a future food source has the **potential to be passed on to the consumer**. Therefore, any drug that is administered to a food source animal must be carefully monitored. The timing of the withdrawal of any medication administered is particularly important. Indeed, timely withdrawal is critical, to ensure that the drug is fully metabolized and excreted out of the animal, and thus is not passed on to the human consumer.

Requisite withdrawal timelines are printed on the outside label of the drug's container. There is also printed material available in other publications to give the veterinarian more information about necessary withdrawal procedures. Drugs which are extra-label, or ELDU drugs, have particularly strict guidelines for early withdrawal from animals to be used as food products. By contrast, ELDU drugs administered to companion or service animals (dogs, cats, horses, mules, etc.) do not have similarly strict withdrawal procedures.

Residual Drugs in Food Source Animals

Residual medications in food source animals may induce a number of negative consequences in human consumers. The **adverse effects** that the human consumer may experience include a number of severe medical conditions. One danger is a **systemic toxicological effect** (a poisonous condition) that impacts the entire body. Another danger is the likelihood of **mutagenicity**, as some residual drugs may cause the cells in the body to mutate or change. Other residual drugs may become carcinogenic, predisposing the consumer to develop cancer. Still other residual drugs may affect the reproductive system. These drugs can prevent pregnancy or cause harmful or even teratogenic (i.e., non-inherited deforming) side effects in the unborn fetus.

Further, some residual antimicrobial drugs may **alter the human intestinal flora** and cause digestive ailments. The overuse of antimicrobials may also cause virulent bacteria such as Salmonella and Campylobacter to become drug resistant. Where withdrawal delays occur, testing can become necessary. However, drug residue studies can be expensive, and there is little incentive to carry out these examinations. Thus, careful adherence to drug administration and withdrawal guidelines is essential. The veterinarian should also exercise caution in the disposal of drugs. Careless disposal could cause the food supplies to become contaminated accidentally.

Surgical Nursing

Surgical Anatomy and Physiology

Major Types of Bone Tissue

There are 2 types of bone tissue, compact and spongy. Compact bones give structural strength and support to the body. Compact bones allow for strenuous movement and weight-bearing activities.

Compact Bone

Compact bone is composed of very tightly grouped osteons (also called "haversian systems"). Each osteon is comprised of a solid matrix of osseous lamellae (concentric rings of deposited minerals and proteins) surrounding a central canal containing blood vessels to nurture the bone. Between the lamellar rings are osteocytes (bone cells) situated in lacunae (small spaces). Channels called canaliculi extend from the lacunae to the osteonic (or haversian) canal. Nutrition is brought in through the canaliculi, and waste is moved out.

Compact Bone & Spongy (Cancellous) Bone

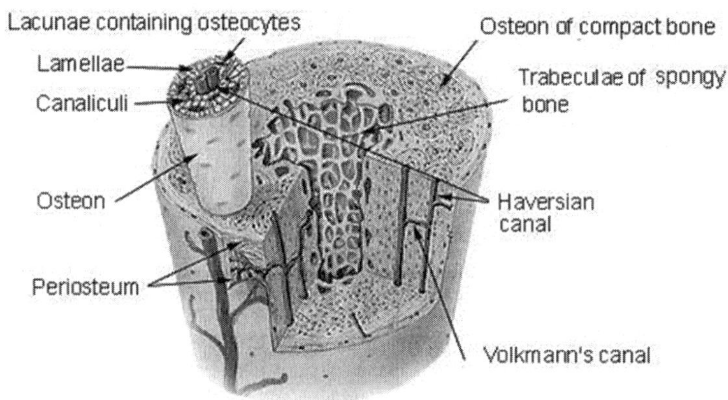

Cancellous Bone

The 2 major types of bone are **compact bone** and **cancellous** (also called "trabecular" or "spongy") bone. Cancellous bone is found inside and at the rounded ends of long bones, in the pelvic bones and breastbone. Its primary purpose is to protect bone marrow, and to provide interior structural support. Cancellous bone is honeycomb-like in appearance, having numerous cavities and spaces interspersed with boney plates and ridges known as trabeculae. Trabeculae are arranged to provide maximum support for stresses and loads incurred, and may gradually rearrange themselves in response to new stresses or burdens.

Cancellous bone does not receive nourishment via osteonic canals (i.e., haversian systems), but rather via canaliculi connecting the various spaces within the trabecular structure. Osseous trabeculae may be composed of mineralized bone or collagen. Collagen is a connective tissue made up of fibrous proteins. The larger trabecular spaces are filled with red bone marrow, where the production of blood cellular components takes place.

Classification and Characteristics of Bones

Bones are typically classified by shape, often using 4 categories: **long, short, flat,** and **irregular**. However, other classification systems use 6 categories: **long, short, flat, pneumatic, sesamoid,** and **irregular** (or "sutural").

Using the 6-category classification system, the first bone type is the **long bones**. Long bones grow primarily through a lengthening of the diaphysis (shaft). The diaphysis is the midsection of the long bone. The diaphysis has 2 rounded ends which are called epiphyses. The long bone also has a marrow cavity, also called a medullar cavity. The medullar cavity is the central section of bone where the yellow bone marrow is kept.

Two examples of long bones are the radius and the femur. The radius in most animals is found in the lower forelimb. The femur in most animals is the upper rear leg bone, and is typically the strongest bone in the body.

The second type of the 6 classifications of bones refers to the **short bones**. The short bones share some similar structural characteristics found in the long bones. However, the short bones do not have a medullar cavity in which to house yellow bone marrow. Short bone examples include the boney digits within the hand and fingers.

The third type of the 6 classification system of bones includes the flat bones, which are thin, level, horizontal bones. **Flat bones** are formed from 2 layers of compact bone with a middle layer of cancellous bone. The skull bones, ribs, pelvis, and scapula are all classified as flat bones.

The fourth type of the classification system includes the **pneumatic bones**. Pneumatic bones have an air-filled cavity or indentation, such as that found in the sinuses.

The fifth type includes the **sesamoid bones**. Sesamoid bones are small, short bones of an irregular spherical or sesame seed–like shape. The sesamoid bone helps to alleviate some of the stress caused by friction, and/or to reduce pressures otherwise applied to a tendon or joint. One example of a sesamoid bone is the patella or kneecap.

The sixth type includes the **irregular bones**. Irregular bones are bones that do not fit into the classifications of long bones, short bones, flat bones, pneumatic bones, or sesamoid bones.

Muscles and Nerves

There are 4 primary tissue types in the human body: **epithelial, connective, muscle**, and **nerve tissue**. The latter 2 are described here. Muscle tissue consists of 3 main subtypes known as skeletal, smooth, and cardiac muscle. Skeletal muscle is described as striated contractile tissue attached to the skeleton. It has a striated appearance – characterized by alternating light and dark bands under microscopic view. Skeletal muscle is responsible for voluntary control and movement.

Smooth muscle is involuntarily controlled muscle, and is found in the walls of the hollow organs. It moves much more slowly, has no striations, and is "autonomically" or involuntarily regulated. Hollow organs, specifically, blood vessels, bladder, uterus, and the gastrointestinal tract derive dilation, contraction, and peristaltic movement from smooth muscles. The third muscle tissue subtype, Cardiac muscle, is located within the heart. It is also striated, but unlike striated skeletal muscle, it is involuntarily controlled.

Structure of a Skeletal Muscle

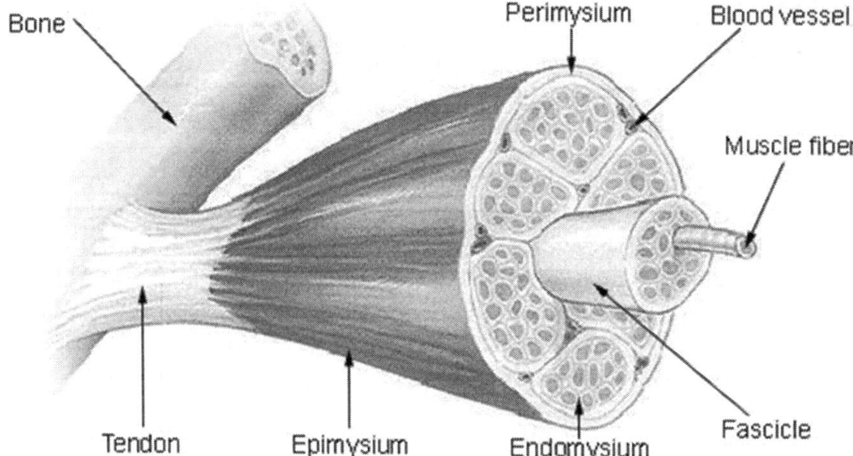

The fourth type of tissue is **nervous tissue**. It is located within the **brain, spinal cord, and nerves**. Neurons and neuroglia are 2 key cell types. Neurons are nerve cells which work to transmit signals or impulses, to react to stimuli, or produce voluntary actions or responses. Neuroglia (or "glial") cells can be described as a network of tissues and fibers found in the brain and spinal column that provide support, protection, and nutrition to neurons, among other functions.

Central Nervous System

The **brain** is the organ within the body that has control over the **central nervous system**. In its most elemental form, the **central nervous system consists of the brain and the spinal cord**. The brain itself consists of the cerebrum (the 2 hemispheres that collectively make up the forebrain and midbrain), the cerebellum (or "small brain"), and the brain stem (connecting the brain and spinal cord).

During embryological development, the **emerging brain** (existing then as 3 swellings in the embryonic neural tube) is divided into the prosencephalon, the mesencephalon, and the rhombencephalon. The prosencephalon becomes the forebrain, the mesencephalon becomes the midbrain, and the rhombencephalon becomes the hindbrain. The brain stem is the lower portion of the brain that is attached to the spinal cord. The spinal cord is comprised of a thick cord of nerve cells that is attached to the bottom of the brain, or the brain stem.

The **spinal cord** has a protective boney covering which is known as the vertebral column. The vertebral column is a part of the skeletal axis. The spinal cord sends out nerve impulses or signals by way of efferent nerve paths, and receives them by way of afferent nerve paths. Thus, afferent nerves transmit signals or sensory impulses to the central nervous system, while efferent nerves send impulses or signals away from the brain to the organs or muscles.

The **meninges** are 3 layers of membranes which function to **protect the central nervous system**. The meninges are dense, fibrous connective tissues that enclose the spinal cord and the brain. The 3 layers are known as the dura mater, the arachnoid mater, and the pia mater.

Cerebrospinal fluid is a clear, water-like fluid found in and around the brain and the spinal cord. The cerebrospinal fluid works to cushion the central nervous system from pressures or outside forces. The cerebrospinal fluid is also a source of nourishment for the brain. The fluid contains essential protein, glucose, ions, and other substances that keep the central nervous system healthy and fit.

The blood-brain barrier (BBB) refers to certain extra-dense membranes lining the capillaries of the brain. This **barrier allows certain liquids or substances to pass through** to the central nervous system while preventing the entrance of many others. It is yet another form of protection for the brain. Blood contains oxygen, glucose, and fat-soluble compounds that are able to pass through the blood-brain barrier. However, the blood-brain barrier keeps out waste products and many drugs.

The Cardiac Cycle

The **cardiac cycle** refers to all **cardiac events that occur from one heartbeat to the next**. The heart rate is largely determined by the demand for oxygen throughout the body – although arousal, stress, anxiety, and other factors may also intervene.

The cardiac cycle may be divided into 2 phases: **diastole and systole**. A four-phase cycle is also sometimes described. Phase 1 is the ventricular filling period, occurring when the ventricles are in diastole. At this time the atria are in contraction, filling the ventricles.

Phase 2 is the isovolumetric contraction period, which begins with ventricular systole initiation. Phase 3 is the ventricular ejection period, when the ventricles contract and send blood into the pulmonary artery and aorta. The fourth and final phase is the isovolumetric relaxation period, initiated upon ventricular return to diastole.

Blood Vessels

Blood is the red body fluid that flows within the body's vascular system. Blood is carried by a **system of vessels** or tubular channels. **Arterial vessels** carry oxygenated blood away from the heart, and venous vessels carry deoxygenated blood to the heart. The pulmonary vein is unique in that it is responsible for carrying oxygenated blood to the heart from the lungs. Oxygenated blood is blood that has been combined with oxygen, and from which carbon dioxide has been removed.

The blood is moved under pressure from the heart. Artery walls are thicker than the walls of veins, as they must sustain direct cardiac pumping pressures. However, on average, veins are larger in diameter and have many one-way valves to facilitate the passive return process. Larger arteries divide into smaller blood vessels known as arterioles. The arterioles distribute blood from the arteries to the capillaries.

The force of blood applied at regular intervals by way of cardiac contraction is known as blood pressure.

Oxygenation of Blood

The **oxygenation of blood** is completed by way of the cardiac cycle, through the heart's 4 chambers. The **right atrium** is the part of the heart that **accepts deoxygenated blood** from the superior and inferior vena cava. The vena cava is the largest vein that carries blood back to the heart. From the right atrium, **deoxygenated blood is sent into the right ventricle**. The right ventricle then contracts, moving the **deoxygenated blood into the lungs**. The lungs are responsible for the diffusion of carbon dioxide out of the blood in exchange for oxygen diffusion into the bloodstream, as gaseous molecular equilibrium is obtained. The **oxygenated blood then flows out of the lungs** and into the left atrium. The left atrium is the upper left chamber of the heart. Once filled with oxygenated blood the left atrium contracts, sending the blood into the left ventricle, where its contraction forces the blood out and into the aorta. From that point, the oxygenated blood moves throughout the body's arteries and then veins to complete the hematic response to the cardiac cycle.

Capillary and Venous Return Systems

Capillaries have walls that are constructed from a single layer of endothelium. This allows the **exchange of carbon dioxide and oxygen gases by molecular diffusion**, as well as the osmotic exchange of nutrient fluids and waste molecules (such as glucose and urea) via the capillary stream. Capillaries are described as the smallest blood vessels found in the body. They also serve as a depressurizing link between the arteries and veins in the body.

Veins are described as any blood vessel that **transports deoxygenated blood** within the body (with the exception of the pulmonary vein, which carries oxygenated blood back to the heart). Venous walls are much thinner than arterial walls, as they accommodate a much lower blood pressure than that of the arteries. Veins have interspersing one-way valves as an essential feature, to prevent any backflow of deoxygenated blood. Backflow could otherwise be caused by low blood pressures in the body. Venules are the venous counterpart to arterioles, and carry blood back to larger venous vessels.

Whole Blood

Whole blood is made up of fluid and cellular substances that join to carry out specific functions within the body. One of the fluids is called plasma. Plasma has a very light yellowish color. **Plasma** is the primary liquid in which hematic cells are dispersed to form whole blood. Plasma is 90% water and 10% blood plasma proteins. There are also traces of other materials in this substance.

The **hematic cells** in whole blood each have a specific function within the body. **Erythrocytes, leukocytes,** and **thrombocytes** make up the cellular components in whole blood. The substance in the plasma that is responsible for **clotting** is known as **fibrinogen protein**. Removal of fibrinogen protein leaves a fluid substance known as serum. Blood is a necessary component in the body. Blood transports dissolved proteins, oxygen, carbon dioxide, hormones, lipids, and metabolic end products within the body. The blood flows within the circulatory system as the heart pumps blood to the lungs and then throughout the body.

Digestive Processes

Digestion is a process that food undergoes so that the **body can absorb** and **use its nutrients**. The digestive process terminates in the **excretion of waste**. The digestive process uses certain substances which can chemically change food into nutrients that the body can absorb. The digestive process incorporates both mechanical and chemical actions in the breakdown and absorption of food. The mouth is the starting point in the digestive process.

Food enters the mouth to be ground up into smaller particles before being swallowed. It is in the mouth that food is first combined with digestive enzymes (such as salivary amylase) as it is chewed or masticated. Digestive enzymes work to further break down the food. The esophagus carries the food down to the stomach. There, the food is mixed with additional digestive enzymes known as gastric juices. Gastric juices are formed from hydrochloric acid, protein-digesting enzymes, and mucus. More youthful stomachs may also contain the proteolytic enzyme chymosin (also called rennin). Chymosin is used to coagulate milk, converting it from a liquid into a semisolid mass.

After being acted upon by the gastric juices, ingested food becomes a softened, semi-solid mass called **chyme**. Chyme is described as a **combination of water, hydrochloric acid, and digestive enzymes**. Chyme is passed from the stomach into the small intestine. The small intestine is responsible for a major portion of the digestion and absorption process. The small intestine is located between the stomach and the large intestine. The small intestine releases pancreatic and intestinal enzymes to be blended with the chyme. Gradually the chyme is separated by the lacteals into chyle (emulsified fats and fatty acids) and excrement. The chyle is taken up by the lacteals and passed into the lymphatic system. From there it is transported into the bloodstream via the thoracic duct. The excrement travels from the small intestine into the large intestine, where excess water is absorbed. The latter part of the small intestine (the ilium) and the large intestine are host to considerable bacteria, many of which act to synthesize niacin (nicotinic acid), thiamin (vitamin B1), and vitamin K, which are then absorbed into the body. Finally, undigested food is transported to the rectum, located between the colon and the anal canal. The body releases this undigested food as feces, which passes through the anus.

Ruminant Digestion

Ruminant digestion is a process of digestion used by animals with hooves. The animal eats raw, unprocessed material and then regurgitates or brings food up from the stomach in a form that has not been completely softened or digested. The food that is partially softened is referred to as a cud or bolus. The animal proceeds to further masticate the **cud**, which allows it to digest the material more thoroughly. This is known as remasticated food. **Remasticated** or chewed food continues to be mixed with a clear liquid known as saliva. The remasticated food is then re-swallowed and split into layers of solid matter and liquid matter in the first 2 chambers of the stomach. This additional swallowing of food is known as deglutition. The first 2 chambers of the stomach are known as the rumen and the reticulum. The ruminant stomach actually contains 4 compartments in total, called the rumen, the reticulum, the omasum, and the abomasum. The abomasum is referred to as the "true" or glandular stomach, as it is where final acidic and enzymatic digestion takes place.

Anatomy and Functions of Ruminant Digestive System

The **rumen** (the first stomach chamber) is the **most spacious of all the chambers** in the ruminant animal. The rumen is responsible for **blending the food with the right amount of pH, temperature, and bacteria in anaerobic conditions**. The second chamber is known as the **reticulum** or the second stomach. **Cows and sheep** have this type of stomach. The lining of this compartment has a **hexagonal honeycomb pattern**. This pattern is beneficial to the process of absorption. Absorption through this expansive surface area allows for the taking in of volatile fatty acids.

The **omasum** is the third chamber in the ruminant stomach, and is responsible for further **crushing of food**. The omasum absorbs or soaks up water, magnesium, and bicarbonate. The omasum is located between the reticulum and the abomasum. The abomasum is the fourth stomach on a ruminant animal. This is the true stomach, as it is responsible for blending the food with digestive enzymes. This blending causes chemical digestion to begin. The chemical digestion allows nutrients to be absorbed by the small intestine.

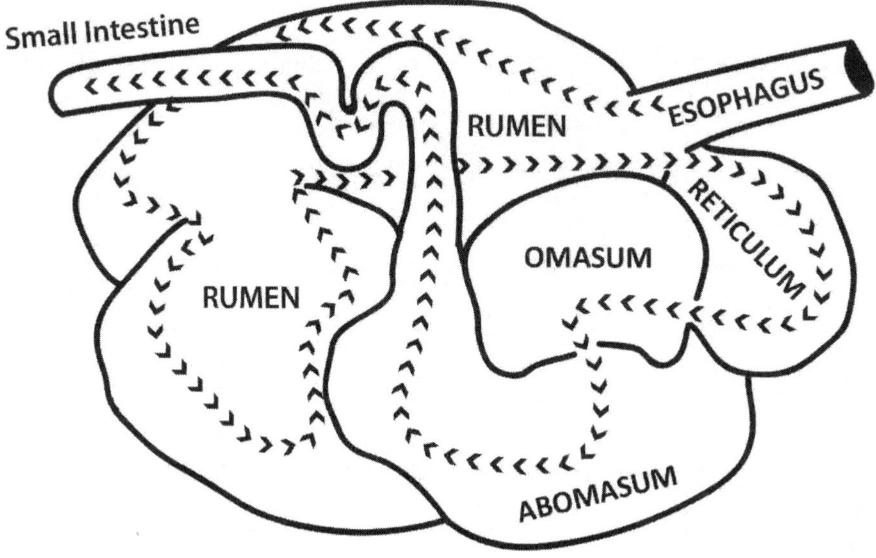

Urinary System

The **excretory system** is a complex network that **discharges waste materials** left over from the metabolic functions of the body. The body can expel waste through the action of **defecating or urinating**. The urinary excretory system is made up of the **kidneys, ureters, urinary bladder, and the urethra**. The kidneys remove liquid waste from the bloodstream. This liquid waste is called urine, which is expelled from the body.

Each species of animal has a specific shaped and sized kidney, although most are shaped in the form of a bean. The ureters are urinary ducts responsible for transporting urine away from the kidneys and into the bladder in mammals. The ureter is fashioned from smooth muscle. The urinary bladder is a hollow, stretchy sac used for urine storage. Urine is collected and stored until it is discharged. Urine ultimately passes through the urethra, which is a tube extending from the bladder to the body's exterior. The urethra is fashioned from smooth muscle, with a sphincter between itself and the bladder that operates under voluntary control for this discharge process.

Urine Production

The **excretory system** incorporates 3 phases in urinary production. The 3 phases are referred to as **filtration**, **reabsorption**, and **secretion**. The filtration phase occurs in one of the many nephrons found in the kidney. Within each nephron is a circular-shaped cluster of capillaries called the glomerulus. It resides under a thin, double-membraned outer covering called Bowman's capsule. High pressures from the renal artery force water, salt, and other small molecules out of the glomerulus. This solution of water, salt, and other molecules is known as glomerular filtrate. This solution is then filtered through Bowman's capsule. Bowman's capsule is responsible for removing waste products, inorganic salts, and excess water.

The second phase of urinary production occurs when nutrients that are left over from this filtration process are reabsorbed into the body through renal tubules. Principally, this reabsorption is carried out in the proximal convoluted tubules or PCTs, with reabsorbed materials entering the surrounding peritubular capillaries. The process of concentrating and absorbing salts is carried out in the nephron tubule known as the loop of Henle. In the third phase of urinary production, blood pH is regulated in the distal convoluted tubules (DCTs) by processes of absorption and secretion, with certain substances released into the DCTs from the peritubular capillaries.

Bilirubin

Bilirubin is a brownish-yellow substance found in **bile**. It is the by-product of hemoglobin, released when aging or superfluous red blood cells are broken down by reticuloendothelial cells found in the liver, spleen, and bone marrow. Other chromoproteins may also contain heme and thus contribute to the formation of bilirubin when broken down. Bilirubin is responsible for the yellowish appearance in bruises, as well as the yellow, icteric appearance of the skin when jaundice develops – typically due to liver dysfunction. Bilirubin is formed by the metabolism of heme, which is the deep red iron-containing pigment found in the blood. As red blood cells die, they are broken down into heme and globins. Eventually the heme is changed into $Fe2^+$, carbon monoxide, and bilirubin.

Elevated bilirubin levels are common in newborns, as high numbers of red blood cells, needed only in the womb (due to low oxygen transfer through the placenta), are rapidly destroyed at birth. Bilirubin can become **toxic in neonates**, as the blood-brain barrier remains immature and may be unable to protect sensitive brain tissues from the deleterious effects of hyperbilirubinemia (jaundice). Bilirubin is rapidly broken down by light; thus newborns are assisted in the breakdown of bilirubin by being placed under special lighting for treatment.

Forms of Bilirubin

In its primary form, **bilirubin is unconjugated** – i.e., not joined together with other substances. This unconjugated form of bilirubin is lipid-soluble and thus can readily attach itself to serum proteins. The resulting solution is transported to the liver for conjugation. The **conjugated form of bilirubin is water-soluble**, which means it can be dissolved completely in water. The conjugated form of bilirubin has the basic structure of glucuronic acid. **Glucuronic acid** is derived from glucose. The combination of glucuronic acid with drugs, pollutants, acids, and other toxins tends to render them harmless through a process known as glucuronidation. Glucuronidation is the body's way of producing water-soluble forms that can readily be discharged from the body through urination.

Finally, bilirubin can be used to **check for hepatic (liver) damage**. Evaluation involves the measurement of the amount of **bilirubin that is present in the urine**. Laboratory tests can measure total bilirubin, along with direct (conjugated) and indirect (unconjugated) levels. With a properly functioning liver, the bilirubin should virtually all be in a conjugated form. However, this is not true when hepatic (liver) damage is present. An excessive amount of unconjugated serum bilirubin indicates prehepatic jaundice or hepatic-induced jaundice. Likewise, this can be determined by the levels present in the urine.

Skeletal Articulations

A **skeletal articulation** exists whenever 2 bones come together for purposes of movement. Another name for an articulation is a joint. A **joint** is structurally created when **tissue binds 2 or more bones together**. The tissue can consist of fibrous, elastic, or cartilaginous materials. Joints can be classified by way of the following kinds of articulations: synarthrosis, amphiarthrosis, and diarthrosis.

Synarthrosis joints are fixed in a permanent position. An example can be seen in the suture joints of the skull. **Amphiarthrosis joints** allow only limited movement, such as the pubic symphysis. Symphysis indicates that the bones merge naturally. **Diarthrosis** refers to a joint that is capable of changing position in multiple of directions. An example would be the shoulder, which allows wide ranging motion.

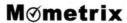

There are 3 additional types of structural joint classifications: fibrous, cartilaginous, and synovial. The first 2 are classified according to the tissues creating the joint (fibers or cartilage). The last refers to the synovial fluid feature that characterizes this joint.

Anatomical Direction

There are 12 descriptive terms of **anatomical direction**. These terms can be grouped according to varying similarities in reference points. For example, a direction can be described in terms that indicate the location of the body part. Therefore, a direction toward the head is referred to as **cranial**. A direction toward the tail is known as **caudal**. The direction that refers to the backbone is called **dorsal**. The direction away from the backbone is known as **ventral**.

The direction that describes the location nearest to the median plane is known as the **medial**. The direction that is the longest distance away from the median plane is known as the **lateral**.

The location that is nearest to the backbone is called the **proximal** — used particularly when one is referring to the nearer aspect of limbs or appendages. The location farthest from the backbone is called **distal** — used particularly when one refers to the more distant aspect of limbs or appendages. The term **anterior** can be applied when one is talking about the direction of the head. The term **posterior** can be used when one is talking about the direction of the tail. The term palmar is used to describe the palm of the hand or bottom of a front foot, hoof, or paw. The term plantar is used to describe the area on the bottom of the foot, or rear hoof or paw.

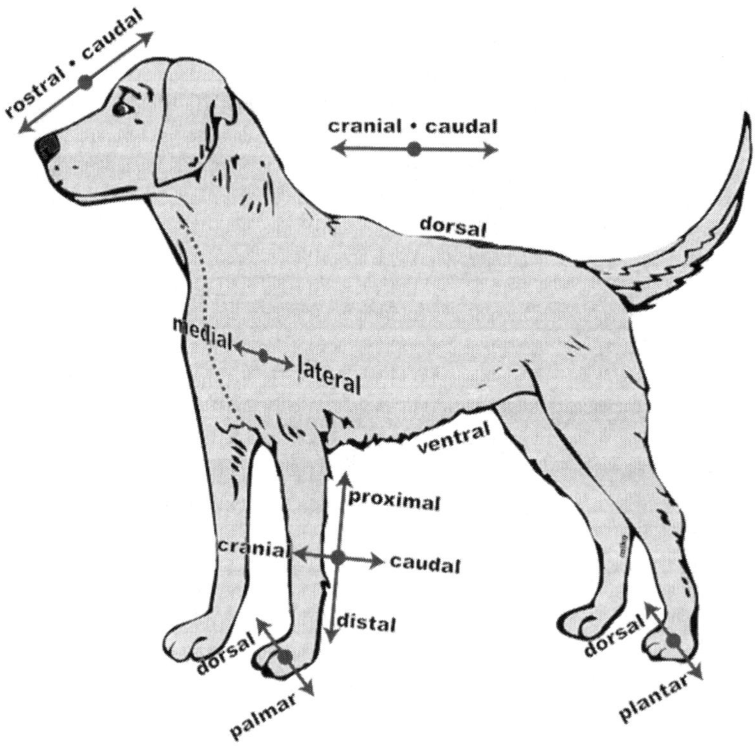

Joint Classification

Three types of **joint classifications** are: **fibrous, cartilaginous,** and **synovial**. Fibrous joints are bony articulations joined by **strong fibers**. These joints are intended to move little if at all. One example of fibrous joints can be seen in the skull sutures. The only time these joints move is during the process of birth, to accommodate the confines of the birth canal. However, they persist in fibrous form as points of subsequent cranial growth. In late adulthood they eventually fuse. Joints that are linked by cartilage without a joint cavity are known as cartilaginous joints. **Cartilage is a strong, stretchy tissue.** Cartilaginous joint examples include intervertebral discs and the pubic symphysis.

Synovial joints are identified by the **presence of synovial fluid** — a clear viscous fluid that provides the joint with lubrication and nourishment. These joints have a joint capsule or sac which contains synovial fluid. The synovial membrane (or bursa) is a thin layer of tissue that encloses both cartilaginous and non cartilaginous surfaces, creating a joint capsule. The synovial membrane is responsible for the secretion of the synovial fluid. The limb joints found within the body are synovial joints. Synovial joints can also be diarthrotic joints.

Anatomy of the Ear

The ear is the organ responsible for **hearing and balance** in mammals. The ear has 3 main parts: the **outer ear, middle ear,** and the **inner ear**. The outer ear includes the pinna (the visible outside ear or auricle), the auditory canal, and the tympanic membrane or eardrum. The middle ear transmits sound from the outer ear to the inner ear via 3 articulating bones called ossicles. The ossicles are named as follows: 1) the malleus or hammer, 2) the incus or anvil, and 3) the stapes or stirrup. Each bone is nicknamed in both Latin and English according to its shape. The small bones vibrate to amplify and relay sound waves from the eardrum to the inner ear. The Eustachian tube links the middle ear to the nasal cavity. The liquid in the inner ear helps maintain balance. The inner ear consists of the cochlea and the semicircular canals. The cochlea is coiled in shape like a snail shell. The cochlea has thousands of hair cells that move in response to sound waves, generating auditory nerve impulses in response. The "organ of Corti," the principal section of the cochlea, translates the neural impulses into sounds. The sound transmission is conducted by an impulse that makes its way from the brain along the auditory nerve.

Common Surgical Procedures

Ovariohysterectomy

A **spay (ovariohysterectomy)** is a surgery that removes the ovaries and uterus from females. The procedure is usually performed between **5 and 7 months of age;** however, in large or giant-breed dogs it **may be performed as late as 12–18 months.** Early spaying of large and giant-breed dogs can cause delayed closure of the growth plates leading to longer and thinner bones, which increases the risk of musculoskeletal injuries such as cruciate ligament tears. Although these are the recommended ages to spay a female pet, it can be done at any time in the pet's life and should always be recommended. Female dogs that are spayed prior to their first heat cycle have a greatly reduced risk of developing mammary cancer, whereas female dogs that have not been spayed have a greater risk of developing mammary cancer.

Castration

Castration is the **surgical removal of the testicles in male animals.** In dogs, an incision is made in front of the scrotum where the testicles are removed, and in cats, the testicles are removed through two incisions into the scrotal sac. Neutered dogs are less likely to display dominant behavior and aggression, along with less roaming after being neutered. Male cats that are neutered are less likely to mark their territory by urinating and are less likely to be aggressive. There is a decreased chance of testicular cancer, perianal tumors, and prostate cancer.

Cryptorchidism

Cryptorchidism (undescended testicles) may occur when one or both testicles do not drop into the scrotum. Both testicles should have migrated to the scrotum by at least 2 months of age; if one or both have not descended, they could be hung up in the belly (abdominal cryptorchid) or in the inguinal area (inguinal cryptorchid). If a dog that is cryptorchid is not neutered, it can cause major health issues including testicular torsion, plus they have a much higher risk of testicular cancer. A cryptorchid neuter is more involved because there may be an abdominal incision and longer surgery time. The veterinarian will palpate the SQ tissue to locate the retained testicle, and if nothing is palpated, then it is an abdominal cryptorchid. If the testicle is felt in the SQ tissue, then an incision is made right above it, and the testicle is removed rather easily. If it is an abdominal cryptorchid, an incision is made into the abdominal cavity, and once the ductus deferens is located, it is followed until the testicle is retrieved.

GI Foreign Bodies

If a dog or cat ingests a foreign object such as toys, string, bones, or any item that will not be able to pass through the GI tract, this causes an **obstruction** and **normally requires surgery** to remove the object. Foreign bodies stuck in the GI tract can perforate the intestinal tract, and there is the risk of the contents of the intestine leaking into the abdomen, which can cause peritonitis (abdominal inflammation) and sepsis, which are life-threatening. Most **GI foreign bodies** require surgery under general anesthesia to remove the object, and this procedure is called an abdominal exploratory surgery. Most foreign bodies will get stuck in the stomach, requiring that a gastrotomy be performed (meaning opening the stomach), or in the intestines, requiring that an enterotomy be performed (meaning opening the intestine). Some foreign bodies may cause enough damage to the intestines such that more than one enterotomy is required. If a part of the bowel cannot be saved, then an intestinal resection and anastomosis will be performed, meaning a segment of the intestine is removed surgically and reattached to the healthy ends.

Enucleation

Enucleations are commonly performed on dogs or cats when the eye must be removed because it is extremely painful and not salvageable. An eye that has a severe corneal or scleral laceration, painful dry eye with corneal scarring, proptosis, tumors, and end-stage glaucoma are all cases that may result in enucleation. There are two surgical options for enucleation: the **transconjunctival approach** and the **transpalpebral approach**. The transconjunctival approach is performed by making an incision around the conjunctiva, which results in less orbital tissue loss, less bleeding during the surgery, and a faster procedure, but it should not be done on an eye that has an intraocular infection. The transpalpebral procedure is done by making an elliptical incision around the eyelids and the globe, along with all of the secretory tissue including the conjunctiva, eyelids, and nictitating membrane being removed.

Cranial Cruciate Ligament and Caudal Cruciate Ligaments

A **ligament** is connective tissue that connects two bones or cartilage. The **cranial cruciate ligament and the caudal cruciate ligament** (CCL) connect the femur with the tibia and cross over each other at the middle of the stifle to stabilize that joint. CCL tears vary in their severity by whether it is a partial or complete tear and if it was sudden or the result of a chronic condition. To determine if the patient has a torn CCL, the drawer test will be performed. The veterinarian stabilizes the femur with one hand and manually manipulates the tibia with the other; if the tibia moves forward, this is a positive drawer effect and indicative of a torn CCL. With a CCL tear, most dogs will not be using the affected leg or toe touching, and it will be painful. If the leg is not treated, it will lead to damaged cartilage and bones, which will cause lifelong osteoarthritis.

Cystotomy

A **cystotomy** surgical procedure is defined as making an opening in the urinary bladder wall. The most common reason to perform a cystotomy is to remove uroliths (bladder stones). Prior to performing a cystotomy to remove bladder stones, an abdominal radiograph should be taken to visualize the stones. The surgical procedure starts with a caudal abdominal midline incision; then the bladder should be isolated from the rest of the abdominal contents and surrounded by laparotomy sponges. Once an incision is made ventrally, the stones and calculi are removed with sterile forceps. Often, a small, sterile spoon will be used to remove the smaller particles. A urethral catheter is flushed multiple times to make sure that all of the stones have been removed, and the stones obtained are sent out to a reference lab for analysis. The bladder can be sutured with 4-0 monofilament, absorbable sutures. Multifilament suture has been known to promote urolith formation, and nonabsorbable sutures are associated with urinary calculi formation. Within 14 days, the urinary bladder regains almost 100% of its tensile strength.

Pyometra

Pyometra is defined as a life-threatening secondary infection of the uterus that must be treated as soon as possible. During the heat cycle, white blood cells (WBCs) that normally protect the uterus from infection are kept from entering the uterus, allowing sperm to enter and not be destroyed. Following the heat cycle, the progesterone hormone levels are still high for up to two months, and this causes the uterus lining to thicken to prepare for pregnancy. The lining will continue to thicken if pregnancy does not occur for several estrus cycles, which will lead to cyst formation in the tissues. Fluid secretions from the thickened, cystic uterine lining allow for an ideal environment for bacteria to grow. High progesterone levels will prevent the uterine muscles from contracting in order to expel any obtained fluid and bacteria. Bacteria from the vaginal area can enter through an open cervix, and an unhealthy uterus with a thickened and cystic lining will not be able to appropriately expel any invaders.

Symptoms of Pyometra

Signs of pyometra include loss of appetite and lethargy, as well as pus discharge from the vagina. Pus will only be seen from the vagina if the cervix is open. If the cervix is closed, then the pus will build up inside of the uterus (called a closed pyometra), and the patient will likely present with a distended abdomen. Dogs that present with a closed pyometra will appear to be very ill very quickly, due to the toxins released into the bloodstream that the bacteria release. More severe clinical signs in a patient with closed pyometra include vomiting, diarrhea, and polyuria (increased urination), due to the toxins from the bacteria affecting the kidneys' function to retain fluids. Polydipsia also occurs (increased drinking) to compensate for polyuria. Diagnostics to confirm pyometra include a high WBC count and globulin levels, which is a protein of the immune system. A urine specific gravity is normally low due to the effects that the bacteria have had on the kidneys. Ultimately, radiographs will confirm an enlarged uterus.

Pyometra Treatment

To **treat pyometra,** it is recommended to remove the infected uterus and ovaries (ovariohysterectomy). Most patients that are diagnosed with pyometra are unhealthy, which makes them high-risk surgical candidates. They will require IV fluids pre-, peri-, and post-surgery and will need a longer hospitalization stay to closely monitor their recovery. There is a medical treatment that is not highly recommended: to give prostaglandins, which are hormones that lower the progesterone level, thus allowing the uterus to contract and get rid of the bacteria and pus accumulation. The use of prostaglandins does not have a high success rate, and it has multiple side effects such as vomiting, abdominal pain, and panting. If left untreated, the outcome is most likely death due to the toxic effects of the bacteria or a ruptured uterus.

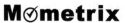

Onychectomy

The **declawing procedure** is also known as an **onychectomy**, and it is normally only performed on the front claws. An onychectomy is the removal of the claw, including the last bone in the digit. There are a couple of different surgical procedures used to perform an onychectomy. One method is to use a size 12 scalpel blade to cut out the claw. Some veterinarians use a more traditional method using a Resco nail trimmer to clip out the nail. The surgical sites are closed normally with surgical glue, and a pressure wrap is placed over the foot for 24 hours. Some veterinarians use a surgical laser to remove the claw. Using the laser results in little to no bleeding because it seals off the blood vessels as it cuts, and there is less swelling because it does not tear or crush the tissue. The laser will seal off the nerve endings as it cuts through the tissue, and this could reduce pain. A tendonectomy can also be done in which the claw is not removed but the tendons under the paw are cut so the claws are always retracted into the paw.

Total Ear Canal Ablation

There are three parts of the ear: the inner, middle, and outer portions. The inner ear controls balance, the middle portion holds the tympanic bulla and the eardrum, and the outer portion contains the ear canal and the pinna. A **total ear canal ablation** is the surgical removal of the whole ear canal and the pinna. This is followed by a bulla osteotomy, which is the opening and cleaning of the infected debris in the bulla. A total ear canal ablation is normally performed once medical treatment for chronic ear infections is not helping and the patient is in constant pain. Total ear canal ablation is also recommended if there is cancer in the external ear canal, and it could be a cure depending on the size of the tumor and if it can be completely removed with this procedure.

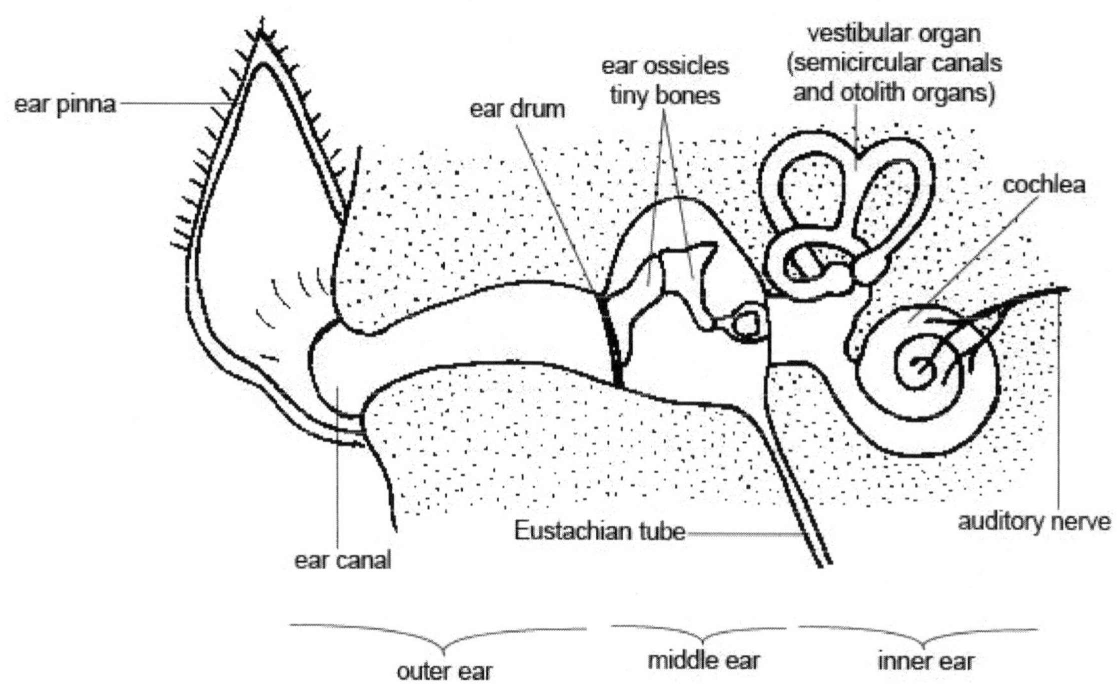

Tibial Plateau Leveling Osteotomy

A **tibial plateau leveling osteotomy** (TPLO) surgery is done to treat a cranial cruciate ligament tear by reducing the tibial plateau angle and eliminating the instability of the joint. Before the TPLO procedure, an X-ray of the stifle is taken for a measurement of the tibial plateau angle. During surgery, the joint is examined and any damaged cartilage is removed in order for the patient to regain normal function. A curved saw is then used to cut a semicircle into the inside top portion of the tibia. This cut portion is rotated to get the desired tibial plateau angle, and then a bone plate is placed on the bone holding the two pieces in the new alignment. After the surgery is complete, post radiographs of the stifle are taken to ensure that the angle is correct and the bone plate placement is correct.

Gastropexy Surgery

A **gastropexy** is a surgery that permanently attaches the stomach to the abdominal wall. It is done to prevent gastric dilatation and volvulus (GDV) or "bloat," which occurs when the stomach fills with air and twists and is life threatening. Treatment for GDV requires surgery to decompress the stomach and repair any internal damage done, as well as perform a gastropexy to prevent it from happening again. A gastropexy is done by attaching the pyloric antrum to the right side of the abdominal wall to prevent further stomach rotation. A gastropexy can be done a few different ways including belt-looped, circumcostal, incorporating, laparoscopic-assisted, or incisional. The incisional gastropexy is done by attaching the muscular layer of the gastric wall's opposite side to the right abdominal wall. Belt-looped gastropexy is done by tunneling a seromuscular flap through the abdominal wall, and circumcostal gastropexy is done by taking a seromuscular stomach flap and wrapping it around the last rib and then attaching it to the stomach wall. Laparoscopic-assisted gastropexy allows for suturing or stapling the stomach securely.

Cesarean Section

There are three surgical options for a cesarean section (C-section), including **C-section**, C-section **plus ovariohysterectomy**, or an **"en-bloc" spay** and C-section. A C-section is done by isolating the uterus in the abdomen so the fetuses and their placentas can be identified, and an incision is made on the great curve of the uterine horns to remove the puppies. Once the puppy is removed, the fetal envelope is opened and the nasal passages are wiped. The umbilical cord is still oxygenating the puppy via the placenta, and the cord will be clamped with two mosquito hemostats and then cut between the two. Some owners may want their dog to be spayed at the time of the C-section; therefore, an ovariohysterectomy is done after the C-section is performed. An "en-bloc" spay and C-section may also be done, which is a procedure during which the ovarian and uterine pedicles are clamped two or three times and no ligatures are done until after the entire uterus is taken out and handed to the technicians aseptically. The technicians open the uterus, remove the puppies, and resuscitate while the surgeon ligates and closes the incision.

Resuscitating Puppies After a C-Section

Three things need to be prevented when **resuscitating the puppies:** hypothermia, hypotension, and hypoxia. To prevent hypoxia, the nasal passages and mouth must be cleared of any secretions. This is normally done by gently using a bulb syringe because too much suction can damage the tissues of the pharynx and larynx. Rubbing the puppy's thorax will **stimulate it to breathe** and help to clear the lungs of fluid, which will result in less heat loss. Once the puppies are moving and breathing on their own, they can be placed in a box with warm towels or towels over a warm water blanket to keep them warm. Administering IV fluids as soon as the mother arrives for surgery will help maintain adequate blood pressure for the mother and the puppies. The puppies should continue to be resuscitated until they have 10 breaths per minute and they are making noise and moving around. Swinging the puppies is no longer a recommended technique for resuscitation.

Square Knot

The **square knot** is applied at the beginning and end of both the **interrupted suture pattern** and the **continuous suture pattern**. The square knot is the knot most preferred by surgeons in tying off a suture securely. The square knot is created by **making 2 casts with the suturing material**. The casts are directed in a reverse route between each cast. The cast is completed by manipulating the tags to exit on the matching side of the loop. The surgeon will put on a constant pressure when the knot is tightened securely. Most suturing material requires that the square knot have at least 3 casts. Some have more than 3, depending upon the material that is used in making the square knot. The surgeon will use as many casts as necessary in typing off a square knot securely. However, the bulkiness of the knot will increase as more casts are used.

Square Knot and Surgeon's Knot

The **square knot** requires that an **alternating reverse direction** be used. This method of tying off the square knot ensures that it is made correctly. Knots tied off without this reversal are considered to be "granny knots" that have the tags on the opposite sides of the loop. The granny knot is not used by most surgeons due to the fact that this knot may slip and lose its hold.

The **surgeon's knot** begins in much the same way as that of the square knot. The difference is accounted for in the way that the strand is passed through the loop **twice on the first cast**. This knot is tied off in similar fashion as that of the square knot. This additional cast creates more friction on the first pass. The increased friction gives the surgeon an advantage. The surgeon's knot is to be applied in instances where the tension on the tissue presents a problem in using a square knot. However, this knot is problematic because of its knot mass. In addition, this knot has an asymmetrical form which is not usually beneficial in surgical procedures.

Buried Knot

The veterinarian will select the buried knot when the application of a subcuticular or intradermal pattern is required. Intradermal describes a space within the skin. The buried knot incorporates a square knot in its tying off pattern. The suture is passed on the nearby side from close to the surface to deeper into the incision and then crossed to the farthest side and passed from deep in the incision to close to the surface. This technique allows the knot to be hidden deep within the skin's tissue. This pattern can be described as an interrupted suture pattern that has been turned upside down.

Three general approaches are evident in the 3 basic knot tying procedures. These approaches can be categorized as instrumental methods, one-hand methods, and two-hand methods. Instrumental tying requires the use of the square knot. This is the most commonly applied knot used by veterinarians in surgery.

General Knot Tying Principles

The **one-hand knot tying method** is applied in procedures where a deep hollow in the body must be reached. The solitary hand is easier to manipulate in the limited space than 2 hands or an instrument. The one-hand method uses the square knot. The two-hand method produces a uniform square knot. However, this method is time-consuming and considered to be quite tiresome.

The relationship between suture security and tying technique has been discussed as 2 variables where one increases as the other decreases, or vice versa. To complete the knot, the veterinarian must apply enough force to each strand to construct a secure square knot. For adequate interrupted sutures, the veterinarian selects a synthetic material with 3-mm tags. However, surgical gut tends to become larger and loosen. Thus, surgical gut is about 6 mm long with long tags. The veterinarian will eliminate any frayed or damaged suture material in the construction of the knot. The veterinarian will only apply instruments on the boundaries of the material. The recommended number of casts meant for a suture material will be used. This will limit the mass of the knot, and reduce ill effects on the tissue.

Suture Techniques

For surgical incisions, absorbable suture is commonly used for **closure**. The sizes of the suture material range from the largest being (0) and in numeric order — as the number rises, the suture gets smaller. Therefore, 2-0 is bigger than 4-0. The tensile strength of the suture compared to the tissue needing to be sutured will determine the suture size needed. **Subcuticular suture patterns** can be done with either continuous or interrupted sutures. Interrupted sutures are performed by each suture strand being tied and cut after the bit giving a more secure closure. Microorganisms are not likely to migrate along this type of suture pattern, which is why it is used for wounds that are infected. **Mattress sutures** are used when there is more of a distance from one side of the wound to the other and tension is needed to bring the edges together. **Surgical adhesive** glue is a liquid wound adhesive that can be used for minor cuts or abrasions, and it is also used in feline declaws. Skin staples are commonly used to reinforce a sutured wound closure to further prevent dehiscence.

Interrupted and Continuous Suture Patterns

There are a number of advantages and disadvantages involved in the procedures surrounding suturing. Sutures can be applied in an interrupted and continuous pattern. Sutures which are considered to be interrupted are those that are cut and tied off at the end of every stitch. Sutures which are considered to be of an uninterrupted and continuous pattern are those cut at the end of the entire suture procedure only. A **closing stitch** is applied at the end of the wound or incision site. The advantages of interrupted suture patterns include the **precision that can be applied to the entire suture line**. In addition, this ensures that the failure of one knot does not result in a significant failure along the entire suture line. The disadvantage in the interrupted suturing method is that it is **time-consuming**. This procedure also **requires more suturing material** than is used in a continuous suturing method. Further, the interrupted method may more easily introduce foreign substances and debris along the incision site line.

Advantages of Continuous Suture Patterns

Sutures can be applied in an **interrupted or a continuous pattern**. Sutures which are interrupted are cut and tied off at the end of every stitch. Sutures which are continuous are cut only at the end of the entire suturing procedure. Continuous suture patterns are less time consuming than the interrupted suture patterns. These patterns are also considered to be more airtight and watertight than an interrupted pattern. In addition, there is a reduced tendency to introduce foreign substances along the incision site line, which is a distinct advantage.

The primary disadvantage is the possible failure of the knot or a break in the line, which could result in a failure of the entire suture line. Another distinct disadvantage of the continuous pattern lies in gauging wound approximation and tension. The continuous suture procedure cannot be regulated and adjusted with precision during the suture procedure. By contrast, interrupted sutures allow for readjustments in tissue margin matching and tension with each new suture.

Simple Interrupted Suture Pattern

The suture material is cut after each suture is tied off in a simple interrupted pattern. This is considered an appositional pattern that allows the veterinarian to adjust and regulate the suture tension used. The stitches are about 5 – 10 mm apart from each other. The skin's density or thickness must be considered in deciding on the distance from the edge of the incision to where the stitch is placed. The simple interrupted pattern is applied by the veterinarian to suture skin, subcutaneous tissue, fascia, vessels, nerves, the gastrointestinal tract, and the urinary tract.

The **interrupted suture pattern** can be applied over cutaneous sutures that are buried. This application **strengthens and supports the skin sutures**. The veterinarian will apply a wider stitch on thin skin or in cases where cutaneous sutures are not present. The suture will be pushed through the fullness of the entire tissue. However, in cases where the skin is too thick a suture will be placed partway into the tissue. This is also true when buried cutaneous sutures are applied. This partway placement is considered a split thickness approach.

Simple Interrupted Intradermal Suture and Simple Continuous Patterns

The **simple interrupted intradermal suture** is placed so that the knot is buried within the skin. This simple interrupted pattern is placed upside down into position. The pattern gains passage deep in the tissue, past the superficial subcutaneous tissue, to the dermis just below the epithelial edge. The pattern runs across the incision site and then gains passage from the dermis to the superficial subcutaneous tissue, where it leaves off. The suture is secured at the base of the tissue with 2 square knots. This pattern ensures contact with the protective layer of surface tissue and the lining of the organs. This is an appropriate method to use for intradermal or subcuticular closures.

The **simple continuous pattern** is initiated with 2 square knots. This is also an appositional pattern. The suture is begun with 4 casts of the suture material. The suture can be cast with 2 different methods.

The Gambee Pattern

The **Gambee pattern** can present a problem for the surgeon. It is an appositional pattern constructed from a modified simple interrupted pattern. The developer of this pattern was attempting to find an ideal suture for use on the intestines. Specifically, the problem was to avoid mucosal eversion where the organ is turned inside out. This may otherwise occur when suturing bladder or intestinal tissue.

The Gambee pattern is an interrupted suture method. The suture is inserted from serous to mucosal surface, then back into the mucosa on the same side of the incision and out into the middle of the cut surface. Then it travels across the incision into the opposite side, down into the open gut lumen, then back through the mucosa and finally through the wall to the serous surface. There it is drawn tight and tied across the incision. In this way the section of the suture within the wall transports the inner mucosa down to the place where it belongs.

Continuous Intradermal Suture Pattern

The **continuous intradermal suture** is created in an appositional pattern that is placed over another layer. This pattern can be referred to as the continuous buried cutaneous suture. This suture is recommended when an **alteration is required in making the horizontal mattress suture**. The continuous intradermal suture starts off in much the same way as the interrupted buried pattern. The surgeon is careful to place each surgical thread on the inner section of the skin. The stitches are set in a pattern that sits at right angles to the skin's borders. The surgeon sets each loop of surgical thread in such a way as to do away with any empty space or void. The surgeon fastens every 4th or 5th loop of surgical thread to the tissue on the bottom.

Suture line ischemia is a consequence of an inadequate supply of blood flow, such as a blocked artery. **Suture line necrosis** or tissue death can also be a consequence of using more thread than is actually needed. The surgeon should place a suture's end ½ to ¾ inches from the seam's border to ensure that the knot is buried.

Simple Continuous Pattern Methods

A simple continuous suture pattern can be cast in 2 different ways. The first method involves casting the suture just beneath the skin. The sutures are visible. The sutures can be placed in a parallel position towards the tissue edges. The suture can be placed towards the front, on the surface of the skin, leaving the visible sutures at an angle near the edge. However, this suture pattern has a **propensity to gather into creases**. Further, the skin's edges may constrict to prevent the proper air and blood flow.

Even so, the simple continuous pattern is sturdy and easily produced. Further, the time-saving application of the simple continuous pattern is an advantage. Likewise, the continuous pattern uses less suture material than the interrupted pattern. This can produce a distinct economic advantage. The continuous pattern creates a watertight and airtight seal or closure. This pattern is particularly valuable in the applications concerning the skin, subcutaneous tissue, fascia, the gastrointestinal tract, and the urinary tract. One disadvantage is found if there is a noticeable break along the suture line. The knot may fail to hold.

Ford Interlocking Suture

The **Ford interlocking suture** can be called the blanket stitch or the continuous interlocking suture. The interlocking loop is created by moving the needle above the trailing suture material after every stitch. The suture is initiated with 4 casts, and requires 4 casts on the end with a final loop to the loose end. The end is tied with a knot. This suture pattern is not economical because of the excessive suture material that is used. However, the suture does provide an airtight and watertight seal similar to the simple continuous pattern. There is a similar disadvantage in the strength and integrity of the suture line. The failure of the beginning or ending knot can cause the suture line to fail in its entirety. Other risks include poor wound margin approximation and potentially marked tension. The precision of the tension given to the sutures cannot be regulated or controlled with certainty using this method.

Continuous Intradermal Suture

In completing the **continuous intradermal suture**, the final suture should be **tacked down with a loop fixed to the loose end**. This knot can be pulled down into the lower tissue and secured. The skin sutures which lie on top should be placed close together in such a way as to reduce the spaces left open in the epithelial closure. These sutures produce a good effect in the stitching of intradermal and subcutaneous closures. This method is an inexpensive use of suture materials. In addition, when using dissolving sutures, there is no need to remove the sutures at a later date.

The Ford interlocking suture is another appositional pattern. The Ford interlocking suture can be called the blanket stitch or the continuous interlocking suture. This suture has many similarities to that of the simple continuous suture. However, one difference is that the failed knot of the Ford interlocking suture will not be as risky as that of the simple continuous suture. The knot found on the Ford interlocking suture is harder to remove. This suture is found on the top side of the skin.

Mattress Suture Patterns

Mattress sutures **lower the stress placed on the skin's boundary or edge**. These sutures are ideal whenever there is a **high level of tension** already present in the tissue. The interrupted horizontal, interrupted vertical, and continuous horizontal suture patterns are all names of specific mattress suture patterns used by a surgeon. However, mattress sutures have a propensity to evert or turn outwards from the boundaries of the tissue.

The **interrupted horizontal mattress suture** should not be applied in **close proximity of the skin**, as this could cause ischemia. Ischemia is caused when pressures displace and compress involved tissues. This may be averted by the use of rubber-tubing stents that keep the arteries and other vessels in the body from being blocked off.

The surgeon will select an interrupted vertical mattress suture for use on tissue with tension. This type of suture is sturdier than the horizontal mattress suture.

The continuous horizontal mattress suture is much like the continuous parallel buried subcutaneous suture. The continuous horizontal mattress suture applies **sturdy quality surgical seams over an existing suture layer**. The sutures are completed by tying a loop to the loose end.

Lembert Suture Patterns

The **Lembert suture pattern** uses an inverting or reversal pattern which is best applicable to hollow closures. This suture is needed in the bladder, stomach, or uterus. The Lembert suture can be used to form either an interrupted or a continuous suture pattern. The serous membrane is the thin external lining around the internal organs of the body. The tissue, serosa to serosa, is physically brought together through the inverted Lembert suture using the interrupted pattern. The serosa is found on the inner chest, abdomen, and stomach. The surgeon places the suture so as not to infiltrate the lumen. The suture must not block off the hollow spaces located within the lumen. Suture stitches are cast in a perpendicular direction towards the boundary's edge of the surgical cut. These surgical sutures will be placed deep inside sturdy tissue. In the case of operations involving the intestines, the submucosa is included in this deeply sewn stitch. Stomach incisions are the most common use of the continuing Lembert suture. Otherwise, this stitch is almost never used. In the case of small mammals, this stitch must be modified so that the lumen of the intestines and the submucosa is part of the stitching process.

Far-Far-Near-Near and Far-Near-Near-Far Suture Patterns

The **far-far-near-near** and **far-near-near-far** suture patterns have been modified from the vertical mattress suture pattern. These sutures are also a blending of the tension and approximating suture and wound approximation suture. The far-far-near-near and the far-near-near-far suture patterns are beneficial for providing a surgical seam that does not require undue direct pressure to be placed along the tissue's edge. These types of sutures are appropriate for **skin, subcutaneous tissue, and fascia closures under tension or stress pressure**.

The far-far-near-near and far-near-near-far suture patterns are applied by surgeons where the **skin that is cut will result in a wide distance between the tissue margins**, from edge to edge. The portion of the suture that is farthest away from the edge will lower the tension from the portion of the suture that is nearest to the opening. The surgeon should be watchful for the skin's propensity to invert along its edges or boundaries. Of additional note, the suture is cast in a twofold overlapping pattern which uses double the amount of suture material.

Choosing the Appropriate Suture Pattern

A good number of veterinarian surgeons utilize just a few suture patterns on a regular basis. However, there are some that can only be selected for use by an expert. The 3-loop pulley or locking loop is selected by the skilled suturing surgeon when other sutures would not be appropriate. In addition, the surgeon expertly selects the appropriate suture materials and sizes of material. In the majority of cases, the surgeon will apply 4 casts and 2 square knots. One suture material known as **polydioxanone requires more casts or throws** to ensure the material has been firmly fixed into place. A continuous suture is finished off with at least one more cast or throw over than what is normally called for in suturing with polydioxanone material. The veterinarian will inspect every single knot to be sure that each one has been firmly fixed into place. The veterinarian will use a square knot for the most part. However, the surgeon's knot is more likely to be used if the tissues are under pressure or stress. The appositional pattern is favored over the use of everting or inverting patterns

Removing Sutures

Sutures that are firmly fixed in place may cause the epithelial cells in the skin to quickly grow down the length of the stitch. The problem occurs when the cells reach the lower tissue. At that point the cells become keratinized, and redness and swelling in the form of an abscess can result. Usually, this happens with sutures that are left in the body for an excessive length of time. Thus, the surgeon will want to remove the skin sutures after a period of 7 to 10 days. In cases where the sutures are buried and have resulted in tissue binding strength, only 7 days is usually required before removal. Sutures that have not succeeded in binding the skin together may need to stay in for 10 to 14 days. The surgeon will remove the skin sutures by grabbing the loose tab attached to the knot. The surgeon uses his fingers or the hemostat to perform this task. The surgeon will pull the buried suture's knot up to expose it for clipping. The surgeon can then begin cutting and removing the clean suture material through the skin.

Surgical Environment, Equipment, Instruments, and Supplies

Describe the Different Types of Scissors Used in Veterinary Surgery.

There are a variety of scissors used in veterinary surgery. The types include operating scissors, Mayo scissors, Metzenbaum scissors, iris scissors, wire-cutting scissors, Littauer and Spencer suture removal scissors, and Lister Bandage scissors. The scissors most routinely used are known as **operating scissors**. These scissors can be used for **cutting sutures** and **drape material**. Scissors can be categorized based on the shape of the blade, the point of the tip, or the cutting edge. Scissors applied in cutting away thick tissue or sutures in dissection are known as Mayo scissors. Scissors applied in cutting away delicate tissue in dissection are known as Metzenbaum scissors. These scissors allow fragile cuts to be accomplished via a longer handle versus a shorter blade. Scissors applied with even more precision in intraocular surgery are known as iris scissors. These scissors are small in size, quite fragile, and have a very sharp pointed tip.

Describe the Different Types of Thumb Forceps Used in Veterinary Medicine.

Thumb forceps include those that can be applied as either tissue or dressing forceps. The difference is found in the blade and tips. Tissue forceps are used to grasp tissue with tips that resemble teeth. Dressing forceps hold the tissue or dressings with smooth or smoothly serrated tips.

Adson tissue forceps provide a strong grip. However, this strong grip does little harm to fragile tissue — largely because the structure of the Adson tissue forceps includes a solitary tooth-like tip.

Brown-Adson tissue forceps are similar to the Adson forceps. However, these forceps have a wide, easy-to-hold handle and a tip with 16 thinly shaped teeth that mesh or engage with each other.

Hollow internal organs can more easily be grasped with the rounded tips of the **Russian tissue forceps**. In the application and removal of dressing material, these dressing forceps are particularly beneficial. These forceps are structured with a smooth blade edge.

Types of Scissors

Scissors applied in cutting away wire sutures are known as wire-cutting scissors. These scissors have short, bulky jaws with a saw-toothed blade edge. Scissors applied after an operation or in the removal of sutures are known as Littauer and Spencer suture removal scissors. The structure of these scissors includes blunt tips and one blade that is shaped like a finely arched hook. Scissors applied in the removal of bandages are known as Lister bandage scissors. These are safe to come into contact with the skin due to the flat, dense end and dull tip of the lower blade.

There are a variety of thumb forceps used in veterinary medicine. These include tissue forceps, Adson tissue forceps, Brown-Adson tissue forceps, Russian tissue forceps, and dressing forceps. Thumb forceps have a structure that incorporates the use of a spring apparatus. The veterinarian should normally hold the forceps as he or she would hold a pencil.

Types of Self-Retaining Forceps

The **Doyen intestinal forceps** are applied in holding the bowel in place. This instrument can also close off the lumen, or the tubular space of the bowel. However, the structure of the instrument prevents the target tissue from being crushed. It has notches like a row of teeth on a saw which extend from the top to the bottom.

The **Ferguson angiotribe forceps** are used for holding a large band of parallel tissues in place.

The **sponge forceps** are applied in surgical procedures or in preparation for surgery. These forceps can also provide hemostasis, which means that bleeding may be stopped by way of this instrument. This instrument has a hole in its end. The hole can be of various shapes including straight, curved, smooth, or serrated.

The **Backhaus towel clamp** is applied to firmly fix in place the drapes or folds of the patient's skin. The structure of this instrument has arched tips.

There are a variety of self-retaining forceps used in veterinary medicine. Self-retaining forceps have a ratchet-like mechanism which turns in one direction. This mechanism allows the veterinarian to move the tissue back inside or retract the tissue in a firm grasp. Other types of self-retaining forceps include: Allis tissue forceps, Babcock tissue forceps, Doyen intestinal forceps, Ferguson angiotribe forceps, sponge forceps, and Backhaus towel clamps.

The **Allis tissue forceps** are applied when tissue needs to be held in place. This instrument has short teeth that fit together and interlock.

The **Babcock tissue forceps** are applied to grasp more fragile areas of tissue without causing additional trauma. This instrument has a structure that is applied without the benefit of gripping teeth. This absence of teeth is easier on the tissue. The instrument has a very wide, flared tip that securely holds the tissue in place.

Hemostatic Forceps

Hemostatic forceps are used to provide hemostasis, which means that bleeding is stopped from flowing by use of these instruments. These instruments are structured to firmly clamp and hold blood vessels closed and/or in place. These instruments have various shapes which include hinged, curved, or straight. There are a number of different types of hemostatic forceps used, which include Kelly and Crile forceps, Halstead mosquito forceps, Rochester-Pean and Rochester-Carmalt forceps, and Rochester-Ochsner forceps. The Kelly and Crile forceps are applied to securely hold larger blood vessels and tissue in place. The structure of these instruments can be long or short in length. However, the standard length of the instrument is measured at 12.5 cm or 4.5 inches long. In the case of the Kelly forceps, the construction has transverse grooves which lay distally or away from the point of the attachment. The Crile forceps are constructed with a complete set of transverse grooves or furrows which lay in a crosswise direction.

Hemostatic forceps are used to provide hemostasis. Halstead mosquito forceps are applied to capillary bleeders. This instrument has a thinly shaped tip that may be shaped as an arch or a straight angle. The entire jaw of the instrument has a series of crosswise serrations. The length of this instrument is 10 cm or 4 inches long. The Rochester-Pean, the Rochester-Carmalt, and the Rochester-Ochsner forceps have some similarities in use and shape. The longest ones are the Rochester-Pean and the Rochester-Carmalt forceps. These 2 instruments are measured at 20 cm or 9 inches long. Kelly forceps are applied to stump and pedicle surgical tying procedures or ligations. Carmalt forceps include grooves which extend from the top to the bottom of the device. Pean forceps have grooves which lay in a crisscross or transverse direction. For every tooth on the Rochester-Ochsner forceps, an additional tooth has been added to the Rochester-Pean forceps.

Needle Holders

Needle holders are instruments that are able to hold **arched suturing needles during surgery**. These instruments are constructed as **hinged forceps**. Mayo-Hegar and Olsen-Hegar are 2 kinds of needle holders applied in surgical procedures performed by veterinarians. Mayo-Hegar needle holders are the heavier of the 2 types of needle-holding forceps used. This instrument does not have a cutting blade. The cutting blade on the Olsen-Hegar needle holders are used when sutures need to be cut. This eliminates the need for an extra set of scissors. This instrument has a needle-holding jaw. However, care should be taken to prevent the unintentional severing of sutures during a procedure. The 2 instruments are constructed with a system of interconnected grooves on the ends. The Mayo-Hegar and Olsen-Hegar needle holders hold the needle in place during a surgical procedure. The Mathieu needle holders open and close by a touch of the fingers, as this instrument does not have loops for the fingers to be placed inside.

Retractors

There are a number of retractors that are beneficial in veterinary medicine. The **purpose of the retractor is to pull back, hold, and secure tissue or organs during surgery**. This allows the veterinarian to establish better unobstructed access to the operation site. Retractors can be either manually operated or self-retaining instruments. The retractors which fall into the manual operation category include: Senn, Meyerding, Hohmann, US Army, and malleable retractors. Senn retractors are constructed with 2 tips consisting of either dull or sharp blade edges. This instrument is applied for superficial retraction purposes on the outside of the skin. The dull blade edge is applied to regions where delicate tissue is held in place. The sharper blade edge is to secure the fascia. Meyerding, Hohmann, and US Army retractors are applied in the securing of larger muscle mass. These instruments also serve to secure more superficial incisions that do not run as deep.

Self-Retaining Retractors

Self-retaining retractors have a locking function and are able to retract and secure tissues without the surgeon or assistant staff having to manually hold the tissues back and away. This is beneficial in surgery, as it allows the surgeon and assistants to focus on other demands. Balfour, Finochietto, Snook, and Covault retractors are all self-retaining devices. Balfour retractors are constructed for use in abdominal surgical procedures which are far from the surface of the skin. This instrument secures a wound's outermost layers, particularly those surrounding the abdomen. The instrument also comes in a variety of sizes. Finochietto retractors are applied when retraction is needed during surgical procedures in the chest (thoracic) area. Snook and Covault are instruments applied in the surgical procedures involving the ovaries. These instruments are often used in ovariohysterectomy. In veterinary medicine, they are also sometimes called spay hooks. The construction of the Snook retractor consists of a broad, level handle. This instrument has a smooth, curved-shaped end. Covault retractors are constructed with a handle that has 8 flat surfaces. These retractors have a circular end that resembles a ball shape.

Malleable Retractors

Malleable (shapeable) retractors are also manually operated, and are constructed to give the veterinarian the ability to bend the instrument to reach down into the deeper cuts or injuries. This malleable feature makes it easier to retract or secure areas which are normally difficult to reach. The retractors which fall into the self-retaining category include Gelpi, Weitlanders, Balfour, Finochietto, Snook, and Covault. These instruments have a locking function and are configured in such a way as to secure tissues without having to be manipulated or held in place by the surgeon or assistants. A Gelpi retractor is constructed with a solitary sharp end that juts outward. This instrument is applied in the retraction of incisions that are not very deep. Weitlanders are instruments which have been constructed with ends that look like the teeth on a gardening tool. These ends can be dull or sharp to the touch. The instrument is also applied in the retraction of incisions that are not very deep.

Basic Types of Orthopedic Surgical Equipment

Orthopedic surgery is applied in connection to bones, joints, ligaments, and/or related muscles. There are a variety of instruments used during orthopedic procedures. For example, during a surgical procedure a veterinarian may need to apply wire twisters to aid in holding the needles. These are large in size. **Jacobs drill chucks** can be applied to move the pins into position during the surgery.

The function of the instrument known as the **Rongeurs** is to split apart and remove the bone from the area. Another tool used in this endeavor is known as the **Lempert**. Yet another forceps instrument used to cut away the bone is known as a **Liston**.

Osteotomes, bone curettes, and mallets are also sometimes applied during an operation to **divide bone into smaller pieces**. Finally, any sharp pieces of bone left in place must be smoothed or sanded down with a **bone rasp**. If the veterinarian should need to free the periosteum or tissue surrounding the bone, then the Periosteal elevator called the Freer and Langbeck would be applied.

Common Orthopedic Instruments

Orthopedic surgery is applied as a medical remedy for diseases, disorders, and injuries involving bones, joints, ligaments, or related muscles. There are a variety of instruments used during orthopedic procedures. These instruments include Kern and Richards forceps, Verbrugge and reduction forceps, wire twisters, Jacobs drill chucks, ostomies, Rongeurs, Lemperts, Listons, mallets, bone curettes, bone rasps, Periosteal elevators, and Freer and Langbecks. The application of the

Kern and Richards forceps is beneficial in securing tissues in the musculoskeletal system. The construction of the forceps includes teeth that can strongly grasp the tissues being retracted. Many of the constructed forceps also function with a ratchet-type mechanism. This mechanism allows the veterinarian to manipulate the bone fractures or breaks. The surgical procedure may involve inserting screws or other fixators in the region. If this is the case, the surgeon will use the Verbrugge and reduction forceps to hold the screws or fixators in place. In this way the bone fragments are held in a state of reduction until full stabilization has occurred.

Types of Scalpels

The **Bard-Parker scalpel handle** is constructed with a blade that can be disconnected and removed. The reattachment of a blade is accomplished by the use of a number 3 or number 4 needle holder. The Bard-Parker scalpel handle is the most widely used in surgical procedures on small mammals. For more delicate incisions, the veterinarian will use a number 15 blade. This blade is paired with a smaller rendering of the number 10 handle. For arthroscopic procedures which delve into the inspection of the inside of the joint, the veterinarian will select a number 11 blade. The number 11 blade works well for stabbing incisions. The pointed tip construction is beneficial. The number 12 blade is constructed with a hooked end. This blade is used to take out sutures and for removal of an animal's claws.

Scalpels for Small Animals

The **scalpel** is a tool that the veterinarian will apply during surgical procedures on virtually all animals. The skilled veterinarian will use a variety of scalpels in this endeavor. A widely found scalpel handle is known as the Bard-Parker. This handle is constructed with a blade that can be disconnected and removed. The reattachment of this blade is accomplished with the use of a number 3 or number 4 needle holders. This is the most widely used handle style in surgical procedures on small mammals. There are some significant pairings that should be noted regarding the handles and the blades. For instance, the numbers 10, 11, 12, or 15 scalpel blades are typically paired in conjunction with number 3 handle. The number 20 blade is commonly paired in conjunction with the number 4 handle. However, the veterinarian may select the number 10 blade more often in conjunction with the pairing of the number 4 handle.

Types of Surgical Needles and Suture Material

The needle point known as the tapered point is not used for cutting. **Tapered point needles** are constructed with and without an eye component. The eyeless needles are constructed with a swaged component. This component allows the suture end to be inserted into a hole drilled or a u-channel in the end of the needle and then crimped or bonded, avoiding the bent suture drag of an eye-insertion format. Eye-insertion, threaded needles leave the suture jutting out on either side of the needle's hole. These threaded needles can lead to some tissue trauma as the needle is passed through.

Veterinarians will select and use non-synthetic suture material known as **surgical gut.** The more widely used absorbable synthetic suture material includes polyglycolic acid, polygalactin acid, polydioxanone, and polyglyconate. Polyglycolic acid is constructed from synthetic polyester which is derived from a chemical process involving hydroxyacetic acid. Polygalactin acid is constructed from a copolymer of lactic and glycolic acids. Polydioxanone and polyglyconate are constructed from synthetic polyester.

Surgical Needle Uses

Surgical needles are found in a variety of **geometric forms and sizes**. The geometric shapes include arched, straight, and half an arch. The veterinarian will use the arched or curved needle most often. These arched or curved needles are gauged according to the size of the circle. The range of the circle is 1/4, 3/8, 1/2, 5/8 in size. The surgical needles are constructed as one-half of a circle with 2 kinds of needle points. The 2 kinds of needle points are known as a cutting point and a tapered point. The needle point known as a cutting point comes in reverse, triangular, or side cutting implementations. These needle points are best applied in the cutting of skin, cartilage, or tendons. The needle point known as the tapered point is not used for cutting. This is due to the rounded or oval shape of the point. The round reverse cutting points are selected for their use with torn or ragged edged tissues.

Sizing Suture Material

The **measurement units for suture material** are provided by USP or Pharmacopeia sizing guidelines. Pharmacopeia refers to a database or book which provides particular information for medical drugs or materials. Suture material sizes are represented by identifying numbers written as 4-0, 3-0, 0, 1, and 2. The suture material 4-0 is referred to aloud as "4 ought", with the word "ought" used in reference to the number zero.

The diameter or the width of the suture material can be determined by looking at the number with reference to zero. The larger the number, the thicker and larger the size. Therefore, a size 2 suture is larger than a size 1 suture. Likewise, the diameter or width of the suture gets thinner as any number paired to the left of a zero enlarges. This indicates a smaller size. Thus, the size 3-0 is larger in size than 4-0. Wire suture sizes are indicated by the wire's gauge, ranging in size from 18 to 40 gauge. The higher gauge numbers indicate a thicker wire and vice versa. The veterinarian performing a surgery should select the best suture material and needle size based upon the surgical site, the recovery needs, and past experience.

Suture Materials

The veterinarian will apply a **non-absorbable suture material** in surgery. These materials are constructed from man-made and natural resources. Natural sources include silk, cottons, linens, and stainless steel. Silk does lose its ability to stretch after a 6-month period. However, silk is still beneficial as material which will not soak up a liquid. Cotton is derived from a spun cotton fiber that originated from a cotton plant.

Stainless steel has limited flexibility, and thus can be difficult to manipulate. However, stainless steel is often used in veterinary medicine.

Non-absorbable synthetic materials include polypropylene, polyamide/nylon, and polymerized caprolactam. Polypropylene is derived from a synthetic plastic. Polyamide/nylon is derived from a polymerized plastic. Polymerized caprolactam has an outer layer that has been coated with a synthetic fibrous material. This synthetic fibrous material is applied by veterinarians in the surgical procedure to close the skin flaps after an operation.

Caring for Instruments and Other Surgical Implements

Surgical implements and other reusable items will need to be **sterilized prior to being used again**. Typically, this is done using an autoclave. **An autoclave is a pressurized container** that superheats water and thereby steam cleans and purges everything placed inside it. Instruments and linens should be packed using a standardized procedure to ensure that optimal sterilization takes place. Perforations in pans or trays should not be blocked. The holes should be left unobstructed to allow better steam flow to occur during the sterilization process. Further, all boxlocks and ratchets should be opened and exposed upon placement into the ultrasonic cleaner. This allows the cleanser access to hard-to-reach locations on the instrument. The ultrasonic cleaner should not be overloaded with instruments. The implements that are to be used first should go on the top of the tray. The heavier implements should be packed on the bottom of the tray. In general, it is not good practice to vary the kinds of metals placed within the same cleaning cycle.

CARING FOR STAINLESS STEEL INSTRUMENTS

The veterinarian must take special care of the stainless steel instruments used in medical practice. Instruments exposed to certain materials can acquire a **residue on the surface**. This residue should **not be allowed to dry** as it may lead to staining, pitting, and corrosion of the instrument. Thus, the veterinarian should keep the implements moist until they can receive a thorough washing. The veterinarian should wash the instruments in distilled water, using approved cleaning products. The cleaning products should have a pH foundation ranging from 9.2 to 11. Tap water is not recommended for use as it can cause mineral deposits to form on the instruments' surface areas. An **ultrasonic cleaner** is recommended for use in the sterilization process. Ultrasonic cleaners have been studied and found to be 16 times more efficient than manual cleaners.

WRAPPING INSTRUMENT PACKS FOR STERILIZATION

The gown and towel packs must be sized to fit into the autoclave for sterilization. There should be enough room for steam flow to **penetrate to all areas**. The size of a gown and towel pack should be approximately 30 x 30 x 50 cm, and weigh no more than 5.5 kg. The density of the gown and towel pack should not be more than 115.3 kg/m^3. A space should exist ranging from 2.5 to 7.5 cm of empty void between packs.

In addition, the packer should have **2 pieces of wrapping material** of the correct size folded like a diamond. The placement of the pack will go in the middle of the uppermost wrap. The corner closest to the packer will be folded over the uppermost region of the pack. A flap will be created by folding a small portion of that corner. Repeat this procedure until all side corners are fashioned in this manner. The final corner will be tucked under the 2 side corners with a small flap left to pull it open. Continue this procedure until all the layers have been folded in like manner.

FURTHER CARE FOR STERILIZING AND STORING SURGICAL INSTRUMENTS

During **sterilization and storage**, some metals are susceptible to **electrolytic corrosion**. This is a chemical reaction that can destroy metal surgical instruments. Therefore, following cleaning these implements should be submerged in "**surgical milk.**" The bath in surgical milk coats the implements with a lubricant which acts as a rust inhibitor. This is followed by a drying process which is accomplished with clean paper. Some instruments may require further treatment with lubricants. The veterinarian should check the condition of each instrument before returning it to service.

Other sterilization considerations require the veterinarian's attention. Surgical gowns, laparotomy sheets, drapes, and skin towels should be folded accordion style. The freshly washed and dried surgical gowns should be examined for tears. If free from damage, the gown can be wrapped inside out with sleeves on top of the gown. The ties should be skillfully folded on the inside. The veterinarian will routinely need a laundered towel to be available. The towel is essential for drying hands after a surgical scrub. Thus, this towel should be positioned in the gown pack.

STERILIZATION MONITORS

Sterilization monitors are classified as follows: indicator tape, chemical indicator strips, Bowie Dick tests, and biological indicators. The veterinarian should utilize more than one sterilization monitor to maintain quality control. The first type of sterilization monitor is known as indicator tape. The lines on this tape will change color upon contact with steam or ethylene oxide. However, this tape cannot be used to determine that a certain temperature has been reached in the sterilization process. The **tape changes color** when any steam comes into contact with the tape. Thus, the veterinarian cannot use this tape to gauge the period of time that the sterilization process has lasted. Instead, the veterinarian would do well to use a chemical indicator tape which has been placed under the folds of a gown. This placement ensures that the steam has reached the inside of the gown. In addition, the chemical indicator changes color after it has had contact with steam or ethylene oxide for an adequate period of time.

Sterilization Monitors

The third type of sterilization monitor should also be applied in the sterilization process. Commercially available tests are available in the form of the **Bowie Dick tests**. These tests come with an indicator tape which can be positioned in an out-of-the-way location in the autoclave device.

The **autoclave** is the steel compartment used to apply steam, pressure, and high temperatures to the packs and instruments. This positioning lets the veterinarian know with certainty that the steam has penetrated that area. However, the veterinarian will also apply a biological indicator to make sure that heat-resistant bacteria have been adequately exposed to the sanitation process. Finally, the veterinarian should also track time, temperature, and pressure in the sterilization process. This process must be exact in order to ensure that the destruction of living microorganisms has been accomplished, to reduce the threat of residual infection. This careful attention will ensure that quality control is maintained in the sterilization process.

Sterilization and Patient Preparation

Preparing a Patient for Surgery

The veterinarian is responsible for **preparing a patient** for surgical procedures. First, the veterinarian must make sure that the **patient is cleared of germs** which trigger disease. This preparation takes place before the patient is admitted into the operating room. Second, the animal should have its **bladder emptied of fluids**. This may be accomplished by walking the animal until it urinates. Another method involves manually pressing on the bladder until the animal releases its contents. Third, the animal's **hair is removed from the incision site**(s) with electric clippers and a number 40 blade. The animal's hair should be removed by holding the clippers at an angle and moving against the direction of the hair growth. Fourth, the surgery site should be **free of loose hair** and scrubbed thoroughly, and then cleansed with a surgical disinfectant. Fifth, the **surface area of the preparatory table must be vacuumed** thoroughly and the operating room disinfected well before patient's entrance. The patient's scrub should not be contaminated during the transferring of the patient to the operation table. Sixth, the final step involves **positioning the monitoring equipment**, with the patient given a reapplication of antiseptic on the incision site.

Common Surgical Clips and Animal Positioning for Surgery

The **standard preparation site** for laparotomies or surgical cuts through the abdominal wall requires that the animal be placed in a **lying position on its back** (i.e., in a dorsal recumbent position). This position is necessary for the veterinarian to perform an ovariohysterectomy or a splenectomy. For abdominal surgeries, removal of the fur is extensive. If the veterinarian is to perform surgery on a cat, then the cat's hair should be removed in a sideways direction. The distance extends one clipper blade past the nipple for cats. The distance extends to at least 4 inches on each side of the midline for large sized dogs. In the case of a canine castration, the hair is removed from the scrotum, prepuce, and continues to the inguinal or groin area. In the case of feline castrations, there is not a need to move as much hair.

Preparing the Surgical Site

The standard preparation site for surgical cuts **requires some removal of hair**. If the clipping is finished, then there may be a need for **additional hair removal through plucking**. The hair can be pulled out by the roots in the testes and the region surrounding the scrotum. In the case of removal of claws in cats and puppies, and for tail docking, hair removal is not recommended. The animal having perineal urethrostomies, rectal fistulas, and anal sac surgeries should be positioned so that the veterinarian can access the lower body in the front of the animal. Therefore, the patient should be placed in a ventral recumbent position. The animal's tail should be securely fastened to the top or side of the patient. The animal's hind legs should be allowed to hang down over the edge of the table. It should be noted that in the case of orthopedic surgeries, it is necessary to prepare a larger surgical site so that the surgeon has a greater range of motion for the limb.

Draping the Patient

The animal having surgery is referred to as the patient. The patient must be securely positioned on the operating table. This patient is given one last surgical site sterilization. The surgical team member should be fully masked and gowned in sterile garments. The team member places a drape over the patient at this time. The **sterilized drape** protects the patient from any contamination along the surgical site. **Field drapes are positioned over unsterilized regions of the animal**. These drapes are placed one at a time on the perimeters of the sterilized surgical site. The surgical team member should not try to move the drapes once they have been positioned, as this could lead to contaminants entering the sterilized surgical site. The surgical team member will use **towel clamps to fasten the 4 corners of the drapes to the skin**. The last procedure includes laying a large drape or laparotomy sheet over the entire region. There should be a gap left for easy access to the surgical site. This gap still covers the site, but can be folded back to reveal the area underneath, with the final drape covering the uninterrupted sterile area.

Surgical Scrubbing Procedures

The veterinarian must use the **proper scrubbing procedures** to prepare a patient for surgery. There are 2 widely used scrub products used by veterinarians. These scrub products are chlorhexidine and povidone-iodophor. The patient requires scrubbing around the incision site before surgery can be carried out. The scrubbing is done in a circular motion, gradually moving outward away from the incision site. The scrub should consist of an ample lather for a thorough cleansing. The surgical site should be cleansed with the scrubbing product a total of 3 times. The second application should be accomplished with brand new gauze. The third application must also be done with a new gauze square. Upon the third scrub, this gauze should have no dirty residue. The procedure should be done again if the gauze is dirty, and should be repeated until the gauze comes away clean. The initial scrubbing procedure may be accomplished with an alternative product such as sterile saline.

Cleansing the Surgical Site

The next stage of cleansing requires that the **incision site be treated with chlorhexidine or povidone-iodine**. These products are used for **further antiseptic purposes**. This stage can be accomplished using 1 of 3 application procedures. The first application procedure involves the use of non-sterile gauze. **Antiseptic** is applied on the medial section along the incision line. Another application of antiseptic is applied to the left or right of the incision site ending at the quadrant's edge farthest from the area. The second application procedure involves the use of non-sterile gauze. Antiseptic is applied on the medial section along only one side of the incision line. A second pass is accomplished with new gauze. This pass is applied to the other side of the incision line. The third application procedure is to apply antiseptic with a spray over the incision site. Either of these application procedures can be used to prepare the patient for surgery.

Numbered Stroke Method

There are further procedures which should be followed before surgery. The staff should **position the sterile scrub brush** and any packs and surgical equipment nearby before commencing the scrub. The staff should dress in surgical scrubs and don the cap, gown, and mask at this time. The staff should remove all jewelry and inspect the fingernails. The fingernails should be cut short and absent of all nail polish. The hands are scrubbed with a **sterile scrub brush** and an application of antiseptic soap. The scrub starts at the edges of the fingertips of one hand using a series of stroking motions. A total of 12 strokes are applied to each finger. The outside (baby) finger marks the beginning of the procedure. This is continued, and ends with the thumb. The staff will move on in a scrubbing motion towards the palm. From this area, the staff will move towards the back of the hand and move along to the side of the hand.

Final Steps of the Numbered Stroke Method

The **scrubbing motion** should be continued by moving from the side of the hand to the 4 surfaces of the wrist. The scrub continues up the arm, but ends 2 inches below the elbow. The staff will completely rinse out the brush before repeating the scrub on the other hand. More antiseptic soap is needed to complete this procedure. A rinse is required of both hands at the end of the scrub with antiseptic soap. The hands should be held in an upward position. The drying procedure is accomplished with a sterile towel. The staff should apply one side of the towel to one side for the right hand and right arm. The other side of the towel should be applied to the left hand and left arm. These specific procedures should be followed for every surgical procedure.

Operating Room Rules

There are a number of rules that apply to general operating room procedures. The purpose of these rules is to maintain aseptic conditions as they apply to the surgical suite and the patient. The staff should always dress in the **proper surgical garments** when present in the operating room. The proper surgical garments are surgical scrubs, a hooded cap called a bouffant, surgical mask, a sterile gown, and foot covers or surgery shoes. The staff should not engage in **unnecessary communication.** The staff should **reduce their movements to necessary actions**. The staff should obey proper procedures when opening sterile equipment packs. These procedures should be adhered to when handing sterile equipment to other staff members. These procedures take into consideration the fact that the front side of the surgical gown, from the waist to the shoulder and down the arms, is sterile. The surgical assistant is responsible for handing off sterile equipment to the surgeon.

Final rules are required to maintain **general operative and postoperative order**. The surgical assistant **monitors and supervises the orderliness of the surgical table.** The assistant will be responsible for cleaning instruments and **maintaining the patient's hemostasis.** The assistant will retract the patient's muscles and tissues during the surgery, and will be responsible for cutting the sutures during the surgery and upon closure. The assistant will be diligent about using implements that are sterile beyond a doubt. Contact with a non-sterilized item will result in the contamination of both the item and the individual.

The operating room rules should be strictly adhered to in an effort to maintain aseptic conditions as they apply to the surgical suite and the patient. The surgical assistant plays a major role in this endeavor. However, all staff members must abide by these rules to ensure that this environment is not compromised by contamination.

Proper Surgical Attire and Assistant Placement

The front side of the surgical gown, from the waist to the shoulder and down the arms, is the person's **sterile field**. However, this **can become contaminated** if proper infection control procedures are not followed. The hands should be held **close to and in front of the body** when not needed for the surgical procedure. The hands should also be kept above the waist and surgery table. The staff should move by passing one another with their backs toward each other. The staff should never move with their backs facing the patient.

Surgical assistants should be positioned to **receive sterile equipment** without intruding upon the sterile field or the patient. The surgical table should be kept orderly. The instruments are kept sterile. The assistant will be responsible for handing over all instruments in response to the surgeon's need. The assistant will tap the surgeon's hand with the instrument to ensure that the proper contact has been made between the instrument and the surgeon.

Sterile Scrubs and Masks

The operating room can become **contaminated by the presence of street clothes**. Therefore, it is critical that staff wear **sterilized surgical scrubs** in the operating room. The staff member that clips the hair on the animal as preparation for surgery should wear a smock over the scrubs. The staff member must also wear a hooded cap that completely covers the person's hair. In addition, hooded caps may be needed to cover beards, moustaches, or other facial and neck hair.

There are 2 types of **surgical masks** that can be worn by the staff: **molded masks and flat masks**. Molded masks are best when there is little need to cover an abundance of facial hair. This mask can permit air to escape from beneath. The flat-style mask has pressed folds with a metal nose band. This construction gives the wearer a more customized fit which does not allow air to escape as readily as the molded mask, but which fully secures any facial hair.

Assisting in Surgery

The assistant is responsible for maintaining the patient's hemostasis. This is accomplished by **positioning the suction near tissue** to accommodate any blood flow. The tissue should **not have suction applied directly to it**. The assistant will also dab the tissue region with gauze. The assistant keeps track of the quantity of gauze squares used. The assistant will dispose of the used gauze properly. The skilled assistant is responsible for drawing back the muscles and tissues with the retractor. The assistant's skill is most evident when the patient has the least amount of trauma or distress. The surgical assistant is **responsible for cutting the sutures** during and after the surgical procedure.

The operating room rules should be strictly adhered to in an effort to maintain aseptic conditions as they apply to the surgical suite and the patient. The surgical assistant plays a major role in the success or failure of the surgical procedure.

Upright Equine Surgical Positioning

Horses can stand even after being given anesthetic medication to bring them into a numb or sleeping state. The surgeon **may require that the animal remain on its feet** in an upright position for some surgical procedures. Typically, these procedures can involve teeth extractions such as the first premolar extractions involving an animal with problems grinding teeth. These molars are also known as wolf teeth. Other surgical procedures employ the **use of an epidural**, which produces a sedation effect on the animal by injecting anesthesia directly into the spine. The anesthesia allows the horse to lose its ability to sense pain in all or part of the body. The pain is a direct result of the surgical procedures performed on the animal. The horse will require anesthesia for the following operations: rectovaginal tears, perianal lacerations, Caslick's, removal of the ovaries or testicles, tendon splitting, and neurectomies. The animal should be monitored throughout the procedure and recuperative period.

Equine Dorsal Recumbency Surgical Positioning

The surgeon will require that the horse be laid on its back for surgical procedures that involve the abdominal area. Laying an animal on its back is referred to as the **position of dorsal recumbency**. Areas involving the abdomen may include surgical procedures of the following types: colic, exploratory, cesarean, laryngeal ventriculectomy, umbilical and inguinal hernia repair, bilateral cryptorchid castrations, and unilateral cryptorchid castrations. Arthroscopies require the use of an endoscope to inspect the joints. The surgeon will require that the horse be placed in a dorsal recumbent position for most arthroscopies, including the carpus arthroscopy. The carpus arthroscopy is an operation on the bone in the horse's front leg joint. Another type of arthroscopy involves the hock stifle. Neurectomies are surgical removals of a nerve. The horse placed in dorsal recumbency requires a thick, soft material to be placed underneath its shoulder and gluteal muscles. The horse that is not given enough cushioning may come down with myositis or muscle inflammation.

Preparing a Horse for Surgery

The horse has to be conditioned for surgery by following a series of steps. The horse should have its **coat neatly trimmed and vacuumed** to reduce the amount of contaminants. It should be noted that arthroscopic surgeries may require the surgical site to be shaved clean.

The staff member should wear a **hooded cap and a mask** to maintain a sterile environment before proceeding with additional preparations on the horse. The staff member will use a bacteriostatic agent on the operative site to reduce the amount of impurities. The most common bacteriostatic products include chlorhexidine or iodine-based soaps.

The staff member should **remove all the dirt by scrubbing the region for at least 7 minutes**. A brush may be used during the scrubbing process. The staff will follow up this scrub with an alcohol rub. This is known as a defatting process that will remove oil from the skin. Surgical procedures involving the eyes or testicles do not require the use of alcohol.

Equine Operations in Lateral Recumbency

The horse is **laid on its side** for some of the following procedures: eye surgery, tooth extractions, mandibular fracture repair, laryngotomy, laryngoplasty, periosteal strips, splint fracture removal, neurectomies that involve 2 or more branches, and condyle fracture repairs. The term **lateral recumbency** refers to this sidewise positioning. Some carpus arthroscopic surgeries, fetlock, and shoulder surgeries also incorporate this sidewise position. The horse should be checked to make sure that there is no pressure on the down elbow, as this could cause some damage to the horse. One way to improve the horse's circulation is by moving the down foreleg into a forward position. This also helps to protect against radial nerve paralysis. The horse's weight should be supported with pads and leg supports in an effort to safeguard the contralateral limbs. The horse's halter and face regions should be padded to prevent injury to the horse's facial nerves when the head drops. The horse's head requires additional padding to keep the facial nerve from paralysis while the horse is lying down. A halter should not be worn during the surgery.

Other Needs for Equine Surgical Procedures

The staff member will cautiously move the horse to the operating room, and will give the horse one more germicidal scrub in the operating room. The germicidal scrub employs the use of a solution known as **tincture of Salvon or iodine**. Attention to the sterilized environment present in the operating room is always on the mind of the veterinary technician.

In addition, the technician will assist the surgeon in the following tasks:

- assisting the veterinarian in putting on the surgical gown
- placing the drape or sterile towels over the horse
- troubleshooting any radiograph equipment that is not working properly
- assisting in monitoring the patient and radiograph.

The **radiograph** is an instrument used for x-rays on surgical procedures employed in the repair of fractures or broken bones.

The veterinary technician can have additional responsibilities involving the monitoring equipment.

Preparing a Horse for Eye Surgery

The staff member will need to follow certain steps to **prepare the eye** before **equine ocular surgery**. The horse's eyelashes must be trimmed off. The staff member must be cautious to avoid getting the lashes in the horse's eyes, as it can cause the horse to experience discomfort, soreness, and inflammation. It may also lead to injury of the eyeball or its surrounding tissue. The staff member **should not apply any standard bacteriostatic agent** to the eye region, as it is too caustic for this fragile area. However, the staff member may employ the use of a weak povidone-iodine and saline solution to the surrounding skin of the eye. If needed, saline can be poured over the eyeball to clear the eye of any hair or debris. In certain situations the staff member may need to sew the eyelids closed. This suturing is performed when the eye is to have a surgical procedure that is enucleate in nature. An enucleate procedure involves the removal of a tumor or other object with or without damage to the eyeball.

Presurgical Preparations for Equine Surgery

Horses must not eat or drink for a period of 12 hours prior to a surgical procedure. Blood tests should be completed prior to surgery, as well. The horse will be made ready for surgery by having any filth or dander removed from its coat. The horse will need to be unshod to prevent self-injury during the recovery period. The hooves will need to be thoroughly cleaned. The jugular vein is clipped and aseptically made ready. The jugular vein is the vein responsible for the flow of blood away from the head. The placement of the IV catheter is settled on by the horse's reclining position. The IV will be placed in a low position when throat operations necessitate it. The horse will be given the following: pre-operative antibiotics, a tetanus vaccine, and pain medication. This is followed by a mouth rinse before any anesthesia is given. The surgeon will instruct how to place the horse on the table. The surgeon will also indicate what regions need to be clipped and prepared after the horse has been given anesthesia. The horse's hooves will be covered in gloves or plastic to prevent any foreign substances from entering a sterile area.

Veterinary Technician Responsibilities During and After an Equine Surgical Procedure

The anesthetist may need the technician to provide **blood pressure readings throughout the surgery**. This can be critical when the horse has been given blood pressure–altering medication such as dobutamine, which can artificially raise the horse's blood pressure. The horse must also be monitored to ensure that the systolic blood pressure does not fall below 80 mm Hg.

The veterinary technician is also responsible for monitoring the horse during **postoperative recovery**. The horse should be safeguarded to prevent self-injury when anesthetics begin wearing off and the horse becomes more alert and aware of its immediate circumstances. The horse will more than likely need to come to its senses in the **same position in which it was sedated**. For instance, horses that were put to sleep in a standing position should wake in that same position. However, this is not true of horses that have been placed in a dorsal recumbent position or in a left lateral recumbent position.

Horses that have been sedated in either the **dorsal recumbent position** or the **left lateral recumbent position** will need to **wake up in a right lateral recumbent position**. The horse in the right lateral recumbent position will wake up on its right side. The horse will also need to be dressed in a recovery helmet to prevent injury. The horse will need to have a thick, soft material placed between the halter and the facial regions. The horse's legs will be restrained by being bound in a thick, soft material to prevent any damage to the leg areas. The endotracheal tube that has been passed through the windpipe area must be firmly fixed into place. The technician may need to ensure that the horse is positioned properly before removal of this tube. The normal procedure for an assisted recovery allows the removal of this tube after the horse shows that the throat is functioning properly. This is exhibited by the horse's ability to swallow. The normal procedure for an unassisted recovery allows the horse to remain standing while this tube is taken out.

General Postoperative Care for a Horse

The horse receiving **postoperative care** should be allowed to return to its own stall and stable, provided that the stall is warm and dry, and the setting is calming and quiet, as the horse should not be subjected to loud or distressing noises. The veterinarian will have suggested the best diet to be followed in accordance with the type of surgery that the animal received. The diet and feeding schedule recommended should be fully adhered to by the caregiver of the horse. The horse can experience a condition known as ileus following the administration of a general anesthetic. Ileus is the horse's inability to empty its intestines due to a blockage or peristaltic (smooth muscle) dysfunction (i.e., a bowel blockage). Thus, the horse should be checked to ensure that it is able to produce a bowel movement. The caregiver should take the vital signs of the horse twice a day throughout the horse's initial recuperation period.

Vital signs that are monitored in the horse involve the condition and **healthy functioning of the stomach and intestines**. A **soft diet** can be given to the horse after the animal has produced a bowel movement. Bran mash is an example of a soft food that can be given to the horse at this time. The horse should stay on a soft diet for a few hours, after which the animal can be allowed hay. The horse can later return to its regular feeding schedule. However, this is done by giving the horse gradually increasing amounts of routine feed throughout the day. The horse's consumption can be allowed to increase as long as the horse continues to exhibit normal bowel movements. In addition, the horse's vital signs should continue to be monitored. The veterinarian should be called in for a rectal examination if the animal is in distress. The distress may be a problem with a bowel that has become impacted with fecal material that the horse is unable to pass.

Postoperative Care for Arthroscopic Surgery and Fracture Repair

The animal recovering from arthroscopic surgery will need to have its **bandages checked periodically**. The wound should be **free from any pus or mucus**. Other signs of infection may appear in the form of heat, swelling, or pain. The animal requires a 5-minute walk with the attendant after a period of 24 hours has lapsed. Animals recovering from a surgical procedure involving the repair of a fracture or broken bone should also be monitored for signs of infection. The region beneath the cast should not have any visible signs of pus or mucus. Any infective discharge could also cause the **cast to become soft and unreliable**. Other signs of infection can be present in the form of peculiar smells or an abnormal swelling on the surface of the cast. If signs of infection persist, the cast may be exchanged for a sturdy bandage at this juncture. The bandage will allow dressings to be changed and the wound to be cleaned and monitored more frequently and readily. The bandage should be strong enough to hold the injured limb in position without breaking or giving way. The veterinarian will be able to determine the type of bandage needed based on the degree of complications associated with the fracture repair.

Treatment Procedure If a Horse Develops an Impacted Bowel Following Surgery

The horse that has been given a general anesthetic can experience complications involving the development of an **ileus**. Ileus is a condition that occurs when the animal is **unable to produce a bowel movement**. The bowels can be blocked from an obstruction in the intestines, usually hardened fecal matter that becomes compressed inside the horse's intestines. This may be sequelae from the surgical anesthesia, which may have transiently suppressed normal peristalsis in the bowel.

The veterinarian will begin to alleviate this problem by administering a **combination of mineral oil and warm water** into the stomach. This solution is given by way of a nasogastric tube passed from the horse's nose into its stomach. The horse may also require intravenous fluids. In addition, the horse may need to be walked by an attendant to try and stimulate the gastrointestinal tract. The veterinarian will want to carefully monitor the horse's vital signs. The vital signs — including pulse, body temperature, breathing, blood pressure, and bowel sounds from the gastrointestinal tract — must be taken 4 times a day until the horse is able to produce a bowel movement.

Bandaging

Basic Principles of Bandaging

The veterinarian should have clearly specified the proper procedures for cleaning and rinsing the surgical wound. The animal should be given a **sterile, dry bandage** (unless wet-to-dry dressings are ordered due to infection) in accordance with the veterinarian's advice for treating the wound. The dressing should be placed **flat against the wound in a smooth layer**. The bandage should not have any creases or rumpled layers to irritate the wound. The standard bandage will consist of the following 3 layers: a) a **primary layer of gauze** which comes into direct contact with the skin, b) a **secondary layer of a thick cotton material** or leg quilt that can soak up body fluids, and c) a **third layer of material at least 1 inch thick**. The last layer should be tightly wrapped, but not so tightly that it restricts the blood flow going into the limb. The third layer may be from a product known as Elastoplast or Vetrap. Importantly, if a bandage falls off the animal may experience a fall. If the bandage is too restricting the animal may suffer with a deformed arch in the connecting muscles attached to the bone. These connecting muscles and tissues include the tendons. Thus, it is important to properly position and fix the bandage in place.

Types of Bandages Used for Open and Closed Wounds

The type of bandage that a horse receives should be considered in connection with the type of injury that the horse has experienced. Bandages may be required to protect the horse's wound and/or to provide **additional bracing to a limb**. A **limb-supporting bandage** may be useful whenever the horse needs to be shipped to another location. In addition, this supporting bandage may help to alleviate problems associated with safeguarding the horse in case of falls during and after surgery. The supporting bandage may even be strong enough to allow a rider to be carried by the animal. The bandage may also be used to hold **medication against the wound site**. This may be especially important when the animal has an open wound. The medication is applied to the first layer that touches the skin of the animal. This first layer is referred to as the "**adherent dressing**." Caution should be taken when removing this layer from the wound, as there is a tendency to pull necrotic tissue off with the bandage.

Complications of Bandages Used for Open and Closed Wounds

Necrotic tissue consists of cells which have **died off due to injury or infection**. The planned **removal of necrotic tissue is called débriding** the wound, and is carefully undertaken with proper preparation. The accidental or unplanned stripping of necrotic tissue can inflame a wound, worsen an infection, and cause the animal unintended distress. The chances of unintentionally stripping a wound are decreased when a non-adherent dressing is applied. A non-adherent dressing is appropriate for use on closed surgical wounds (i.e., wounds that have been sutured or stapled closed).

A **closed surgical wound** is appropriate to be dressed with medicated gauze on the first layer. However, the application of non-medicated gauze may be used after the initial bandage has been removed. The subsequent bandages should only be non-medicated when the wound shows **no sign of infection**. Infection can be present in wounds that are warm to the touch or swollen. In addition, the wound may have pus or mucus oozing from it. The next layer is called the secondary layer. This layer consists of a thick, absorbent material that can cushion the limb. The application of a standard bandage can be employed to securely fix this padding into place. The third layer is determined by the type of wound and its location. Typically, some products used in this application include Elastoplast, Vetrap or a woven cotton material.

Applying a Bandage to a Horse's Leg

In applying a bandage to a horse's leg, the caretaker should **remove any filth or contaminants** from the injured leg. This cleansing is followed by a **thorough rinsing and drying** of the leg. Careful attention to these details can eliminate the risk of infection, skin irritation, and dermatitis. The horse's wound should be carefully attended to in adherence with the veterinarian's advice. The wound should be dressed with **clean gauze**. This dressing may be applied with an **antibiotic cream**, if directed by the veterinarian. However, this may not always be advisable.

This primary layer is followed by a secondary layer of **malleable, hygienic, cushioned material**. This layer is placed tightly enough to be secure, but not enough to reduce the adequate flow of blood to the limb. The secondary layer goes on just underneath the primary bandage. This padding should be at least one inch thick. The layer should not be creased nor have folds or crinkles that could irritate or abrade the wound. If the attendant places the bandage directly on a joint, then the likelihood that movement will loosen the bandage is high. Where such placement is necessary, particular caution should be taken to ensure that the bandage extends well above and below the joint, to better secure it in place.

Completing the Placement of a Bandage on the Horse's Leg

For a **lower-leg equine bandage**, the attendant should begin the bandage at a level that is higher than the fetlock joint on the interior of the cannon bone. The attendant should use a spiraling pattern beginning at the front towards the back of the limb. The bandage should be long enough to be wrapped down the leg and back up the leg. Each layer must be given a consistent pressure, and be applied in such a way as to cover an expanse of at least 50% of the underlying support bandage. These layers must be evenly positioned and smooth to the touch. The limb will need to be given a replacement bandage in this same manner every 1 to 2 days throughout the recovery period.

Careful attention to detail should alleviate any problematic issues from occurring during recuperation from the wound. If complications do occur, they tend to be circulatory problems, skin rashes, or inflammations.

Postoperative Bandages for the Carpus, Hock, and Foot

The **hock** is the horse's joint in its hind leg. The **carpus** is the bone in the horse's joint between the forelimb and its hoof. These 2 areas require the application of a bandage that incorporates a figure eight pattern in its design. Elastoplast is the material of choice for wounds located in these areas. The bandage should be positioned so that it adheres to the hair over the top and underneath the joint.

There is a **risk of pressure sores** with a bandage of this configuration. However, this risk can be lessened by excluding the accessory carpal bone and point of the hock from the bandage. Further, the bandage can also be given a small cut a little higher than the Achilles tendon. This cut will prevent the bandage from arching and putting additional stress on the tendon. Some caregivers also place additional padding on either side of the tendon to increase the contact surface area and reduce pressure on the tendon. This is important as skin and tendon erosions and necrosis can occur from an overtight bandage in this area. The bandage should be placed directly below the carpus or hock in an effort to keep it from moving down the joint. Careful attention should be given to keep the horse from finding this bandage too restrictive, and making undue efforts to remove it for greater freedom of movement.

In most cases, a **foot bandage** is needed to protect a puncture wound or an abscess. An abscess is a pus-filled pocket that can be the result of bacterial infection. The foot bandage is used to **hold antibiotic creams and other medications over the wound**. The foot bandage can also hold a poultice over the wound. A warm poultice can be any moist preparation that is used to ease the animal's pain, extract pus, or increase circulation. The most widely used bandage is called Animal Lintex. The patient should have a clean dressing applied at least once a day. The subsequent bandages should be applied after the wound has been inspected for infection. The poultice or the medication may need to stay on the horse through the night to provide the most benefit to the animal. The condition of the puncture wound or abscess will determine whether or not more medication or poultices are needed to continue treating the animal.

Casting

Preparing a Patient for the Placement of a Cast

There are a number of steps involved in **applying a cast** to a patient. Initially, gauze that is free from any infective organisms is positioned on the injury. This gauze can be pretreated with a medication. This gauze is covered with a wrap that is capable of soaking up any body fluids that are released from the injury. This wrap is held firmly in place with a conforming bandage. The leg must be covered with a clean, stretchy, knitted fabric that serves as a protective non-porous layer between the cast and the other bandages. This stocking extends down the limb to the toe or hoof area. The next application includes a Gigli wire for casts that need to stay on the horse for only a short period of time. Gigli wire is actually a flexible wire saw, named after its Italian surgeon inventor, Leonardo Gigli. It can be used to cut away the cast with a minimum of invasion. The Gigli wire saw is used in casts that are intended to be removed from a horse that remains on its feet. There is no need to lay a horse down for cast removals that have been created with the incorporation of a Gigli wire saw.

Types of Casts Used Postoperatively

The **full cast** is a padding-lined, rigid plaster or fiberglass-resin casing that holds the injured limb in place. The plaster should extend over the limb to the region beneath the elbow or stifle. The stifle is the upper hind leg of the horse, with the stifle joint comparable to the human knee. The full cast is described as a plaster that extends to the foot region. A **partial cast** is described as a plaster that encloses a part of the leg. However, a partial cast does not include the foot region. Partial plasters or partial casts are also known as sleeve or tube casts. Casts that are only applied to the foot are known as short casts or foot casts. These types of casts are initiated under the fetlock joint and enclose the length of the foot. The fetlock is the lower part of the horse that is located slightly above and in back of the horse's hoof. The cast should stabilize a break, protect the healing process, and ensure that the horse's broken bone will heal correctly, in the proper position.

Application of Rigid Casting Material and Monitoring After Casting

The stocking is covered with a Vetcast plaster roll (actually, it is usually a polyurethane resin–impregnated fiberglass roll, rather than traditional plaster). This roll must be submersed in a warm water solution to prepare it for application to the limb. The application of the roll should be done in alternating vertical and horizontal directions, as this will increase the resiliency of the cast. However, casts that will remain on the animal for an extended period of time should also be padding-wrapped at the top of the cast. This extra wrap will reduce friction caused by movement and rubbing. A cast-cutting saw or cast spreaders are employed to remove the cast from the limb. Horses that have been casted should be monitored on a daily basis. The horse may exhibit intolerance in wearing the cast. A horse having problems adapting to the cast may require extra support and attention by the attendant.

Digit Amputation for Cattle

Digit amputation is a procedure used to remove an **infected claw** from a cow's lower leg. The veterinarian will require that the cow be placed in a lateral recumbent position for this surgical procedure. The cow will be laid on its side with the infected claw facing in and right side up. The claw and the mid-metacarpus to the hoof will need to be thoroughly shaved and sterilized. This is crucial, as this claw comes into contact with manure and other substances which can lead to infection. The animal will receive an anesthesia to reduce the pain. This is given to the animal by way of a ring block or intravenous local. The cow will require a tourniquet applied distal to the carpus or hock to stop excessive bleeding. The tourniquet consists of a rubber tube. The veterinarian will use obstetrical or Gigli wire to sever the claw from the animal. The cow will need to have its bandage changed on a regular basis to prevent infection. The cow that is healing properly will not need the bandage if a 2 to 3 week period has passed without complications.

Preparing for a Laparotomy

The surgeon will perform a **laparotomy** on an animal that requires further **internal inspection of the abdomen**. Typically, this is exploratory surgery performed when significant diagnostic concerns warrant it. The surgeon will be better able to diagnose and treat the animal after further inspection has been made. It is common for this procedure to be performed on cattle. The cow can remain on its feet during the procedure, safely contained in a narrow passageway known as a chute. Otherwise, the cow may be placed in stocks intended to house livestock. The cow will be given a local anesthetic to reduce any pain. The paralumbar fossa is shaved and cleaned thoroughly. It is critical to maintain a sterile field at the surgical incision site. Therefore, the cow's tail is secured to its hind leg. The tail binding can be made from rope or the animal's halter, but under no circumstances should the cow's tail be fixed to any immobile object. Fastening the tail to an immobile object can cause the tail to be pulled loose from the animal. The surgeon will remove the laparotomy sutures in 2 or 3 weeks, after the incision site has had a chance to heal.

Teat Laceration Repair in Cattle and Goats

Female cattle and goats can experience **trauma to a teat**, leaving them unable to fully release milk from the udder and limiting the nourishment they are able to provide their offspring. This trauma can be caused by a cow or another animal accidentally **stepping on the animal's teat**. Animals kept in booths inside a barn are often exposed to this type of accident. The tip of the teat is the area most likely to be injured. It is not as common for the animal to experience trauma to the total teat region. The healing of this injury can be slow and difficult because it is supple tissue that is in perpetual motion throughout the animal's daily activities. Surgical intervention is required when an animal sustains a teat laceration or tear. The cow or goat can be operated on in a variety of positions. The most common are those where the animal is placed on its back or allowed to remain standing, depending on the animal's size, health, temperament, and the extent of the injury, etc.

The placement of the animal on its back is referred to as the **dorsal recumbent position**. The cow or goat undergoing surgical repair will need to be sedated, typically with the application of a ring block. The animal will need to be washed and sterilized to prepare the surgical site. The animal can have a tourniquet applied to the region. The tourniquet is needed to stop any unnecessary bleeding or milk seepage. Rubber tubing is the typical material used as a tourniquet. The teat of the animal may also need to be fitted with a prosthetic device (i.e., a drain). This device will allow the injured teat to release its contents without any milking action taken. Hand-milking the animal postoperatively is not recommended, as it can disrupt the sutures. The animal can return to its milking schedule in about 2 weeks, or as recommended by the veterinarian. This will usually occur shortly after removal of the sutures.

Preparing Cattle for Eye Enucleation

The **animal's eyeball** is described as the round mass that is located within the bony eye socket. The surgeon will often **extract the entire eyeball**. This will allow the surgeon to remove any diseased tissue or tumor from the eye's region. The animal may require the application of an antibiotic following the surgery. The antibiotic is given to reduce the risk of infection. In addition, the animal may need a wound spray to be applied to the incision site following the eye surgery. Eye tumors, called ophthalmic neoplasms, are a major concern for cattle owners. Cattle are noted for their propensity to develop malignant tumors arising from ocular squamous cells. The animal with this condition can be unfit for consumption. This can lead to a loss of income for those who raise animals for slaughter. This condition may also shorten the animal's life span considerably.

Performing Eye Enucleation for Cattle

Enucleation surgery refers to taking out all or part of the eye while the eye muscles and related surrounding components remain intact. The animal in need of enucleation surgery should be placed in its halter in such a way as to firmly fix the head to the side of the chute or stall. The head should not be able to move during the eye surgery. The animal's eyes should be closed fast with needle and thread. The animal's hair must be shaved and the animal should be prepared for surgery using proper sterilization procedures. It can be difficult to cleanse the area thoroughly around the tissue that is diseased, but it is necessary to be thorough to reduce contaminants on the animal. The cow or goat should be given a Peterson eye block or a four-point retrobulbar block prior to the operation. These are 2 types of anesthesia that can be applied as a local anesthetic to the eye region.

Castrations on Cattle and Small Ruminants

In **castration**, the scrotum is incised, the testicles removed, and the spermatic cord and testicle-supplying blood vessels are crushed and thereby closed. Cattle are normally castrated when they reach one to 4 weeks of age. Cattle that have this procedure done at a young age suffer less, due to the diminished size of the testicles at this early developmental juncture. It is recommended that the calf be fully vaccinated before scheduling the castration. The vaccinations will be beneficial in preventing clostridial infections like botulism, tetanus, or gas gangrene. Typically, the calf does not receive any pain-numbing medications as this is considered to be expensive and unnecessary. The same reasoning is applied to the absence of a sterile field before the surgical procedure. The veterinarian can perform either an open castration procedure or a closed castration procedure — sometimes referring to the presence or absence of scrotal incisions and/or suturing following the procedure.

Castration procedures are either "**open**" or "**closed**." The calf that has an open castration will receive a surgical incision through the scrotum. An emasculator device is then applied to cut away and crush the spermatic cord (which includes the vas deferens that carries the animal's semen). The surgical site is left open to drain without any suturing. Open castrations are quicker and less expensive, and can usually be done on the farm. In some situations "open" castration refers to incising (i.e., opening) the tunica vaginalis covering the testicle when removing it. The calf receiving a closed castration will have the scrotum cut for testicle removal and then "closed" with sutures. Alternately, it may refer to the testicles being removed with the tunica vaginalis still intact, followed by suture closure. Or, it may refer to an emasulatome device crushing the spermatic cord in a bloodless procedure that causes the testicles to atrophy and wither away. Other non-surgical methods can be applied. For example, an elastrator is a device that places a strong rubber band around the testicles, depriving the area of blood. This method is efficient in removing the testicles, but not recommended for older animals. Small ruminants (hoofed mammals that chew cud) can be castrated using the elastrator. This is normally performed on wool-producing lambs at 1 to 2 weeks of age. It is rare for a lamb to receive an open or closed castration. The tail is also docked (shortened) at this time.

In an **open castration**, the emasculator is applied to crush and cut away the cord which carries the semen. The lamb receiving a bloodless form of closed castration need not be cut at the scrotum. The Burdizzo emasculatome is applied in such a way as to only crush the cord carrying the semen, causing the testicles to atrophy and wither away without surgical intervention or loss of blood. This is similar to the emasculatome procedure performed on a calf during closed castration. However, most lambs headed for meat markets are not subjected to a castration. These animals are slaughtered before reaching sexual maturity. Even so, the lambs will still need to have their tails docked or shortened. Kids are young goats, typically castrated when 1 to 3 weeks old. It is recommended that lambs and kids be given vaccinations before scheduling the castration. The vaccinations will be beneficial in preventing clostridial infections like botulism, tetanus, or gas gangrene. Small ruminant animals will also receive an injection of Vitamin E and selenium at this juncture.

Castration on Pigs

Pigs require an injection of iron dextran prior to the castration procedure. This injection is beneficial for a number of reasons. Primarily, it will keep the animal from becoming anemic. The pig's tail must also be docked at this stage.

This species of animal does have a propensity to cannibalize. Thus, the pig's milk or needle teeth are cut back, as these teeth can hurt the sow or the mother pig if left unchecked. The young male pig should be checked for an inguinal hernia during the castration process. This appears as a bulge that abnormally sticks out through the wall of the scrotum.

The immature pig can be hung up by its forelegs and shaken lightly during the detection process. Detection is made easier in this position, as even the smallest of hernias will expand outwardly with a significant-sized bulge. The inguinal hernia can be repaired following a cleansing with antiseptic. The recovering animal should be housed in a small enclosure that is well maintained and kept clean.

DEHORNING CALVES

Cattle must have their **horns removed** to keep them from **harming themselves and others**. The process of dehorning an animal at a young age is known as **disbudding**. Calves that are disbud range in age from 1 to 2 weeks old. The process is accomplished using an appliance known as an electric dehorner. It is not recommended to use caustic pastes, as this could burn the animal. A gouge-type dehorner can be employed when the horn buds are 1 to 2 cm long. The Barnes instrument is classified as a gouge-type dehorner. Horns that have been allowed to reach a more mature length will need to be removed with a Keystone dehorner or a saw. Typically, the tools employed for this purpose include a hardback saw or wire saw. The animal should be given a cranial nerve block or ring block for local analgesia. As horn removal is painful, adequate anesthetic is essential.

DEHORNING GOATS

Dehorning can be a painful experience for the animal. Therefore, **pain management** is critical. In addition, the animal should be prevented from hemorrhaging or bleeding excessively from a ruptured blood vessel. The animal will need to have a bandage placed over the dehorned wound to safeguard the animal from infections and irritants brought about by insects.

Goats can be dehorned as soon as the horn bud makes itself visible. The dehorning process should be performed with the use of an appliance known as an electric dehorner. Goats have a low threshold for pain. Therefore, analgesic pain management is critical to the success of this procedure.

The goat is susceptible to shock. Physiological symptoms of shock, combined with heightened fear and anxiety, can lead to the animal's untimely death.

The horn removal appliance should not be allowed to reach an excessive degree of heat, as this can lead to cerebral burns. The goat can be significantly harmed when brain tissue near the surface is damaged by the hot iron.

PREPARING A PATIENT'S PREANESTHETIC DRUG PROTOCOL FOR AN EMERGENCY C-SECTION

Careful assessment of **preanesthetic drugs** to be used for a C-section (hysterotomy) is important in that they should not be able to cross the placental barrier and should be short-acting and metabolized rapidly. Certain drugs that DO cross the placental barrier that affect the puppies' survival and should not be used include ketamine, barbiturates, and atropine. Anesthetic protocol should include drugs that aren't metabolized by the liver or excreted by the kidneys because these organs are deficient in the puppies as well. The patient should be preoxygenated prior to surgery, and the procedure should be done as efficiently as possible to move on to resuscitation of the puppies.

PERFORMING A SURGICAL SCRUB ON A PATIENT AND WHAT SUPPLIES ARE NEEDED

To perform a **surgical scrub,** the surgical area needs to be shaved over where the incision will be made and approximately 4 inches around the incision using a 40 blade. After the area is shaved, use a small vacuum to get the excess hair off of the surgical site. Then take a gauze square and pour chlorhexidine scrub onto the gauze and clean the area to get rid of any dirt and debris on the skin.

Next, take a gauze square, pour chlorhexidine solution on it, and make a firm swipe counterclockwise around and down over where the incision will be. You do not want to go back and forth over the incision with the solution because you should be wiping the bacteria AWAY. Go back and forth between the chlorhexidine scrub and solution, making one swipe around and down, then toss. End with the chlorhexidine solution, and then you will spray Betadine over the surgical site, which is an antiseptic microbicide.

Choosing the Correct Size Endotracheal Tube (ET) for a Patient

The **endotracheal tube** (ET) allows oxygen/gas anesthetic or just oxygen to pass to and from the lungs via the trachea of the patient. The technician can palpate (feel) the patient's trachea to determine which size may fit best, or another method would be to measure between the patient's nares and compare to the bevel end of the ET tube. If it fits between the nares, then that is a good indication it will fit in the trachea. For each patient going under anesthesia, three ET tubes should be picked out: the one that the veterinary technician believes will fit the best, one a size smaller, and one a size bigger. This way, if the ET tube thought to be the best fit doesn't fit, another one is close by. Brachycephalic breeds can have deceiving tracheas compared to their face size and shape, and usually their tracheas are smaller. Intubating with the correct size ET tube is crucial because if it is too small, the patient may breathe around the tube and not stay adequately anesthetized. The largest ET tube that can be placed without causing trauma to the tissues is ideal.

Prepare a Patient for a C-Section

A **C-section** is a surgical procedure done to remove puppies from the mother's uterus. A hysterotomy is often done in the event of an emergency such as the dog had previous dystocia or is likely to have dystocia. Premedications for the mother will lower her stress, and premedications that can be reversed are preferred. Often, the patient having a C-section will be dehydrated, so any animal going under anesthesia for this procedure should be administered IV fluids. Dogs presenting in late pregnancy are prone to hypoxemia, so preoxygenation is required five minutes prior to induction and during induction because induction agents commonly cause apnea. The patient will be dorsal, and the abdomen will be surgically shaved, cleaned of any hair, and surgically scrubbed. The veterinarian will remove the puppies from the uterus, clamp and cut the umbilical cords, and hand the puppies to the technician to resuscitate.

Cleaning Instruments and Maintaining Cleanliness

Microbial Control

Degrees of Microbial Control

Microscopic organisms are responsible for the **transmission of diseases** in animals and people. Pathogens are described as the bacteria or viruses that people come into contact with prior to contracting a disease. These organisms are not visible to the naked eye, but can be viewed only with a microscope. Much study has been done on the eradication of infectious disease. Infectious diseases can be substantially reduced when the proper hygiene and sterilization techniques are applied. Sterilization techniques involve microbial management sufficient to eradicate the life form. The absence of any infectious organism and its contaminants represents a state known as asepsis. The sterilization process involves a complete and thorough disinfection method that employs chemicals to eradicate the microbes. These chemicals have a microbicidal component. In addition, bacteriostatic chemicals are often used to prevent further microbes from developing.

Steps Taken to Promote

It should be noted that antibiotics kill pathogens within the body, while **antiseptics** kill pathogens on living tissues. Further, **disinfectants** kill pathogens on inanimate objects. Disinfectants may be classified in accordance with their primary functions. The term **bactericide** is indicative of a solution that is able to eradicate (kill) bacteria. Additional classification as a sporicide indicates a solution that is able to eliminate bacterial spores.

A **virucide** is able to eliminate viruses. A **fungicide** is able to eliminate fungi. However, it should be noted that some pathogens may not respond to the chemical solutions specifically intended to eradicate them. Many pathogens have developed the ability to resist certain control methods. The pathogens that have developed the strongest resistance to microbial control are the protozoan cysts or oocysts, which are single-celled organisms. Some bacterial spores are also able to resist microbial control methods by staying in dormancy until the environment is again hospitable. Other resistant pathogens include certain viruses, TB organisms, various fungi, and vegetative bacteria.

Dry Heat Method

Some **physical antimicrobial control methods** include: desiccation (dehydration), filtration, freezing, moist heat (boiling, autoclaving, etc.), dry heat (incineration), ionizing radiation, and radioactive radiation. Dry heat oxidizes (burns) organic compounds. This sterilization method can be achieved with fire or a hot air oven.

It is usually not enough to dry contaminated surfaces, as the drying process may simply reduce humidity levels and some organisms may continue to thrive and develop rapidly.

A hot blaze can incinerate any microbe that exists on the surface of an object. In addition, infected tissues and carcasses can be reduced to cinders from the process of incineration.

The **hot oven sterilization method** requires the oven's temperature to be set at 170 °C or 340 °F for a period of one hour. The hot oven method is most useful for substances that are in a dry or powdered form, or petroleum-based substances such as paraffin and Vaseline products. Many animal care facilities are known to use dry heat as part of their process for microbial management.

Factors That Affect Efficacy

Most microbial management techniques only produce the desired results for **short durations of time**, and then only under proper conditions. Many control methods are **more effective in situations where the temperature is raised.** The correct concentration of the microbial product must always be utilized to produce the desired results. Disinfectants can lose their strength when mixed with other solutions. Therefore, dilution is not recommended as an effective microbial control strategy. Rather, the disinfectant that is most effective on the organism should be used full strength. In addition, the stage of development of the organism should be noted before the application of an antimicrobial agent to ensure selection of the proper product. The disinfectant must also be applied in quantities large enough to eradicate the organisms present. However, some chemicals may harm certain surfaces or cause harmful chemical reactions to occur on certain surface materials. The reaction may also weaken or render the chemical useless. Thus, the chemical should be applied to surfaces and in situations and settings according to established procedures, to ensure that the desired results are achieved. Some procedures allow for the administration of the chemical by spray, swabs, or immersion. The chemical should also be stored according to the instructions on the package. This will allow the chemical to retain its potency.

Use of Pressurized Steam and an Autoclave

Boiling requires a **3-hour period to fully destroy microorganisms that can cause infection**. The first 10 minutes of the boiling method should eradicate the vegetative bacteria and viruses. However, additional time is needed to eradicate the more resistant bacterial spores. A 2% calcium carbonate or sodium solution can improve the sterilization efficacy. This supplement will also reduce rust.

Another method that destroys pathogenic microorganisms is steam. Steam is reached at the same temperatures that are needed to bring a liquid to a boil. Therefore, steam can be used for sterilization. However, a longer period of time is required to achieve the same effect. **Steam requires a 90-minute period to fully eradicate vegetative bacteria.** However, steam alone is not an effective measure for eradicating bacterial spores from the surface of an object being sanitized. The best and most reliable method of moist heat sterilization is accomplished with vaporized water that is applied under pressure or force. The **autoclave** is a steel vessel that applies steam and pressure to sterilize the equipment used in most veterinary facilities.

Efficacy of Moist Heat (Boiling and Steam)

Damp heat can be used to manage microbial growth and development. A **microbial protein** is released during this process which causes the **organism's biological properties to be reduced or lost**. This process is known as **denaturing**. However, the application of heat and steam vapors is not adequate for a complete sterilization process. The water should be brought to a boiling temperature. In addition, the steam must be trapped inside with a heavy lid covering the boiling water. The weight of the lid gives the steam enough atmospheric pressure to complete the sterilization process needed for successful microbial control. The application of hot water can also be employed to the cleansing and decontamination of superficial external surfaces. This sanitization process is made more effective when hot water and detergents are combined. The detergent causes grease and dirt to disperse within the cleaning solution. This makes clean up much more efficient.

Sterilization

Gamma Radiation and Fluid Filtration

Gamma radiation sterilization is used in the manufacturing of products sold by pharmacies. Gamma radiation is also used in the making of **disposable plastics and some biological goods**. The process is able to produce ionization that disrupts the stability of pathogens on the molecular level, altering the tissue and the DNA during the sterilization process. The result is the death of any exposed organism.

The penetrating effect of gamma radiation should be centralized to prevent any contact with tissues that are not meant to be disrupted by the discharge.

Fluid filtration employs a filter which works to prevent the passage of organisms. The organisms are thus **trapped inside the filtering material**. The filter can apply a positive or negative pressure to allow the fluids to gain access. Bacteria can be trapped inside a filter with a pore size of 0.45 micrometers. Microplasms and viruses can be trapped inside a filter with a pore size of 0.01 to 0.1 micrometers. Larger pathogens will need a filter with pore filters that are smaller in size. A prefilter can be employed to improve the effects of the sterilization process.

Radiation

Radiation is a sterilization method. This method employs an energy wave or ray that is able to disrupt cell enzyme systems and DNA. There are 2 types of radiation applied in the sterilization process.

The first method uses **ultraviolet or UV rays**. This method is only effective for sterilizing objects that are in **close vicinity and fully exposed** to the UV rays. UV rays should be used on surfaces that do not have multiple layers needing to be made germ free. Although the UV ray has a low energy capacity, some transparent surfaces can be treated with UV radiation. However, not all transparent surfaces can be penetrated by UV rays. Eyes should be protected when UV radiation is used, as the eyes are sensitive to its effects.

The second method uses gamma radiation. Gamma radiation is produced by an electromagnetic supply source that generates a cobalt 60 wavelength. Gamma radiation is a very effective sterilizing method, as it can pass through multiple layers of solid or fluid matter.

Chemical Disinfectants

The most effective **chemical sterilization methods** require the use of a variety of chemicals applied as **disinfectants**. Many types of chemicals can be employed to **eradicate and disrupt the cell growth of harmful pathogens**. The chemical reactions on each involved surface and pathogen should be thoroughly understood by the person using the disinfectant. The classification of disinfectants includes low, medium, and high rankings. Chemical compounds given the highest rank are used to eradicate a wide range of organisms. High-ranking disinfectants can kill viruses that have an affinity for either lipids (fats) or fluids (water). In addition, these high-ranking disinfectants are able to eradicate bacterial spores, which can otherwise merely remain dormant on exposed surfaces.

Those disinfectants which receive a medium rank can eradicate the bacterial strain which causes tuberculosis. Disinfectants that receive a low rank can eradicate harmful vegetative bacteria.

The selection of a disinfectant should involve consideration of surface materials. The surface should not be harmed when the disinfectant is applied, nor should adverse chemical reactions occur upon contact. Finally, low-ranking disinfectants should not be overtly toxic to humans or animals. Nor should they be a fire hazard.

Air Filtration

Antimicrobial air filters allow air to pass through but omit harmful microorganisms. Animal care facilities employ this form of sterilization in many ways, including through the use of surgical masks, laboratory animal cage tops, and air duct filters. The most effective filtration screens incorporate a very dense filter that has been manufactured from a variety of products and fibers.

The 3 components that impact the effectiveness of an air filter include: air velocity, relative humidity and electrostatic charge. Any fragment that is larger than 0.3 micrometers will be trapped in a "high efficiency particle absorption" (HEPA) filter. HEPA filters function at an efficiency rate of 99.97 to 99.997%. The masks used in surgical procedures prevent the patient from becoming contaminated by the person wearing the mask. If it is necessary to prevent an infection from being transmitted to the person wearing a mask, then a mask specifically designed for that purpose should be worn. These masks are not interchangeable, and should not be expected to function in the same way. Both types of masks should be replaced after a few hours use with a clean, dry, well-fitting mask.

Advantages and Disadvantages of Using an Autoclave

An **autoclave is a sterilization device.** It is a steel container that uses pressurized steam as an inexpensive, effective sterilization agent. The machine is easy to operate. The autoclave has a dependable record in providing safe, complete sterilization. In addition, existing operation standards help ensure a high level of quality control beneficial to both the veterinarian and the patient.

Objects commonly sterilized in an autoclave include **surgical instruments and equipment, drapes and gowns, suture materials, sponges, and selected plastics and rubber**. However, not all materials can be sterilized with an autoclave. Some plastics can melt in the high, damp heat. The staff should be trained and kept up to date on the use of the autoclave, as this will reduce the risk of improperly sterilized objects being presented to the patient.

Disinfectants

Quaternary Ammonium Compounds

Quaternary ammonium compounds are also referred to as **quats**. Quats include nitrogen compounds that have 4 alkyl radicals linked to a principal nitrogen atom. Quats have 1 acidic radical. Some other names for quats include Cetrimide, benzalkonium chloride, Zephiran, Quatsyl-D, and Germiphene.

Quats function to **disinfect surfaces and objects contaminated with both gram-positive and gram-negative organisms**. In addition, quats can be used to disinfect surfaces and objects contaminated with enveloped viruses. However, individuals applying these disinfectants should wear gloves and avoid contact with the skin, as these compounds can produce ill effects. They can also harm the lining of internal organs within the body. However, quats can be used safely. Quats do not usually cause irritation when safety measures are used and they rank low on the toxic scales. It should be noted that some organic compounds and hard water salts can deactivate or reduce the effectiveness of quats. Conversely, quats can be strengthened by increasing the pH level. Surface areas should be rinsed thoroughly before the application of a quats solution. This should allow the quats to work on the surface without the interference of other compounds.

Soaps and Detergents

Soap can be made from potassium or sodium hydroxide mixed with natural oils. This anionic cleansing agent is a subs**tance that is able to reduce the surface tension found in liquids such as water.** However, soap is not effective in a highly mineralized liquid, such as that commonly referred to as "hard" water. Soap mixed with quaternary ammonium compounds loses its effectiveness. In addition, soap can reduce the strength of a halogen element like chlorine or iodine. Lacking true bacteriocidal properties, soaps should not be employed as antimicrobials or disinfectants.

Detergents are synthetically produced soaps. Detergents are classified as anionic, cationic, or nonionic. The blending of anionic and cationic detergents will counteract each other and produce an unproductive combination. Anionic and nonionic detergents function to cleanse a surface. However, the cationic detergents are the best for providing a more sterile cleanse. Detergents can be improved upon by the addition of wetting agents (surfactants), along with substances to alter the pH levels, enzymes, and non-surfactant materials. The detergent may also be supplemented with chemicals that will either eliminate or enhance the detergent's ability to produce foam or bubbles.

Glutaraldehyde and Formaldehyde

Aldehyde-containing substances can be **bactericidal**. Aldehydes consist of substantially reactive organic compounds which work against both gram-positive and gram-negative bacteria. Aldehydes are also effective against nearly all acid-fast bacteria, bacterial spores, fungi, and a good number of viruses. **Aldehydes** include glutaraldehyde or Cidex, formaldehyde or Formicide, biguanide, and chlorhexidine gluconates such as Hibitane and Precede. The compound glutaraldehyde is not aggressively caustic, but can still damage the skin and respiratory system. A more caustic form can be produced by adding sodium bicarbonate to the commercially available acidic product. This product allows a cold sterilization process to take place. In addition, this product can be applied to surfaces like plastics, rubber, and lenses. However, this product can be inactivated by blending it with organic substances or hard water. Formaldehyde releases a colorless gas. However, there is a 37% to 40% aqueous product that is mixed with water or alcohol. The colorless gas is released from the surface that has been disinfected. Therefore, safety equipment must be worn to reduce toxic contact to the respiratory system and tissues.

Phenolics

Phenol is perhaps the **earliest disinfectant/antiseptic** known, having been used by Joseph Lister when it was called carbolic acid. Phenolics include carbolic acid, coal tar phenols, and cresol. Phenolics have an active ingredient which is able to disrupt gram-positive bacteria and enveloped viruses. Synthetic phenolics are blended with soaps that are not poisonous or bothersome to the body.

Quaternary ammonium compounds can reduce the active ingredient found in the phenolics. However, phenolics will not be deactivated by organic compounds like soap or hard water. The person applying phenol should wear gloves and protective clothing to avoid prolonged contact. Phenolics have been known to produce skin lesions. Cats do not have the necessary enzymes to rid themselves of these toxins. Cats, rabbits, and rodents can suffer harmful effects from this toxin. The mucous membranes are susceptible to burns from exposure to phenolics. Severe ulcerations can result from accidental contact with the eyes. In addition, swallowing this chemical can result in respiratory distress, including hyperventilation. This is due to the toxic effect on the brain that occurs from consumption. Toxicity can result from dosages a low as 0.22 g/lb in dogs. Cats require even less of a dose to produce disastrous results.

Tinctures, Iodophors, and Chlorine

Tinctures are created when **iodines are mixed with alcohol (ethanol)**. **Iodophors** are made when **iodines are mixed with detergents**. It is not expected that iodophors or tinctures will produce a stain or irritate the skin. However, water-based forms of iodine (certain iodophors) are known to be caustic enough to produce stains and irritate the skin. These products can also be corrosive on metallic surfaces.

Chlorine or bleach is found in many homes. The product sold commercially is known as sodium hypochlorite. This is a common and inexpensive disinfectant. However, chlorine mixed with organic substances can be rendered inactive. Chlorine can be corrosive on skin, mucous membranes, metallic surfaces, and clothing materials. Bleach can be harmful when mixed with many unspecified substances. Therefore, caution must be used in its application.

Biguanide, Halogens, and Iodines

Biguanide is an aldehyde-based antiseptic employed as a **surgical scrub or in washing the hands.** This solution has disinfectant/antiseptic properties that can be reduced when mixed with organic substances or hard water. A saline solution will render the disinfectant useless. Biguanide is not a high toxic risk.

Halogens are produced by an electronegative chemical element. The 5 types of halogens include fluorine, chlorine, iodine, bromine, or astatine. Halogens are effective against gram-positive and gram-negative bacteria, as well as acid-fast bacteria, viruses, and fungi.

Iodine and chlorine are widely used to **disinfect surfaces**. Iodine is universally employed in blended solutions made from water or alcohol. Iodophors are disinfectant solutions. An iodophor can be dissolved in another substance to increase its wetting properties (i.e., to make the liquid spread out more readily across a surface). This not only extends the topical product's shelf-life, but also makes the product milder on the skin.

Iodophors are slow to release iodine. A widely used version is known as Betadine. This is commonly used in medical facilities as a scrub prior to a surgical procedure. Betadine is produced with a detergent blended with iodophor.

Peroxygen Compounds

Peroxygen compounds have a strong tendency to cause a chemical reaction with oxygen. However, this oxidization process is also reactive with anaerobic bacteria. Oxidization is completed with the release of oxygen. Two types of peroxygen are called peracetic acid and peroxide. Peroxide is widely sold in stores as hydrogen peroxide in concentrations of 3% and 6%. The manufacturer uses a brown container to reduce the rate at which the product breaks down or decomposes. Peracetic acid is also available for purchase in many stores. This product is sold in its liquid form. It should be emphasized that these products are not effective against viruses. Peroxygen compounds are only effective against gram-positive and gram-negative bacteria, acid-fast bacteria, and fungi. They cannot eradicate pinworm eggs. Peroxygen compounds are most effective for time periods under 30 minutes. The humidity levels in the application area should be at 80%. The concentration levels should be at least 2%. Peroxygen compounds should not be applied to steel, iron, or rubber, as these surfaces may react to create an explosion. Peroxide can be blended safely with a low concentration of bleach. Gloves should be worn to protect the skin.

Alcohols

Alcohols used as disinfectants include ethyl alcohol, isopropyl alcohol, ethanol, and methyl alcohol. Alcohols are effective as a disinfectant against **gram-positive and gram-negative bacteria and enveloped viruses.**

Alcohols can be the solvent base for a variety of antiseptics and disinfectants. Alcohols are inexpensive and do not have a high risk of toxicity. Alcohol is widely used as a **topical antiseptic**. The recommended concentration of isopropyl alcohol is 60% to 70%. The recommended concentration of ethyl alcohol is 70% to 80%. They are generally produced in a 70% solution, as water is also needed to denature the bacterial proteins sufficient for the bacteria to die.

Alcohol will produce a burning sensation if placed on open wounds or irritated skin. Alcohol also has a tendency to dry the skin. A clotted or coagulated mass can form when alcohols are used in areas where the wound has a fluid discharge. This can also present a risk of leaving bacteria alive under the coagulum or clotted mass. Alcohol can cause a vapor-like fog to form on the outside of lenses. Alcohol will cause some plastics to become hard and unyielding. Some cement will soften under the application of alcohol. Finally, the blending of some organic substances can render alcohol ineffective.

Ethylene Oxide

Ethylene oxide is used as a disinfectant in the fight against gram-positive and gram-negative bacteria, lipophilic and hydrophilic viruses, fungi, and bacterial spores. **Ethylene oxide** is abbreviated as EO. EO can be applied to surfaces that cannot be heated. EO has no color and very little odor is given off during its application. However, this substance can be dispersed quickly. It is also a fire hazard that can result in an explosion under certain conditions. EO is kept at a temperature of 70 °F to 140 °F. Application humidity levels should range from 30–40%. Higher levels of humidity produce the best result. This product can be applied in a vacuum type compartment. Ethylene oxide should be blended with CO_2, ether, or Freon. This product should produce optimum results within 1-18 hours of its use. Always dry the sterilized objects, and circulate the surrounding air for a period of 24-48 hours to dissipate any EO residue. This reduces the likelihood of contamination, as there are carcinogenic and other toxins present in EO residues. Finally, the sterilized objects should be covered in a muslin, polyethylene, polypropylene or polyvinyl wrapper.

Autoclaves

All autoclaves utilize a **pressurized steam system** to **eradicate harmful organisms** from the surfaces of objects. Gravity displacement autoclaves (type "N") allow gravity to exchange the air in the sterilization chamber for steam (air is heavier than water vapor and is displaced through a port in the bottom as steam enters the top). Some autoclaves use positive pressure, venting steam into the chamber only after it has been pressurized in a separate chamber sufficient to blow all existing air out. Some use negative pressure (type "S"), provided by a vacuum pump that removes the air — achieving among the highest sterility assurance levels (SAL).

The steam is able to **penetrate multiple layers of material** placed within the confines of the steel vessel. The increased pressure inside the vessels keeps the heated water at the boiling point. The boiled water releases vapor (steam). The usual time required for sterilization is 9-15 minutes. The temperatures should be at 121 °C or 250 °F to properly accomplish full sterilization. The pressure can be decreased to that at sea level to bring the temperature of the steam down to 100 °C or 212 °F. Additional pressure of 15 pounds per square inch (psi) will produce steam at 121 °C or 250 °F. Some autoclaves can be set at 35 psi to reach a steam temperature of

135 °C or 275 °F. The objects should be placed in the autoclave for the recommended amount of time to allow the steam to penetrate all surfaces.

Gravity Displacement Autoclaves

Gravity displacement autoclaves function to gradually displace and replace the air inside the sterilization vessel using gravity as the motivator. In these devices, the water is brought to a boil with electricity. This produces steam and pressure inside the vessel. The steam then intensifies and the pressure builds. The temperature is raised further with still more steam from the boiling water. At this point, the gravitationally lighter water vapor will begin to displace the air inside the autoclave by way of an underside vent. The vent closes when the exiting air is at the proper sterilization temperature. The interior of the autoclave will ultimately reach a temperature of 121 °C or 250 °F. At that point, the sterilization will begin to be timed for the requisite exposure period.

Following the recommended time for sterilization of the contents, the heated water vapor will be released through a small narrow opening into a reservoir. The steam inside the vessel's interior will then be displaced with air that has been sanitized and filtered of impurities. Correct loading of the chamber will prevent any materials from obstructing the proper movement of steam, heat, and air. This is important, as pockets of air can limit the penetration of heated steam, keeping it from reaching all layers and surfaces inside the autoclave. Object surfaces should not be wet when taken from the autoclave if the process has been carried out properly.

Preparing Linen Packs for Sterilization in an Autoclave

Linen packs are used to pack instruments and other items that need to be sterilized. The instruments should be washed and rinsed in deionized water. The instruments should then be broken down into constituent pieces. The staff should also open and unlock the ratchets for thorough cleaning. Disposable linens should be discarded. However, linens that are in good condition should be washed. The linen pack should include a sterilization indicator that can be checked after the sterilization process has been completed. This sterilization indicator will be used to make sure that surfaces inside the pack have reached the appropriate temperatures for the recommended lengths of time to allow proper sterilization to occur. At least 2 layers of material are applied in wrapping each pack. A variety of materials can be used as the outer wrap, depending on the shelf-life required of the sterilized pack. The pack is sealed with autoclave tape that has been marked with the date, contents, and operator. Each pack is marked with its own temperature-sensitive seal. This allows verification that the proper temperatures were reached during the sterilization process. The pack must measure no more than 30 x 30 x 50 cm or 12 x 12 x 20 in. It should weigh no more than 5.5 kg or 12 lbs. The pack density should not exceed 115.3 kg/m^3.

Prevacuum Autoclaves

A **prevacuum (negative pressure) autoclave** can be more expensive to purchase than a gravity displacement autoclave. However, the prevacuum autoclave can hold more objects due to its larger size and greater effectiveness. The prevacuum autoclave works to produce steam from a boiler or water heating tank. Then a **vacuum pump works to remove the air** from the loaded sterilization chamber. This allows steam to fill the empty chamber. The steam's temperature is measured at 121 ºC or 250 ºF or more. The exposure period is timed at this point. When the exposure period is ended, the **steam is vacuumed from the chamber**. This allows heated, dry, sterilized air to enter the chamber to begin the drying process that takes place inside the autoclave. The vacuum action prevents air pockets from forming during the air-steam exchange process, and it also reduces the time that is required for the drying process. It is not uncommon for a prevacuum autoclave to come equipped with a digital display screen. Most prevacuum autoclaves can also print out the interior temperatures and pressures that are reached in the sterilization cycle.

Loading the Autoclave

The **autoclave** requires **routine inspection** and **maintenance**. The autoclave provides the best performance when it is loaded in such a way as to **allow steam to flow freely** inside its chamber. **Wire mesh or perforated shelves** are recommended to promote good circulation. The packs should be arranged with a distance of 2.5 to 7.4 cm or 1 to 3 in from another linen pack. Multiple packs should be positioned on their sides in a vertical position. Containers that are made to hold paper or plastic pouches should be used. The containers hold the pouches in place so the plastic side of one pouch is facing the paper side of the adjacent pouch. Solid pans are laid upside down or on their side. Wrapped goods are arranged on the top layer with other hard and wrapped goods. It is best to operate the autoclave with only one type of metal on the inside. This prevents the likelihood of electrolysis. Thus, it is not recommended to collectively autoclave metals like aluminum, brass, and steel in the same lot.

Prepping Pouch Packs, Hard Goods, and Liquids in an Autoclave

Pouch packs serve the purpose of **securing single instruments**, **sponges**, and a variety of **other** objects. The packs are arranged so that steam can penetrate the layers inside. The loose ends of the pack are fastened with a heat seal or taped down. The ends should be folded over so that the autoclave tape shows the date, contents, and operator.

Hard goods are utensils made from stainless steel or other sturdy materials. Syringes should be separated (pulled apart) in preparation. Trays, bowls, and laboratory cages are typically made from these same hard materials. Hard goods should be washed thoroughly, followed by a rinse with deionized water. It is not necessary to wrap hard goods for sterilization.

Liquids can be autoclaved in a flat container made from Pyrex that is triple in size as compared to the volume of liquid inside. The container requires a loose-fitting lid or a paraffin cover with a needle inserted in the cover to allow air to flow. There are some concerns that infective organisms may remain in autoclaved liquid. Staff should use caution in removing these liquids to prevent injury.

Autoclave Cycles

The autoclave can be set on one of the following settings: wrapped goods, hard goods, and liquids. These settings can be employed for surgical packs, fabrics, liquids, or glass. Another option that can be selected is the gravity or fast exhaust setting.

The wrapped goods setting begins with steam flowing through the chamber. The setting allows for a predetermined temperature to be sustained over a measured time period. The cycle completes when the steam is withdrawn from the chamber. Normal atmospheric pressure will resume after the steam is released. An optional cycle can be selected to provide a drying period.

The hard goods setting is utilized when trays, bowls, and cages are placed in the autoclave. The setting is also employed to rapidly sterilize utensils for immediate use in urgent care situations. Another name for this setting is the flash autoclave.

The liquid setting allows the heated water vapor to be exhausted before the internal pressure is returned to atmospheric levels. This gives the superheated liquid a chance to cool off, thereby keeping the liquid from boiling until it resumes a normal temperature.

Recording Thermometer, Thermocouple, and the Chemical Indicator Quality Control Techniques

The **recording thermometer** keeps track of the autoclave's temperature during each cycle. This device is used to make sure that the appropriate sterilization temperatures are attained. Some types of autoclaves are capable of making a printout of the recorded temperatures and pressures attained during a cycle.

A **thermocouple** is a device which can measure the temperature in moist or dry heat or chemical sterilization applications. The thermocouple is arranged in such a way as to be able to measure the temperatures in the remotest region of the test pack.

Chemically treated paper strips are employed as **temperature confirmation indicators.** These strips change colors when the specified temperature has been achieved. Post-autoclave analysis of these strips can confirm that sterilization temperatures were achieved. They can also be utilized when the toxic gas ethylene oxide is used in the sterilization process instead of steam or dry heat. The paper strips are arranged outside and within a test pack in such a way as to confirm that sterilizing conditions were reached – i.e., that sufficient heat, steam, or gas was able to reach and penetrate into the remotest interior region of the pack. The thermocouple and the chemically treated paper strips ensure that full sterilization has been attained.

The Bowie Dick Test, Surface Sampling, and Biological Testing Quality Control Techniques

The **Bowie Dick test** employs test sheets that have been designed to **indicate a consistent color change whenever air has been effectively evacuated** from the sterilization chamber. It also measures when full steam penetration has been attained. This test shows immediate results via indicator tape and test sheets. However, it does not prove that complete sterilization (time duration) has been achieved.

A surface can be evaluated for sterility by using surface sampling quality control techniques. For example, the surface may be swiped with a sterile applicator. The swiped applicator is then used to transfer any growth to a suitable growth media in a culture plate. This plate should be incubated and observed for any target growth.

The surface or object being tested can also be rinsed down with a sterile solution. The solution can then be collected and examined for any contaminants that may be present.

Surface sampling is an accepted technique for ensuring that the appropriate disinfectant procedures are applied to surfaces found in surgical zones in veterinary clinics.

A biological testing quality control technique can also be employed to determine if the autoclave is functioning appropriately. Biological testing strips are test strips in which bacterial spores have been embedded. These strips have a bacterial population ranging in numbers from 104 to 106 organisms. The strip most likely will have a population of bacteria known as Bacillus stearothermophilus.

The strips will be placed in various locations inside a fully loaded autoclave. The usual operation of the autoclave will be carried out as a full cycle, but under its minimum setting. The strips are next removed from the autoclave when the steam has been evacuated. The bacteria strips should then be incubated as directed by the manufacturer. The incubation period should be determined, and the follow-up process carefully adhered to and recorded, as detailed in any scientific infection control study.

If a prevacuum autoclave is used, other tests are required. This is because it functions properly only if full evacuation of air is achieved from the sterilization chamber. The Bowie Dick test can be employed to test the functioning capabilities of a vacuum system in the prevacuum autoclave. The Bowie Dick test requires indicator tape or test sheets.

Anesthetic Machine

Function of Soda Lime on the Anesthetic Machine

Soda lime is a mixture of **calcium hydroxide and potassium hydroxide**. Soda lime is an important part of the anesthetic machine because it **absorbs carbon dioxide (CO_2).** Soda lime contains ethyl violet, which turns purple when the granules have reached their limit on absorbing CO_2. You must change the soda lime granules after every 8–12 hours of use, and if 8–12 hours of use is not reached in approximately a week, the soda lime should be replaced because moisture is required for the chemical reaction to occur so it could be drying out if it is not used. If the soda lime is exhausted and has reached its capacity to absorb CO_2, gases recirculate to the patient, which can lead to hypercapnia and the patient will require more gas anesthetic and oxygen to stay in the right plane of anesthesia. This can lead to hypotension, organ perfusion, renal failure, and even death. Replace the soda lime by unscrewing the soda lime canister from the anesthetic machine, dump out all of the used granules, fill the canister with new granules, and replace it snug to the anesthetic machine.

Performing a Leak Test

Prior to each anesthetic procedure, the veterinary technician must perform a **leak test** on the anesthetic machine. First, close the pop-off valve along with the end of the breathing tube with your thumb so it is sealed. Push the O_2 flush valve to fill up the reservoir bag. Hold the pressure at around 20 centimeters H_2O on the pressure gauge for up to 45 seconds, and if the pressure holds and the reservoir bag stays full, then there are no leaks. If the reservoir bag slowly deflates and the gauge shows a decrease in pressure, then there is a leak that may be coming from the reservoir bag or the rebreathing tube. If neither of these is causing the leak, then take a spray bottle with soapy water or glass cleaner in it, close the pop-off valve, hold off the end of the rebreathing tube, and flush the O_2 to fill the reservoir bag. Spray certain areas of the machine such as the neck of the bag, areas where hoses connect to the machine, and areas where the soda lime connects to the machine. Squeeze the reservoir bag, look for bubbles to form on the machine, and listen for leaks.

Scavenging System Maintenance

Three passive **scavenging systems** include the floor drop, absorption via charcoal, or a scavenge hose directed out of a window. Passive scavenge systems work on the oxygen flow creating positive pressure during exhalation. Active scavenging systems have a central vacuum using negative pressure that connects to an interface near or on the anesthetic machine. Scavenging systems collect, remove, and dispose of up to 90% of waste anesthetic gases away from the building and staff members. There should be regular inspection and maintenance of the scavenge system. Active systems should be regularly checked for leaks and should be repaired when needed. An activated charcoal canister, such as an F-air canister, must be replaced after 12 hours of use or once it reaches 50 grams of use, whichever comes first. The F-air canister should be weighed on a gram scale after each use and discarded after it reaches 50 grams.

Crash Cart Supplies and Drugs

The **crash cart** should be in a central location in the hospital close to an anesthetic machine in case the patient needs to be under anesthesia or receive oxygen support. Some supplies that should be available in the crash cart are catheters, tape, syringes, needles, fluid bag, Ambu-bag, and emergency drugs. Emergency drugs that are vital to include in the crash cart include epinephrine, atropine, naloxone, lidocaine, and doxapram. Epinephrine is used to treat anaphylactic reactions, and it is also used to stimulate the heart in cardiopulmonary resuscitation (CPR). Atropine is used to treat an abnormally slow heart rate and is an important drug used in CPR. Lidocaine is used to treat cardiac arrhythmias. Doxapram is used to stimulate breathing in a patient under anesthesia or after, as well as to help initiate breathing in newborn patients after a C-section. The crash cart should also include a drug dosage chart for each emergency drug.

Dentistry

Anatomy and Physiology and Dentistry

The Triadan System

Numbering Teeth

Veterinarians employ the **Triadan system** to number the teeth. In this system **each tooth is given a 3-digit number.** The first digit indicates the **quadrant**. The mouth of the animal is divided into 4 quadrants or sections. For permanent or adult teeth: 1 = upper right quadrant; 2 = upper left quadrant; 3 = lower left quadrant; 4 = lower right quadrant. For deciduous or baby teeth: 5 = upper right quadrant; 6 = upper left quadrant; 7 = lower left quadrant; 8 = lower right quadrant. The **second and third digits indicate the particular tooth** in the quadrant, numbered 01-11, starting with the teeth nearest the midline and progressing toward the outside. In dogs, for instance, the incisors are numbered 01-03; the canines are numbered 04; the premolars are numbered 05-08; the molars are numbered 09-11 (09-10 in the upper quadrants). The lower right canine would be designated with the number 404.

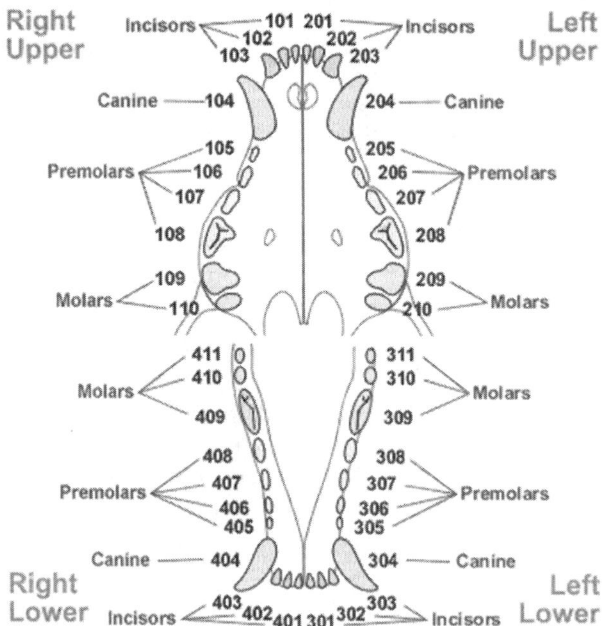

The Triadan System in the Canine

The **Triadan system** divides the canine's mouth into four separate quadrants, with the upper right maxillary being quadrant 100, the upper left maxillary quadrant is 200, the left mandibular quadrant is 300, and the right mandibular quadrant is 400. Then starting between the first incisors, the teeth are counted distally (away from the center). The first incisor on the upper right is number 101, for example. The canine teeth are always 04, so the maxillary right canine is 104. The first molars are always 09, so the maxillary left first molar is 209. As for deciduous teeth (baby teeth), the numbering system keeps going back to the right maxillary quadrant being 500, the left maxillary quadrant is 600, the left mandibular would be 700, and the right mandibular is 800.

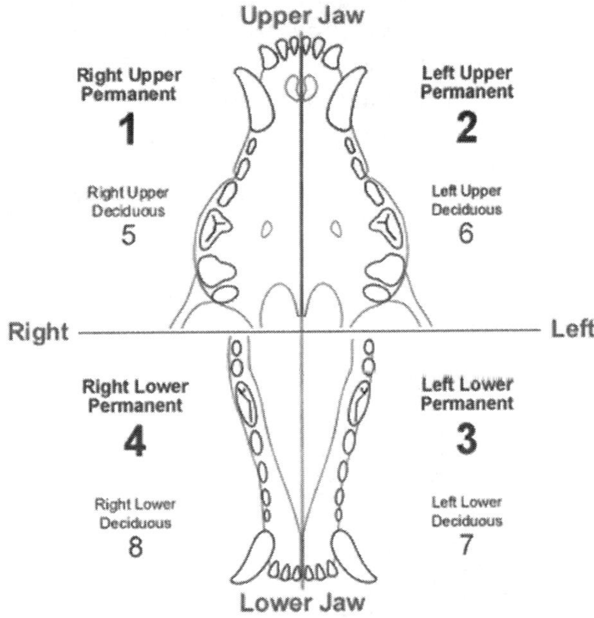

The Triadan System in the Feline

The **feline Triadan tooth numbering system** is comparable to the canine system, except the feline has fewer teeth. Using the carnassial teeth as landmarks in cats will help to identify other teeth because it will vary from a full canine Triadan numbering system. Adult cats have 30 teeth including 4 canines, 12 incisors, 10 premolars, and 4 molars. There are four quadrants identified in the feline Triadan system with the right maxilla being the 100s, left maxilla is the 200s, the left mandible is the 300s, and the right mandible is the 400s. The upper feline carnassial teeth are the last premolars and end in 08 on the Triadan numbering system, so the upper right last premolar (carnassial) would be 108. The lower feline carnassial teeth are the first molars and end in 09 on the numbering system. Therefore, the lower right first molar is 409. Canines on the feline Triadan system always end in 04, so the lower left canine tooth is 304.

Incisors, Canines, Premolars, Molars, and Carnassials

Incisors (the front teeth) have a **sharp edge ideal for cutting and tearing food** into pieces. Incisors are particularly useful for animals that eat plants. Canines or dogs also have teeth that are pointed known as the **cuspids**. These are the fearfully long and sharp "eye teeth" – so called for their orientation under each eye. These teeth serve to grasp food, anchoring it in the mouth or tearing it into pieces. **Premolars** are also called **bicuspids**. These teeth are found adjacent to the canines (cuspids, or eye teeth) and the molars. The premolars cut, sever, and hold the animal's food. Food is chewed or broken up in the mouth by the canines and the premolars. The **molars** work to grind the food into a form that can be easily swallowed. Molars are found at the back of the mouth. Molars are fashioned with 4 cusps in the shape of a four-sided figure. The **carnassial** teeth are the largest of all the sharp teeth used for cutting flesh. These teeth are found in carnivorous animals and are fashioned to cut and tear meat from the bone of the prey. Dog carnassial teeth are the upper fourth premolars and lower first molars. Cat carnassial teeth are the upper fourth premolars and lower molars.

Anatomy of the Tooth

Starting from the middle of the tooth is the pulp, which is made up of connective tissue, nerves, and blood vessels. The dentin covers the pulp and makes up most of the tooth. **Dentin** is a harder tissue that can detect if something is hot or cold. The **cementum** is the calcified tissue that covers the dentin, and the enamel is the hard outer layer of the crown of the tooth. Enamel is actually the hardest tissue in the body. The **periodontal ligament** helps hold the tooth in the socket as it attaches to the cementum and the **alveolar bone**. The alveolar bone forms the jaw and surrounds the tooth roots. The **gingiva**, also known as the gums, is the soft tissue that covers the rest of the periodontium, and the space by the gingiva and the tooth is labeled the gingival sulcus.

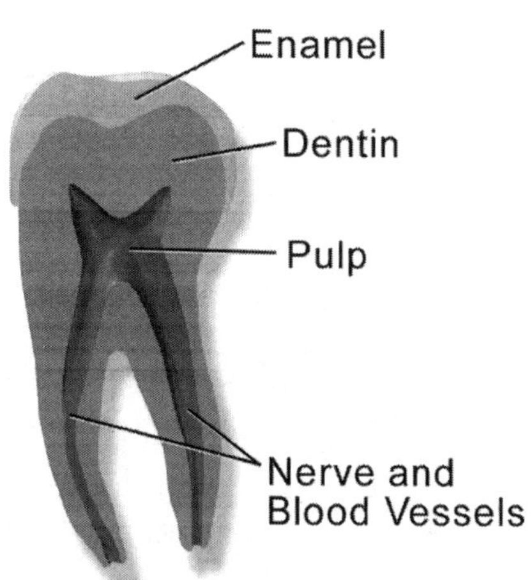

Tooth Anatomy

Four Stages of Periodontal Disease

Periodontal disease is infection and inflammation of the tissue supporting the teeth (periodontium) caused by bacteria, plaque buildup, and the animal's response to the bacteria present. There are **four stages of periodontal disease**: Stage one involves gingivitis with no attachment loss. Stage two is early periodontitis with less than 25% attachment loss along with stage one furcation in multirooted teeth meaning that the periodontal probe fits less than halfway under the crown of the tooth. Stage three is moderate periodontitis with 25-50% attachment loss along with stage two furcation of multirooted teeth meaning the periodontal probe extends more than halfway under the crown of the tooth. Stage four is advanced periodontitis, attachment loss is greater than 50%, and there may be a stage three furcation in multirooted teeth in which the periodontal probe will fit under the tooth's crown from one side to the other.

Anatomy of Equine Teeth

A **foal** is a young horse with 24 temporary or deciduous teeth. An adult horse will develop 40 to 42 permanent or adult teeth. A **stallion** is an uncastrated adult male horse. A **gelding** is a castrated adult male horse. A **mare** is an adult female horse. An **adult** horse has the following dentition formula: (2 times I3/3, C1/1, P3/3, M3/3).

The 3 sets of incisors in the horse's mouth have a specific function. **Incisors** are used to grasp, nip, and tug food found growing in the pasture. The horse's cheek teeth include 3 premolars and 3 molars. The **cheek teeth** function to grind up the animal's food. Only the mare is found without

canine teeth (also called tushes). The small upper **premolars** (if present at all) are referred to as "wolf teeth". These teeth may have benefited prehistoric horses, but appear to have since gone through a transformation causing them to be less developed than earlier versions. Thus, it is not uncommon to have the wolf teeth removed to allow for more comfort and to reduce any interference when the horse's bit is worn.

Tooth Resorption in Cats

Tooth resorption is very common in cats, affecting nearly 60% of them and is defined by the erosion of the dentin on one or more teeth. The tooth contains the root canal, which holds the blood vessels and nerves, and this is surrounded by dentin, which is a calcified tissue covered by enamel. Resorption starts with the breakdown of the enamel, and given enough time, the root will be affected or the crown may be missing. Tooth resorption will begin to look as if the gingival tissue is growing into the tooth, and in some patients, there will be a hole in the tooth where the tooth meets the gum line. The tooth resorption process is very painful; clinical signs may include excessive drooling, pain response when the affected tooth is touched, difficulty eating or not eating at all, and even bleeding in the mouth. The only treatment would be to extract the entire affected tooth.

Function of the Enamel on the Tooth

Hydroxyapatite is the chief mineral found in the **enamel of teeth**. This mineral is one of the hardest and most plentiful found in the body. Enamel is composed of 96% mineral and 4% water and organic substances. The 2 proteins found in enamel are called amelogenins and enamelins. Enamel is the exterior layer that is used to wrap the uppermost part of the tooth or crown. **Ameloblasts** function to shape the enamel when the tooth is being formed. This process is stopped when the tooth breaks through the gums in the mouth. The enamel functions to prevent bacteria from damaging the tooth. The enamel does not possess any sensitivity, as used in the sensory processes.

Dog tooth enamel can range in thickness from <0.1 to 0.6 mm. The cat tooth enamel can range in thickness from <0.1 to 0.3 mm. The enamel in hypsodont teeth of herbivores both covers and exists in complicated folds within the dentin. In this way the durability of the tooth is increased for animals that must constantly chew hard, cellulose-based foods. The dentin is a part of the tooth that is hard and calcified, albeit not as hard as enamel. It lies underneath the enamel and envelops the pulp and root canals. The extensively folded enamel in hypsodont teeth is evident in horses and cattle, among other herbivores.

Dental Pulp and the Cementum

Dental pulp is located on the inside of the tooth. It is formed from **living tissue, odontoblasts, fibroblasts, and other cells**. The **pulp** is plentiful in blood vessels, nerve endings, and lymphatics. The dental pulp is also the region where the root canal joins the root. The pulp comes into the tooth through the apical delta. The **apical delta** is the tiny opening found in the tip of the root. The pulp cannot be exposed or it will become contaminated, and necrosis and inflammation will develop. A high level of pain will accompany this condition. Direct trauma may harm the pulp yet still leave the uppermost part of the tooth uninjured. This uppermost part of the tooth is known as the crown. Pulp necrosis must be treated by removing the tooth or by performing a "root canal" cleaning.

Cementum is a mineralized tissue that covers the dentin of the root and the neck of the tooth. This bony tissue is composed of inorganic matter (45% to 50% hydroxyapatite), about 33% organic constituents (mostly collagen fibers, along with Sharpey's fibers and other organic substances), and about 22% water.

DENTIN IN THE TOOTH

The **dentin** is formulated as the **greatest bulk of the tooth**. The dentin is located beneath the enamel and cementum of the tooth, and over the pulp chamber. The dentin is formed by a cell inside the tooth known as odontoblasts. The cells form a biological role in creating the dentin in a process called dentinogenesis. The dentin is a strong substance like that of bone but softer than enamel and cementum. However, dentin has a tendency to decay rapidly. Exposed dentin can lead to severe cavities when left untreated. The dentin provides an extra barrier of protection from the bacteria that would attack the pulp. Dentin is porous, and is yellow in color. Dentin permits the movement of fluids to pass through its pores. Dentin is composed of about 72% inorganic material, 18% organic material (mostly collagen), and 10% water. Heat, cold, touch, and changes in osmotic pressure can result in physically painful sensations. The collagen in the dentin gives the tooth the flexibility needed to absorb shock. This keeps the tooth from breaking or fracturing. The dentin can be mended when tertiary dentin is created.

ALVEOLAR BONE, THE GINGIVAL, GINGIVAL SULCUS, AND THE SULCULAR FLUID

The bone enveloping and sustaining the teeth is known as the **alveolar bone**. This bone undergoes constant internal repair and regeneration processes. The alveolar bone provides a consistent deposition and resorption process throughout the lifetime of the adult tooth. Entrenched deep inside the bone are Sharpey's fibers. These fibers are incorporated into the cementum and aid in anchoring and supporting the tooth.

The **gingiva** or gums are formed from soft mucosal tissue that envelops the jawbone. The gingiva provides the teeth with protection from harmful bacteria. The gingival tissue is reddish in color due to the blood that is visible beneath the translucent outer epithelial covering. The 3 sections of the gingiva consist of the marginal gingiva, the attached gingiva, and the interdental gingiva.

The section of gingival tissue immediately beside the tooth and forming an adherent pocket is known as the **gingival sulcus**. The gingival sulcus can be probed between the marginal gingival tissue and the tooth, and is typically measured at a depth of 1 to 3 mm in dogs. This section is measured at a depth of 0.5 to 1 mm in cats.

The **sulcular fluid** runs through the sulcar epithelium. It is produced from secretions from the gingival connective tissue. The fluid bathes the sulcus. The fluid is abundant in immunoglobulins and has other antimicrobial properties. The production of secreted sulcular fluids is multiplied whenever the gums are reddened and inflamed.

CEMENTUM, THE CEMENTOENAMEL JUNCTION, AND PERIODONTAL LIGAMENTS

Cementum functions as a structural system that attaches the tooth to the stabilizing periodontal ligaments. Enamel and dentin are both formed from harder substance than cementum. Cementum is yellow. Cementoblasts secrete the cementum into place. It is constantly reabsorbed and mended. Periodontal ligaments fasten the gingiva to the cementum. However, the gingiva cannot be readily secured back to the cementum if disturbed.

The **cementoenamel junction** is at the base of the enamel where the crown meets the cementum enveloping the tooth's root. The cementoenamel junction fastens the tooth with periodontal ligaments at the gingiva.

The **periodontal ligaments** consist of collagen, elastic fibers, blood vessels, nerves, and lymphatics. The periodontal ligament anchors each tooth in the alveolus or socket by fastening the cementum of the tooth to the alveolar bone. This support system provides the teeth with enough strength to undergo large compression forces used in chewing without damage to the bones. The teeth are not directly attached to the bone. The periodontal ligaments can absorb shock and protect the nerve endings. The sensory nerve endings located in the ligaments function to provide a pain sensor and pressure sensor used by the brain in responding to changing pressures in chewing, among other forces impacting the teeth. These ligaments also help supply the alveolar bone and cementum with nourishment.

Dentition

Dentition Formula for Dogs

The growth, location, and type of teeth are known as the **dentition**. All animals have a total of 4 types of teeth that have been divided by rows representing the upper and lower jaws in the mouth. In each formula the location of the first number tells how many incisors should be present. The second number indicates how many canines. The third indicates the number of premolars. The fourth number indicates how many molars. These numbers will be multiplied by the number 2 to give a total that represents both sides of the mouth. Deciduous teeth or baby teeth are lost when the animal is young. However, adult teeth are grown in place of the baby teeth that are lost.

Dogs produce 28 deciduous teeth. Dogs have 42 permanent or adult teeth. The dentition formula for the number of teeth a dog has is given as follows: 3 1 4 2 and 3 1 4 3. The dog has 3 incisors, 1 canine, 4 premolars, and 2 molars on its upper jaw. The lower jaw has 3 incisors, 1 canine, 4 premolars, and 3 molars. Thus, the dog has a combined total of 42 teeth.

Dentition Formulas for Cats, Horses, and Swine

Cats produce 26 **deciduous teeth**. Cats have 30 permanent teeth or adult teeth. The **dentition formula** for the number of teeth a cat has is given as follows: 3 1 3 1 and 3 1 2 1. The cat's upper molars can be determined by looking at the numbers 2, 3, and 4. The cat's lower molars can be determined by looking at the numbers 3 and 4. The upper molars are labeled 2, 3, and 4, while the lower molars are labeled 3 and 4.

Horses produce 24 deciduous teeth. Stallions are uncastrated male horses (otherwise called geldings after castration). They have 40 to 42 permanent teeth or adult teeth. Mares are female horses. They have 30 to 36 permanent teeth or adult teeth. Commonly, horses do not develop canine (eye) teeth. The dentition formula for the number of teeth a horse has is given as follows: 3 1.3 3 and 3 1 3 3. Swine or hogs produce 32 deciduous teeth. Hogs have 44 permanent teeth or adult teeth. The dentition formula for the number of teeth a hog has is given as follows: 3 1 4 3 and 3 1 4 3.

Ruminants, Hamsters, Guinea Pigs, and Rabbits

Ruminant animals are those that have hoofs and chew cud. Sheep, cattle, and goats are ruminant animals. The ruminant animal produces 20 deciduous teeth. The ruminant animal has 32 permanent teeth or adult teeth. The dentition formula for the number of teeth a ruminant animal has is given as follows: 0 0 3 3 and 4 0 3 3.

Hamsters belong to the **rodent family**. Hamsters produce 16 permanent teeth or adult teeth. Gerbils, mice, and rats are all members of the rodent family. They also produce 16 teeth. The dentition formula for these rodents is given as follows: 1 0 0 3 and 1 0 0 3. Guinea pigs are also a member of the rodent family. However, this particular rodent produces 20 permanent teeth or adult teeth. The dentition formula for the guinea pig is given as follows: 1 0 1 3 and 1 0 1 3.

Rabbits or hares are **small mammals**. Rabbits produce 28 permanent teeth or adult teeth. The dentition formula for the rabbit is given as follows: 2 0 3 3 and 1 0 2 3.

Crown, Root, Buccal, Lingual, Labial, and Palatal

Crown: The section of the tooth that is visible from the gum line and above. This portion of the tooth is enclosed under a layer of enamel.

Root: This term refers to the section of the tooth that is not visible to the eye. The root lies underneath the gum line. It is deeply lodged within the surrounding tissue and bone.

Buccal: Refers to the surface of the tooth or gums that is closest to the cheek within the mouth.

Lingual: Refers to the tongue or the fleshy organ found on the interior of the mouth and the regions within its vicinity (i.e., the lingual tooth surface).

Labial: Refers to the lips and the region within their vicinity.

Palatal: Refers to the region in the mouth that is closest to the palate or the roof of the mouth.

Tooth Roots for Dogs and Cats

Dogs have 4 kinds of teeth. They include the incisors, the canines, the premolars, and the molars. A single root is deeply lodged beneath the incisors, the canines, and the first premolars and the third molar of the dog's lower jaw. Two roots are found under the second and third premolars, the fourth premolars of the lower jaw, the first and second molars on the lower jaw, and possibly the third molars on the lower jaw. Three roots are underneath the jaw line supporting the fourth premolars of the upper jaw and the first and second molars on the upper jaw.

Cats also have one root supporting the incisors, the canines, the second premolars of the upper jaw, and the first molars on the upper jaw. Either 1 or 2 roots that have merged offer support to the molars on the upper jaw. Two roots support the third premolars on the upper jaw, the third and fourth premolars on the lower jaw, and the lower molars. Three roots support the fourth premolars on the upper jaw.

Mesial, Distal, Rostral, Occlusal, and Furcation

Mesial: Refers to the region in the mouth that forms the anterior midline, or forward middle dental arch near the middle of the forward section of the mouth.

Distal: Refers to the direction moving toward the last tooth in each quadrant of a dental arch, or the edge of an incisor located near the midline of the jaw.

Rostral: Refers to the portion relating to or oriented toward the nose of an animal.

Occlusal: The section of the tooth's molar or premolar that functions to chew or grind food.

Furcation: Refers to the break or dividing point between the roots of a tooth that are joined at the crown.

Administering Nerve Blocks Prior to Tooth Extraction

Four **nerve blocks** can be used in dogs to provide a local block prior to extractions. These include the infraorbital, maxillary, middle mental, and inferior alveolar. In cats and brachycephalic dogs, the infraorbital foramen is too short, allowing for the whole maxilla on the corresponding side to be affected so that nerve block is not used. The infraorbital nerve block (rostral maxillary) provides analgesia to the incisors, canine, and first three premolars on that side, along with the soft tissue and adjacent maxillary bone. The maxillary nerve block affects the branches of the maxillary nerve including the infraorbital nerve, pterygopalatine nerve, and palatine nerves. The bones, teeth, and soft tissues of the maxilla will be blocked. The middle mental nerve block (rostral mandibular) affects the canine, incisors, and soft tissues and bone of the corresponding side. The inferior alveolar nerve block (caudal mandibular) blocks all of the mandibular teeth, bone, and soft tissues on the corresponding side rostral (toward the nose) to the injection.

Feline Stomatitis and Treatment

Stomatitis is an extremely painful inflammation of the cat's mouth and gums caused by periodontal disease or certain viruses such as feline immunodeficiency virus, feline leukemia virus, and feline calicivirus. A lot of times, the cause may be immune mediated where the body's immune system attacks the oral cavity in response to bacteria in the mouth. Stomatitis causes ulcers to form inside the cat's mouth, on the tongue, gums, lips, and in the back of the throat. Common clinical signs of stomatitis include the cat's mouth being too painful to eat, drooling, bad breath, weight loss, and an unkempt hair coat because it is too painful to groom. To treat stomatitis, the pain must first be controlled with medication, followed by a thorough dental cleaning with radiographs to see the extent of the periodontal disease. Extraction of molars and premolars tends to help because bacteria attach to the surfaces of the teeth and removing them will help minimize bacteria that may be causing the immune system to attack.

Formation and Effects of Plaque and Tartar

Plaque is a mix of bacteria and their by-products, salivary components, inflammatory cells, and oral debris that can form within hours on the teeth. As the pet eats, the food particles stick in between and, on the teeth, and once bacteria in the mouth start to digest these food particles, plaque forms. After time passes, the bacteria die and the calcium in the saliva can calcify the dead bacteria, forming a hardened form called **tartar**. As plaque spreads, it leads to inflammation of the gums called gingivitis, and as the plaque and tartar continue to develop underneath the gum line, it can infect the tooth root and a dental scaling will be needed to clean the teeth. In the later stages of periodontal disease, the surrounding tissues of the tooth break down and are destroyed and the bony socket holding the tooth in place becomes eroded, loosening the tooth.

Equine Teeth and Their Purpose

Male **horses** will have 40 teeth, and females will have 36–40 teeth by maturity due to the fact that some female horses do not develop canine teeth. Horse's teeth erupt an estimated 3 mm a year to replace the tooth length that wears as they eat. Starting at the front of the mouth, horses usually have 12 incisors, which are also called nipper teeth, which are used for biting and cutting the food from the pasture; these teeth give a general idea of the horse's age. A horse's permanent canines do not erupt until around 5 years of age, and these teeth do not continue to erupt and do not serve a purpose. The horse normally has 12–16 premolars that erupt around 2 years of age that are used for grinding and crushing food. Wolf teeth are found in front of the horse's first premolar, and they may emerge between 6 months and 2 years of age or not at all. Wolf teeth have no purpose and can cause pain and discomfort to the horse because they can be pointy. The horse normally has 12 molars that erupt at around 1 year of age and will be finished erupting by age 3.

Oral Examinations and Treatment

Dental Hand Instruments

The veterinarian will utilize 2 varieties of hand-held instruments in dental work. These instruments are categorized as cutting or non-cutting implements. The **cutting instruments** are fashioned with the following: the cutting edge, the blade, the shank, and the handle. The **non-cutting instruments** are fashioned with the following: the point or face, the nib, the shank, and the handle. The shank is found on both varieties of instruments. It functions to connect the handle of the instrument to the blade of the cutting instrument or to the nib on the non-cutting instrument.

The veterinarian will grasp the handle utilizing an adapted pencil grip. This allows the middle finger to remain at rest along the shank. The middle finger can feel vibrations that flow through the instrument when it is moved over a rough surface. This movement is directed with the additional support provided by the middle finger. A fulcrum (i.e., a point of rest, typically on an adjacent jaw) provides a steady handhold on the instrument. This fulcrum can also help direct the movements of the instrument with more precision. The third or fourth finger can be used to hold the fulcrum.

Hand Instruments Used in Dental Procedures

There are three parts to a **dental hand instrument**: The handle is the part you hold, and the shank is the part that connects the handle to the working end, which is the blade or probe end of the instrument that touches the teeth. The working end may be curved or straight depending on what it is used for on the teeth. Scalers have sharp tips and edges and are used to remove supragingival (above the gum line) calculus from the teeth. Curettes have two sharp edges, a blunt tip, and a curved back, and they are used to remove calculus from under the gumline (subgingival) on the root surface and on the gingival tissue on the opposing side (gingival curettage). Explorers are used to examine the surface of the tooth with its flexible steel tip that can detect any abnormalities such as a furcation. Periodontal probes measure the pocket depth of the gingival sulcus and are used to measure gingival recession to help determine the stage of periodontal disease.

Dental Hand Instruments That are Used for Extractions

A **periosteal elevator** is used to lift the gum tissue to help remove some of the alveolar bone in an extraction with the flat side of the blade pressing against the tooth's surface and the curved side against the soft tissue to decrease tearing. **Dental elevators** are used by placing the concave side of the instrument along the tooth's surface and the curved side between the tooth and the alveolar bone to stretch and tear the periodontal ligament in order to loosen the tooth for easier extraction. Extraction forceps are used to grip and remove the tooth after it has been loosened and can also be used to crack off heavy calculus. **Root tip picks** are used to stretch and break the periodontal ligament to obtain a fractured root tip if necessary.

Periodontal Probe and the Shepherd's Hook

The **periodontal probe** can have a lone end, but some come as double-ended implements. The probe is moved down the length of the long axis of the tooth between the gingiva and the surface of the tooth root. The probe is directed in such a way as to run along the perimeter of each tooth on all 4 sides. All abnormal sulcus depths are carefully written in the patient's chart.

The **Shepherd's hook** is also known as the explorer. This dental instrument is applied as a probe. It functions to investigate the condition of the tooth's enamel. The veterinarian will also check out any decay or broken teeth that are found in the animal's mouth. The instrument is shaped with a pointed tip which helps relieve any discomfort that may be experienced. The tool can be applied with a light touch which does not hurt the gums. The explorer can be beneficial in exposing any subgingival calculus or loose teeth. Cats can also be examined with the explorer. In particular, the explorer can help detect external feline odontoclastic resorption lesions, or FEOR's, in the feline species. This condition is found in approximately 28 to 67% of all felines.

Sickle Scaler and the Curette Scaler

The sickle scaler is fashioned in the form of a triangle. This instrument has 2 cutting edges with a sharp tip. Sickle scalers function to remove tartar or supragingival calculus from the teeth. The straight shank can be applied to the anterior or front teeth. The contra-angle shank can be applied to the posterior or back teeth. The sickle scaler should be pulled in a direction away from the gum line. The cutting edge of the sickle shank should be positioned just beneath the raised strip of the calculus. This will allow the calculus or tartar to be scraped away from the tooth without harming the gingiva.

The curette scaler is fashioned in the form of a spoon with a curved back. The architecture of the curette scaler utilizes a half circle in cross section. The curette scaler comes in 2 forms, the universal and the area specific.

Curette Scaler and the Periodontal Probe

The **curette scaler** functions to remove tartar or subgingival calculus from the mouth. It is also useful for root planing and for removing the soft tissue found in the periodontal pocket. The veterinarian will position the cutting edge adjacent to the tooth. The handle should be held in a parallel direction towards the root of the tooth. The curette scaler should be moved in a direction that pulls away from the root of the tooth. The veterinarian will need to make multiple strokes as the calculus is removed from the tooth. This is done until the tooth's surface begins to appear as shiny and even.

A **periodontal probe** is an example of a non-cutting instrument. The periodontal probe is shaped in a form that is extended, slender, and curved along one end. The veterinarian will use the probe to determine the depth of the gingival sulcus. The veterinarian will also use this probe to come to a diagnosis about the condition of the periodontium.

A periodontal probe is used to measure the pocket depth of the gingival sulcus (pocket) during each and every dental procedure to evaluate how much periodontal support there is. The probe has tiny marks etched in millimeters on the blunt end, it is placed parallel to the long axis of the tooth, and with slight pressure it is run around the tooth to measure the pocket depth. The pocket depth is the distance between the base of the pocket and the gingival margin. In dogs, it should not exceed 3 mm, and in cats, 0.5–1 mm is normal. If there is gum recession, it can be measured with the periodontal probe. This is important to document at each annual dental cleaning and keep in the patient's record to see trends and diagnose stages of periodontal disease.

Ultrasonic Scalers

Ultrasonic scalers take off the gross calculus or tartar found above the gingival line. A gentle pressure on the tooth is all that is necessary. This light touch will ensure that heat is not allowed to become intense. Heat can cause the enamel to become rutted, which can result in injury to the pulp. The area beneath the gum line should not be treated because of the likelihood of heat buildup. This is caused by the inability of the tip to be cooled off by water when under the gum line. The application of an abundant supply of water is recommended. The water keeps the teeth cool in the ultrasonic cleaning process. The water should be demineralized or filtered to keep reduce problematic buildup in the tubing. The veterinarian should only work about 5 seconds on each tooth. The tips require replacement on a regular basis. The tips should be checked for proper length, as they have a tendency to wear and shorten with use. This will reduce the efficiency of the equipment. The patient should be given an oral rinse frequently. It should be a disinfectant, preferably a 0.12% chlorhexidine solution.

Ultrasonic Scaler Tips

Veterinarians will employ ultrasonic scalers as an efficient method to **remove calculus** from the surface of the tooth. The instruments function with a vibration that moves along the end of the scalers at a frequency rate of 20 to 45 kHz or 20,000 to 45,000 cycles per second. This is an

ultrasonic frequency rate. The instrument is available with a variety of power ratings. The tips can be oval or egg-shaped, formed as a bowed line, or in the shape of a number 8. There are 3 tips available: magnetostrictive, piezoelectric, or sonic. The magnetostrictive tip pulsates at a frequency of 18 to 29 kHz in an oval pattern. The piezoelectric tip keeps a linear pattern and pulsates at 40 kHz. The piezoelectric tip is the tool of choice, as its linear vibration does not produce a high degree of trauma or stress in the patient. The sonic tip can pulsate with a frequency of up to 18 cycles per second. It operates on an oval-shaped pattern. The units function at a lower temperature, giving off little heat. Some commercial units work better than others. Therefore, the veterinarian should be an informed shopper before purchasing this equipment.

Sharpening Hand Instruments

Hand-held instruments should be given a good sharpening before they are sterilized. The instrument can be checked for dullness by placing it in the light. The light will reflect off the immediate cutting edge on dull objects. However, if the cutting edge has no reflection then it will appear as a fine black line, indicating a sharp edge. The veterinarian can apply a sharpening stone to the instrument's edge to improve its ability to cut. Stones are available in coarse or fine textures. An example of a coarse texture is found in the ruby stone. The ruby stone requires water as a **sharpening lubricant**. An example of fine texture is found in the Arkansas stone. The Arkansas stone requires oil to be used as a lubricant in the sharpening process. A fine or medium texture can be found in the India stone. The India stone also requires the use of oil as a lubricant during the sharpening process. An additional coarse texture can be found in the carborundum stone. The carborundum stone requires water as a lubricant. A fine or medium texture can be found in the ceramic stone. The ceramic stone requires water or dry lubricant to be used during the sharpening process.

Air-Driven and Roto-Pro Bur Scalers

The veterinarian will employ the use of a low-speed handpiece, high-speed handpiece, and a three-way air and water syringe when using a basic air-driven scaler. The more complex units will have a variety of available options, including piezoelectric scalers, sonic scaler outlets, suction, fiberoptic illumination, extra electrical outlets, and electrosurgical outlets. Compressors will be required to supply the air. However, this can be alleviated by the use of compressed air tanks. The compressors can be used with low noise, oil-cooled compressors or with the noisier oil-free dental compressors. The oil-free dental compressor is more expensive. The maintenance of the compressor requires a weekly check on the oil level. The oil must be changed at least every 6 months.

The veterinarian will employ the use of roto-pro bur scalers when mechanical scalers are needed. It can operate at 300,000 to 400,000 rpm. The mechanical scaler is beneficial in the removal of tartar and calculus that is deeply built up on the teeth. However, caution should be used due to the risk of injury to the enamel, dentin, and soft tissue.

Measuring the Gingival Sulcus

The depth of the sulcus can be gauged by inserting the periodontal probe. This measurement should be taken after the teeth have been polished. The normal measurement for felines is measured at a sulcus depth of 0.5 to 1 mm. It is important to rid the teeth of plaque. Otherwise, the plaque will blend with the saliva to create tartar or calculus on the teeth. Calculus is a hard crust that can tightly adhere to the teeth. Calculus will lead to gum inflammation and gingivitis. Gingivitis is a condition that causes the gums around the roots of the teeth to become red and swollen. The veterinarian will apply treatment above and below the gum line to remove gross calculus using dental extractors. Cats require a light touch, as they have delicate teeth that can be broken or cracked with little difficulty. The next step in treatment requires the application of a mechanical scaler to eliminate supragingival calculus and plaque. The last step requires the use of a hand curette to remove any residual subgingival calculus that is left on the teeth.

Examining a Patient

The veterinarian will need to find out about the patient's history in the initial steps of the examination, and then closely inspect the animal's face and head for symmetry. The nasal and ocular regions should be inspected for any secretions, lumps, or swollen areas. The lips, mouth, tongue, teeth, and gums should also be checked. The gingival sulcus will need to be measured around the perimeter of the tooth. The veterinarian should apply the scaler above and below the gingiva. Minuscule ruts created by the scaling process will require a thorough polishing to even out the teeth and remove any plaque. The veterinarian will then wipe down the teeth. The teeth should be allowed to air dry. The veterinarian should then place fluoride solution on the teeth, which should remain on the teeth for the recommended time period. The veterinarian should record the services performed on the teeth at the time of each patient's visit.

Applying Fluoride to the Patient's Teeth

A fluoride treatment is spread over the teeth as soon as the teeth have been thoroughly polished. This topical solution should be left on the teeth for up to 4 minutes. The residual topical fluoride is wiped from the teeth after that time. Some prophy paste already has a fluoride base, alleviating the need for an additional treatment with fluoride. However, most veterinarians prefer the second application of fluoride so as to increase the protection offered to the patient.

Fluoride offers protection to the teeth in the form of an antibacterial agent. Fluoride also desensitizes the teeth to feelings of pain from cold, heat, or touch. Fluoride increases the defensive ability of the enamel by fostering the tooth's mineralization development. The fluoride left in the animal's saliva will be absorbed in the spots on the tooth surface that are absent of minerals. These bare spots will also entice other minerals to the tooth's surface, like calcium. Fluoride is turned into a substance known as fluorapatite when it becomes part of the tooth in this absorption process. Fluorapatite is more resistance to acids than hydroxyapatite, and will not dissolve easily.

Instruments and Equipment Needed for a Tooth Extraction Procedure

The dental instruments that will be needed for a **tooth extraction** will depend upon which tooth is being extracted. Single-rooted teeth such as incisors and canines will require an appropriately sized elevator, forceps, a blade, and small sutures (4-0). In order to extract multirooted teeth, a flap is created with the use of an elevator and a surgical blade. The high-speed handpiece will be used to drill the bone with a round burr from the alveolar crest and then using a taper fissure burr to cut the tooth into two, so that each root is separate. Forceps will be used to pull out the roots, and a small suture will be used to close the area. Canine tooth extractions will require the use of a periosteal elevator to lift the flap if the tooth is well attached, then a taper fissure burr will be used to cut around the tooth. An elevator will then be used to loosen the tooth, and forceps are used to extract the root. A bone rasp can be used to remove any remaining bone pieces. Radiographs will be needed for all pre- and post-extraction films.

Importance of Polishing in Every Dental Procedure

Polishing is a very important step in the dental cleaning procedure. A low-speed handpiece and prophy paste are used. At the end of the handpiece is a prophy cup that holds the prophy paste. With pressure, polish all surfaces of the teeth that have been scaled. Polishing will leave a smooth surface on all teeth that will prevent plaque and bacteria from adhering to a rough surface. It is much easier for bacteria and plaque to build up after a dental cleaning due to scaling, so polishing well is very important. After polishing, use the rinse handpiece to rinse excess prophy paste from the mouth. Polishing must be done well, but not for too long on each tooth, and the polisher should spin no faster than 4,000 rpm to avoid increased friction on the tooth's surface. The polishing handpiece can cause thermal damage and enamel loss to the tooth if held in place for too long with too much pressure. It is recommended to polish using light pressure for only three seconds on the crowns of all teeth starting at the most caudal teeth, ending with the incisors.

Polishing a Patient's Teeth After Scaling

Patients that go through the scaling process to remove calculus and plaque will usually have grooves left on the teeth. This is caused by both the hand and mechanical implements used in the scaling process. **Polishing** will take off any **plaque that has not been removed** in the scaling process. In addition, the polishing process will create a smooth and shiny surface on the teeth. The veterinarian should only polish each tooth for 5 seconds. The heat that is generated can be reduced with the use of a **fine grade tooth polishing paste** or flour. Water will also reduce the temperature. The prophy cup (a rubber cup-like endpiece used in polishing teeth) should be kept in motion throughout the process. The veterinarian should apply enough pressure on each tooth to cause the polishing cup to widen or flare outward. However, the veterinarian should be gentle and apply the pressure at a setting below 3000 rpm. The veterinarian should work diligently to give the teeth a fine polish on the surfaces of the supra- and subgingival regions. Cats are cleaned with a Cavi-jet type system. This system has small prophy cups which are appropriate for the small sized teeth found in cats.

Positioning a Patient for a Dental Exam

The handling of the animal requires precise, directive movements. One such movement involves **lifting the animal by the sternum**. This cuts down on the likelihood of the animal experiencing gastric torsion. In addition, it is not a good idea to turn the animal an excessive amount of times as this increases the likelihood of more stress. The veterinarian should finish the dental procedure on one side of the mouth before moving on to the other side. The labial region (the region of the lips) on the animals should be scaled and polished before the other areas are addressed. The second surfaces to be addressed are the palate and the tongue section behind the lips. The veterinarian will finish one side before the animal is turned for work on the other side of the mouth. The scaling and polishing should then be completed on the remaining labial, palatal, and lingual sections of the mouth.

Dental Charts

The veterinarian should check the patient's file and dental chart at the outset of each visit. The dental chart is the written record of every visit that the patient has made. The design and layout of the chart will be determined by the facility's selection among the chart formats available. The chart should include a section to verbally describe each tooth and tooth surface.

The written record should be organized in such a way as to give sufficient space to document the condition of the teeth. This section should include a listing of all known calculus, caries, fractures, gingivitis index, malocclusions, resorptive lesions, and oral lesions.

The chart in the animal's permanent record should make note of any dates that the animal received dental care. In addition, the chart should describe the treatment and prognosis given at the time of the visit. The veterinarian will rely on the accuracy of this record in treating the patient on the next visit. The veterinarian will need to make an assessment of the overall treatment success or failure in comparison with the state of the mouth on the initial visit.

Routine Dental Examination Precautions

There are a number of **risks involved in a routine dental examination**. One risk involves the **temporomandibular joint**. This joint is subject to harm if the proper size mouth gag is not applied during the examination. Another more common risk involves **fluid aspiration**. Fluid aspiration can occur when the dental exam is not conducted with the correct dorsal positioning of the animal. Moreover, this aspiration can be prevented when a cuffed endotracheal tube and a pharyngeal pack are applied. The patient's head should be positioned with its face down. This allows the fluids to drain properly from the mouth. The table should be inclined to promote this drainage.

Hypothermia is also another risk associated with a routine dental examination. The patient can have a heat pad placed underneath its body to minimize this possibility. Another method to maintain body temperature calls for a circulating water blanket.

The patient should have its eyes covered to prevent any injury from occurring. The turning of the patient should be conducted in such a way that the sternum is rolled under. Large-breed animals are particularly susceptible to harm if turning is not done correctly.

Controlling Oral and Environmental Bacteria

The staff seeks to **control cross-contamination** that would negatively impact the health of the patient and the staff. This cross-contamination prevention requires the staff to take advance measures that would provide protection from any contaminants. The staff should only use equipment and implements that have been completely sterilized. In addition, all implements and equipment must first be thoroughly washed and rinsed. The removal of gross fragments must be accomplished during the wash. The implements are washed with a detergent-based solution. The implements and detergent are placed within an ultrasonic bath and covered. The sharp and hinged instruments are given a surgical milk wash to reduce the contaminants hiding within the crevices.

The **autoclave** is incorporated in the next part of the sterilization process. The use of autoclave film or envelopes will reduce the time needed for the autoclave process. However, for those items that cannot be placed in the autoclave it is recommended to use plastic infection barriers. The staff should maintain sterilization procedures that ensure sterile areas remain uncontaminated. Staff members should follow the directions suggested by the manufacturer of the product to ensure that sterilization procedures are maintained.

Dental Radiography

Dental radiographs are instruments which supply the veterinarian with x-ray images of the animal's mouth. The animal's dental needs can be assessed based on the **condition of the teeth** and **gingival sulcus**, **spot cavities**, **resorptive lesions**, and **retained roots**. In addition, the x-ray can give the veterinarian the ability to judge the severity of any intraoral neoplasia present. The x-ray can also be useful in assessing the condition of the bone and root system of the teeth. The veterinarian can use the x-ray to count the teeth in the mouth. Any periapical abscesses present within the mouth are also exposed by the x-ray images.

The veterinarian will recommend the practice of giving **scheduled dental radiographs** to young animals. This routine practice should provide the veterinarian and other caregivers a means of reviewing the permanent dentition recorded in the animal's charts. The animal with periodontal disease should be scheduled for radiographs at a rate of every 12 to 24 months.

Protecting the Technician During a Dental Examination

There are certain procedures that the dental technician should use for **protection against injury during a dental examination**. The first area of concern involves the technician's clothing. The equipment that provides the **most protection against bacteria** include a surgical mask, glasses, and disposable gloves. Further reduction of bacteria can be accomplished by an application of spray in the patient's mouth. This spray consists of a solution that is 0.12% chlorhexidine.

In addition, the technician should work on the animal from a **sitting position**. This position reduces stress on the technician's back. The animal should be at a height where the technician's forearms and wrists can rest on the table. The technician's knees should be able to fit comfortably under the table that the animal is resting upon. The technician's thighs should be in a horizontal position facing the table. The technician's hand should be able to rest on the surface of the table to gain support.

The dental examination should be performed in conditions where the **lighting is good**. The best lighting conditions include head-mounted halogen lights and/or a directional light mounted to the ceiling.

Radiography

Types of Film and the Parallel Technique Used

Film types used to take images of the incisors and canines (eye teeth) in dogs are known as **occlusal films**. A benefit in using size 2 film is its common use in human dentistry. Products used widely are usually far less expensive and are available for purchase in bulk quantities. The film can be purchased in speeds ranging from A-F. However, the film ranging from D-F is rated at a greater speed. The most widely used speed is the film rated as E.

The parallel technique for radiographs requires that the veterinarian position the film in the animal's mouth in a parallel relationship to the long axis of the tooth, and perpendicular to the entering x-rays. Thus, the film is placed in front of the tongue next to the tooth or teeth to be captured on film. The technician will move the x-ray tube so that the tip of the tube and the elongated extremity of the tooth are perpendicular to each other. Then, the beam of the x-ray will irradiate in a perpendicular direction to the film. The image will be made with the midsection of the film parallel to and directed at the targeted tooth or teeth. The image may also include other related structures found in the animal's mouth.

Benefits of Dental Radiography and Types of Film Used

The veterinarian should take a **dental radiograph** prior to any extraction of a tooth. This gives the veterinarian the ability to ascertain the condition of the root system and the number of teeth involved in the procedure. Endodontic procedures applied in the treatment of dental pulp diseases are established as effective when radiographic images are consulted. The veterinarian will also use these images to follow-up on root canal procedures. The radiographs are employed in the determination of the file depth.

Intra-oral film used in dental radiography is available in different sizes. However, the most widely used is for the treatment of dogs and cats. The sizes of intra-oral film applicable for cats are those which number 0 or 2. The sizes of intra-oral film applicable for dogs are those which number 2 or 4. The application of size 4 film is required to take images of the incisors and canines (eye teeth) in dogs.

Film Placement Using the Bisecting Angle Technique and Tube Shift Technique

The **bisecting angle** technique can be applied to gain other specifically distorted (but potentially advantageous) images. If the tooth is imaged on the film with a longer appearance, it is known as elongation. This result can be achieved by aligning the x-ray beam to the tooth (rather than to the film) at a 90 degree angle. The veterinarian may take the images using an intraoral or an extraoral film type.

The **tube shift technique** is applicable for obtaining radiographs in conjunction with the bisecting angle technique. The tube shift technique can be referred to as the localization technique, the buccal object rule, or "SLOB". All of these refer to the same technique. The acronym SLOB indicates the following: S for same; L for lingual; O for opposite, and B for buccal. Two radiographs capture the image of the target and the reference object. Lingual to the reference point are those objects that have the appearance of moving in a similar direction to the direction in which the tube head was aligned. Buccal to the reference object are those objects that have the appearance of moving in an opposing direction than the direction in which the tube was aligned.

Film Placement Using the Parallel Technique and the Bisecting Angle Technique

Any film placed in an animal's mouth should be held firmly in place with a section of gauze that has been pressed between the upper part of the film and the teeth's occlusal surfaces. This exacting placement allows the veterinarian to target specific areas in the mouth, like the mandibular molars or the premolars. Other techniques can be applied to gain the dental radiographic images needed.

If the space between the tooth and the film is larger than a 15 degree angle, then the bisecting angle technique may be needed. The veterinarian will place the film behind the targeted tooth at an angle that divides the space that exists between the film and the long extremity of the tooth in half. The technician will then position the tip of the long x-ray tube perpendicular to the bisected angle. The tooth will be imaged on the film with a shorter appearance known as foreshortening. This result can be achieved by aligning the x-ray beam to the film (rather than the tooth) at a 90° angle or perpendicular position.

Chew Toys and Hard Food

Chew toys are beneficial in **maintaining a healthy mouth with clean teeth**. The benefits are derived by the chewing action which reduces the buildup on teeth and periodontal ligaments. The dog should not be given chew toys or chew bones that are harder or more resilient than the dog's teeth, as these could cause the dog undue trauma or fractures. The dog should not be given any dried hooves or nylon chew bones. These types of products have been associated with injuries involving slab fractures in the animal. Nylon rope toys can also cause injury to gingival tissue. Tennis balls can lead to the exposure of dental pulp. Dense rubber toys or rawhide strips allow the jaw bones to be exercised while the plaque and calculus is removed from the teeth. Rawhide absorbs the animal's saliva during the chewing process. Consequently, the strip becomes soft and removes further debris from among the teeth's crevices. The dog can safely swallow the rawhide pieces. Hard food should be given to the animal to reduce the soft food debris that can adhere itself to the teeth. The caregiver should make chew toy and hard food selections based on products that have received the approval of the Veterinary Oral Health Council or VOHC.

Home Dental Care

Home dental care can be managed by conscientious animal owners. Instruction regarding the importance of managing plaque and tartar buildup can support and encourage proper home dental care. The caregiver should be instructed on how to brush the animal's teeth, and should check the mouth before brushing. This oral examination may detect painful areas or other problematic areas in the mouth. The caregiver should not brush the teeth if problems are detected, so as to keep additional trauma from occurring to diseased areas. Brushing should not be done along teething gums as this can be painful on the animal. Veterinary products can be applied in daily tooth brushing. Home care applications can include antibacterial or fluoride products. Daily cleaning, emphasizing the teeth's crown, helps prevent problems from developing. Some benefits are also found in products like chew toys and hard food that help reduce the buildup of food and debris found on the teeth. However, there is still a need to provide the animal with expert care by licensed veterinarians. This care includes routine oral examinations.

Normal Cat or Dog Occlusions or Bites

Normal occlusion is the act of bringing the upper and lower teeth to a **closed position or bite**. The normal bite that is recommended for cats and dogs is a **scissor bite**. In general, a scissor bite means that that the upper carnassial teeth overlap the lower carnassials. A scissor bite is also described as a closing of the lower incisors just behind the upper incisors, along with the closing of the lower canines between the upper incisors and canines, without touching each other. This bite pattern differs some in dogs. The carnassial teeth are fashioned from the upper fourth premolars and the lower first molars. All meat-eating or carnivorous animals will have carnassial teeth fashioned from the last upper premolar and last molar in the animal's mouth. Studies reveal that the canine (eye) teeth and the maxillary fourth premolar teeth (carnassial teeth) appear to be at a greater risk of fracture than other teeth. Thus, they deserve careful and regular examination.

Vocabulary Terms

Malocclusion: This term is used to describe the condition existing when the teeth in the maxilla do not make proper contact with those in the mandible, when biting down.

Prognathism: This term is used to describe the physical position of the maxilla to the lower jaw. In this case, the lower jaw projects out past the maxilla or upper jaw. This is also known as "undershot" or "bulldog bite". This physical malformation is more common in brachycephalic breeds that have short, broad-shaped heads. This condition can occur in conjunction with animals that display an anterior crossbite.

Brachygnathism: This term is used to describe the physical position of the upper jaw projecting out past the lower jaw. This malformation is due to the mandible being shorter than the maxilla. This is also known as overshot jaw or parrot mouth.

Level bite: This term refers to a situation where the upper and lower incisor teeth meet each other end to end, rather than the upper (maxillary) incisors just overlapping the lower (mandibular) incisors as they should.

Wry mouth: This term refers to the animal with half of its jaw somewhat longer on one side than on the other side. This condition is not easily treatable. In addition, this condition tends to be hereditary.

Posterior crossbite: A condition in which the maxilla is narrower in width than the mandible in the back, positioning the upper fourth premolar inside the lower first molar. This is a rare occurrence, particularly in dogs that have long noses.

Oligodontia: This term refers to the animal that has fewer teeth than normally found in the animal's breed.

Anodontia: This term refers to the congenital absence of teeth.

Edentulous: Refers to having lost all teeth (typically later in life).

Polydontia: This term refers to the animal that has more teeth than is normally found in the animal's breed.

Dental interlock: A condition in which the growth of one jaw can be restricted by the eruption of deciduous teeth that have developed in an abnormal fashion. The mandible may stop developing in a normal fashion when other deciduous teeth interrupt the process. One illustration is when the upper deciduous canines emerge rostral to the lower canine teeth to "lock" or prevent the mandible's normal forward development.

Retained deciduous teeth: A condition in which the deciduous tooth's root system is not reabsorbed to allow growing space for the permanent or adult teeth. When this growing space is not given, then the permanent tooth will be unable to grow and erupt properly. Typically, this changes the tooth's position in the mouth and results in malocclusion. This condition is more commonly found in toy breed dogs.

Fibrosarcoma and Epulis

Fibrosarcoma is the third most common cancerous tumor found in dogs. This cancer can quickly develop, and it has a tendency to spread. The tumor has an abnormal formation which presents as a firm nodule. Tumor-induced ulcerations and/or necrosis can sometimes also appear. The veterinarian will need to perform a biopsy before being able to make a clear diagnosis. However, the veterinarian may well give the caretaker a guarded prognosis once the diagnosis of fibrosarcoma has been determined. The veterinarian will surgically resect (remove) the cancerous tumor. However, it should be expected that a large mass of surrounding muscle and bone will also require removal. In addition, the patient will more than likely require follow-up treatment with chemotherapy and radiation.

Not all tumors are malignant. One type of nonmalignant tumor is known as epulis. This oral tumor can be found in dogs and, rarely, in cats.

Gingival Hyperplasia

The animal that has **gingival hyperplasia** can experience a gradual enlargement and overgrowth of the gums. The enlarged areas of the gums can trap plaque and calculus below the gum line.

This condition can be attributed to genetic factors or it can be attributed to the excessive administration of drugs. The following drugs are particularly prone to inducing this condition: diphenylhydantoin, nitrendipine, nifedipine, and cyclosporine.

Animals having this condition will exhibit gradually **expanding mass or masses near the gum line, bleeding gums, and mouth tenderness**. Large and giant breed dogs more commonly present with gingival hyperplasia. Boxers are also more prone to gingival hyperplasia. Other dogs associated with gingival hyperplasia include the Great Dane, Collie, Doberman Pinscher, and Dalmatian. The enlarged mass or masses can be surgically removed by the veterinarian. The application of a scalpel blade can be used as long as the animal is under anesthesia. However, this condition may need to be repeated as these growths can come back in the future.

Gemini, Fusion and Enamel Hypoplasia

Gemini (dental): This term refers to a single root with 2 crowns. This abnormality is a result of 2 teeth that did not properly divide into 2 fully developed teeth.

Fusion: This term refers to the development of a single larger tooth from 2 teeth buds. This large tooth is developed by a joining or merging of 2 or more teeth including the crowns, roots, and dentin.

Enamel hypoplasia: This term refers to a state where tooth enamel does not form correctly or is damaged during development. Either mishap will cause portions of the enamel to be omitted or diminished. The weakened enamel may wear or chip away, leaving the dentin open to the elements. The dentin cannot hold up to oral events and exposures without proper enamel protection. Therefore, these teeth will deteriorate more quickly than teeth that have developed normally. Another name for enamel hypoplasia is distemper teeth, in reference to young dogs with enamel hypoplasia due to a distemper virus infection prior to the eruption of their permanent teeth.

STOMATITIS

Stomatitis is a condition in which the **mucous membranes lining the mouth become red and irritated**. This inflammation often involves cheeks, gums, tongue, lips, and the roof or floor of the mouth.

Stomatitis may form as a consequence of poor oral hygiene, iron deficiency anemia, foreign bodies, and thermal, chemical, or electrical burns (chewing on electrical cords, indiscriminate ingestions, etc.). It usually represents an inefficient immune response. Cats may contract stomatitis from coming into contact with a bacterial plaque that induces hypersensitivity or an allergic reaction. Animals having stomatitis may exhibit a number of symptoms, including a change in behavior, severe pain, irritability, aggressiveness or depression, excessive drooling, or changes in appetite. The appetite changes may be attributed to problems associated with chewing and eating.

The veterinarian will check for a series of multiple lesions around a tooth or an entire gum line. The lesions appear as broken or infected skin. The veterinarian that detects such lesions can diagnose the patient with stomatitis, indicating the mouth inflammation in the animal.

ABSCESSED TOOTH

The veterinarian should check animals with serious, **progressive periodontal disease** on a regular basis. Animals can develop accelerated decay and root abscesses as a result of this disease. The most common location for an abscess is the fourth premolar. This is the carnassial tooth in canines. The fourth premolar is unique in that it has 3 roots attached to the tooth. Out of these 3 roots, the one nearest to the surface is the one most likely to become abscessed.

To develop an **abscess**, infectious bacteria must work past the gum line and into the root. This will be easier in situations of serious decay or broken teeth. As soon as the bacteria arrive at the root system, they begin attacking the tissues. The root has little resistance to the attack. Thus, the attack will ultimately lead to the formation of an abscess (i.e., a pus pocket), trapped at the base of the tooth. In situations of considerable swelling, the abscess may present as a lump underneath the skin. In the case of a carnassial tooth, the lump is located right beneath the eye.

CONDITIONS ASSOCIATED WITH MISDIRECTED TEETH AND RETAINED DECIDUOUS TEETH

Misdirected teeth are created when an animal's deciduous teeth impede the intended positioning of the animal's permanent teeth.

Deciduous or baby teeth may also be called "milk teeth", "primary teeth", "temporary teeth", and "first set" teeth.

Occasionally, an animal will not lose its deciduous teeth. When this occurs it is referred to as "**retained deciduous teeth**". When deciduous teeth are retained, any emerging adult tooth brings pressure to bear on the root system at the base of the deciduous tooth. The 2 teeth fight for the same space, typically causing the permanent tooth to develop and emerge on one side or another of the pre-existing deciduous tooth. Thus, with a deciduous tooth still in place, the normal eruption of a permanent tooth is redirected to a different location in the mouth. This misdirection gives the condition its name.

The double sets of teeth trap food and thus lend to dental decay. The double sets of roots prevent normal development of the tooth socket, and ultimately erode gum support around both teeth. The animal suffering from this condition may present with abnormal wear, periodontal disease, and/or premature tooth loss. Pulling retained teeth early on is the solution.

Impaction, Worn Teeth, Caries, Eosinophilic Ulcers, and Dental Trauma

Impaction: Refers to a tooth that that fails to emerge from beneath the gums. It stays inside the tissue or bone and causes the animal pain.

Worn teeth: Teeth that are worn down badly. It is most apparent when the brown center of dentin is exposed. This can be detected with a dental explorer. When applied as a probe, it may reveal flaws in the dentin.

Caries: Refers to cavities or hollow erosions in the teeth at points of decay. Coronal caries do not occur as often in meat-eating animals. This can be related to the high pH found in the carnivorous mouth. The pH level is higher than that found in human mouths. Even so, bacteria in the mouth emit acids, and thereby produce the progressive dental decay called caries.

Eosinophilic ulcers: These non-life-threatening ulcers typically appear on the lips and tongue. Normally healing quickly, they may sometimes persist 12 months or more. Trauma (injury) is the usual causative factor. When occurring on the upper lips of cats, this condition is also known as rodent ulcers (from the old belief that cats contracted the ulcers from hunting rodents). The ulcer is formed when a localized invasion of white blood cells disrupts microcirculation to tissue cells. This destroys the healthy cells and causes a sore to form.

Trauma (dental): Sudden injury from an object or event that impacts the teeth and surrounding tissues.

Abscessed Tooth, Oronasal Fistula, and Tetracycline Staining

In some situations, the **abscessed tooth** may exude a yellow or green discharge, which further indicates an infection is present. The abscess may also stop the discharge and close up. However, the potential for further complications is high for abscesses not given the proper medical attention. An **untreated abscess can lead to an infection in the head or in an ey**e, resulting in subsequent blindness. In addition, the animal may suffer from a widespread loss of its teeth as the infection disperses throughout the root system.

The maxilla is the upper jawbone. It can also become abscessed, resulting in a condition known as **oronasal fistula**. A fistula is a narrow passageway between 2 spaces. An abscess-induced oronasal fistula is the result of erosion between the oral cavity and the anterior respiratory tract. This fistula can allow food and fluids to enter the respiratory tract, resulting in chronic inflammation and infection. The dog may exhibit symptoms such as nasal discharge, a protuberance on top of the tooth root, sneezing, and a persistent cough.

Tetracycline is an **antibiotic that may be used in cases of abscess**. The veterinarian should be aware that tetracycline can cause a pregnant dog or young puppies to have teeth that are yellow in color. This is a result of tetracycline staining.

Gingivitis Indices GI2-GI3 and the Periodontal Index

Moderate gingivitis is designated as GI2 and is characterized by gums that bleed during the exam, and by the presence of edema or fluid (i.e., puffy gums). However, the gums will still have a normal gingival sulcus depth.

The last designation is described as GI3. This designation is given for advanced gingivitis. The gums will be inflamed and be edematous and will present with excessive bleeding. The animal may already have attachment loss, with some teeth loose or missing.

Ultimately, the animal can also experience **periodontal attachment loss**. This is measured by degrees. The percentage or proportion in one-hundredths of the periodontal support destroyed by the gum disease is known as the periodontal index. The periodontal support is the connective tissues that enclose the tooth and its root system. A periodontal probe is used to make an assessment of the degree of attachment loss in the animal's mouth.

Gingivitis and the Gingivitis Index

Gingivitis is a term referring to general inflammation of the gums. It can be localized to one tooth, or it can be widespread. It is caused by a buildup of food debris and bacteria called plaque. Left uncleaned, plaque hardens into tartar, making it even more difficult to keep the teeth clean of plaque. Most bacteria found in plaque are aerobic, gram-positive rods and cocci. Treatment of gingivitis may cure or alter the course of the gum's condition. Untreated, gingivitis can spread into the ligaments and bone that support the teeth and cause them to eventually fall out.

The gingivitis index is used to measure the amount of inflammation present within the animal's mouth. The designation of GI0 is given to describe normal, healthy gingival tissue. This state is characterized by fresh breath, pink gum coloration, and a normal gingival sulcus depth. GI1 is described as marginal gingivitis. Marginal gingivitis will have some edema, but will not bleed during the probe. The gums will have a normal gingival sulcus depth.

Mobility Index

The veterinarian will employ the **mobility index** to determine the **amount a tooth has moved**. This measurement calculates the change of a tooth in relation to its socket. This can help in determining the extent of disease present. This is needed to indicate a tooth's stability given the progression of periodontal disease. The designation of M0 indicates no movement. The designation M1 indicates movement measured at less than 1 mm laterally and with no apical mobility. M1 designation is given when small sideways movements can occur with pressure. It also indicates that no upward (outward) movement is permitted. M2 is given to designate moderate tooth mobility. The measurement indicates 1 to 2 mm of movement laterally, but still without either apical or upward mobility. The designation M3 indicates both lateral and apical mobility. The tooth is moving to the side and in an upward direction. Typically, the veterinarian will recommend extraction of a tooth with an M3 designation.

Periodontal Disease

Periodontal disease attacks the support system of the mouth. This system includes the gingiva, ligaments, cementum, and supporting bone. The gingiva is the flesh that encloses the roots of the teeth. The ligaments are made of tough fibrous tissue that connects the tooth to the bones in the mouth. The cementum is the bony tissue that encloses the root system of the teeth. The supporting bone is made from collagen fibers and calcium phosphate.

Periodontal disease first appears as red and swollen gingiva (gums). Dogs and cats usually do not develop periodontal disease until after the age of 4. However, at least 85% of all dogs and cats over the age of 4 will have early periodontal disease. The animal that has this disease will initially exhibit a buildup of plaque on the teeth. Plaque is described as a soft deposit caused by the residue that builds up on the teeth from saliva, mucus, bacteria, and food debris. Left uncleaned, plaque will eventually harden and mineralize into calculus or tartar on the teeth.

Periodontal Index and the Mobility Index

The **periodontal index** is measured in millimeters. The measurement is taken from the **cementoenamel junction (CEJ) to the lowest point of the problem**. The designation given for healthy gingiva is PI0. Healthy gums will have deep, solid structures. The gums will have no evidence of inflammation or disease. The designation of PI1 is described as an absence of attachment loss. However, PI1 does indicate that the animal suffers with gingivitis. The designation of PI2 will be given to animals that have less than 25% attachment loss. The designation of PI3 will be given to animals that have 25 to 50% attachment loss. The designation of PI4 will be given to animals that have a 50% or greater attachment loss.

The periodontal support system includes the gingiva, ligaments, cementum, and supporting bone. This support system works to keep the teeth in position inside the mouth. The gingiva is the flesh that encloses the roots of the teeth. The ligaments are tough fibrous tissue that connects the bones in the mouth. The cementum is the bony tissue that encloses the root system of the teeth. The supporting bone is made from collagen fibers and calcium phosphate.

Periodontal Disease and Treatment Methods

The **plaque** will eventually transform into a mineral known as **calculus (or tartar).** The development of calculus will escalate the periodontal disease process, making it easier for bacteria and debris to accumulate around the teeth. In addition, the bacteria now accumulating will be anaerobic, gram-negative rods and various filamentous organisms. Endotoxins and exotoxins will be created. Endotoxins are released when bacteria decompose. Exotoxins that are released by bacteria can have negative impacts on the central nervous system. These toxins further damage tissues and undermine the support structure of the tooth. Periodontal disease is progressive in nature and cannot be cured. However, animals with this disease do respond positively to dental management and care.

The severity of the disease can only be diagnosed by a veterinarian. The veterinarian may employ a number of treatments in the care and management of the disease. Treatment that can have beneficial impact to the animal includes: a) complete scaling and prophy (tooth polishing), b) root planing, c) antibiotics, d) gum surgery, e) tooth extraction, f) home care, and g) products like dry food and chew toys, as recommended by the Veterinary Oral Health Council or VOHC.

Gum Diseases

Causes of Gum Disease and First 2 Classifications (Grade 0 and Grade I).

Gum disease can be prevented with proper care of the animal's teeth. This care requires daily maintenance due to the nature of the mouth. Plaque can build up on the teeth within a 6 hour period. Plaque is formed from organic debris and bacteria which can be transformed through a mineralization process to produce a hard deposit on the teeth after only 24 to 48 hours. This hard deposit is called calculus or tartar. The flesh around the gums becomes further inflamed in response to the calculus on the teeth. Other changes in the body can negatively impact the health of the gums. Some factors include imbalances in the blood or hormones. These factors are secondary aspects to be considered in the prognosis and treatment plan, but are not the originating cause of the disease.

There are a total of 4 grades used in **classifying gum disease**.

Healthy gums have the following classification and characteristics: Grade 0 gingival tissues show a sharp gingival margin, pink coloration, and emit no unpleasant smells. Grade I gum disease has marginal gingivitis, physical evidence of gram-positive aerobic cocci and rods, a minor red coloration to the gums, a mildly unpleasant smell, but no evident swelling.

Gum Disease From Grade II to Grade V.

Grade II gum disease has moderate gingivitis, a deep red coloration, and inflamed and swollen gums. The veterinarian should expect the gums to bleed during the examination. The designation of Grade III gum disease has severe gingivitis, early periodontitis, deep red and purple coloration to the gum margins, and swollen pockets along the gums. The veterinarian should expect bleeding of the gums during examination.

Grades I, II, and III can be resolved. Grades IV and V are irreversible in nature.

Grade IV gum disease has moderate periodontitis, intensely reddened and irritated gums, deep pockets with swelling, and minimal tooth movement. Grade V gum disease has severe periodontitis, prominent tooth movement, tooth loss, 50% or more loss of bone, evidence of anaerobic gram-negative rods, and a profuse quantity of infectious mucus.

Feline Odontoclastic Resorption Lesions

Feline odontoclastic resorption lesions, or FORL, are common observations made when treating cats. Other names for FORL are feline cervical lesions, neck lesions, or enamel erosions. These lesions should not be mistaken for caries. The lesion originates at the CEJ (the tooth's cemento-enamel joint). There will be **evidence of missing enamel**. The granulation tissue (fibrous connective tissue found in healing wounds) inside the lesions has small lumps with a rough, grainy texture. Cells inside of the lesions differentiate into odontoclasts along the periodontal ligament, causing dentin and root replacement resorption as they attack and take in the nutrients or chemicals found in the dentin and enamel. The lesions will work into the pulp. The outward appearance of the tooth can be misleading, as the root may be small or nonexistent. There may also be one or more lesions on both the lingual or buccal side of the tooth. These lesions should be considered progressive in nature. Not all lesions are visible. Some lesions are found beneath areas of plaque or inflamed gums. The veterinarian should particularly examine multi-rooted teeth and the molars and premolars for resorption lesions. However, there is a possibility that these lesions will appear on the canines and incisors.

Causes and Signs

The reason an animal develops **feline odontoclastic resorption lesions** (FORLs) is not known. Some theories state that the inflammation is a consequence of plaque that incites odontoclast cells to break down the enamel. Nutritional hyperparathyroidism could also be a contributor to FORLs. Another contributing theory involves a chronic calcii virus. Some believe that another viral infection during the tooth's growth and development is the reason behind FORLs. Still others believe that long-term regurgitation of hair balls is a contributing factor. Another theory holds that the animals have a diet lacking essential pH. Of note, FORLs have a propensity to attack purebred felines. These purebreds include Persians, Abyssinians, Siamese, Russian blue, Scottish fold and

Oriental shorthairs. This propensity may point to genetic factors as contributing to the onset of the disease.

Regardless of the cause, the animal will experience severe pain. The lesions produce even more pain when they have been allowed to eat away at the enamel. The animal suffering with FORLs will react negatively to this intense pain. Some symptoms to look for include change in appetite, change in food preference, difficulty chewing, irritability, aggressiveness, tenderness in the jaws, bleeding around the mouth, and/or excessive salivation.

Classifications

Feline odontoclastic resorption lesions, or FORLs, are designated in 5 stages. These designations are given in relation to the degree of identified deterioration. Stage I addresses minimal loss. Stage I FORLs are diagnosed when erosion into the tooth's enamel is measured at less than 0.5 mm at the neck. Stage II FORLs are diagnosed when the lesions have been able to enter and spread through the dentin. Stage III FORLs are diagnosed when the lesions have been able to spread into the pulp canal, but have not yet had significant impact upon the tooth's structural foundations. Stage IV FORLs are diagnosed when the lesions have been able to enter and spread through the pulp canal so drastically that the tooth's structural foundations have been negatively impacted. This results in a significant tooth loss. However, Stage V is so severe that it is only diagnosed when the roots are still attached, but the tooth's entire crown is missing. At this point, the root may have become "ankylosed" (or fused) to the adjacent bone, as the periodontal ligament will likely have been replaced with the bone-cementum tissue.

Diagnosis and Treatment

The veterinarian should only examine the cat after the application of anesthesia. This will cause the animal to lose sensitivity to pain during this otherwise difficult examination. The veterinarian should first check the feline for evidence of noticeable lesions. The inspection should include a thorough perusal of every tooth. The veterinarian can use a dental explorer to inspect above and below the gum line. Lesions may be detected underneath sections of plaque or inflamed gums. Therefore, it is advised to **remove the plaque to increase the chance of detection**. Dental radiographs can then be obtained to isolate neck lesions. Dental radiographs can also aid the veterinarian in diagnosing the severity of the disease.

There is some controversy surrounding **tooth restoration in animals with lesions.** Restoration of a tooth with lesions will not stop the progression of the disease but may prolong the retention and use of the tooth. In general, restoration should only be done on teeth that have Stage I lesions. Teeth with lesions that are Stage II to V are usually extracted.

Characteristics and Benefits of Local Anesthesia for Animal Dental Procedures

Local anesthesia can be given when there is no evidence of infections or abscesses. Local anesthesia is usually short in duration, but can be effective for a period of 6 to 8 hours. Amide agents, derived from ammonia, can begin working after 3 to 5 minutes. The anesthesia is best administered via the nerves entering and exiting the bony foramina. The veterinarian should take precautions to prevent injury to the nerves when giving this drug through an injection.

Epinephrine is found in some types of anesthesia. This drug is a **synthetic form of adrenaline** that works to relax the airways and constrict the blood vessels. However, epinephrine is not recommended for use on some patients due to certain associated risks. Thus, the type of anesthesia should be selected in conjunction with the needs of the individual patient.

The benefits surrounding the use of local anesthesia include: a) a lower rate of postoperative discomfort; b) induced loss of sensitivity to pain can be sustained and adjusted at lower levels; and c) fewer complications in the recovery period.

Feline Lymphocytic-Plasmacytic Stomatitis

Cats are susceptible to a serious condition known as feline lymphocytic-plasmacytic stomatitis. This disease is associated with an irregular and severe immune reaction to the presence of bacteria-bearing plaque. There is no direct research that identifies any specific cause for the condition. However, specialty-bred cats like Siamese, Himalayans, and Abyssinians seem to contract the disease more often than other cats. One of the symptoms of the disease is extreme allergenic sensitivity to the plaque found on the teeth. This sensitivity may lead to an acute allergic reaction. The reaction is described as significant inflammation at the point where the teeth encounter the gum line. Typically, the disease will quickly progress to include the following symptoms: intensely red and swollen gums, inflamed lesions located along the back side of the throat or esophagus, difficulty chewing, loss of appetite, and significant weight loss. The entire oral cavity may eventually become painfully inflamed. The animal will stop grooming itself. This is due to the pain associated with the disease. Thus, the animal's fur will have an unkempt and untidy appearance. The veterinarian can perform an oral biopsy to confirm the diagnosis. The diagnosis may lead to the decision to remove some or all of the cat's teeth. Any teeth remaining in the cat's mouth should be cleaned daily.

"Floating" a Horse's Teeth

There are times when it may become necessary to "**float**" a horse's teeth. However, a veterinarian should be consulted before this decision is made. The term "floating" refers to a **file** (called a "float") which is used to **smooth a horse's teeth.** The goal is to make the horse's bite level and consistent. Unlike humans, an **adult horse's teeth continue to grow throughout its lifetime**. However, the upper jaw's structure causes the narrower, lower jaw to move in a sideways direction when the horse is eating. Thus, the horse will grind its food using a slanting chewing motion. The effect can produce pointed edges on the horse's teeth — on the upper cheek teeth toward the outside of the mouth, and on the bottom cheek teeth toward the inside of the mouth. The condition may become bad enough to cut at the horse's cheeks and interfere with the horse's eating, and the horse may even be noted to accidentally drop food and lose weight if the problem is severe. Consequently, the veterinarian will check the condition of the horse's mouth, including symptoms such as halitosis, lacerations in the mouth, and difficulty eating as noted by an inability to keep hold of its food, the presence of head tilts when wearing a bit, and undigested food present in the horse's fecal matter. All of these symptoms could lead the veterinarian to suggest that floating a horse's teeth is necessary. The horse should be examined on an annual basis by a veterinarian.

Why Floating the Teeth in Horses is Necessary

Horses will regularly have to have their **teeth floated**, meaning to file their teeth with an instrument called a float to provide them with a flat and smooth chewing surface. If a horse does not have a flat surface to chew, then it cannot digest properly, which will lead to weight loss and a decreased absorption of nutrients. A horse's upper jaw is wider than the lower jaw, which causes their teeth to wear and the edges of the upper teeth will become longer on the outside of the horse's mouth where they overhang the lower jaw. Also, the lower teeth that go into the upper jaw will wear as well. A horse's teeth are unique in that they continually emerge from the gums for the majority of their adult life and are not ground down naturally when they chew to create a flat surface due to the unequal upper and lower jaw widths, so an annual oral exam and float are necessary.

Mouth Gags for Dental Procedures

Mouth gags are used to prop open the patient's mouth during a dental procedure. Using spring-loaded mouth gags between the canines to prop the mouth open is not recommended because they produce a constant pressure that can cause bulging of the soft tissues between the mandible and the tympanic bulla of cats. The force from the mouth gag can also compress the maxillary arteries, which are a cat's main route of blood supply to the retina and the brain, which can cause temporary blindness. Another option to hold the mouth open would be to cut off the end of a 25-gauge needle cover and place it between the upper and lower canines.

Proper Safety Measures While Performing a Dental Procedure

The veterinary technician must take certain precautions during a **dental procedure**. First of all, the technician must wear a mask that includes a face shield or a mask and goggles to protect the mouth, nose, and eyes from bacteria in the patient's mouth. The technician should have appropriate seating so they can obtain proper posture while performing the dental cleaning. The patient should be intubated with an appropriately sized ET, which should be adequately cuffed to prevent aspiration. The patient's mouth should be rinsed with a diluted chlorhexidine solution or brushed with it to decrease the bacterial aerosolization of the mouth. Another major factor to consider with the dental patient is temperature regulation. The patient's head will be consistently doused in water from the cleaning as well as if there are any extractions making the patient colder. Wet towels must be consistently exchanged for dry ones under the patient's head, and the patient's temperature must be monitored closely.

Dental Home Care that Owners Can Use to Help Prevent Plaque and Tartar Buildup

It is very important that members of the veterinary team explain **dental home care** with owners. There are numerous ways to perform home dental care in between annual dental cleanings. The number one way to keep dogs' and cats' teeth clean is to brush their teeth by using a finger brush or pet-friendly toothbrush and pet-friendly toothpaste. Avoid human toothpaste. Also, food additives work by preventing further plaque buildup on the teeth by sprinkling the correct amount per body weight of the pet onto their food once daily. Water additives work by reducing the bacterial count in the pet's mouth by adding the correct amount of additive per body weight of the pet to their water daily. There are a variety of dental chews and specialized dental diets that are designed to scrape plaque off of the teeth as the pet chews.

Routine Dental Cleanings for Dogs and Cats

It is important for owners to bring their pet into the veterinarian for an annual exam, which will include a full oral exam, checking for any fractures, furcations, oral lesions, ulcers, periodontal disease, as well as gingivitis. After a dog or cat turns 1 or 2 years of age, it is time for them to have their first dental prophylaxis (**dental cleaning** to halt the progression of periodontal disease and gingivitis) if their teeth have started to develop tartar. A routine dental cleaning includes dental radiographs, ultrasonic scaling of the teeth to remove any calculus, and polishing to smooth over where the scaling took place. While the pet is under anesthesia, a thorough oral exam is performed, including checking pocket depths and assessing any tooth resorption or abnormalities seen on radiographs. Dental disease can cause pain, tooth loss, and bad breath. Any bacteria caught under the gums can travel to the vital organs such as the heart, kidneys, and liver.

Properly Maintaining the Dental Machine Before and After Each Use

There are a few components to the **dental machine** that need to be properly maintained in order for it to work properly. First, the scaler tips must be regularly checked for wear before they are used and changed out if there is more than 2 mm of wear. The high- and low-speed handpieces must be lubricated and cleaned only with alcohol after use. Lubricating the high- and low-speed handpieces prevents them from sticking. The compressor will need to be drained after each use to get rid of the extra moisture and pressure buildup. Always use distilled water for the dental machine because tap water will cause clogging, corrode the valves in the dental system, and introduce bacteria.

Caring for High-Speed Handpieces

The **high-speed handpiece** must be properly maintained so that it works properly and does not stick. The spray nozzle is the front of the handpiece head with a small hole where the water sprays out onto the teeth, and this water line can become clogged, so a gauge wire can be inserted into the hole to loosen debris, and it also should be oiled after each use. The rubber gasket on the bottom of the handpiece helps make a seal so that water and air will not leak out; this gasket needs to be replaced when it becomes worn. The head of the handpiece contains a turbine that spins, and when a lot of debris accumulates inside, it will make the turbine stick, which makes it difficult to remove the dental burrs. If the turbine begins to stick, it must be removed and the head chamber should be cleaned out with a swab of alcohol and then it should be oiled.

Maintaining Low-Speed Handpieces

The **low-speed handpiece** should be cleaned daily with hot water and a nonabrasive cleaner on the outside of the handpiece. The handpiece should be lubricated daily by rotating the pins on the bottom of the handpiece and placing oil in the smaller of the holes called the air inlet, then running the handpiece to distribute the oil for a few seconds. Every week, the nose cone, which is the removeable part of the handpiece that holds the motor, the chuck housing ring that locks and unlocks the handpiece so the prophy angle can be set in place, and the speed direction ring located in the bottom of the handpiece that changes the rotation direction to forward or reverse and control the handpiece speed should all be lubricated.

Charting During a Dental Procedure

Charting during a dental procedure is useful in that it allows the technician to make notations pertaining to every portion of the patient's mouth. The dental chart goes into the patient's medical record, so it must be organized, and charting methods must be consistent. The chart normally represents the mouth with a picture of the full dentition of the patient, and there is an area on the dental chart for notes, diagnosis, and the preferred treatment plan. Charting is normally the first step to the dental cleaning process; that way, if there is a suspected extraction, that tooth will require less scaling; therefore, less anesthesia time will be needed. The degree of calculus and plaque will be noted in the chart as well as any missing or fractured teeth. Worn teeth can be notated either by attrition (tooth-on-tooth contact) or abrasion (tooth-on-object contact). Important abnormalities to include in the dental chart would be tooth mobility, pocket depth measured by the periodontal probe, degree of gingivitis (0–3), and stage of periodontal disease. Any furcation exposure, abnormal bite, and tooth resorptions should be noted as well.

Dental Radiography

Importance of Dental Radiographs

Dental radiographs play an important role in helping the veterinarian evaluate the pet's teeth. Radiographs can show problems such as fractures, tooth root abscess, tooth resorption, bone or soft-tissue tumors, bone loss, retained deciduous teeth, and impacted teeth. A lot of patients that present for a routine dental cleaning may have other underlying oral problems. Radiographs allow the internal tooth structures, such as the roots and the bone that surrounds the roots (the alveolar bone), to be examined. Common findings seen on dental radiographs include fractures, tooth resorption, oral masses, and pockets greater than 3 mm in dogs and greater than 2 mm in cats. It is also recommended to take radiographs after tooth extraction to ensure that the entire root has been extracted and that the surrounding bone is intact.

Views and Positioning Techniques

Dental radiographs need to include the entire crown and root of each tooth to allow for an accurate diagnosis. A full-mouth set of radiographs consists of rostral maxillary and mandibular views as well as right and left maxillary and mandibular views. The maxillary canines should be imaged on their own separate oblique views to prevent superimposition of the first and second premolars on the canine roots. Parallel technique is used for imaging the caudal mandibular premolars and molars. For parallel technique, the patient is dorsal, the sensor is placed parallel to the tooth, and the X-ray head will be perpendicular to the tooth. Bisecting angles are used for all maxillary teeth and rostral mandibular teeth. For the bisecting angle technique, the patient is in sternal positioning for the maxillary teeth and dorsal positioning for imaging the mandibular teeth. The sensor is placed in the mouth under the root and tooth being imaged, and then the X-ray head is angled at a certain degree to bisect the tooth.

Laboratory Procedures

Anatomy and Physiology

Components of Whole Blood

Whole blood is formulated from a mixture of fluid and cellular substances. The substance described as fluid is referred to as plasma. **Plasma** is a yellowish liquid which contains the blood, proteins, and lipid particles in the bloodstream. Plasma makes up 55% of total blood volume. Blood plasma can be broken down into the following substances and amounts: 10% dissolved proteins, hormones, lipids, enzymes, salts, carbohydrates, vitamins, and waste materials and 90% water. Cellular components are suspended within the plasma. Upon closer examination of the cellular components, one will find erythrocytes, leukocytes, and thrombocytes (also called platelets). **Anticoagulants can be added to plasma to prevent clotting from occurring**. This becomes necessary whenever plasma is separated from whole blood anticoagulants. Serum is plasma after coagulation has already occurred. It is collected via a centrifugation or separation process that removes the clotted and solid materials from the residual fluid.

Issues Associated with Different Types of Anticoagulants

Many kinds of blood tubes are utilized in the serum separation process. These tubes have been specifically designed to perform a unique function. Whole blood and plasma are in need of a tube containing an anticoagulant. However, the technician should be aware that some types of anticoagulants in plasma can hinder the results of certain tests. Thus, the technician should be aware of the type of anticoagulant found in each tube.

For instance, Heparin is derived from a salt of sodium, potassium, lithium, or ammonium. Heparin is often the best choice to use in plasma samples. This is due to its low propensity to alter the chemical analysis done in tests. The measurement for a supplement of this anticoagulant is given at 20 units of Heparin per milliliter of blood. The anticoagulant ethylenediaminetetraacetic acid or EDTA has a low propensity to cause changes in the structure of an organism. EDTA is usually applied to hematological-based tests. However, EDTA is not a good choice when used for plasma-based tests that require chemical analysis. Finally, sodium fluoride is a glucose preservative with additional anticoagulant properties.

Separating Serum from Whole Blood Samples

A **blood sample should be allowed to reach room temperature** before attempting to separate serum from a whole blood sample. The blood requires about 20 to 30 minutes for complete clotting. The next step requires a wooden applicator stick, which is used around the rim or inside edge to separate the clot from the sides of the tube. Next, the blood goes through a centrifugation process set at 2000 to 3000 rpm for 10 minutes. The speed and time should be carefully monitored to prevent hemolysis from occurring. Hemolysis is a particularly problematic outcome of prolonged centrifugation. Next, the serum at the top of the tube is poured into another container. Another method allows the serum to be removed with a pipette or a small tube that draws the liquid out from the centrifuged tube. The liquid or serum in the pipette should also be transferred into another tube. The carefully marked tube should be placed in a refrigerator or freezer, depending upon the subsequent need.

Hemolytic and Icteric Serum

Iatrogenic conditions are events, situations, or outcomes caused by medical staff. For example, the veterinarian or assisting staff may cause hemolysis through poor specimen procurement or handling procedures — potentially requiring further blood drawing. However, in other instances hemolysis may occur for reasons outside staff control. Regardless, the technician should be aware that higher levels of phosphorus, potassium, total protein, and aspartate aminotransferase can be found in tests performed on hemolytic serum.

Serum that has a tinge of yellow color may be indicative of a more serious problem in the animal. The yellowish color is associated with a condition known as jaundice. The term "icteric" is used to describe something pertaining to or affected with jaundice. A yellow-tinged blood sample could therefore be described as icteric in appearance. Jaundice implies the presence of some form of liver disease in the animal.

The technician should also be aware that icteric serum has a tendency to produce high Bilirubin readings during the chemical analysis of the specimen. The technician should also be aware that other aspects of the test results may be impacted by these increased levels.

Lipemic and Hemolytic Serum

Describing blood serum as "**lipemic**" is to say that it has **high triglyceride or lipid levels**. These high levels are associated with 1 or 2 contributing factors. The first contributing factor involves the animal's diet. The second involves the presence of a disease that affects the animal's normal metabolism.

Lipemic serum has a murky or opaque appearance, due to the high concentration of suspended fat present. Serum that is described as lipemic may hinder accurate chemical analysis in some tests performed. Blood samples from lipemic serum–prone animals should be collected after a fast of 12 hours or more, so as to reduce the likelihood of a lipemic serum specimen.

The technician should be **alert to any serum that is pink or reddish in color**. This coloration indicates that hemolysis has taken place. Hemolysis is a condition that results whenever red blood cells have been ruptured or "lysed" (i.e., disintegration of the cell membrane). With hemolysis, hemoglobin will be released into the surrounding fluid. Other cell contents will also be released that can alter laboratory tests and findings.

Causes of Increased or Decreased Urea Output

Urea (or carbamide) is a nitrogenous byproduct of protein, and it must be eliminated from the body.

However, although urea is a waste product it also helps produce an important countercurrent system in the kidneys. This system allows for crucial reabsorption of water and essential ions. Specifically, as some urea is reabsorbed it raises the osmolarity in the kidney. The greater the osmolarity, the more water that will be reabsorbed. This is important to maintaining both blood pressure and a proper concentration of sodium ions in the blood plasma. Thus, the tubules in the kidneys work to reabsorb up to 40% of the urea (the remainder being excreted in urine and sweat). The level of excreted urea is one measure of the health of the kidney's glomerular filtration system.

Most organisms have to deal with the excretion of nitrogen waste from protein metabolism in one form or another. In aquatic organisms the most common form of nitrogen waste is ammonia. In birds and reptiles, nitrogen waste is excreted as uric acid. In other species, including mammals, nitrogen waste is excreted as urea.

Function of Creatinine in the Kidneys

A primary source of **cellular energy** is the **aerobic breakdown of ATP** (Adenosine-5'-triphosphate) to ADP (Adenosine diphosphate), by which energy is released. When sufficient oxygen is not available for this normal energy production process, the body draws upon stores of creatine phosphate (or phosphocreatine) found in the muscles and brain. This molecule is used to anaerobically generate ATP from ADP in situations of intense energy demands or low oxygen availability. A byproduct of this process is "creatinine."

The **glomeruli** in the kidneys filter almost all creatinine out of the blood. Therefore, an animal that has high blood serum levels of creatinine usually has low or non-functioning glomeruli.

Other factors that can lead to a high serum creatinine include dehydration and other pre-renal or post-renal causes. Thus, the technician should collect a serum or plasma sample for necessary testing. However, the technician should be aware that hemolytic serums can impact the results of this test. Hyperbilirubinemia (high bilirubin levels) may also provide misleading results.

Types of Samples Needed to Assess the Increased or Decreased Urea Excretion Levels

Serum samples allow the technician to **perform blood urea nitrogen (BUN)** tests on an animal. However, the use of plasma samples will not be beneficial. These samples are taken with ammonium oxalate, which creates an artificial rise in the BUN level. Likewise, plasma samples taken with fluoride will artificially lower the BUN levels. Further, samples that are **lipemic** will produce biased results.

Lipemic serum will have **high triglyceride or lipid levels**. These high levels are associated with an animal that has 1 of 2 contributing factors. The first contributing factor involves the animal's diet (i.e., a high fat diet can lead to high lipid levels in the blood). The second contributing factor involves the presence of a disease that affects the animal's metabolism.

Lipemic serum has a **murky or opaque appearance**. Serum that is described as lipemic may hinder the chemical analysis of some tests performed. Therefore, the animal should not be fed for at least 12-18 hours prior to the collection of the sample. The technician should also test the sample promptly to reduce the likelihood of bacterial contamination.

However, a **rise in serum urea nitrogen levels** can be attributed to a number of factors beyond kidney function alone. For example, dehydration and heart failure can both result in elevated blood urea nitrogen (BUN). Further, urea excretion levels can be impacted when the animal increases protein consumption. Medications and health changes, such as corticosteroids and fever, can also impact the quantity of urea expelled from the body. These factors are considered non-renal factors because they have no relation to the kidneys' performance. However, the kidneys are nevertheless impacted by various pre-renal, post-renal, and non-renal factors. Shock can be considered either a pre-renal or a post-renal factor. Other post-renal problems may involve a blockage of the ureters, bladder, or urethra.

Animals that have anorexia, liver disease, or renal tubular damage may exhibit lower levels of urea excretion. Urea levels that are high can be instrumental in the diagnosis of a low- or nonfunctioning kidney.

Causes for Increased Glucose in the Blood

Hyperglycemia is indicated when an animal has a **high level of glucose present in the bloodstream**. This is often an indication of the disease known as diabetes mellitus. The pancreas is an organ that is found near the stomach. It works to secrete hormones (including insulin), glucagon, and somatostatin into the bloodstream. Insulin is responsible for moving glucose out of the blood and into the cells, where it is burned for energy. Diabetes mellitus occurs when the pancreas produces insufficient insulin, thus allowing glucose levels in the blood to rise.

However, there are other diseases and factors unrelated to the pancreas that can produce this same condition. For example, cats can experience high levels of stress when going for a vet clinic visit. This **level of stress may induce abnormally high glucose levels**. This abnormal reading is referred to as stress-induced hyperglycemia. Other abnormal readings can be attributed to conditions such as malabsorption, chronic liver disease, etc. Thus, the technician may want to conduct a more definitive "glucose tolerance test" to gauge how well the animal makes use of carbohydrates and sugars over a longer period of time.

Virus Replication and the Signs Relative to Viral Infections

Viruses have unique need of a host. The host cell accomplishes what the virus alone cannot do. The virus is unable to generate its own nucleic acid in the replication phase. After infection, the host's cell membrane is compromised and starts to fail. This failure produces an immune response in the cell. This response is hindered due to the location and integration of the virus within the host cell. A **virion** is a form of living, infectious virus that exists within an infected host's cells. Once fully formed, each virion will leave the cell without delay in the assembly-release phase. In this phase the replicated virus releases further virus particles in the host. These particles escape the cell either by cell lysis or by "budding" outward on the cell wall. Upon complete maturation, they are ready to invade a new cell host.

Viral infections produce negative conditions in the host. These conditions can be defined by clinical analysis. The first negative condition occurs when the virus produces a disease. The disease can be described as beginning in a milder, subacute (unnoticed) form and extending into a peracute (aggressive) form, and potentially culminating in chronic, long-term illness. This virus has resulted in an apparent infection that is both clinically evident and burdensome.

Viruses Replication Process

Viruses are very different from bacteria. The replication of viruses into genetic copies of each other happens in the following 4 phases. On most occasions the virus gains entry into the host via 1 of 3 points: a) the mucosal surface of the respiratory tract, b) the urogenital regions, or c) the gastrointestinal tract. In the attachment phase, the virus will fasten itself to a host cell membrane. Then, the virus seeks to erode the nucleic acid core of the host cell membrane. This weakening of the core supplies the virus with an entry point directly into the cell. The capsid is defined as the protein-based, coiled or polyhedral structure that constitutes the shell of the virus. The shell or outer coat surrounds a virus's nucleic acid. The shell containing viral RNA or DNA is called a "viral particle" and constitutes a virion, or the infective form of the virus. The uncoating phase happens at the same time that the virus accomplishes the penetration phase. The virus then refocuses the DNA of the host cell to make a replica of its own viral nucleic acid.

Reducing the Effects of Viral Diseases

Major Factors

There are 3 critical issues that must be addressed in a viral infection. These are **health measures, immunization, and medical care**. Those coming into contact with the viral infection should make every effort to use appropriate hygienic measures. Viral infections can be reduced when hands and surfaces are disinfected on a regular basis. In addition, the bodies of deceased animals must be properly and hygienically disposed of quickly and appropriately to prevent further infection.

General principles of health maintenance are also important. Animals should be given an appropriate diet that nourishes the body with minerals and vitamins. This diet is essential in maintaining a healthy balance in the animal. In addition, clean water should be made available in a plentiful supply. The animal may experience stress when overcrowded conditions occur. Therefore, it is also essential to maintain a balance in the population. Further, newly acquired animals should only be introduced to the herd after an appropriate period of quarantine.

Other Factors That Can Help

Quarantine procedures are recommended to maintain the health of the other animals. A quarantined animal should be fully isolated from all available people and animals. This isolation should prevent the spread of a viral or other infection, and reduce all healthy animals' exposure to any diseases caused by infective processes.

Immunizations and **vaccinations** are important deterrents to infectious diseases. The client should be encouraged to maintain all recommended immunizations in order to keep each animal in optimum health. Immunizations help the animal to develop resistance to specifically targeted diseases.

Where infections nevertheless do occur, prompt **attention to symptoms** should be given. The animal should always be given an appropriate regimen of medical care upon the detection of an infection.

Signs of Viral Infections

The first negative condition occurs when the virus results in a clinically identifiable disease. This is defined by the **noticeable symptoms of infection** present in the host. However, not all diseases have immediately noticeable symptoms. Some are described as silent, nonapparent, or subclinical infections. The danger in these infections lies in the ability of the host to infect others with the disease. The host becomes a carrier for the virus. This creates a less than efficient identification and defense process.

A few models of **apparent and nonapparent infections** are found in rabies, FIV, and equine infectious anemia viruses. Some viral infections are most readily apparent when the infected cells stop functioning. This is the case where the neurons in an animal infected with rabies stop working. This also occurs in cats that have been with the FIV virus.

In addition, a host can experience an **impaired immune system** due to an infection. This is true of the horse that has been infected with the equine infectious anemia virus (EIAV). Sometimes the detrimental impact to the immune system may actually produce conditions more problematic than those caused by the virus alone.

Cellular Organelles Within the Cytoplasm and Their Functions

There are numerous **organelles** found in **cellular cytoplasm**. They include ribosomes, mitochondria, endoplasmic reticula, chloroplasts (chlorophyll, in plant cells), and Golgi bodies. **Ribosomes** are cellular organelles which manufacture cellular proteins. They can be found freely floating in the cytoplasm, arranged in small clusters, or attached to endoplasmic reticula (intracellular tubular membranes which transport materials). Ribosomes manufacture essential proteins by "reading" the RNA produced by genetic DNA, and translating it into the kind of protein indicated.

Mitochondria are specialized organelles which make up as much as 25% of the cytoplasm. Mitochondria transform organic substances from foods into a useable source of chemical energy.

The **endoplasmic** reticulum is a network of tubes that alters and transports proteins, produces and stores macromolecules (i.e., glycogen and natural steroids), and sequesters calcium.

Golgi bodies process cellular products, releasing them back into the cell or excreting them as needed.

Prokaryotic Cells and Eukaryotic Cells

Prokaryotic cells are simple organisms without a nucleus (i.e., a central structure that contains chromosomes and genes). Bacteria are a common form of prokaryotes. A typical bacterium is a single celled, parasitic microorganism. Bacteria are parasitic in that they live in or on and feed off of other organisms.

Eukaryotic cells are characterized by multiple complex structures enclosed within cellular membranes. Most eukaryotes have 3 main parts. The first part is the outer cell membrane or protective shell that allows oxygen and food particles to pass through, and waste to be excreted. The second part is the inner cytoplasm – an organic compound with the consistency of jelly – that contains cytosol and organelles. In animal life, cytoplasm occupies over half of the cell's volume. Cytosol is the watery portion of the cytoplasm, excluding all structures and organelles.

Cellular organelles, such as mitochondria, chloroplasts, and Golgi bodies, perform specific functions within the cell. The third part of the eukaryotic cell, also found in the cytoplasm, is the nucleus. It contains genetic material and controls cell growth and reproduction processes.

List and Define Epithelial and Connective Tissues as 2 of the 4 Primary Types of Tissues.

There are 4 primary tissue types in the human body: epithelial, connective, muscle, and nerve tissue. The first 2 are described here.

Epithelial tissue lines the exterior of the body, as well as all cavities and surfaces of solid structures within the body. This tissue is composed of either a single-cell layer (i.e., simple squamous or columnar cells) or several "stratified" layers of cells. Primary epithelial tissue functions include: secretion, excretion, absorption, protection, sensation detection, and selective permeability.

The second type of tissue is known as **connective tissue**. This tissue is located in a variety of places within the body. Connective tissue types determine the function that is carried out. Some types of connective tissues work to connect, support, and protect the structures and organs within the body. Other types of connective tissues work to insulate. Still others are responsible for the transportation of fluids and for energy storage.

Cell Structure, Material Processing and Routing, and Certain Enzymatic Functions

The **cytoskeleton** is the framework of the cell, and allows movement within the cell. Further, this structure protects the cell. Intracellular transportation is carried out as organelles and vesicles move about within the cytoskeleton framework.

Within each cell is a "center" called the **centrosome**. It organizes cellular microtubules, and regulates cell-cycle progression. Within the centrosome are centrioles. **Centrioles** organize and replicate the mitotic spindle for successful cell division and reorganization. The **Golgi complex** (also called the Golgi body, apparatus, or dictyosome) serves as a processing and routing system for the cell. This organelle packages proteins for use in the cell or for secretion outside the cell. The

Golgi complex also builds **lysosomes**, which are responsible for breaking down and recycling molecules within the cell. Non-working organelles, intracellular bacteria, lipids, carbohydrates, and proteins are also contained in the lysosomes.

Arising from the endoplasmic reticulum are "**peroxisomes**," which are responsible for removing toxins from the cell. Peroxisome enzymes known as oxidase and catalase carry out this elimination process. Peroxisomes can self-replicate through a process of enlarging and division.

Common Specimens

Dirofilaria Immitis

Dirofilaria immitis is the term given for a parasitic heartworm commonly associated with canines. This parasite can sometimes be seen in wet smears and in Giemsa stained smears. However, when the parasite is not present in considerable quantities, it can be overlooked. The buffy coat method should be employed to increase the chance of an accurate diagnosis and identification of the heartworm. The veterinarian should also employ the modified Knott's method and the filter technique. These 2 techniques will aid in the detection and screening of microfilaria. However, it should be noted that low quantities of filarial or afilarial organisms cannot usually be detected using these methods. Other sensitive tests like the immunological techniques should be employed instead. The antigens can be identified in cases of gravid female infestation. The animal will construct a multitude of antibodies that can be recognized with the application of ELISA techniques. ELISA is an acronym for enzyme-linked immunosorbent assay. Antibody testing is perhaps the most frequent method of diagnosis.

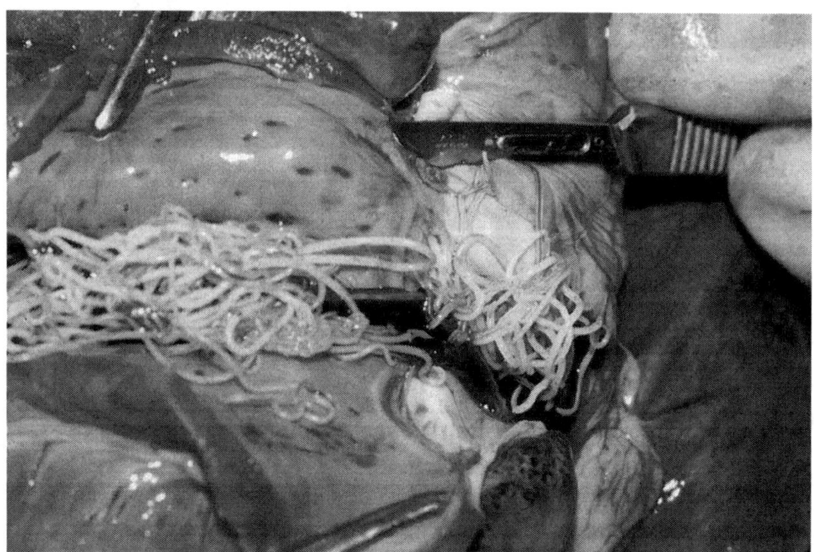

Diagnostic Characteristics of Dirofilaria Immitis

The presence of Dirofilaria immitis, or heartworm, is evident in a variety of symptoms exhibited by the host. This parasite takes up residence within the heart and pulmonary artery of the host animal. Heartworms can infect dogs, cats, and other non-domestic animals. Most animals become infected through a **mosquito bite**. Another method of transmission is through a transplacental infection of microfilaria. The prepatent period is described as the time between the initial infection and the maturation of the parasite into an adult (typically, when the parasite begins laying eggs). From infection to maturation requires a period of 6 to 8 months.

Animals that have been infected by heartworm will exhibit symptoms of **lethargy**, **exercise intolerance**, and **cough**. The cough can be more noticeable when the animal is exercising. Animals that have had heartworms for a lengthy period may exhibit additional problematic symptoms. These symptoms include: severe weight loss, fainting, coughing up blood, and congestive heart failure. Animals that are more active can exhibit symptoms of heartworm infection earlier than those less active. Likewise, animals that are heavily infected may also exhibit earlier symptoms of heartworm infection. Preventive medicine can reduce the likelihood of infection by heartworm. In particular, animals should receive limited exposure to mosquito bites.

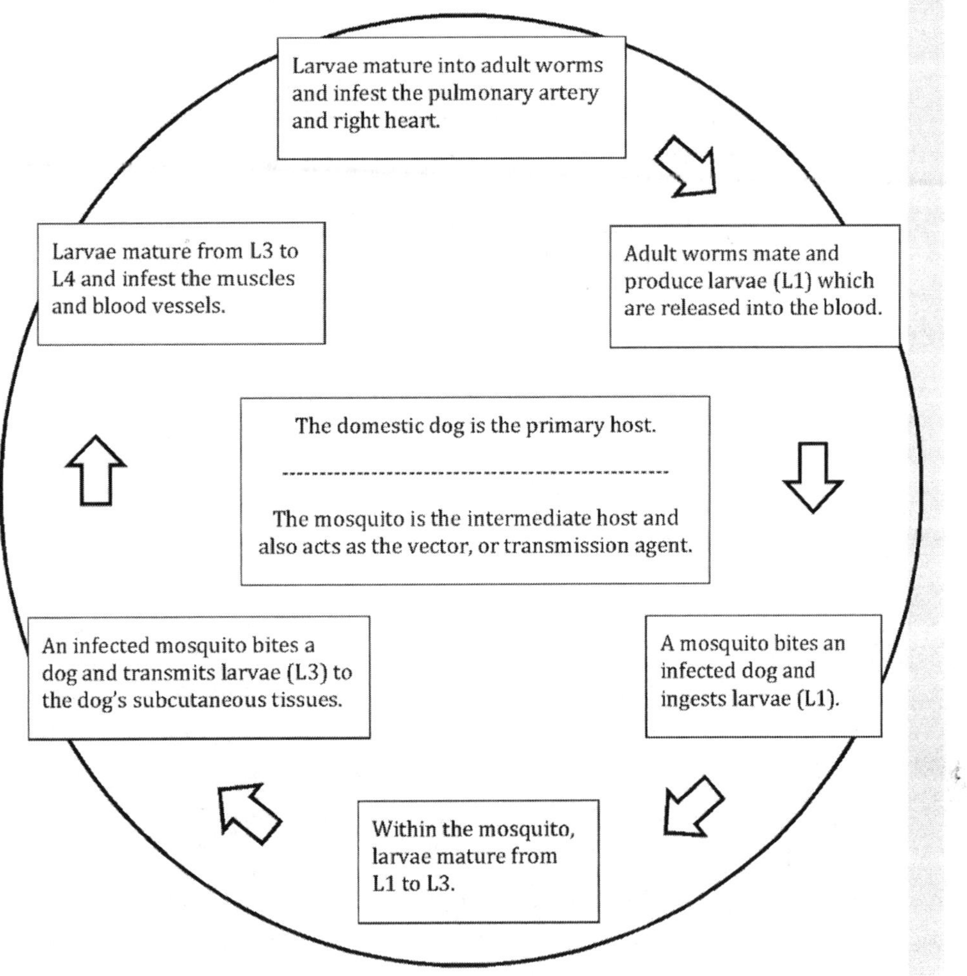

Complete Blood Count (CBC)

A **complete blood count** (CBC) gives information on the patient's RBCs, WBCs, and platelets (thrombocytes). Information provided by the CBC about RBCs is the hematocrit results, which tells how many RBCs are present, and the hemoglobin, showing how much is available. If these readings are low, it can mean that the patient is anemic, and if they are high, that points toward dehydration. A CBC also shows the total number of WBCs along with the numbers of certain types of WBCs including eosinophils, neutrophils, monocytes, lymphocytes, and basophils. An abnormal increase or decrease in WBCs can indicate severe infection going on in the body because WBCs are there to protect the body and fight infection. Platelets are another important section of the CBC because they are the first to respond to any wound, whether it is microscopic or large. If platelet numbers are reading low on the CBC, that indicates that the patient cannot form blood clots appropriately. This may be caused by an immune disorder or a serious systemic illness.

Dipylidium Caninum

Flea or **louse larvae** may ingest the eggs of Dipylidium caninum, whereupon the insect becomes infected. The potential cat or dog that ingests the adult louse or flea will become infected. This **tapeworm parasite** is able to grow into adulthood inside the animal's body. Eventually the animal discharges fecal matter that contains gravid (egg-bearing) tapeworm segments known as proglottids. These proglottids have a complete reproductive system. A clinical inspection, in the form of a fecal flotation examination, can expose proglottid segments.

The animal that has this type of infestation may be seen scrubbing its bottom across the surface of the ground. The animal may find this scrubbing action brings relief to itching and irritation in the area around the anus. This discomfort may be caused by active segments of the parasite found near the anus. Sometimes, detection can be made through inspection of the feces for more obvious segments of the tapeworm. The infected animal should be treated with medications. However, a preventive stance is recommended — principally to reduce the animal's exposure to fleas or lice infestations.

Life Cycle and Infection Routes

The diagnostic characteristics of **Dipylidium caninum tapeworm** can be seen in both dogs and cats. The prepatent period for Dipylidium caninum (the time between the initial infection and reproductive maturation) is about 3 weeks. This form of tapeworm resides in the small intestines of infected dogs and cats. The tapeworm itself presents with a long ribbon-shaped body. These worms have a head, neck, and segmented body parts. The segmented body parts are formed unceasingly in the neck region of the worm.

The older segments are found on the tip of the worm's body. These older segments (gravid proglottids) are discarded at maturational intervals. The discarded proglottid segments are able to independently reproduce, as each contains both male and female reproductive organs. The segments stay active as long as host warmth is retained. Finally, the segment opens up in order to release the eggs that are inside. These eggs are eaten by an adult louse or flea larva, ultimately to infect or be ingested by another animal.

Ancylostoma Caninum

The dog **hookworm** parasite (**Ancylostoma caninum**) can be detected by fecal flotation testing. The parasite's eggs can be observed as clear, smooth, thin-walled eggs found in the feces. The worms are not usually seen by the naked eye due to their small size. The worms range in size from about ½ to ¾ inches in length. Further, the hookworm is capable of fastening itself firmly to the wall or lining of the small intestine, and thus is not normally dislodged.

Ancylostoma caninum can have very detrimental effects on the host animal. Some of the more severe symptoms include anemia, weakness, and melena. Anemia is a condition in which the blood is deficient. Melena is a condition in which the body produces black, tarry, blood-bearing feces. The blackened, tarry feces indicate that there is bleeding in the bowel region (rather than up higher, where it would have been all or at least partially digested). This parasite infection can be treated with proper medical care. However, a preventive stance is recommended, reducing the animal's exposure to feces within its immediate surroundings.

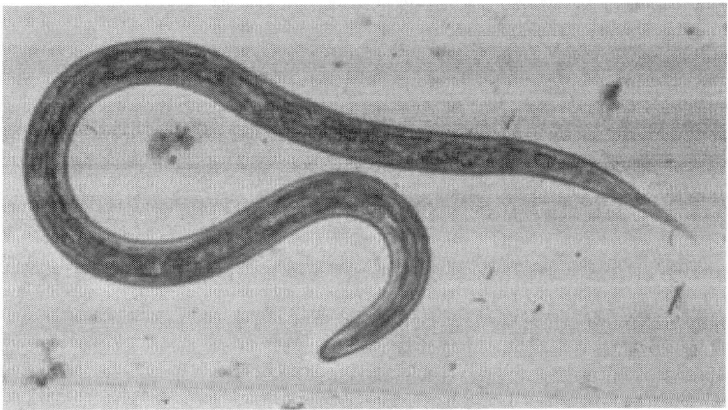

Life Cycle and Infection Routes

Ancylostoma caninum (or "dog hookworm") is defined as a hookworm that takes up residence in the small intestines of canines. Hookworms are blood-sucking parasites that can cause significant disease in the host animal. The hookworm fastens itself to the wall of the small intestine. There, the hookworm proceeds to feed on the animal's blood. Feeding is accomplished via intestinal wall penetration using its hook-like mouth.

In most cases, infection occurs when an adult dog ingests the eggs or larvae by consuming food or water that has been contaminated. The soil around the animal may also become contaminated with the larvae of the hookworm. Another method of infection occurs when a dog consumes an infected host. The canine may also become infected by larval penetration through the animal's skin. Further, young canine pups may become infected through mammary glands by drinking its mother's milk. Finally, the fetus may be infected through the uterus via the placenta. The parasite can be detected 2 to 3 weeks after the initial infection.

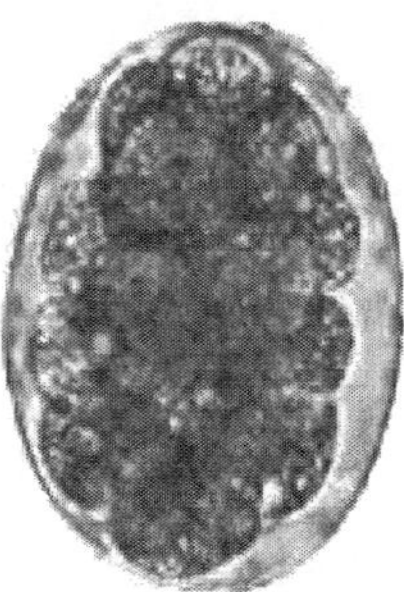

Giardia Duodenalis Life Cycle and Infection Processes

Giardia duodenalis, or simply "**Giardia**," is a single-cell protozoan that can intestinally infect an animal. Infection occurs when the host ingests dormant cysts found in contaminated water, or by consuming food contaminated with moist feces that host the parasite. As the cysts can survive for months in a moist environment – even in cold, clean-appearing water, including water treated for city drinking – infections are difficult to avoid. Once ingested, the Giardia parasite fastens itself to the surface of an animal's small intestines. These protozoans may also be found moving freely along the mucosal lining of an animal's intestines.

Giardia can infect a number of mammals, including dogs, cats, cattle, horses, sheep, goats, and pigs. Infected animals develop severe symptoms of diarrhea. Giardia duodenalis has 2 basic life cycle states: trophozoite and cystic. In the metabolically active (feeding) stage the Giardia protozoa are known as trophozoites. Possessing a flagellum, the trophozoite is motile – meaning it can move freely as it seeks nourishment. The other life cycle state is the non-motile cystic stage. At the conclusion of the trophozoite life stage, the protozoa rapidly replicate via binary fission, and then transform themselves into inactive cysts. Upon expulsion from the host, the cysts quickly become infective and thrive in any moist environment for several months.

Detection and Treatment

The cycle of **Giardia duodenalis** infection continues when a new host is attacked. The new host typically consumes water or food that has been contaminated with Giardia cysts. The infection spreads rapidly, as the infective cysts break open in the intestines of the new host animal. These broken cysts release the now metabolically active trophozoite into the new host animal. The prepatent period, the time period from initial infestation to reproductive maturity, for Giardia is 7 to 10 days.

The fecal flotation method is usually effective in making a diagnosis of the infection. Another method used is the direct smear technique. A diagnosis is confirmed when either the cysts or the trophozoites are viewed. The cysts present a smooth, thin-walled protective covering which protects the parasite held inside. The trophozoite has a piriform (pear or teardrop) shape. The trophozoite has bilateral symmetry and a light coloration of green. Giardia can be effectively treated with medication and proper follow-up medical care.

Trichuris Vulpis Life Cycle and Infection Routes

Trichuris vulpis, or **Whipworm**, is a type of **nematode** or **roundworm** that can be found in human and canine intestines. The whipworm gets its name from its shape, similar to a whip. The whipworm resides in the cecum and large intestines of canines. The prepatent period (from infestation to maturation) is about 3 months.

An animal is infected by whipworm through the consumption of food or drink that has been contaminated with infective eggs. In the process of digestion, the eggs hatch, and migrate into the cecum where they grow into larvae and then develop into adulthood. This development process within the cecum (which marks the start of the large intestines) takes a period of 3 months. The whipworm migrates out of the cecum and into the large intestine of the animal. There, the whipworm attaches itself to the intestinal wall. Once attached, the whipworm finds nourishment from blood drawn through the intestinal wall and capillary penetration.

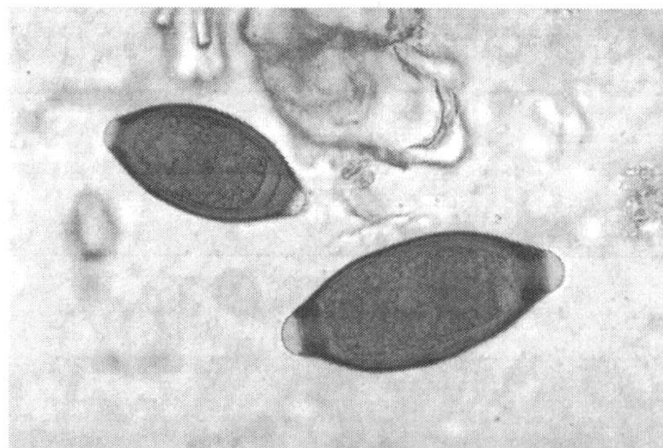

Diagnostic Characteristics

The **Trichuris vulpis** worm is detected by viewing the **eggs in the feces**. This viewing is accomplished through the fecal flotation technique. The animal may experience a range of symptoms depending upon the amount of worms present in the animal. A small number of worms may not produce any observable symptoms. Animals with a large infection of worms may have more severe symptoms. Symptoms include: extreme and severe watery diarrhea, bright red blood in the stool, rapid dehydration, and even death.

The immature larvae may be resistant to certain medical interventions. However, most medications are effective in the treatment of adult whipworms. The animal can be expected to need medical treatment for a period of several months. This allows all the larvae to mature so that they can be effectively eradicated in adulthood. Preventive care is recommended, and involves the removal of feces from the animal's surrounding area. The fecal matter can increase risk of infection as it may have active eggs that have been excreted from an infected animal's body.

Toxocara Cati Infection, Detection, and Treatment

Mature Toxocara cati roundworms produce eggs. These eggs are discharged or expelled from the body in the fecal waste released by the feline. The development period outside of the body lasts for about 10 to 14 days, at which point the eggs are actively infective. An unsuspecting feline will become infected by eating the infective eggs, usually in another food product that is consumed by the animal. The process then has begun all over again in this new unsuspecting host.

Kittens can be infected by drinking the **infected milk** of a mother cat. The infected cat's vomit will often have visible signs of the worms. The recommended treatment for roundworm or toxocara cati is the use of an appropriate medical deworming agent.

Laboratory and physical symptoms of Toxocara cati include: 1) for visceral (intestinal) larva migrans – hypereosinophilia, hepatosplenomegaly, pneumonitis, fever, and hyperglobulinemia; and 2) ocular (eye) larva migrans (endophthalmitis) – leukokoria, loss of vision in the affected eye, eye pain, and strabismus. Cats are the primary host, but humans can become infected.

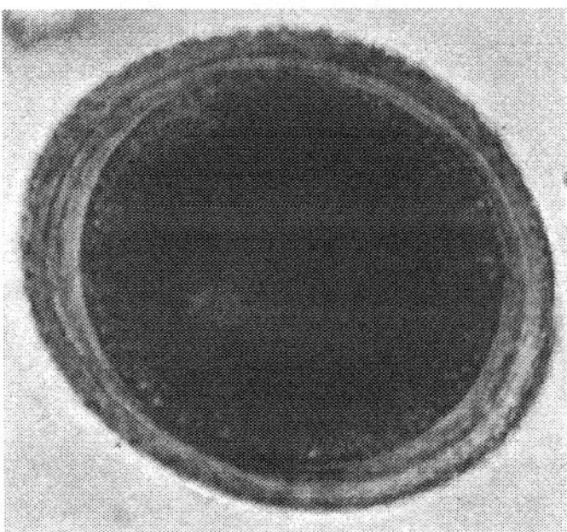

Life Cycle, Infection, and Diagnosis

The Toxocara cati or **feline roundworm** may sometimes be visible in the vomit of an animal. Toxocara cati roundworms inhabit the small intestines. It takes about 8 weeks from initial infection until this parasite can be detected through clinical means. The fecal flotation method can be used to expose the dark brown, thick-walled, pitted eggs of Toxocara cati. However, the eggs are not always present in the feces. Therefore, it is entirely possible that the results of a fecal flotation test will produce a false negative result.

The Toxocara cati has a complex life cycle. Infection occurs through eating an infected host (rodents, beetles, earthworms), through ingesting infected maternal milk, or by direct ingestion of eggs (via vomitus, fecal matter, etc.). The ingested eggs hatch inside the cat. After emerging from their eggs, the larvae enter the small intestines of the host animal. From this juncture, the larvae enter the circulatory system of the feline, and then migrate to the pulmonary system, where they are coughed up and swallowed into the stomach. There, the larvae mature and reproduce more eggs to be discharged from the body in the feces.

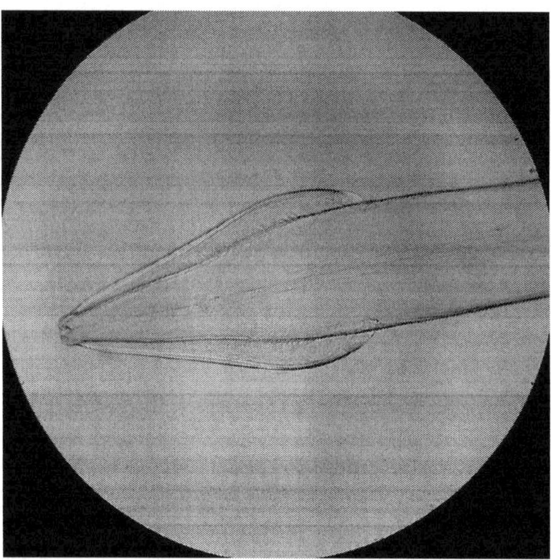

Struvite and Calcium Oxalate Crystals in Dog and Cat Urine

Struvite crystals (triple phosphate crystals) are commonly found in a dog or cat's urinalysis and are normally not an issue unless there is also a bacterial urinary tract infection. If there is no bacterial infection, struvite crystalluria is not related to struvite urolith (bladder stone) formation. Struvite crystals look like coffin lids under the microscope. **Calcium oxalate crystals** may result in the formation of calcium oxalate uroliths especially when there is a large amount of these crystals. Calcium oxalate dihydrate crystals look like little envelopes, and calcium oxalate monohydrate crystals look like dumbbells. In a case of ethylene glycol toxicity, a different form of calcium oxalate crystals form that look like colorless picket fence posts and are found in neutral to acidic urine.

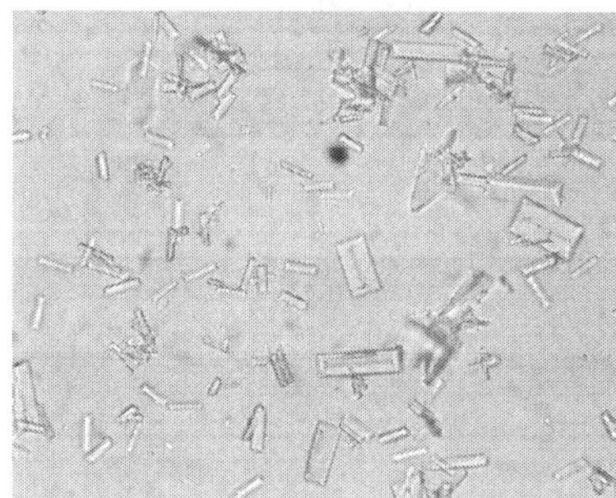

Common WBCs and Their Role in Inflammation

Neutrophils, sometimes referred to as the first responders, are the first to arrive at the site of **inflammation** and will continue to come to the site as long as the inflammation lasts. Neutrophils will engulf microorganisms and destroy them; they also signal the other WBCs to the site. Eosinophils are slightly larger than neutrophils and have segmented nuclei with eosinophilic cytoplasmic granules. They are often seen associated with mast cells, allergies, parasitic disease, and fungal infections. Lymphocytes arrive at the site of inflammation a few days after it started. They have a round nuclei that is about the same size as an RBC. Lymphocytes present in two categories: T cells or B cells. T and B cells spring into action when they come across antigens. Monocytes remove damaged cells and microorganisms and are usually plentiful during inflammation. Basophils increase due to an allergic or parasitic response, but they are normally very scarce.

Isospora SSP

The canine or feline with **Isospora ssp** (subspecies) coccidiosis has been infected by the consumption of the parasite's eggs. The most prominent symptoms are frequent and excessive bowel movements consisting of soft, fluid-laden diarrhea. The severity of the diarrhea may be indicative of the acuteness of the infection. Because of the copious fluids expelled in an effort to flush the parasites out, the animal experiencing acute symptoms may be in danger of dehydration and death.

The **fecal material** contains active eggs or oocysts that have been excreted with the feces from the infected animal's body. Upon proper examination, it will be noted that the infected stool contains many clear, spherical to ellipsoid, thin-walled oocysts that can best be detected by the fecal floatation method. Once coccidiosis is confirmed, the disease should be properly treated with medications and appropriate follow-up medical care. Preventive care is also highly recommended, and involves the removal of feces from the animal's surrounding area, as the continuing presence of infected fecal matter can increase risk of recurrent infection.

Life Cycle and Infection Processes

Isospora ssp (subspecies) is one of many sporozoan intestinal parasites of the order Coccidia. As a Coccidian, it is a spore-forming single-celled (protozoan) parasite. This parasite infects both cats and dogs. Coccidia parasites typically take up residence in the small intestines of an animal. Diseases that occur as a result of these protozoa fall under the descriptive header of coccidiosis.

Puppies and kittens that range in age from birth to 6 months of age are susceptible to the disease. Adult animals that have a suppressed immune system can also be susceptible to this disease. Stress can cause the immune system to be weakened to a point that the animal finds itself more susceptible to this infection. The prepatent period, the time of infestation to maturation, can range from 4 to 12 days. Puppies or kittens are usually around the age of 2 weeks or more when they contract coccidiosis. This disease can be detected by the fecal flotation method.

Ctenocephalides SSP

There are 2 common species of **Ctenocephalides spp** (subspecies). A widely found species is the cat flea known to pulicologists (those who study fleas) as **Ctenocephalides felis**. Another species is the dog flea, which is known as Ctenocephalides canis. While the dog flea is rarely found, the cat flea is routinely found on both cats and dogs. An animal that has been infected by the cat flea may be diagnosed through readily visible evidence. Adult fleas take up residence and grow on the host's skin. Adult fleas lay eggs, which fall off the host in areas that the host frequents (bedding, living areas, etc.).

Upon hatching (in 1-6 days) the larvae live on organic debris and adult flea feces (requisite to their continued development). The larvae range in size from about 1.5 to 5 mm in length. Upon larval maturation they spin a cocoon in which they reside as a "pupa" – an insect in a metamorphosis stage. After 1-2 weeks the pupa is a fully developed adult flea. However, the pupa will not leave the cocoon until adequate environmental stimuli indicate they are near a suitable host (e.g., heat, physical pressure, carbon dioxide, or movement). If no stimulus prompts emergence, the flea can remain in a quiescent cocoon state for up to 350 days.

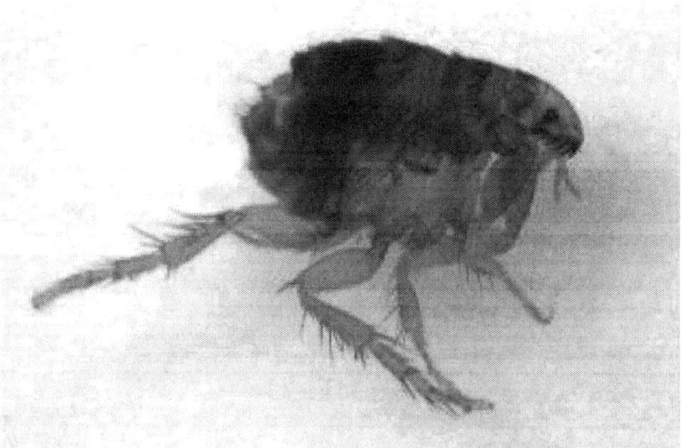

Infestation Activities and Symptoms of Ctenocephalides SSP

Adult flea coloration is reddish-brown to black in appearance. The adults do not have wings, but are able to jump great distances. The adults have a life span that ranges from about 4-25 days in length, receiving nourishment by biting and drinking the blood of the host. The flea is a parasitic insect which can rapidly spread by leaping onto other hosts and surfaces. The animal that has been infected by fleas may experience flea allergy dermatitis (as may humans who sometimes briefly become secondary hosts).

Dermatitis is an inflammation that appears as redness, itching, and/or swelling of the skin. Animals with this condition may exhibit symptoms such as scratching excessively. This scratching can further damage the animal's skin.

The animal should be closely observed in order to detect fleas or residual flea feces. Flea feces appear as small specks of dirt on the animal. Where discovered, treatment should take place. The bedding and living environment of the animal should also be checked and treated, if necessary. Preventive care is recommended to reduce exposure to the infection.

Diagnostic Characteristics of Cheyletiella SSP

Cheyletiella (the name used by acarologists – those who study mites and ticks) has long been called "walking dandruff" for the mite's propensity to carry skin scales around with them as they move about. **Cheyletiella mites** can infest dogs, cats, and rabbits. Mites are creatures with 8 legs that extend beyond the margins of their bodies. The adult mite is oval in shape, and can take up residence on the host's skin surface or on hair shafts or in hair follicles. The mite's stages of development require approximately 21-35 days for completion. The entire life cycle takes place on the host.

The adult mite is capable of living for 2-14 days off the body of the host. When off the host, mites have the ability to infect an animal through environmental contacts. Even so, mites normally infect an animal through more direct contact (i.e., moving among animals that come into physical contact with each other). Walking dandruff has the following symptoms: obvious scurf or dandruff scales, visible mites on the surface of the skin, pruritus (itching, resulting in scratching for relief), inflammation of the skin, crusts, and small swellings or spots.

Walking dandruff is detected by skin scrapings, the cellophane tape method, combings, or via microscopic study. Once diagnosed, walking dandruff can be treated with appropriate medications.

LICE

There are 2 kinds of lice. The **sucking lice** are called Anoplura. The **biting lice** are called Mallophaga. Different species of Anoplura attack different species of animals. The species known as Haematopinus spp will infect cattle, pigs, and horses. The species known as Linognathus spp infects dogs, cattle, and sheep. The species known as Solenopotes spp infects cattle. The species known as Pediculus spp infects humans. Likewise, different species of Mallophaga attack different species of animals. The species known as Damalinia spp (subspecies) infects horses, cattle, and sheep. The species known as Felicola subrostratus infects felines. The species known as Trichodectes canis infects dogs.

These 2 different kinds of lice have certain commonalities. For example, the adult lice have similar shapes — dorsoventrally flattened with the head narrower than the thorax. "Dorsoventral" refers to the belly-to-back anatomical axis.

Those animals that become infected may have lice on their skin and in their hair.

LIFE CYCLE, SYMPTOMS, AND TREATMENT

Lice lay eggs, which are known as **nits**. The nits are typically glued to the hair shaft so as not to fall from the host. Lice are also transferred from one host to another through **physical contact**. Lice have the ability to spend an entire life cycle on a single animal or host. Lice infestation is typically readily evident through close observation. The parasites are visible on inspection. Further, the animal may exhibit excessive itchiness, accompanied by a scruffy, dry, or brittle hair or fur coat.

When infestation is evident, the animal or human should be deloused. Delousing will free the person of lice through the application of a medication. This treatment is designed to kill the lice. Preventive care is highly recommended. Medication should be applied to all the surfaces with which the animal has had contact. This includes the animal's bedding and surrounding living area. Failure to fully treat the animal and all the infective surfaces can readily result in a reinfestation of the lice. Reinfestation will likely require yet another thorough treatment to be applied to the animal and all surfaces involved.

STRONGYLUS VULGARIS

Strongylus vulgaris is an **equine intestinal worm** ranging in length up to 25 mm. This worm takes up residence in the large intestine of a horse. The prepatent period of the equine worm can range from about 6-12 months in duration. Non-infective eggs are discharged in the feces when a host animal defecates. Following excretion, the eggs go through a developmental process in stages.

The eggs move from first stage larvae, or the L1 stage, to the second or L2 stage without becoming infective. This is followed by the third or L3 stage. It is in this last stage of development that the larvae become infective. After the L3 stage and upon ingestion, the larva sheds its protective sheath or covering (called "ex-sheathing"). This allows the larvae to migrate and eventually to pierce the walls of the intestines at or below the cecum. The cecum is the first intestinal pouch, at the point of which the large intestine originates.

DIAGNOSIS, TREATMENT, AND PREVENTION

Once the **Strongylus vulgaris larva** has penetrated the intestinal wall, it travels further until it enters the submucosa. The submucosa is the layer of connective tissue directly beneath the mucus membrane of the intestine. Horses that have been infected by the equine worm will experience a range of clinical signs. The signs of infection include colic, fever, diarrhea, weight loss, and death.

Colic is a pain that occurs in the abdominal region, typically due to spasm, obstruction or distention of the viscera.

A Strongylus vulgaris infection can be detected via the fecal flotation method. The larvae in stages 1 and 2 can be killed easily. At these stages the larvae exist largely in residual manure. Thus, the spreading and breaking up of manure is an effective deterrent to the growth and development of the larva. There is also treatment available for larvae that reach stage 3 and then become adult worms. Treatment can be found in the form of antiparasitic medications that can be administered to the horse.

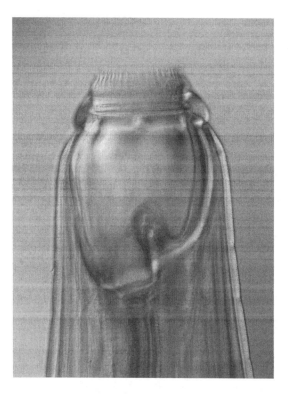

Preparing and Maintaining Specimens

Maintaining Hematology Specimens That Will Be Sent out to a Reference Lab

Hematology samples, including plasma, serum, and whole blood, must be kept in the refrigerator until they are sent to the lab and with cold packs. Blood cytology slides should be kept out of the refrigerator to avoid lysing of cells. To obtain a blood sample for clotting factors, a sodium citrate (anticoagulant) blue-top tube would be used. Draw enough blood needed for the coagulation profile, spin the sample down in the centrifuge, and draw off the serum to place in a red-top tube. Either store the sodium citrate sample in the freezer, or send it to the lab within a half an hour of obtaining it. All samples must be clearly labeled with the patient's name, client's last name, and date, as well as all necessary paperwork sent with the sample to the laboratory.

Proper Storage and Handling of Microbiologic Samples to Be Sent to an Outside Laboratory

Certain tests available for **microbiologic** examination include bacterial cultures, fungal cultures, western blotting, virus isolation, and many others. Most of these tests rely on the growth of intact viable organisms or the detection of the nucleic acids and proteins of these pathogens. Most tests require that each tissue or fluid specimen be obtained aseptically and shipped in sterile, clearly labeled bags. Tissues and fluids for most assays can be kept frozen until shipment, but if the sample can be delivered within 24 hours, then keeping the sample chilled is preferred. Degradation of certain toxins such as *Clostridium perfringens* and *C. botulinum* can happen if not frozen right after collection.

Maintaining Feces for In-House Fecal Tests

Fecal samples can be kept in the fridge for up to a week without affecting the parasites, but getting them to the clinic to be evaluated quickly is ideal. If an owner is obtaining the sample, they can store it in a tightly sealed container (Tupperware) and store it in a cool, dry place such as the refrigerator and out of sunlight. When collecting feces from a litter box, it is important that the owner collects the sample from the correct pet if multiple cats are using the litter box, and the sample must be fresh and not hard. If giardia is suspected, then the sample must be obtained directly from the rectum for the SNAP test, and because trophozoites will not survive storage, a fecal floatation sample must be evaluated right away.

Proper Blood Sample Handling

Patients should be prepared in advance whenever blood work is anticipated. Most tests require the patient to have **fasted** (to go without normal food intake) prior to taking the sample. The technician that collects the sample should be familiar with the criteria and procedures involved. These include: 1) the correct sizes of needles to be used, 2) dry syringes of proper dimensions, 3) appropriate evacuation tubes to prevent hemolysis and clotting, etc, and 4) the volume of blood needed for testing.

Hemolysis is a condition that ruptures and destroys red blood cells. Hemolysis often arises from improper specimen collection. Contamination, poor line connections, incorrect tube mixing or tube filling, and incorrect needle size may all cause hemolysis.

Serum is the post-clotted liquid part of blood that is used to conduct certain tests. Serum will often be beneficial in preventing unwanted chemical interactions. Tests requiring whole blood or plasma samples should be mixed with an anticoagulant when collected. However, the technician should verify that the tests being conducted will not be hindered by the presence of the anticoagulant. The technician should place samples in the refrigerator if the test is not performed promptly. In addition, the technician should collect enough samples to conduct all the tests being requested. The technician should compare the normal values for a given test procedure to each sample collected in the laboratory. Conventional laboratory quality control procedures should be maintained.

Collecting Cells for Microscopic Examinations

Solid Mass Imprinting, Scraping, and the Swab Technique

Cells to be examined under a microscope may be collected with the **solid mass imprinting technique**. This technique can be employed when exposed tissues of concern shed a thin outer layer without difficulty. Likewise, some tissues removed by surgical procedures can undergo the imprinting technique. The veterinarian will need to expose the center of the mass leaving a fine cut along the edge. The excess fluid and blood should be blotted clean. The veterinarian should always employ a separate sterile microscope slide with each imprint taken.

Collections can also be made with the **scraping technique**. This technique employs a mild, scraping or rub from a sterilized scalpel blade. This rub allows the cells to be gathered on a film. The cells are then scattered out onto the sterilized microscope slide for examination.

The third type of collection is known as the **swab technique**. A swab is a small stick with cotton used to gather the cell samples. It is rubbed or stroked gently over the target area, and then applied to a microscope slide or culture dish for further evaluation.

FLUID ASPIRATION

There are a multitude of names for **fluid aspiration** (withdrawing fluid by suction, i.e., a syringe, etc.), largely based on the aspiration sites. These are categorized under the following terms: abdominocentesis (abdominal), thoracocentesis (chest), cystocentesis (bladder), cerebrospinal fluid (or CSF tap), and arthrocentesis (joints). The veterinarian will clean the site with a surgical scrub before taking a sample. This is required for all samples dispatched for microbiology testing, and is essential to maintain proper aseptic conditions. The veterinarian will more than likely allow the patient to stay on its feet in a standing position during these procedures. There are 2 exceptions to the standing position option. The first arises when the animal requires cystocentesis (urinary bladder aspiration). This procedure requires that the animal be placed in a dorsal or lateral recumbency position. Likewise, and second, the animal must be placed in a lateral recumbency position when a CSF aspiration or "tap" is required. The veterinarian will next seek a bacterial culture of the fluid, and/or centrifugation for inspection of the sediment. This gives the veterinarian the opportunity to inspect the fluid and its contents more closely.

THE SWAB TECHNIQUE

The **swab technique**, involves a swab (a small stick with a cotton tip) used to gather the cell samples. A swab is particularly helpful when applied in the gathering of cell samples used for diagnosing problems associated with the female organs. These samples are collected to assist the veterinarian in making judgments about the estrous cycle stage, using uterine and vaginal discharges. The veterinarian will use a speculum when gathering vaginal samples. A speculum is a medical instrument used to hold a body passage such as the vulva open. In addition, the veterinarian will employ the swab technique when gathering cells from the ears of an animal. The swab technique is also useful in the examination of fistulated lesions. A fistulated lesion (a lesion producing an abnormal passageway) requires cleaning of the tube or passage where the sample is collected. This cleaning should be done prior to use of the swab technique. This technique should also be followed by cleaning of the affected area after the sample has been collected.

CHARACTERISTICS OF FLUID SAMPLES THAT SHOULD BE NOTED

The veterinarian should note any specific characteristics found in fluid samples. The fluid samples should be examined for the following: color, odor, and turbidity. Turbidity refers to the opaque qualities found in the fluid, such as particles and sediment. The veterinarian should note the total nucleated cell count or TNCC. In addition, the veterinarian should make note of the total protein found. These amounts will be used to further categorize the type of fluid sample taken.

There are 3 types of fluid: **transudates, exudates** and **modified transudates**. The fluid samples categorized as transudates are those that are found to have less than 500/mL of TNCC in conjunction with a total protein measuring less than 3 g/dL (typically, extracellular fluids that have filtered through membranous tissues). The transudates are further categorized if it is a sample lacking in color, as with ascites. Ascites are described as fluid in the abdominal region. The fluid samples categorized as modified transudates include total protein counts between 2.5 and 7.5 g/dL. Modified transudates have an opaque or pink coloration. The veterinarian can make note of the exudate samples that are categorized by their total protein counts which are higher than 3 g/dL. A count of this type is helpful in determining that inflammation is present in the patient.

Preserve Parasitic Samples for Outside Laboratory Testing

There are a number of steps to take in the preservation of parasitic samples that will be sent away for diagnostic testing. It is essential that the sample be kept in an unchanged condition for accurate diagnostic confirmation. The first step requires that fresh samples be packed in leak-proof containers. These containers should be sealed securely.

The containers with the fecal samples require a label with the following information: date, site from which the specimen was acquired, the animal owner's name, the species of the animal, an identification number for the animal and/or the name of the animal, the referring veterinarian, the address of the clinic, and the telephone number.

The fecal sample can be sent for outside laboratory testing in its pure form. The fecal sample may also be mixed with a solution of 10% formalin at a ratio of 1:3. Formalin is a solution of formaldehyde in water. The use of a diluted alcohol or formalin solution is recommended to preserve whole parasites or segments of parasites for proper laboratory microscopic examination, identification, and relative concentration or "parasitic load" indices.

Maintaining Laboratory Equipment and Supplies

Light Microscope

One optical instrument used for specimen evaluation is known as the **light microscope**. This instrument has a number of eyepieces, a light source, a light condenser, a stage, objective lens, and a focus. The term **monocular** is used to describe an instrument with one eyepiece. The term **binocular** is used to describe an instrument with 2 eyepieces. In a microscope, the eyepiece allows further magnification of the viewed field. The magnification or enlargement is normally set at 5, 10 or 15 times. This is written as the following: 5x, 10x, or 15x. The light source can be adjusted to provide the viewer with varying shades of concentrated luminosity. The instrument comes with a condenser that allows the light to be diminished or increased. Slides are placed on the stage or platform for inspection purposes. The stage or platform can be adjusted or moved horizontally or vertically by turning one of 2 knobs. The specimen on the slide is magnified or enlarged by using the objective lens. The microscope employed in clinical microbiology requires the following available settings: 10x, 40x, and 100x objectives. The focus is adjusted for coarse focus or fine focus by moving one of 2 knobs.

Proper Use and Maintenance of a Microscope

Some supplies needed for cleaning the **microscope** include cotton-tipped applicators, distilled water, suction bulb, Kimwipes, optical cleaning solutions, and a soft brush. After each slide, the ocular lens, objective lenses, stage, and stage clips should be cleaned, as well as the entire microscope daily. To clean the objective lens, a cotton-tipped applicator dampened with an adequate cleaning solution can be used, and then it is dried with a Kimwipe. Distilled water should be used to wipe away any debris from the lenses and the microscope body and then dried with lens paper. Inspect the cord for frayed wires or any damage, and then lower the stage or raise the arm to gain access to the objectives for cleaning. A suction bulb can be used to suck tiny hairs that get stuck in the eyepieces, then wiped with Kimwipes and 70% ethanol and dried. Kimwipes moistened with water should be used after fecal solution gets onto the stage to prevent pests and dust from adhering to it. A microfiber cloth and warm water can be used to wipe down the microscope body and then dried.

Cleaning and Maintaining the Ultrasonic Cleaner

Ultrasonic cleaners use high-frequency sound waves to create high- and low-pressure waves inside the machine, creating tiny bubbles that will burst. When these bubbles burst, it creates a gentle scrubbing sensation (cavitation) when they contact soiled instruments. To clean the ultrasonic cleaner, the appropriate cleaner is added to the distilled water filling the chamber and the machine is turned on so that once cavitation occurs it pushes the cleaner into the tiny, hard-to-reach areas of the machine. Cavitation erosion happens over time as a natural wearing process of the surface of the chamber, but it can happen faster if there are dirt particles on the bottom of the chamber that can wear the metal enough to cause leaks, Instruments must always be placed into the basket in the ultrasonic cleaner and should not be put onto the bottom of the chamber. The metal and other dirt particles from soiled instruments can create rust films in the tank, as well as if tap water is being used to fill the chamber instead of distilled water. Certain cleaning chemicals are available to remove rust films.

Caring for and Maintaining the Centrifuge

The **centrifuge** is used to spin a substance such as urine, feces, or blood and separate their components based on density. The inside of a centrifuge is normally made of either ceramic, aluminum, or stainless steel and should be cleaned daily with the appropriate cleaner, which may vary depending on the material on the inside of the centrifuge. To thoroughly clean the centrifuge, the rotor and sample tube holders should be removed and washed with warm water and liquid dishwasher soap, along with the inside of the centrifuge. Full-strength bleach and other caustic cleaners shouldn't be used because they can damage stainless steel. Steel wool and wire brushes can also damage the interior coating and create corrosion, so they should be avoided as well. Water should never be poured into the centrifuge because that can cause damage to the motor, gaskets, and sensors.

Calibrating and Maintaining the Refractometer

The **refractometer** is used to measure the urine specific gravity as well as the plasma total protein. The refractometer can be calibrated by placing a drop of distilled water on the prism, closing the lid, and reading it while holding it to the light and looking through the eyepiece; it should read 1.000 for distilled water. If the reading is off for calibration, then the instrument can be adjusted by turning the screw on the bottom counterclockwise, which moves the dividing line under 1.000, and then turn it clockwise until it reaches 1.000. The refractometer should be stored at 60-100 °F for accurate readings. After each use, the refractometer needs to be cleaned with a soft cloth moistened with a little water to wipe the prism and lid and then dried, or else the next reading will appear blurred.

Culture Incubator

In clinical microbiology, the use of a **culture incubator** may be necessary to cultivate organisms outside a normal host environment. The incubator can maintain very exact temperatures to successfully support organism growth. These temperatures serve to duplicate the optimum growth conditions found in natural circumstances. One of the more commonly used temperature settings is 37 °C (centigrade or Celsius) or 98.6 °F (Fahrenheit) which duplicates the temperature found in humans. In certain incubators, oxygen concentration and humidity can also be varied for optimum conditions. Veterinarians normally use cultures derived from specimens grown at 37 °C. This includes specimens from reptile and amphibian cultures. This temperature allows a majority of the organisms to grow. However, the body temperatures of reptiles and amphibians can fluctuate with the temperature of the creature's environment. This form of fluctuation is referred to as poikilothermia. The veterinarian should note that most standardized tests require a temperature of

37 °C. One standardized test that the veterinarian may use is known as the Kirby-Bauer sensitivity test.

Media Types

Trypticase Soy Agar, MacConkey II Agar, and Columbia Colistin-Nalidixic Acid

Many microorganisms can be cultured in the medium known as **Trypticase Soy Agar**, abbreviated as TSA. Bacterial hemolytic reactions can also be studied with this medium. A similar medium contains 5% Sheep Blood and is referred to as a Blood Agar Plate (abbreviated as BAP). TSA plates enriched with blood or other specialized growth media are intended to propagate the so-called "fastidious" organisms (i.e., those with complex nutritional needs).

The veterinarian will select a **MacConkey II Agar** (abbreviated MAC) for gram-negative organisms. It employs crystal violet and bile salts to hinder gram-positive bacterial growth. This medium also incorporates a neutral red indicator. This indicator is able to turn another color (pink to purple, based on developing pH) in the presence of lactose fermentation. Lactose fermenting bacteria are abbreviated as LFs. The altered coloration differentiates the LFs and non-lactose fermenters. Non-lactose fermenters are abbreviated as NLFs. The medium is expected to inhibit the growth of the bacteria known as Proteus spp.

Colistin is an antibiotic employed in intestinal infections that arise from a wide assortment of organisms. The medium that combines this antibiotic with nalidixic acid is known as Columbia Colistidin-Naladixic Acid Agar. It is able to pick out gram-positive organisms. Columbia Colistidin-Naladixic Acid Agar is abbreviated as CAN. It contains 5% Sheep Blood.

Salmonella-Shigella Agar, Trypticase Soy Broth, and Campylobacter Agar

The **Salmonella-Shigella Agar** culture medium is abbreviated as SS. This medium is selective for specific enterobacteria. The specifications of the selection include those organisms which are defined as pathogenic and gram-negative. This medium can employ lactose fermentation–generated color changes to allow various distinct colonies to be brought into view. This medium also employs ferric citrate to differentiate the bacteria that generates H_2S (hydrogen sulfide). The ferric acid brings about a black coloration when H_2S-producing bacteria are active.

Trypticase Soy Broth is a medium abbreviated as TSE. This medium has an all-purpose function. It is able to nurture most bacteria within its solution. Even most fastidious bacteria will find this medium to be more than sufficient for its needs. The veterinarian will employ this medium for most blood cultures and sterility confirmation tests.

When a veterinarian requires a particularly sensitive medium, then Campylobacter Agar with 5 Antimicrobics and 10% Sheep Blood is a good choice. This is often referred to as Campy BAP. The veterinarian will employ this medium most often when developing Campylobacter spp. These organisms can be obtained from fecal specimens in a microaerophilic setting.

Bunsen burners, Electric Heating Elements, and Alcohol Lamps

Veterinarians also use an appliance known as a **Bunsen burner**, usually fueled from a wall gas outlet. The burner's gas is ignited by a spark striker. A metal inoculating loop is used to transport microorganisms from the specimen sample to a culture dish. It is typically flame-sterilized in the Bunsen burner between culture applications. The Bunsen burner is also employed to "heat fix" bacteria to a microscope slide. This is critical, as the bacteria might otherwise be washed away during the staining process.

An **electric heating element** can also be used to sterilize metal transfer (i.e., inoculation) loops. The electric heating element is normally made from ceramic and operates electrically. Thus, natural gas is not required with this device. The electrical device gives a consistent burn to the applied surfaces. This is an advantage of an electrical device over a gas fueled Bunsen burner.

Another sterilization device is known as an **alcohol lamp**. This device is less expensive, but it does require more time in the sterilization process — i.e., the metal loops take longer to be sterilized using an alcohol lamp than a Bunsen burner. An alcohol lamp is fashioned from glass. A wick extends into the alcohol held in the base. The lamp is ignited with a match or other combustible source.

Sterile and Non-Sterile Areas of the Body for Obtaining a Specimen for Microbiological Culture

A **sterile region** in the body is defined as one that does not typically contain bacteria or fungi within its regions or hollow spaces. While not absolutely sterile, blood samples, urine samples, spinal fluid samples, joint fluid samples, solid organ samples, milk samples, and lower respiratory tract samples should not normally contain bacteria. These types of samples are frequently cultured to determine whether or not bacteria are present. Various non-sterile zones are found in the hair or fur regions, skin, sputum or saliva, intestinal tract, feces, ears, upper respiratory tract, nostrils and associated nasal regions, and the trachea. As non-sterile zones, these areas are expected to be full of resident bacteria and normal flora. Thus, specifically, various organisms are customarily present in these areas in healthy animals. By contrast, it is a potentially serious problem when disease-causing bacteria are found in the sterile areas of an animal.

Collect and Culture Swab Specimens

The veterinarian will apply a **sterile cotton swab** or a **culturette** to collect a specimen from an animal. The swab will be used to swipe the ears, nares, and abscesses. Fluid directly from the specimen may be squeezed directly onto the swab, if possible. There is a small measure of liquid or gel placed in the prepackaged swab containers. This gel can be used in conjunction with the sterile swabs to operate as a transport medium. This transport medium allows the organisms to remain in a state that can best be used for germination or further development when transported to another location. This viable state can last for a period of up to 48 hours, if the swabs are maintained in a proper environment in the interim.

A swab is typically used to inoculate a third of the surface region of the culture plate with microorganisms. The culture media potentially consists of BAP, CNA, and/or MAC. After the microorganisms have been introduced, then the swab is positioned in a THIO broth (a culture media for anaerobic and microaerophilic bacteria and sterility tests).

Next Steps in the Collection and Culture of Swab Specimens

The technician will either break or cut the end of the swab off. This is dependent upon the type of material from which the swab is constructed. It can be constructed of wood, plastic, or metal. The length of the swab should not extend beyond the opening of the tube in which the swab is stored.

The **inoculated plates** are streaked to give the bacteria a linear growth pattern on the surface of the medium. This streaking is created when a contaminated needle, swab, or inoculation loop is drawn across the medium. The streak pattern also gives the bacteria needed isolation. The veterinarian may next select a flamed, sterile slide. This sterile slide can be inoculated with a gram stain. Then, the inoculated plate is stored for incubation over 24 hours. The incubation period allows the cells or microorganisms to develop under a controlled temperature. This steady development is necessary so that the microorganism can continue to grow and multiply within the medium. The veterinarian is able to control the environment in which the microorganism is grown.

Culturing Solid and Urine Specimens

Solid specimens require alternate collection and culture techniques. These specimens can be defined as those collected from hard lumps, solid matter, and tissue samples. **Tissue samples** are derived from organs, skin and scales. These samples must be cultured in order to allow the biological material to grow under special conditions. This is performed by placing the collected substance in a small volume of liquid base or broth over a period of 24 hours. The liquid base or broth is then subcultured. **Subculture** means that the bacterial growth is transferred from another culture medium onto a plated media. Aseptic techniques designed to prevent infection from pathogens are applied in the collection of tissue samples. Necrosis or tissue death is a grave concern that must be prevented from occurring.

Two methods used to collect urine samples are cystocentesis and catheterization. **Cystocentesis** (needle aspiration) is the technique used to collect the most optimum urine specimens for culture purposes. In particular, extraneous contaminants are virtually eliminated. However, a sterile **catheterization** tube inserted through the urethra can also be applied with equal success, when due care is taken.

Collecting and Culturing Liquid Specimens

Specimens with a fluid base can be extracted with a syringe or sterile tube. These items are useful in aspiration of the following: abscesses, tracheal washes, bronchial washes, nasal discharges, joint fluid, or spinal fluid. The extracted fluid from the specimen is used in the inoculation of the culture plates. Typically, BAP, CNA, and MAC plates are employed in this task. Some extracted droplets from the sample are also united with a thioglycollate ("Thio") broth. A third of the surfaces on the microscopic slides are inoculated by use of a pre-flamed, somewhat cold to the touch, inoculation loop. The inoculated plates are streaked to give the specimen a linear growth pattern on the surface of the medium. This streaking is created when a contaminated needle or inoculation loop is drawn across the medium. The streak also gives the bacteria needed isolation. Some of the remaining specimen collected from the syringe or tube is then used for a gram stain.

Gram Stains

There are a number of steps that must be taken when using **gram stain kits**. The first step involves the specimen. One method involves taking a colony from a suspended plate positioned in water. The other method involves placing a droplet of thioglycollate broth onto a microscope slide. The veterinarian will allow the specimen to air dry. This is followed by subjecting the slide to heat, in order to "heat fix" the specimen to the slide. The slide will then be ready for inundation in Gram's iodine for a one-minute period. This is followed by a thorough rinsing with tap water. The slide is next inundated in a decolorizer for a period of 10 seconds. This is followed with another tap water rinsing. However, if the slide remains overly dark-toned, then the procedure should be repeated. The slide is then inundated in a safranin counterstain for a period of 30 to 50 seconds. This step is followed by a final tap water rinsing.

Subsequent Steps for Completing a Gram Stain

The purpose of the **safranin counterstain** is to reveal features in the specimen that may not have been visible through application of the primary stain. Once the safranin counterstain has been thoroughly rinsed, then the next step is taken. The rinsing is finished when no stain residue is apparent in the rinse water. The slide should be allowed to air dry. The veterinarian may decide to blot the slide dry with a paper to hurry along the drying process.

At last the slide should be viewed beneath an oil immersion (100x) objective lens. Bacteria with a coloration ranging from purple to dark blue are gram-positive. Bacteria with a pink coloration are gram-negative. The bacteria are thus identified in accordance with Gram's classification methods. The result of completing the steps correctly gives the veterinarian the opportunity to make a diagnosis using the results of the gram stain process.

Performing Laboratory Tests and Procedures

Obtaining and Set Up a Fine Needle Aspiration

To obtain a **fine needle aspirate**, you will need a 25-gauge needle and a 10 ml syringe. Insert the needle into the mass or lesion, apply a small amount of suction through the syringe, and redirect a few times inside the mass while suctioning back to get a good-sized sample. Release the syringe plunger to release the suction, and then pull the syringe with the needle out of the lesion. Remove the syringe from the needle, pull back the plunger to fill the syringe with air, and then replace the needle. Push the plunger to express the sample that is most likely just small enough to be in the needle and not the syringe onto a clean slide. Too much force or pressure will rupture the cells, so obtain and prepare the sample gently. Air-dry the sample on the slide. Once dried, the sample must be stained using either a modified Wright or rapid stain. Once the slide is stained, it is examined under 40× magnification, a drop of immersion oil is placed on the sample spot identified under 40×, and then moved to 100× to evaluate.

Performing a Differential Blood Smear Evaluation

Once the slide is prepared for a **differential blood smear**, it is stained and then examined under 100× magnification with immersion oil. Three portions are evaluated, including RBC morphology, WBC differential count, and an estimated platelet count. First, examine the RBCs and note any abnormalities in size, shape, or color as well as any inclusions (Heinz bodies or Howell-Jolly bodies). Using a manual counter, the technician will perform the WBC differential and count the monocytes, lymphocytes, neutrophils, eosinophils, and basophils starting from one side of the slide on the start of the monolayer moving to the other side of the slide, up and repeat (the "battlement pattern") until you have counted 100 WBCs. To get the absolute value of each WBC type, the total counted for that specific WBC (e.g., eosinophils) is multiplied by the total WBC count. Last, the platelets are estimated by examining 10 fields in the same pattern as the WBC differential count and count all the platelets in each field. Then add all of the platelet counts together from all 10 fields and divide by 10. Then take that result and multiply by 20,000 to get the estimated platelet number per microliter of blood.

Low-Dose Dexamethasone Suppression (LDDS) Test

A common test that is run to diagnose Cushing's disease is the **low-dose dexamethasone suppression** (LDDS) test. With this test, a sample of blood is drawn to determine the dog's baseline cortisol level, and then a small dexamethasone (synthetic cortisol) injection is given to the dog intravenously. Another blood sample is taken at 4 and 8 hours after the dexamethasone injection was given to measure the dog's cortisol levels. As blood cortisol levels increase after the dexamethasone injection is given, the pituitary gland should be lowering the production of ACTH (the hormone that stimulates the adrenal glands to produce cortisol) and there should be a drop in cortisol levels in the blood in the post-dexamethasone blood samples. The LDDS test can tell you if Cushing's is of pituitary or adrenal origin. If there is a pituitary tumor, there is a slight decrease is cortisol production noticed in the 4- and 8-hour post-dexamethasone samples. If there is an adrenal tumor present, then there will be no reduction in blood cortisol at either the 4- or 8-hour blood sample.

ACTH Stimulation Test

An **ACTH stimulation test** is run to detect Cushing's disease. ACTH is the hormone produced by the pituitary gland to tell the adrenal glands how much cortisol to produce; as the blood cortisol level increases, the pituitary gland will decrease ACTH hormone production. With the ACTH stimulation test, a baseline blood cortisol will be drawn and then an injection of synthetic ACTH is given intravenously. Another blood sample is taken an hour after the injection and will be compared to the baseline sample. The ACTH stimulation test will tell if the patient has Cushing's disease. A dog with Cushing's disease will show an increase in cortisol production in the hour after the blood sample because the body is not being alerted to the slow cortisol production.

Testing for Heartworm Disease in Dogs

There are a couple of ways to test a dog for **heartworm disease**. Testing for microfilaria (baby heartworms) is usually done using the modified Knott's test, which uses a centrifuge to spin the blood sample quickly enough to concentrate the microfilaria that are identified under the microscope. SNAP tests are also used to detect the antigens (proteins the body recognizes as foreign) of adult female heartworms. The SNAP test is performed with a drop of blood and a few drops of conjugate. If the dog tests positive for heartworms, radiographs of the chest will be taken to assess for any damage caused to the heart and lungs, as well as additional blood work to determine kidney and liver function. Dogs should be tested for heartworms before they start on heartworm prevention to be sure that they are negative. Also, dogs already on heartworm prevention should be tested annually. Puppies will start on heartworm prevention right away, because the prepatent period for heartworm disease is 6 months and puppies would not be tested until after that.

Water Deprivation/Urine Concentration Tests

The **water deprivation test** is given to an animal that has been gradually denied water over a period of 3-5 days on an escalating basis. This test will allow the urine to be assessed for the concentration of an endogenous hormone known as ADH or **antidiuretic hormone** — hence the full name "water deprivation/urine concentration" test. ADH is released by animals that are in a dehydrated state. This hormone helps increase renal reabsorption of water, so as to better conserve what little water is remaining in the body. The gradual restriction of water over a 72-hour period should produce the desired ADH release effect. The animal is expected to lose mass, at about 5% of total weight, due to dehydration.

The reference measurement is given as the specific gravity of urine at a normal concentration. This measurement is 1.025 for normal levels of ADH. Insufficient ADH or tubular dysfunction may be detected when the test indicates that ADH concentrates are low. Previously dehydrated animals should not be given this test. Azotemic animals (those with preexisting high serum urea levels) should also not be given this test.

Causes for Increased Serum Amylase Levels

Amylase is a digestive enzyme. This digestive enzyme functions to break down carbohydrates and starches into sugars, beginning with its presence in saliva. It is also found in the pancreas, where it metabolizes stored glycogen into glucose.

There are a number of factors that may precipitate a **rise in serum amylase** levels. Indeed, elevated levels may be directly related to the following conditions: acute, chronic, and obstructive pancreatitis; hyperadrenocorticism; upper gastrointestinal inflammation; obstructions in the digestive system; and/or kidney failure.

Some tests used in veterinary evaluations are adapted from tests originally intended for humans. These tests may require some revision to be successfully applied in animal populations. Serum amylase testing is one of these. The serum should be diluted with a prescribed amount of normal saline prior to running the test. This will compensate for the higher rate of serum amylase activity found in animals as compared to humans.

Maltose does not impact the test results. Therefore, dogs are good candidates for **amyloclastic** tests. However, the same tests used for humans or dogs are not always compatible in testing cats. The tests will require a non-lipemic serum and heparinized plasma samples to produce accurate amylase results. Hemolysis present in the samples can cause the amylase rates to artificially rise.

Type of Sample Needed for Serum/Plasma Glucose Testing

The technician should take precautions when collecting samples for the purpose of **glucose testing**. These precautions should include special handling methods to prevent any variability in the blood glucose levels measured. One precaution involves separation of the cellular components in blood from the plasma or serum. This is necessary to **prevent continued metabolic interactions** from occurring. If continued interaction is permitted, the glucose in the blood will continue to be used up at a rate of 7 to 10% for every hour contact is maintained. Thus, the technician should divide the plasma or serum from the cellular components almost immediately. Further, cats and dogs should not be fed for a period of 16 to 24 hours prior to phlebotomy (blood drawing), to obtain the more definitive "**fasting" glucose level**. This fasting period is not necessary for ruminant animals. Serum is the preferred blood sample. However, the technician should be aware that serum will test at a 5% higher glucose level. Again, the technician should place the sample in the centrifuge without delay. If delays are unavoidable, then the technician should use fluoride to stop the red blood cells from further metabolizing the glucose. It should be noted, however, that fluoride requires at least an hour to completely address this dilemma.

Serum Trypsin-Like Immunoreactivity Test

Animals with **Exocrine Pancreatic Insufficiency** (EPI) do not secrete sufficient digestive enzymes to properly digest their food. However, the diagnosis can be difficult to make. Serum **trypsin-like immunoreactivity** (TLI) is considered the definitive testing standard for an EPI diagnosis. The test measures the levels of certain enzymes in the blood (trypsin, trypsinogen, and particularly TLI).

The digestive enzyme known as **trypsin** is able to break down proteins. Trypsin is normally retained in the pancreas, and only enters the bloodstream if the pancreas is inflamed. The pancreas also produces a forerunner enzyme known as trypsinogen. However, there is normally only a very small amount of trypsinogen found in the circulatory system. The **trypsin-like immunoreactivity test** or TLI is able to detect both of these enzymes, and thus has a high rate of success in identifying EPI in canines. The enzymes should be analyzed with a ligand assay technique. The enzyme levels are calculated to determine if the animal has EPI. The animal should not be fed for a period of 12 hours prior to sample collection. From 5.2 to 35 μg/L is considered a normal canine TLI range (12 to 82 μg/L for cats). TLIs lower than 2.5 μg/L are indicative of EPI (8 μg/L for cats). Chronic pancreatitis can also result from EPI. Juvenile atrophy and pancreatic hypoplasia are also linked to EPI or exocrine pancreatic insufficiency.

Modified Knott's Technique for Blood Parasite Examination

Modified Knott's technique is used to identify and name the blood parasites. There are many kinds of blood-borne parasites (commonly classified as: rickettsial, protozoal, helminth, and viral). Two types of blood parasites that infest dogs are the Dirofilaria immitis (dog heartworm), and Dipetalonema reconditum. The latter can sometimes be mistaken for the former, but Dirofilaria is much more dangerous. The genus Dipetalonema has recently been reorganized, and the new name is Acanthocheilonema reconditum. However, use of the old name persists. The modified Knott's technique requires 15 mL centrifuge tube and centrifuge, 2% formalin solution, methylene blue stain, Pasteur pipettes and bulbs, and microscope slides and coverslips. A centrifuge tube is used for the sample of EDTA (anticoagulant) blood (1mL) and 2% formalin or water (9 mL). The solution disrupts the red blood cell's bonding membrane, causing it to "lyse" or burst. This mixture is placed in the centrifuge at 1000 rpm for 5 minutes. An alternative allows the solution to remain still for 1 hour. The supernatant or liquid on the surface is gently decanted off, so as not to disrupt the sediment. Next, 2 drops of methylene blue is applied to the undisturbed sediment. Aspirating gently with the pipette mixes the solution. A miniscule sample is positioned on a microscope slide and covered with a coverslip. The microscope is set at a ten-power objective. This setting is used to examine the entire slide for microfilariae or larva of an infesting parasite.

Different Collection Methods Used to Perform a Urinalysis

There are a few ways to collect urine for a **urinalysis**. Free-catch (voided) urine samples can be obtained by holding a clean container or tray underneath the pet and catching the urine midstream. A cystocentesis is performed by a veterinary professional by withdrawing the urine directly from the bladder via a sterile syringe with needle; this is the most sterile sample obtained and can be used for culture and sensitivity. **Catheterization** is performed easily on male patients by a veterinary professional. To perform a catheterization, don gloves and clean the prepuce with a chlorhexidine solution, apply sterile lubricant to the end of the catheter, introduce the catheter into the penis, and advance it until there is urine visible in the catheter. Connect a syringe (without a needle) to the other end of the catheter, pull back the urine into the syringe, and finally pull out the catheter.

Documentation Needed When Sending Blood Samples to an Outside Lab

When sending out a blood sample, it is important that the sample is collected into the correct blood tube and that it has the correct corresponding **documentation**. The tube must be labeled with the patient's name, client's name, date, clinic name, and the test to be run. There will be a corresponding form from the reference lab that will be filled out with the same information along with the age of the patient, sex including if the pet is neutered or spayed, if the patient has fasted, and the doctor's name. The reference form will normally list a variety of tests that they have available, and the one requested needs to be marked. Always use a pen with black or blue ink when labeling sample tubes and forms. The sample tube is then placed into the bag provided by the reference lab along with the form.

Documentation Needed When Sending Out Biopsies or Masses to a Reference Lab

A tissue sample such as a **biopsy** or **mass** that has been removed from a patient is sent out to a reference lab for histopathology. The sample is placed into an appropriately sized formalin jar, labeled with the patient's name, client's name, type of specimen, date, and clinic name. A corresponding reference lab form will be filled out that will include all of that same information plus the location of where the mass was on the patient and the size and diameter of the tissue that was excised.

Preparing Hematology Samples to be Sent to an Outside Lab

Blood smears should be **prepared immediately after the sample is collected** to minimize cell deterioration, and they should be stored at room temperature until sent to the reference lab. **Ethylenediaminetetraacetic acid** (EDTA) is the anticoagulant of choice for a complete blood cell count because it best preserves the cellular components of the blood and prevents platelet aggregation. EDTA samples do need to be inverted multiple times, and they must be kept in the refrigerator until shipping. Blood for coagulation testing should be collected into a blue-top tube that contains sodium citrate, and then it is centrifuged for 5 minutes. After the sodium citrate tube is spun down in the centrifuge, the plasma should be removed and transferred to a clean tube without anticoagulant and kept frozen until it is analyzed. Whole blood samples should not be frozen because this causes cell lysis and gross hemolysis, which interferes with testing.

Prepare Cytology Samples to be Sent to an Outside Reference Lab

Cytology samples are normally obtained by fine-needle aspiration (FNA), scraping, or an impression smear. Samples obtained via FNA should be smeared immediately onto a slide before drying using the traditional smearing technique. Highly cellular fluids obtained via FNA can be smeared directly onto a slide, whereas low-cellularity fluids should be centrifuged first to concentrate the cells to create a more adequate smear. Samples that are being sent out to a reference lab must be air dried and labeled with the patient's name, client's name, and the date; then they are placed into a slide holder to be shipped along with the reference lab form.

Creating a Blood Smear

The supplies needed to create a good **blood smear** are two glass slides with a frosted edge, a microscope, immersion oil, and the blood sample. Place a small drop of blood (usually one drop from a 1 ml syringe will be sufficient) on one of the slides right under the frosted edge. The second slide is the spreader slide. Hold the spreader slide at about a 45-degree angle in front of the blood sample on the sample slide. Bring the spreader slide up to meet the drop of blood (still at a 45-degree angle), and allow the blood drop to spread along the short edge of the spreader slide. Next, push the spreader slide in the opposite direction quickly and gently, dragging the blood across the sample slide in a single motion to create a perfect smear. The blood smear is done correctly if it has a feathered edge on the end. The slide should air dry and then be fixed and stained.

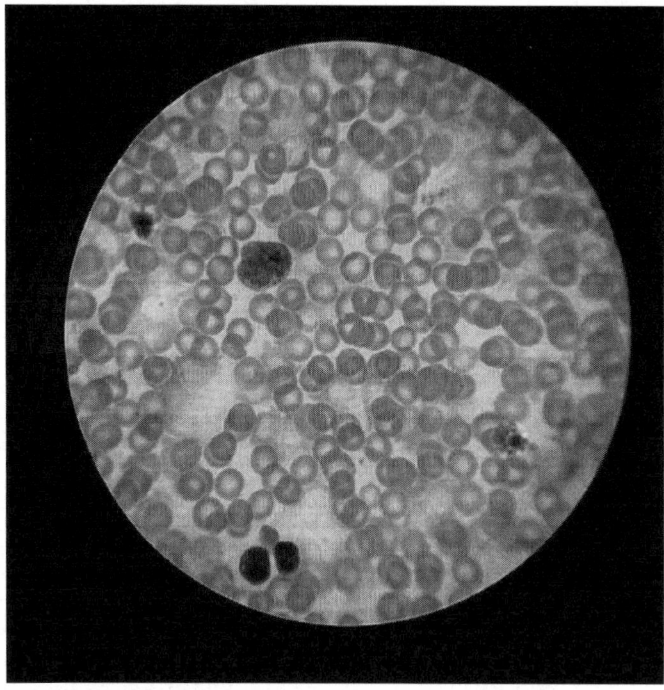

Collecting Hematology Samples

The test that is to be run will determine which **blood tube** will be used to send the sample to the laboratory. To obtain a serum sample, 3 ml of blood (which normally produces ~1 ml of serum) must be drawn and placed into a serum separator tube then allowed to clot. The sample is spun down in a centrifuge, and the serum should be drawn off of the sample within an hour and placed into a red-top tube. To obtain a plasma sample, 3 ml of blood will be drawn and placed into a green-top heparinized (anticoagulant) tube. To obtain a hematology sample for a blood smear, draw 2 ml of blood and place into an EDTA (anticoagulant) purple-top tube.

Packed Cell Volume (PCV)

The **packed cell volume (PCV)**, also known as the hematocrit, measures the percentage of RBCs to the total blood volume. This result is obtained when a small blood sample is drawn into a microhematocrit tube, spun down in a centrifuge where the RBCs are separated from the plasma, and then measured to get the percentage of the sample that is made up of RBCs. The normal PCV is between 35% and 45% in canines and between 25% and 45% in felines. An abnormally low PCV reading, also known as anemia, could result from hemorrhage possibly from ulcers or trauma, hemolysis meaning the destruction of RBCs possibly from an enlarged spleen, or lack of RBC production from bone marrow as in cases of cancer. An increased PCV reading normally results from dehydration or an increase in RBC production.

Materials Needed and Testing for PCV

The materials and equipment needed to perform a **PCV** test are two microhematocrit tubes, a clay stopper, a PCV analyzer card, a microhematocrit centrifuge, and a microscope. By inserting one end of the microhematocrit tube slightly into the blood sample, the blood will flow into the tube. Place a finger at the top of the hematocrit tube to plug it and keep the blood inside. Insert the other end of the hematocrit tube into the clay to plug that end completely so you can remove your finger from the other end. Do this with the second microhematocrit tube as well. Place them into the microhematocrit centrifuge opposite from each other to balance each other. Once the tubes are spun down, line up the bottom of the blood in the microhematocrit tube with the bottom of the card reader. The area in the microhematocrit tube where whole blood stops and plasma starts is where you get your reading; log that number as the PCV value.

Performing a Specific Gravity Test on a Urine Sample

The **urine specific gravity test** is the ratio of the weight of a volume of liquid to the weight of an equal volume of distilled water. The specific gravity will show how concentrated the urine is, which means how much water it contains as well as show how well the kidneys are working. The kidneys function to remove waste products through the urine as well as regulate the body's fluid balance. If the specific gravity is too high, this means that abnormal amounts of water are being eliminated through the urine; if the specific gravity is too low, this can mean that too much water is lost through the urine. If the urine is too diluted, this indicates that the kidneys cannot retain enough water to prevent dehydration. Urine specific gravity is measured by using a refractometer. A drop of urine, either before or after being spun down in the centrifuge, is placed on the prism of the refractometer. The lid is closed over the drop of urine, and by looking through the eyepiece and holding it up to point at the light, you can read the specific gravity reading on the right side. A normal specific gravity value for a cat ranges between 1.020 and 1.040; for a dog, normal readings range from 1.016 to 1.060.

Performing a Fecal Centrifugal Flotation

In order to perform an accurate **fecal centrifugal flotation,** you will need at least 2 grams of feces mixed with at least 10 ml of fecal solution. The feces should be strained through a strainer into a small cup, and then the strained sample is placed into a centrifuge tube and spun at 1,200 rpm for 10 minutes. Create a meniscus by adding a drop of flotation solution to the top of the sample until it is slightly rounded, and place a cover slip on top. Try not to overfill the tube because floated eggs can be lost once the cover slip is put on and fecal material spills over. Let the tube with the cover slip on it sit for 10 minutes, and then remove the cover slip and place it on a microscope slide with the liquid sample side down. Examine the entire area under the microscope at 10× magnification.

Three Types of Demodectic Mange and How it is Diagnosed

Demodex canis is a mite normally found in dog hair follicles and the sebaceous glands of the skin. Canine demodicosis (**demodectic mange**) is when a great deal of these arise due to the body's immune system becoming compromised due to illness. There are three types of demodectic mange: localized, juvenile-onset generalized, and adult-onset generalized. Localized demodectic mange usually affects dogs less than a year old and consists of up to five small lesions of alopecia, scaling, and redness found around the face and forelimbs. The localized form may develop into the juvenile-onset generalized form due to a hereditary immune system abnormality. Adult-onset generalized demodectic mange is the result of a compromised immune system due to an underlying disease that will need to be identified and managed in order to treat the demodectic mange. *D. canis* is diagnosed by performing a skin scraping to look for mites. To perform an accurate skin scraping, squeeze the lesion and apply a small amount of mineral oil on a blade, scraping parallel along the edge of the lesions until the capillaries bleed. Transfer the scraping to a slide, and examine under the microscope on low power.

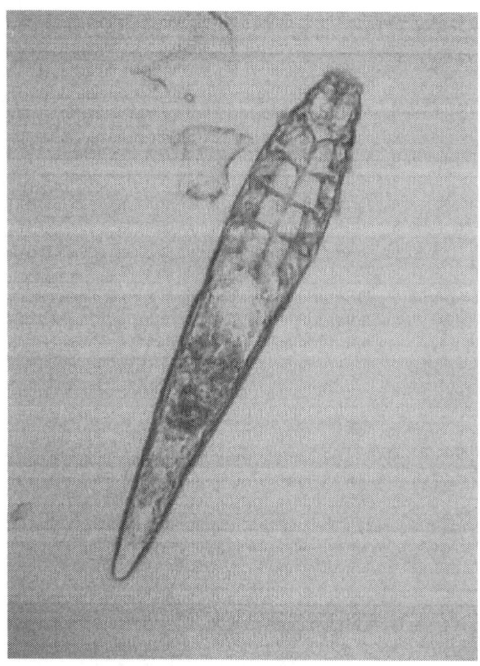

Diagnosing Ringworm in Small Animals

Diagnosing ringworm is done by using a dermatophyte test medium (DTM) culture. Dermatophytes metabolize protein in this culture medium and release alkaline metabolites that turn the medium a red color. Obtaining a sample from the patient's lesion can be done by using a new toothbrush to brush over the lesion or plucking some hair from the lesion with a pair of sterile hemostats and placing the sample into the medium. The DTM plate must be kept in a dark place with the lid closed loosely for up to two weeks. Examine the sample daily, and record if there is growth or color change; after two weeks, place a strip of clear tape over the sample in the DTM to obtain a sample on the sticky side of the tape. Place a drop of new methylene blue stain on a slide, stick the tape on top of the stain, and then examine the slide under 40× magnification.

Causes of Increased Serum Lipase Levels

The digestive enzyme **lipase** works to decompose the long-chain fatty acids that constitute lipids. This process produces reduced fatty acids and alcohols. Normally, only a small amount of lipase can be detected in the serum. However, when serum lipase levels rise it may be indicative of a problem associated with acute or chronic pancreatitis.

Other factors that may contribute to elevated lipase include kidney failure, hyperadrenocorticism, dexamethasone treatment, and bile tract disease. More recent testing products include colorimetric and dry chemistry kits. These products can be used to make an initial assessment regarding lipase levels. However, it is a tedious measurement process.

If a veterinarian believes an animal's symptoms point to acute pancreatitis, serum amylase and lipase tests should be conducted on the patient. However, a cat with pancreatitis should not be diagnosed solely on the basis of serum lipase levels. The serum lipase levels in cats can be low despite the presence of disease in the animal.

Regardless, the testing sample collected should be nonhemolyzed and nonlipemic serum or heparinized plasma.

Bilirubin in the Liver

Bilirubin is a byproduct of the **metabolism of hemoglobin**. Hemoglobin is broken down into heme and globin by the mononuclear phagocytic system (sometimes called the reticuloendothelial system). Heme is then further broken down into bilirubin. The liver functions to modify byproducts and toxins such as bilirubin, reducing them into a form that can be readily excreted from the body. Bilirubin not yet modified by the liver is called "unconjugated" or "indirect" bilirubin. Bilirubin that has been modified has been attached to a glucuronide (creating glucuronic acid), allowing it to be excreted in the bile. This bilirubin is called "conjugated" or "direct" bilirubin. Added together, indirect and direct bilirubin serum levels provide a "total bilirubin" measure.

If bilirubin builds up faster than the liver can metabolize it, or if the liver is not functioning properly, a condition called "**hyperbilirubinemia**" may develop. When the concentrations of bilirubin are particularly high, it can discolor the skin, mucus membranes, and whites of the eyes to make them appear yellowish — a condition called "jaundice" (from the French word jaune, meaning yellow).

In such situations, the liver's own enzymes are sometimes measured to determine whether or not the liver is functioning properly.

Increased Amounts of Unconjugated and Conjugated Bilirubin

Bilirubin levels can be measured in either **blood plasma or serum**. Total and direct levels of bilirubin can be measured specifically in the blood. The **level of indirect (or "unconjugated") bilirubin** is the difference between these two. When bilirubin levels are high (due either to liver damage or rapid RBC hemolysis), significant amounts of bilirubin may pass into the urine (instead of being excreted largely through the bile, passing through the bile ducts and into the intestines). In the intestines, direct bilirubin is further broken down by bacteria into a substance called "urobilinogen," which ultimately gives stool its normal yellowish-brown color. All bilirubin in the urine is of the direct or conjugated form, as indirect or unconjugated bilirubin is not water soluble and thus cannot readily pass out of the body.

The term "**hepatic**" is used in reference to anything involving the liver. Prehepatic jaundice is defined as the liver's failure to process unconjugated bilirubin. Hepatic jaundice and post-hepatic jaundice are directly linked with a rise in conjugated bilirubin levels. Post-hepatic jaundice typically involves partial or full obstruction of the biliary and cystic ducts (cholestasis), keeping the conjugated bilirubin from leaving.

Increased Amount of Urine Urobilinogen

Urobilinogen is produced by bacteria in the intestines. The bacteria utilize conjugated bilirubin to produce urobilinogen. Insignificant levels of urobilinogen are released in the urine.

Cats and dogs are the only animals that are subjected to **routine urobilinogen testing**. In these animals the test indicates particularly unhealthy liver conditions. Abnormally high levels of urobilinogen are indicative of hepatocellular disease. Lower levels may indicate that there is a barrier in the bile ducts. This is true for both humans and dogs.

It is common for normal dogs to have no or very low amounts of urobilinogen in the urine. The urine urobilinogen analysis requires a urine sample to be analyzed promptly. Timely analysis will prevent any urobilinogen from being changed into urobilin. Urobilin is not identifiable in the analysis used to detect urobilinogen. Therefore, the results of the test will not produce accurate information regarding the sample if the sample is allowed to sit for a lengthy period of time.

Test Methods Used for Detecting Bilirubin and the Types of Samples Required

Diazo reagent is a **plasma** or **serum analysis technique for the presence of bilirubin**. Ictotest tablets have a form of diazo reagent and are employed to identify the presence of bilirubin in the urine. Ictotest tablets are able to detect as little as 0.05 to 0.1 mg of bilirubin/dL, and thus are very unlikely to produce false negative results. When the urine is diluted by known increments and re-tested in a serial fashion, the analysis may reveal semi-quantitative results. The rate of the color formation (blue to purple) and the color intensity are both proportional to the amount of bilirubin in the urine. A pink or red color indicates a negative result.

Reagent strips like Ictostix and Multistix can also be employed in testing. These reagent strips also contain a form of diazo reagent. However, the Ictotest tablet is more useful, due to its higher sensitivity to bilirubin in urine. False-negative results may occur if a test sample has been left out too long, as bilirubin rapidly breaks down, especially with exposure to light. False-negative results may also occur if the urine contains large quantities of ascorbic acid or nitrites (released via bacterial growth). In addition, some medications can result in a false-positive reading.

Instruments and Tests Used to Measure TSP

The **Goldberg refractometer** is a device which can gauge total protein levels in serum. The Goldberg refractometer can be obtained from the American Optical Company in Greenwich, CT. This instrument is beneficial in screening a variety of metabolic processes, including Electrolytes, lipids, hemolysis, urea, and glucose. These measurements gained in the screening process can point to other conditions in the patient. Other tests may be necessary to obtain more accurate results.

The **Biuret method** is also used to determine the total amount of serum protein in a sample. This method can be employed in both wet and dry chemical analysis. The method requires that an automated or computerized serum analyzer be used. This analyzer applies a total dye binding process to calculate the serum proteins present in the serum.

The sample collected should be nonhemolyzed and nonlipemic. The serum or plasma samples can be collected with EDTA or heparin preservatives, but heparin will produce a measurement that is somewhat lower. Of additional note, proteins can be denatured or changed on a molecular level when detergent or UV light is introduced, so detergent and UV light should be kept away from the sample.

Conditions That Can Affect the Levels of Serum Proteins

Total serum protein can be abbreviated as **TSP**. Protein levels in serum are calculated based upon the amount of albumin and globulin found in the blood. Albumin and globulin are the 2 primary kinds of protein contained in the blood. The amount of serum globulins can be compared to the amount of serum albumin. While there is generally slightly more albumin, the ratio should be close to 1:1. Any substantial variation could be indicative of other health problems.

Serum protein changes may be shock induced. Further, high albumin levels may be caused by severe dehydration. **High globulin** levels may be caused by: 1) diseases of the blood (leukemia, hemolytic anemia, etc.); 2) autoimmune diseases; 3) certain kidney and liver diseases; et cetera. **Low albumin levels** may be caused by: 1) malnutrition; 2) severe burns; 3) other kidney and liver diseases; 4) gastrointestinal malabsorption syndromes; 5) Hodgkin's lymphoma; 6) uncontrolled diabetes; 7) hyperthyroidism; and 8) heart failure. Thus, the veterinarian can check the level of each serum protein to explore many aspects of an animal's health. However, pregnancy, injuries, infections, prolonged bed rest, chronic illness, and certain medications may also affect blood protein levels.

Globulin Fractions and Increases in Globulin Levels

Electrophoresis involves the electrically induced movement of molecular particles. It can also be applied to protein molecules, such as globulin or albumin. Electrophoresis is a technique used to divide globulin from albumin. **Fibrinogens** are soluble proteins that allow blood to clot. Fibrinogens are also present in the globulin fraction. Fibrinogen can occasionally be calculated from the total protein present. The amount of fibrinogen equals approximately 4 g/L of the total plasma protein fraction. This measurement requires a plasma base.

Electrophoresis can reveal any comparative larger or smaller quantitative differences in protein particles. Upon separation, observation, and measurement, these differences may indicate the presence of particular diseases in the animal. However, each species of animal should only be compared with normal levels in relation to that specific species.

Globulin levels may be raised when **antigenic stimulation** occurs. In addition, other factors, including inflammation or infections, neoplasia, or abnormal immunoglobulin production can contribute to this rise in levels.

Increases or Decreases in Albumin

Animals may sometimes present with one or more diseases that will contribute to **altered albumin or globulin concentration**. However, it is important to note that, generally, the total serum protein (TSP) will remain the same. The reason that the TSP level does not change is because **globulin levels tend to rise as the albumin level lowers**. Even so, certain infections, stressors, malnutrition, and other factors can sometimes affect TSP levels (usually then seen in an overall decrease).

The globulin level can be used to derive the albumin level by subtraction. The globulin level is determined by taking the albumin away from the total TSP level. The serum albumin levels can be calculated by applying the albumin dye binding technique.

The veterinarian should be aware that there is a chance that the animal suffering from shock will experience a rise in albumin levels. More frequently, the animal will have a lower albumin count due to the presence of other conditions, including acute liver disease, starvation or undernourishment, malabsorption, enteritis, colitis, parasites, pregnancy and lactation, persistent fever, improperly managed or untreated diabetes, shock, nephritis or nephrosis, ascites, and loss or reduction in blood volume.

Significance of Elevated Levels of Alanine Aminotransferase in the Serum

The **enzyme alanine aminotransferase** is abbreviated as ALT. This enzyme has been more recently referred to as serum glutamic pyruvate transaminase (SGPT). Yet another name for this enzyme is alanine transaminase.

It has been noted that more than 90% of all ALT activity is found in the hepatocytes of dogs, cats, rats, rabbits, and primates. Thus, in these animals, an elevated level of ALT is generally diagnostic for liver disease. Therefore, the veterinarian will measure the ALT level in these animals whenever the status of the liver's function is in question.

However, birds, horses, pigs, and ruminants have a much lower level of hepatocellular ALT activity. In these animals, ALT enzymes are more active in various muscle tissues. Therefore, increased levels of serum ALT in these animals is typically indicative of skeletal muscle injury or necrosis, rather than liver disease.

Testing for Non-Plasma Specific Enzymes

There are particular enzymes that are not normally present in either plasma or serum. The levels of these specific enzymes can be raised by certain conditions. These conditions include destruction of tissue cells, intensified tissue cell production, barriers in the excretory path, or poor circulation.

A **non-plasma specific enzyme test kit** will consist of the following items: substrates, coenzymes, and cofactors. The enzymes should be analyzed under specified temperatures. The veterinarian should take particular care in sample collection, especially regarding samples that contain anticoagulants.

The international unit of measure is abbreviated as IU. The international unit is also used to display the quantitative measurements obtained through enzyme analysis. The IU is the standardized index used for this practice.

In general, the older unit indices are no longer used. However, occasional deviations from this reporting standard may still occur, whether due to specific machine calibration, operator preference, or residual operating policy. Regardless, the laboratory has the responsibility to include any laboratory-specific reference ranges and standards with any enzyme level reports issued from that facility.

Type of Sample Required to Test for Aspartate Aminotransferase

The **enzyme aspartate aminotransferase** is abbreviated as AST. Another name used is aspartate transaminase. In former years, the term serum glutamic oxaloacetic transaminase was also used. The abbreviation for serum glutamic oxaloacetic transaminase is SGOT, and this acronym is still occasionally used.

AST enzymes, along with other enzymes, facilitate many intracellular processes and functions. Thus, they are **only found in the bloodstream when cellular damage has released them into extracellular fluids**, by which they are drawn into the vascular circulation.

The level of AST has not been linked with any particular organ in the body. However, this enzyme has been linked to various tissues of the body, including cardiac muscle, diaphragmatic muscle, skeletal muscle, and the liver. Therefore, whenever these tissues sustain any injury, then a rise in AST levels in the serum or plasma can be expected.

The veterinarian should perform a test for AST levels using a plasma or serum sample that is not hemolyzed or lipemic. The specimen should be properly centrifuged, allowing the AST to be separated from the red blood cells. This will give a more accurate reading of the AST level.

Significance of Changes in the Levels of Alanine Aminotransferase in the Serum

ALT/SGPT enzymes are specific to liver and muscle tissue. Injury to any of these cells releases this enzyme into the bloodstream. Therefore, knowing where this enzyme is most active can reveal where tissue damage may be occurring in the body, when the levels of this enzyme are elevated.

The level of ALT can be measured in both plasma and serum samples. There may be a high ALT level measured in initial tests, but that lowers when further tests are performed over time. That would indicate either that the first test was simply out of the norm, or that a transiently injurious event occurred that is quickly resolving. Unfortunately, when the levels increase or remain high over time, it is likely that a serious disease is involved. In animals in which ALT enzymes are more active in the liver, the veterinarian will need to explore the liver's functioning capacity and health. In animals where ALT enzymes are more active in muscle tissues, the veterinarian will look to skeletal muscles for sources of disease and damage.

In some cases canines are given medications that can unintentionally and artificially increase ALT levels. However, medications are less likely to produce this side effect in cats.

Characteristics of Alkaline Phosphatase

Practically **all the organic tissues within the body are constructed with the involvement of the enzyme alkaline phosphatase**. This is an enzyme that catalyzes and synthesizes phosphoric acid. **Alkaline phosphatase** is produced primarily in the liver and bone, with some made in the intestines and kidneys — and by the placenta during pregnancy. Alkaline phosphatase is abbreviated as AP. AP is usually found in low quantities in the serum. Abnormally elevated AP levels may point to the presence of certain conditions in the body. These conditions include: intrahepatic or posthepatic cholestasis, medication-induced liver damage, bone tumors, osteomalacia, and parathyroid hormone overproduction, etc. The rise in AP levels will not usually be linked to reduced rates of enzyme metabolism and discharge. Rather, a rise in AP levels can usually be attributed to a rise in production of AP. Young animals may have a rise in AP that can be linked to bone growth. However, the same high level of AP in older animals may be from a different cause. For instance, the rise in AP levels can be directly linked to a bone injury or obstructive liver disease. In addition, certain medications will cause this rise for about 2 weeks after the drug has been given to the patient. These medications include some anticonvulsants and glucocorticoids.

Significance of Elevated Levels of Aspartate Aminotransferase (AST) in the Serum

Aspartate aminotransferase is abbreviated as AST. The significance of high levels of AST in serum can be linked to a number of potential health issues. These issues can include an impairment of the liver, destruction of red blood cells, or damaged heart or skeletal muscle tissue.

Even so, the veterinarian should not rely on the results of the AST analysis alone. The veterinarian should also administer ALT enzyme tests. The ALT and AST tests should be used in conjunction when considering a diagnosis, particularly when assessing the liver.

However, there are some types of animals that will not benefit from this combination of tests. For these species, the AST can be used as a solitary measure to detect liver disease. Regardless, the veterinarian should continue to explore the possibility of other contributing factors that could be linked to the rise in AST levels, as changes in these enzymatic levels are not diagnostically definitive.

Characteristics of the Enzyme Known as SDH

The abbreviation for the enzyme **sorbitol dehydrogenase** is SDH. Sorbitol dehydrogenase is produced in liver cells. The veterinarian will often be able to detect liver cell damage by making an appraisal of the SDH levels in the serum.

In veterinary applications, SDH has been found to be a particularly **effective indicator of acute hepatocellular (liver cell) damage and disease**. It also has a high sensitivity to toxins, and thus is a very early indicator of toxin- or medication-induced liver damage.

Likewise, necrosis (the death of cells) in the liver can be associated with higher levels of SDH in the serum. Necrosis is a result of injury or disease in the patient.

SDH levels should be analyzed to determine if a large animal has a liver disease. The SDH test is more appropriate for use with larger animals than is ALT testing. However, the SDH enzyme is known to be unstable and can lose its ability to react after about 8 hours. Therefore, the sample should be analyzed as soon as possible after collection. The practice of sending samples to outside labs to be analyzed may be problematic if the tests are thereby delayed. Thus, the veterinarian may need to use a local laboratory or one within the clinic to alleviate this problem.

Characteristics of the Enzyme Known as GGT

GGT is the abbreviation for the enzyme known as **gamma-glutamyltransferase**. This enzyme can be located in elevated concentrations in some of the body's organs. Primarily these organs include the liver, pancreas, and kidney.

High concentrations of GGT in the serum **point directly to liver maladies**. In particular, the liver disease known as cholestasis can be detected when GGT levels are high. However, there can be other liver diseases that can contribute to the higher GGT levels. Therefore, the veterinarian should monitor both ALT and GGT in the smaller-sized animals. The veterinarian that notes a rise in ALT levels and a rise in GGT levels should actively explore potential causes of liver disease in the small animal.

Another type of disease found in small animals that elevates GGT enzymes is fatty liver disease. In addition, the veterinarian should rule out any medication side effects that can cause increased levels of GGT.

Increases and Decreases in Serum Levels

Serum Bile Acid Levels and Serum Cholesterol Levels

Animals with liver disease will have **higher serum bile acid levels** due to the liver's inability to filter the acids from the blood (diseased hepatocytes have a decreased ability to extract bile acids from the blood). Thus, higher levels of serum bile acid are found in these animals. Postponed emptying of the stomach and fasting will lower these levels. An animal with ileal or lower (post jejunal) small intestinal disease will have a lower serum bile acid level. **Cholesterol** is a steroid alcohol created through a liver synthesis process. **Hypothyroidism** can result from higher levels of serum cholesterol in an animal. Hypothyroidism is a deficiency in thyroid hormone production.

High cholesterol levels may also indicate lipemia. **Lipemia** is an unusually high level of lipids or fats in the blood. Higher levels of cholesterol may portend some serious maladies in a patient. These serious maladies include diabetes mellitus, hyperadrenocorticism, nephrotic syndrome, certain liver diseases, bile duct obstruction, and pregnancy complications.

The test for serum cholesterol levels cannot be used alone to diagnose liver dysfunction, but should be used in combination with other diagnostic indices and liver function tests. Prior to collecting a blood specimen, the patient should not be fed for a number of hours. In this way a more accurate base level can be determined. A non-hemolyzed serum or heparinized plasma sample should be utilized for testing.

Serum Bile Acid Levels

Bile is produced by the liver, and is very important in the digestive process. Bile acids are both hydrophobic (lipid, or fat soluble) and hydrophilic (polar, or water soluble). This means that bile is able to break down water-insoluble fats in a water-saturated environment (i.e., the intestinal tract).

Bile is **synthesized from cholesterol** — more than half of which comes from diet, with the remainder created by synthesis in the body (in the liver, intestines, and other cells). Cholesterol synthesis is facilitated by acetyl-CoA. **Acetyl-CoA** is derived from an oxidation reaction. Oxidation is a chemical reaction that incorporates oxygen into atoms or molecules. In bile production, the oxidative process converts pyruvate into acetyl-CoA, by which cholesterol is synthesized, then from which bile is produced in the liver. Bile is stored in the gall bladder in humans and most domestic animals, except in horses and rats.

Usually, serum bile acid levels are low. This is due to the body's bile reabsorption process in the ileum or lower small intestines and the filtration of blood through the liver. Low serum bile acid levels "post-prandially" (after a meal) may indicate ileal dysfunction. High levels are indicative of liver disease (even when other liver function tests may appear normal).

Serum Potassium Levels

The **potassium cation** (positively charged ion) contributes to sustaining the fluid and electrolyte balance within the body. This balance is maintained by fluid dynamics, 90% of which take place within the cells of the body.

The normal range of both serum and plasma potassium levels is 3.5 to 5.5 mEq/L — and they are the same whether reported as milliequivalents per liter (mEq/L) or millimoles per liter (mmol/L). Higher levels of serum potassium are indicative of a number of potential concerning conditions. These conditions include adrenal cortical hypofunction, acidosis, and late-stage renal failure. A high potassium levels is referred to as hyperkalemia.

An abnormally low level of serum potassium is referred to as **hypokalemia**. Conditions that are attributed to hypokalemia include alkalosis, insulin therapy, and surplus fluid loss associated with diuretics, vomiting, and diarrhea.

The best test results are generally obtained with a plasma sample. However, the sample may be either non-hemolyzed serum or heparinized plasma. Blood cells must be separated from the fluids within 2 hours or the testing values may be altered. This is particularly critical when analyzing samples taken from cattle and horses, as their blood cells continue to release potassium over time.

SERUM SODIUM LEVELS

Sodium is essential to the body's fluid balance. Sodium also gives support to the movement of water within the body and its cells. Sodium helps sustain osmotic pressures and fluid balances within the body. Sodium is key to the extracellular positive ion attraction that primes the "sodium-potassium-ATPase pump" responsible for moving vital nutrients and materials into and out of cell structures.

Patients will not normally have a high level of sodium in their blood serum. When a high level is noted, then the patient may suffer from **hypernatremia**. However, this may occur in part because the patient is dehydrated. The veterinarian will most often diagnose hyponatremia in patients with a sodium imbalance. This condition is marked by low sodium levels. Problems associated with hyponatremia include kidney failure, vomiting or diarrhea in association with diuretics, disproportionate ADH, congestive heart failure, and water toxicity.

Patients with sodium imbalances should have their fluid intake monitored to prevent them from ingesting more liquids than needed. The veterinarian should use a **nonhemolyzed serum specimen** for the serum sodium test. Plasma samples can be tested, provided they are collected with lithium or ammonium heparin. However, both serum and plasma specimens must be centrifuged to remove cellular components from the residual fluid used for testing.

SERUM CALCIUM LEVELS

Calcium is the principal element found in the body's skeletal system. Approximately 99% of all calcium found in the body is contained within the bones. The remaining calcium is employed to help move inorganic ions and fluids throughout the body. Calcium is needed in the function of cell membranes, blood coagulation, muscle contraction and nerve impulse transmission, as well as in the activation of certain enzymes.

Parathyroid hormone is abbreviated as PTH. PTH, calcitonin, and vitamin D work together to control the calcium and phosphorus levels within the body. Serum protein, albumin levels, and serum calcium levels should all be appraised simultaneously. This gives the veterinarian the opportunity to observe how the serum calcium levels fluctuate together with the protein and albumin levels.

A rise in serum calcium is referred to as hypercalcemia. **Hypercalcemia** can point to other serious conditions, including pseudohyperparathyroidism, hyperparathyroidism, excessive vitamin D intake, and cancerous bony metastases. An abnormally low level of serum calcium is called **hypocalcemia**. Hypocalcemia can point to serious conditions such as malabsorption, eclampsia, pancreatic necrosis, hypoalbuminemia, and hypoparathyroidism.

SERUM CHLORIDE LEVELS

Chloride is formed when the element chlorine combines with an additional electron to become a negatively charged anion. Working with other positively charged electrolytes (sodium, potassium, calcium, etc.), this chemical helps equalize the balance of electrolytes in the body. The kidneys are responsible for controlling the levels of chloride ions found in the body.

Hyperchloremia is the term used to describe an abnormally high serum chloride level. The patient with hyperchloremia may have serious health issues, including metabolic acidosis or renal tubular acidosis and overactive parathyroid glands.

The patient with an **abnormally low level of serum chloride** (hypochloremia) may have other issues, including vomiting, anorexia, malnutrition, and diabetes insipidus.

A blood sample for testing should be **nonhemolyzed serum** or **heparinized plasma**. Blood cells must be separated from the plasma or serum promptly in order to avoid biased test results.

Serum Calcium Levels and Serum Phosphorus Levels

Low levels of serum calcium in ruminants may indicate gastrointestinal stasis. Female cows, dogs, sheep, and horses may experience calcium-related peri- or post-parturient health events with the onset of lactation, as the demands of milk production for nursing overwhelm the body's calcium supplies. It is often called parturient paresis or milk fever, but may also be referred to as puerperal hypocalcemia, hypocalcemic tetany, and milk or lactation tetany. To test for calcium disorders, the veterinarian should obtain a nonhemolyzed serum or heparinized plasma sample.

Phosphorus is another important bodily element. The skeleton contains 80% of the body's phosphorus. **Parathyroid hormone** (PTH) helps regulate the balance of both calcium and phosphorus.

Serum phosphorus levels should be monitored along with serum calcium levels due to the inverse relation that these substances have to each other. Hyperphosphatemia is an abnormally high level of phosphorus which can point to kidney failure, anuria, and hypoparathyroidism. It can be induced by ingestion of an excessive amount of vitamin D, or poisoning with ethylene glycol. Abnormally low serum phosphorus is called hypophosphatemia. It can sometimes arise from a diet low in phosphorus, and may be related to primary hyperparathyroidism, malabsorption, hyperinsulinism, diabetes mellitus, lymphosarcoma, and hyperadrenocorticism. Nonhemolyzed serum or heparinized plasma is needed for laboratory testing.

Urine Sample Containers and Clean Catch Sample Collecting Technique

There are often unique requirements that should be followed in the collection of various kinds of samples. In some situations, a specimen container should be opaque in order to protect the specimen from light. This keeps light from breaking down the components within the sample. Samples that should be protected from light include bilirubin and urobilinogen. Every container should be sterile to keep samples free from contaminants.

Urine samples for bacterial culture require collection using specific techniques such as **cystocentesis** or **catheterization**. Both remove fluids like urine from inside the body—cytocentesis by needle aspiration and catheterization by insertion of a tube. Urine collected in this way is more sanitary than the clean catch samples otherwise obtained. Although **clean catch samples** are not invasive, they are less useful for bacterial cultures. Other names for clean catch samples are free flow or voiding samples. These samples should be taken when the patient is at midstream in the release of urine, as the beginning and final release are not as free from contamination. In addition, the patient's vulva or prepuce (foreskin) requires cleaning beforehand.

Manual Expression and Tabletop Sample Procedures

Urine can also be obtained through a procedure known as "manual expression." This procedure involves the application of light pressure on the bladder, which is continued during the animal's mid-stream expulsion of urine. This procedure adheres to the criteria required for a clean catch specimen. However, the veterinarian cannot use this sample for a bacterial culture, as bacterial cultures require more sterile collection techniques. The animal's vulva or prepuce should be sanitized prior to the procedure.

The veterinarian should not attempt manual expression when it is suspected that the animal has some type of obstruction, as it could lead to bladder rupture. In all cases, the veterinarian should not become impatient or apply too much pressure on the bladder, as this could harm the animal.

"**Tabletop samples**" (spontaneous micturition or voids on the examination table) are appropriate for use given the following conditions: a) the surface of the table is clean, and b) immediate testing of the sample is performed. However, tabletop samples do not meet the requirements for bacterial cultures.

URINE TESTING

CYSTOCENTESIS AND CATHETERIZATION URINE SAMPLE TECHNIQUES

The veterinarian will use **cystocentesis** to collect urine from the urinary bladder. This is accomplished by inserting a needle through the ventral abdominal wall and into the bladder. Aseptic techniques to prevent infection should be applied. In an effort to avoid harming the other internal abdominal organs, the veterinarian should make sure that the animal has a full bladder. The benefits involved in this procedure are associated with the avoidance of contamination derived from the lower parts of the urinary tract. The cystocentesis technique is particularly appropriate for the collection of a urine specimen for bacterial culture.

The veterinarian may otherwise use the catheterization technique to collect urine from the urinary bladder. This is accomplished by using a rubber, plastic, or metal catheter (tube) to allow the passage of urine from the urinary bladder through the urethra with little risk of contamination. The animal's species and sex should guide the selection of the correct catheter type and size to be used in the procedure. Proper aseptic techniques should minimize the risk of infection in the animal and contamination of the sample taken. The veterinarian should also ensure that the animal does not experience any undue stress.

PROPER URINE SAMPLE PRESERVATION TECHNIQUES AND THE CLIENT-COLLECTED URINE SAMPLE

Room temperature is necessary for samples involving specific gravity and crystal evaluations. The urine sample should be placed in a centrifuge. This allows the veterinarian to carry out a cytological evaluation. The veterinarian may prolong the integrity of these cells by the addition of certain chemicals. Preservation chemicals applied include the following: formalin, toluene, or phenol.

Often, client-collected samples are not appropriate for testing. Indeed, client-collected samples may be associated with a multitude of disadvantages. These include: 1) insufficient and unskilled collection techniques, 2) inadequate and unsanitary containers used to receive and transport the sample, and 3) the lengthy time that may pass between collection and testing. These inconsistent variables will allow questions to be raised regarding the validity of the test results. Therefore, the veterinarian should endeavor to personally apply controlled collection techniques in retrieving a sample.

The veterinarian should be aware that room temperatures can change the urine in as little as 2 hours or less. Conditions that may induce a breakdown of the urine sample include the following: a) a rise in ammonia levels; b) the presence of hemolyzed erythrocytes (as opposed to intact red blood cells); c) the presence of a pH level which allows bacteria to grow; d) lower levels of bilirubin, glucose, ketones, leukocytes, and urobilirubin; e) the disappearance of casts; f) an alteration in crystals; g) a darker discoloration; h) the appearance of nitrites; i) a harsher smell; j) a lower or higher concentration of protein; and k) an opaque and muddy appearance.

The veterinarian should place the collected urine sample in the refrigerator. The veterinarian can place the sample in cold storage for a period of 6 to 12 hours. These refrigerated samples should return to room temperature before a test is performed.

Color of Urine Output

The **coloration of urine** ranges from pale yellow to a pale yellowish-brown. This coloration is normal in most animals. The color is directly related to the presence of urochromes. Urochromes are responsible for the yellow pigment found in urine. The specific gravity (the ratio of the liquid's density as compared with water, abbreviated SG) is responsible for the intensity of color. Urine with a reduction in SG will appear lighter in color than urine with a higher SG. In addition, bile pigments are associated with colorations noted as yellowish-brown or greenish. Urine with bile pigments present will also froth when shaken.

Red blood cells are abbreviated as RBCs. The presence of these cells is indicated by a reddish tint to the urine. This condition is called hematuria. Hemoglobin is abbreviated as Hb, and is reddish brown in color. Urine tinted reddish brown indicates a condition known as hemoglobinuria. Myoglobins are brown in color. Thus, brown-tinted urine is associated with a condition known as myoglobinuria.

5 Variables That Control the Volume of Urine Output

The **volume of urine output is controlled by 5 variables**. These include: 1) the **amount of water** that an animal drinks, 2) the **temperatures** within the animal's environment, 3) the animal's **physical activity levels,** 4) the **animal's size**, and 5) the animal's **genus or species**. The animal that has a frequent need to urinate could be diagnosed with pollakiuria (abnormally frequent urination). This is not to be mistaken with polyuria (voiding excessive quantities of urine). Polyuria is often found in patients with undiagnosed diabetes. Other conditions associated with polyuria include nephritis and polydipsia (abnormal thirst). Patients that are in shock, dehydrated, conserving water, or in kidney failure will not produce normal amounts of urine, and consequently will not have a desire to urinate as much. Oliguria (abnormally limited urine production) is a result of these declining conditions. If the patient becomes unable to urinate, then a diagnosis of anuria can be made. Anuria can be a direct result of renal or kidney shutdown. This condition can also be attributed to an obstruction which prevents urine from passing out of the body.

Odor of Urine

Urine is typically associated with some unpleasant smells. Odor in and of itself should not be used to directly derive a diagnosis. However, odor may help the veterinarian to further explore certain likely problems. For example, **odors may be caused by a type of bacterium** likely present in the urine. In addition, the presence of an excessive quantity of ammonia can often be detected from the odor. Certain animals like cats, mice, goats, and pigs can put off a quite pungent odor when urinating. If the animal's urine gives off a sweet or fruity smell, it may be due to ketones present in the discharge. This can point to a number of problems like diabetes mellitus, pregnancy toxemia in sheep, or acetonemia in cows. The excessive quantity of ammonia can often be traced to a rise in bacteria levels. The smell of ammonia will be strong in this case. However, this bacterial proliferation may also emerge in standing, improperly stored urine. The rise in bacteria levels can intensify the overall strength of the smell.

Transparency of Urine Samples

The **transparency of urine samples** is defined in 3 levels or degrees. These 3 degrees include: **clear, cloudy, or flocculent**. The term **flocculent** is often used to describe urine that appears pathologic, containing easily visible particles, mucus, and other debris — often due to the presence of crystals and/or infection. Many animals will produce clear, transparent urine at the time of voiding. However, the horse, rabbit, hamster, and gerbil do not. The horse has mucus and calcium carbonate crystals present in the urine at the time of voiding. The rabbit, hamster, and gerbil have calcium salts present in the urine at the time of voiding. The presence of these components will produce a cloudy transparency in the urine voided. **Cloudy urine** can be created from RBCs, WBCs, epithelial cells, crystals, bacteria, casts, mucus, semen, or lipids. In addition, bacteria or crystals present in the urine can turn voided, standing urine a cloudy color. This is a problem associated with bacterial proliferation and crystal formation that can occur when urine is not stored correctly after collection. Thus, samples should generally be tested promptly to avoid these problematic changes.

Specific Gravity and Reagent Strip Measurements

The veterinarian will place a few drops of urine on a prism cover glass before using the refractometer. The **refractometer** is designed to emit a bright light, refracted through the urine in the analysis process. The veterinarian will read the number from the scale located in the light-dark margin of the instrument. This number will be the SG (specific gravity) approximation for the sample taken. The veterinarian can also determine the total quantity of solids present in the analyzed sample.

The veterinarian will need a larger sample to use the **urinometer**. This device is calibrated at room temperature. The urinometer is placed inside the container holding the urine, and floats upright with the assistance of a weighted bulb. The urinometer has a scale attached to the bulb, which can be read when the index has stopped moving. The SG is read at the meniscus or upper surface of the urine.

The least reliable (but often quick and useful) urine testing involves the use of **reagent strips**. These strips offer inconsistent results when the reading of the SG is over 1.030. The reagent strip is set in the urine until it becomes totally soaked. The strip will change colors. The color of the strip will then be matched with a color scale to determine the approximate SG of the sample.

Specific Gravity and Its Function in Analyzing and Measuring Urine Samples

Specific gravity is abbreviated as SG. SG gives the ratio of the density of urine in relation to the density of distilled water. This number is important when trying to calculate how efficiently the kidneys can concentrate the urine.

Different species of animals will have different urine SG values. The average SG value for a dog is 1.025, ranging from 1.001 to 1.060. The average SG value for a cat is 1.030, ranging from 1.001 to 1.080. The average SG value for a horse is 1.035. The average SG value for cattle and swine is 1.015. The average SG for sheep is 1.030. Higher levels of SG are attributed to animals suffering from dehydration or shock. These animals may not be drinking enough water. In addition, these levels can also be attributed to acute renal disease. Lower levels of SG can be attributed to larger sums of water intake. Other causes can include renal and other diseases.

Thus, the veterinarian will need to obtain an accurate measurement of the specific gravity or SG levels. The devices used to obtain this measurement include a refractometer, urinometer, or reagent test strips.

Proteinuria and Its Detection

Protein is normally absent or present only in trace amounts in the urine. **Proteinuria** can indicate disease in the animal. This condition is associated with excessive quantities of protein or protein metabolites within the urine. The veterinarian will employ the use of a reagent strip to determine the level of protein within the urine. The strip's reading is accomplished by comparison of the urine- soaked strip's colors with a color chart. However, these results can be inconsistent. Furthermore, false positives, false negatives, and human error are all associated with the use of reagent strips.

There are many factors that can contribute to proteinuria. Some have to do with issues surrounding the onset of a kidney disease. Others occur after renal diseases have already commenced.

Proteinuria is often associated with **urogenital system malfunctions**. The veterinarian should also consider the outcome of the test in conjunction with any blood found in the urine. In addition, any microscopic residue should be taken into account. Very alkaline urine may produce a false-positive protein reading. If the specific gravity is very low, a false-negative reading may occur. Further, reagent strips tend to react to albumin and less to globulin. Where urine protein levels are excessive, a follow-up sulfosalicylic acid turbidity test (sensitive to both albumin and globulin) may be helpful.

Measuring Levels in Urine

Measuring Glucose Levels in Urine

Urine glucose levels should also be measured. Higher quantities of glucose can indicate glucosuria or glycosuria. **Glucosuria** can be a sign of diabetes. Further, elevated urine glucose can occur if the kidneys are unable to properly reabsorb glucose in the renal tubules, indicating that the patient may be developing renal disease.

Glucose levels are usually measured at approximately 170 to 180 mg/dL. The veterinarian can use a reagent strip to test the levels of glucose in the urine, choosing either Clinitest or Ames products for this purpose. Reagent strips are useful in the identification of glucose. However, reagent tablets are able to identify all of the various forms of sugars.

The patient with high urine glucose may have an **insulin deficiency** which contributes to the condition known as diabetes mellitus. The patient may also have a history of hyperglycemia that should be considered along with glucosuria.

Thus, the precise measurement of blood glucose levels can provide warning of the onset of **diabetes mellitus**. However, it is important to also recognize that glucosuria can be caused by many other factors. These factors include anxiety, nervous tension, agitation, intravenous fluids containing glucose, and other additional diseases.

Measuring Bile Pigments in Urine

Examples of bile pigments include **bilirubin** and **urobilinogen**. The urine normally contains some conjugated bilirubin and a tiny amount of urobilinogen that has been synthesized by bacteria within the intestines. The veterinarian will be able to use a reactive test pad on a cat to derive a positive bilirubin measurement. However, dogs have been known to produce both false-positive and false-negative results by this method. Thus, these test pads are not recommended for measuring bilirubin in dogs. Urobilinogen test pads have been found unreliable for both dogs and cats. In these situations, bile pigments can be successfully measured using reagent test strips.

Bilirubinuria can be attributed to **biliary obstruction, hepatic infections, toxicity, and hemolytic anemia**. The veterinarian should take care to keep urine samples out of the light. Prolonged exposure to light may cause a false-negative result. This negative result is due to light's oxidizing effect upon the bilirubin. Furthermore, the biological makeup of dogs and cats may predispose an indication of bilirubinuria. This has been linked to an enzyme within the kidneys and livers of dogs and cattle which conjugates excess bilirubin.

Measuring Ketone Levels in Urine

Ketones are described as organic compounds such as acetone, acetoacetic acid (also called diacetic acid), and beta-hydroxybutyric acid. The body produces acetone and beta-hydroxybutyric acid through a process known as **catabolism** (breaking down fats and/or muscles in the body for energy). In this process, initially, fat in the body is converted into energy. The metabolic processing of fat will create ketones. Small amounts of ketones in the body and bloodstream are normal, but large amounts can be toxic to the animal. A high ketone level is known as ketonuria. The ketones are the result of a rapid rate of fat metabolism. In addition, the carbohydrate metabolism is lowered. This can occur simultaneously or as a single process. This causes carbohydrates to discharge into the urine. This can be the result of ketosis or ketonemia.

Hyperglycemia (high glucose levels in the blood) is attributed to an inadequate absorption of glucose. The condition can be exacerbated by a high carbohydrate diet. Hyperglycemia can contribute to ketosis, especially in large mammals.

Ketostix, Acetest, and Ames are reagent strips or tablets used to test for the presence of Ketones. Ketone concentration and reagent strip color strengths are comparative. These tests react efficiently to acetoacetic acid.

Blood Components in Urine and the Process of Urine Sediment Evaluations

Myoglobinuria is a condition that gives the urine a brown tint. This condition may or may not change the color of the urine. However, occult blood in the urine indicates a disease condition that is often hard to identify. Urogenital tract disease can often be linked directly to hematuria. Hemoglobinuria is sometimes linked to intravascular hemolysis or the destruction of red blood cells and the release of hemoglobin. Muscle disease is often linked to hemoglobinuria and myoglobinuria.

The sample preparation for microscopic evaluation of **urine sediment** requires that the specimen first be meticulously blended to ensure equal distribution of all sample contents. This blended fluid is then poured into a centrifuge tube with a conical tip. The centrifuge is then set in motion at 1500 to 2000 rpm for a period lasting from 3-5 minutes. Careful removal of excess supernatant should result in approximately 0.3mL of residual supernatant. The sediment is next dispersed within the residual liquid in a suspended form. Then, the microscope slide receives 2 to 3 drops of liquid for visual examination.

Testing for Blood Components in Urine

The veterinarian should use reagent test strips or tablets when trying to determine if blood is in the urine. RBCs, or red blood cells, are visible under a microscope.

In addition, the animal should be subjected to an examination, as the microscope provides no explanation for blood's presence within the urine. The veterinarian should take into account the animal's medical history and current presentation in seeking an identifiable cause for hematuria. The veterinarian will often require a new sample to further assess the urine for leukocytes. This sample should also be analyzed with a microscope. The use of leukocyte test pads is not recommended, as these pads will frequently result in a false-positive in cats and a false-negative in dogs.

Hematuria is a condition that gives the urine a reddish-to-black cloudy tint, indicating the presence of intact RBCs. Hemoglobinuria gives urine a brown or black tint, indicating the presence of free Hb in the urine.

WHITE BLOOD CELLS AND RED BLOOD CELLS THAT ARE FOUND IN URINE SEDIMENT

Urine sediment typically has a small amount of leukocytes present. **Leukocytes** are also known as white blood cells (WBCs). However, when leukocytes are numerous, then the condition of **pyuria** (pus in the urine) and/or **leukocyturia** (white blood cells in the urine) is indicated. This can be due to an active inflammatory disease in the animal. This disease can be located along the entire length of the urinary tract, or only in the genital tract. The veterinarian should examine the animal closely and collect another urine specimen when more than a few leukocytes (5-8) per high power field (HPF) are observed. Any bacteria observed should also be noted.

When numerous red blood cells (RBCs) or erythrocytes are present in the sediment, the condition of hematuria is indicated. **Hematuria** has been associated with the following: trauma, calculi, infection, and benign or malignant neoplasia. RBCs can readily be seen in a microscopic examination. RBCs are subject to changes in color in certain circumstances. However, the coloration of RBCs is typically that of a light red with refractive disks. The red in blood is due to hemoglobin — but not to the iron in hemoglobin, which is a popular belief. The red tint actually arises from the porphyrin moiety of hemoglobin (to which the iron is bound), and not from the iron itself. RBCs should have a consistent shape and form. If there are more than a few RBCs in the urine (5 or more per HPF), then the veterinarian should explore possible causative factors.

ADDITIONAL URINE SEDIMENT EVALUATION PROCEDURES

The veterinarian may or may not apply stain to a slide during a microscopic urine examination. The veterinarian will examine the slide under reduced illumination with a setting of 10x magnification (i.e., a low-power field objective). This allows the slide to be scanned over its complete coverslip area, and allows for the identification of most crystals, casts, squamous cells, and other large objects. These objects are usually reported according to the number of each type found per "low power field" (LPF).

The setting is then changed to 40x, or a high-power field objective. This allows the veterinarian the opportunity to recognize and name the objects now visible on the slide. These will include crystals, cells, sperm, and bacteria. The various types of cells identified are then recorded as the number of each type found per high power field (HPF).

The veterinarian will submit a summary report of these findings. The count of crystals and casts can be fairly exact in each power field observed. Likewise, these same observations are applied to counts of epithelial and blood cells. The veterinarian will make note of the number of bacteria or sperm under HPF. The report should summarize all the numbers based on these terms: few, moderate, or many.

URINE SEDIMENT FINDINGS

RENAL CELLS AND TYPES OF CASTS

Renal cells originate from the renal tubules, and are not normally found in large quantities in urine sediment. Renal cells are somewhat larger in size than white blood cells (WBCs). The renal cell has a circular shape and a sizeable nucleus, and somewhat resembles the appearance of WBCs. **Renal tubal disease** can be diagnosed when these cells are found in large quantities in the urine.

The tubules and distal portion of the kidneys are the areas in which casts are formed. These manifestations are created out of cells and debris.

The active processes of a particular renal disease may be confined to the renal tubules. This circumstance is often associated with large quantities of casts. However, the specific extent of the disease cannot be measured solely against the quantity of casts found. Casts come in a variety of types including the following: hyaline, granular, epithelial, fatty, and waxy.

Epithelial Cells

There are 3 kinds of **epithelial cells** associated with the sediment found in urine: **squamous, transitional,** and **renal**. **Squamous cells** originate from epithelial membranes in the urethra, vagina, and vulva. They are the largest type of cells found in urine sediment. They have a flat, uneven shape with sharply defined edges and a small, round nucleus. The presence of squamous epithelial cells in urine sediment is not typically a clinically significant finding. However, these cells are not normally found in samples taken using cystogenesis or catheterization methods. This is because the urine exits through a medically inserted device and does not have exposure to the long natural passages lined with epithelium through which the urine normally passes.

Cells which come from the bladder, ureters, renal pelvis, and some sections of the urethra are known as transitional cells. These cells will be spherical in shape with a tail or appendage resembling a tail. This tail is known as the cell's caudate. The caudate and the cytoplasm both appear granulated (i.e., grainy in appearance). High quantities of transitional cells may be an indication of inflammation.

Amorphous Phosphate, Amorphous Urate, Calcium Carbonate, and Calcium Oxalate Crystals

Amorphous phosphates are observed in alkaline urine samples, while amorphous urates are observed in acidic urine samples. These 2 types of crystals look like a precipitation with a grainy texture. In addition, these slightly brownish or pinkish crystals tend to appear in clusters but without any specific shape (i.e., amorphous = without shape). The color is attributed to the ammonium biurate compounds involved. The presence of these crystals may indicate some form of liver disease or portal caval shunts.

Calcium carbonate crystals have a shape that resembles a dumbbell used in weight lifting. These crystals have no color. The presence of calcium carbonate crystals in the urine of horses and cattle is quite common.

Calcium oxalate crystals can be recognized by the X structure found in the center. These crystals are colorless and have a ring shape. The calcium oxalate crystal is usually located within acidic urine samples. However, these crystals may be found in alkaline or neutral urine samples, as well. Dihydrate calcium oxalate crystals are usually observed in urine. Monohydrate calcium oxalates are associated with ethylene glycol toxicity. Likewise, these crystals can be found in the urine of large animals that have ingested these oxalates. Monohydrate calcium oxalate can be associated with calcium oxalate urolithiasis.

Cast Types and Crystals

Cast types include hyaline, granular, epithelial, fatty, and waxy. **Hyaline** is found in the least severe cases of renal irritation. The presence of **granular casts** is only significant when they are found in large quantities. This understanding can serve to prompt a more thorough examination of an animal for kidney disease when substantial numbers of casts are found.

Acute nephritis and **renal tubule degeneration** is associated with **epithelial type casts. Fatty casts** are indicative of renal disease in cats. **Fatty casts** are also indicative of **diabetes mellitus** in dogs. **Acute levels of tubular degeneration** are most frequently associated with **waxy casts.**

Triple phosphate, amorphous phosphates, calcium carbonate, calcium oxalate, leucine, cystine, tyrosine, and uric acid crystals are all types of crystals which are found in urine sediment. Typically, the **triple phosphate crystals** are observed in alkaline urine. However, triple phosphate crystals may be visible in modestly acidic samples of urine, as well. The name of these triple phosphate crystals is associated with their characteristic three- to six-sided prism shape. The crystals have no color. The prism shape brings to mind the shape of a coffin. Triple phosphate crystals can sometimes lead to the diagnosis of urinary tract infection in the animal.

Leucine, Cystine, Tyrosine, and Uric Acid Crystals

Hepatic disease is associated with the observations of leucine, cystine, and tyrosine crystals in urine sediment. **Leucine crystals** can be described as circular-shaped crystals with concentric patterns. **Tyrosine crystals** have a yellowish to brownish appearance. The tyrosine crystal has a spindle-shaped cell structure. These tryosine crystals are flat, 6-sided, crystalline amino acid components which are indicative of a metabolic flaw. This defect is associated with cysteine metabolism and can be connected with uroliths (urinary bladder stones).

Uric acid crystals observed in alkaline urine are also linked with **metabolic flaws**. Regardless of alkalinity or acidity, it is not normal to find uric acid crystals in the urine of dogs, with one notable exception. Uric acid crystals are normal in the urine of Dalmatians. In other dogs a finding of uric acid crystals in the urine may indicate the presence of uroliths. However, Dalmatians are unable to convert uric acid to allantoin in the liver, leaving them to excrete uric acid in their urine. Poorly water soluble, uric acid tends toward crystallization and stone formation in the bladder — which is why 80% of all uric acid bladder stones come from Dalmatians. The presence of **bilirubin crystals in the urine** may be indicative of an animal with a serious condition. The animal may well be experiencing hepatic dysfunction, and may warrant a diagnosis of bilirubinuria.

Erythrocyte PCV Evaluation

Erythrocyte packed cell volume is abbreviated as PCV. PCV can also be referred to as **hematocrit** (HCT) or as erythrocyte volume fraction (EVF). PVC, EVF, or (more commonly) hematocrit is a measure of the percentage volume of whole blood that consists solely of red blood cells (RBCs or erythrocytes). It is normally about 46% for men and 38% for women.

One process for deriving the hematocrit is as follows. A **microcapillary or hematocrit tube is used to collect brand new, anticoagulated blood**. The tube is sealed. Next, the tube is placed in a centrifuge. The **centrifuge** is set at the correct time and speed. The centrifuge should be equipped with a scale that works as a hand-held card or a mechanical reader. The results are calculated in terms of a total volume percentage. Smaller RBCs are found in goat or sheep blood. Thus, these animals will have more red blood cells in their blood, albeit a likely similar total volume percentage.

The **plasma fraction** (i.e., separated portion) of the hematocrit tube is suitable for use in screening out microfilaria. This screening is accomplished by **direct microscopic examination** of the "buffy coat" (middle white blood cell layer) and plasma fractions for evidence of microfilaria and other blood-borne parasitic infestations. Other diagnostic consideration is given to the color pigmentation and clearness of the plasma.

Erythrocyte Indices and Tests for Mean Corpuscular Volume

Erythrocyte indices are established by RBC (red blood cell) counts, Hb (hemoglobin) content, and PCV (packed cell volume). These amounts will be automatically added to the outcomes derived from the electronic counting tools. Erythrocyte indices can be applied for identification in various types of anemias or blood deficiencies.

Particularized erythrocytes or RBCs are given as an average of the mean corpuscular volume (MCV). To calculate the MCV, the PCV is multiplied by 10, and that figure is divided by the RBC (in millions). The outcome is specified as femtoliters or fL. These measurements are determined by the kind of animal and the standard for that animal.

The PCV is measured in units of L/L (i.e., liters of RBCs obtained divided by the total whole blood liters) to give a percentage. These units are divided by the total RBC count. The outcome of this calculation is multiplied by 1000. The result of this final calculation is given in terms of SI units (meaning the International System of Units, abbreviated SI from the French "Le Système International d'Unités").

Measuring Erythrocyte and Hemoglobin Total Numbers

One important measure of **erythrocytes** is the total count of cells found in a given sample. The cells can be counted using a tool that is operated manually or mechanically. The tool will require calibration based upon cell size. The size of the cell may vary based upon the kind of animal from which the sample was taken. These calibrations are critical in the settings used for automatic counters. One type of manual counter is known as a **hemacytometer**. It is not as accurate in obtaining a cell count as an automated counter, but it is economical and readily available for use. Both the manual counter and the automated counter require a diluted sample. RBC indices can be obtained from the total erythrocyte numbers compared to the PCV.

Hemoglobin is abbreviated as Hb. The Hb in RBCs consists of **iron metalloproteins** (i.e., a ferroprotein, or iron in a porphyrin moiety, otherwise called a macromolecule complex or molecular functional group). These **metalloproteins can carry oxygen and carbon dioxide** to other parts of the body. This allows hemoglobin to assist in balancing the acidic/basic structure of the blood. Hemoglobin can be measured by means of photometric methods or automated cell counters. These measurements are recorded as g/dL or g/L. Erythrocyte indices can be obtained from the hemoglobin. A rapid qualitative assessment takes the animal's Hb by computing one third of the PCV.

Measuring the Mean Corpuscular Hemoglobin Concentration

The **mean corpuscular hemoglobin** (MCH), sometimes called mean cell hemoglobin, is the **average amount of oxygen-carrying hemoglobin** found inside the red blood cells in terms of mass.

The value of the MCH can be calculated by the following series of steps. The Hb (hemoglobin) concentration is divided by the total RBC count. The outcome of this calculation is multiplied by 10. The result of this final calculation is reported in units called picograms. Picograms are abbreviated as pg. Therefore, the MCH is a picogram or pg unit measurement.

The measurements associated with Hb and RBC counts are not considered to be as precise as those used to determine the measurement of PCV (packed cell volume). Thus, the mean corpuscular hemoglobin index is considered to be a less than precise, but useful, reference.

The **mean corpuscular hemoglobin concentration** (MCHC) represents the **average concentration of hemoglobin** (Hb) in a given volume of packed red blood cells. Hemoglobin is an iron-containing protein found in red blood cells. Hemoglobin functions to carry oxygen from the lungs to tissues within the body. The mean corpuscular hemoglobin concentration is derived by taking the Hb concentration and dividing it by the PCV (packed cell volume). Then, the result of this calculation is multiplied by 100. The final result is the mean corpuscular hemoglobin concentration. The MCHC will also indicate the average shade of red for the red blood cells — with a lower value indicating cells that appear paler. The mean corpuscular concentration is reported in units of g/dL. The conversion of this number to SI units (i.e., the international standard) is derived by taking the g/dL value and multiplying it by 10 to obtain the SI index of g/L. This calculation does not employ the total RBC count. Therefore, this measurement can be considered to be one of the most precise, in terms of RBC indices.

Measurement of the Reticulocyte Count

Reticulocytes are **immature red blood cells**. The name refers to the reticular (mesh-like) network of ribosomal RNA found in these cells and absent in mature RBCs. It is visible only when properly stained for viewing. RNA stands for the ribonucleic acid found in living cells which helps to produce proteins. RNA is also found in the bone marrow, where most animals produce red blood cells. The Reticulocyte Production Index (RPI) can be used to determine how rapidly reticulocytes are released into the bloodstream, which can be indicative of certain health problems.

To better identify reticulocytes during microscopic examination, the blood is stained with Wright's stain, which gives a bluish-gray color to immature RBCs, indicating the presence of cytoplasmic RNA. If stained with NMB (New Methylene Blue), the ribosomal RNA becomes directly visible and reticulocytes are more easily counted.

Cells or cell components that are stainable with more than one format of stain (i.e., Wright's alcohol-soluble and NMB's water-soluble stains) are referred to as "polychromatophilic." Thus, a few drops of blood and NMB stain are blended together in like amounts. The NMB/blood mix is checked to obtain the amount of reticulocytes visible. The results are extrapolated to produce a percentage of reticulocytes per 1000 RBCs. This percentage can be noted as an absolute count when measured as reticulocytes per milliliter. Reassessments may be needed, as automated counts routinely miscount reticulocytes by as much as 20%.

Measuring the Reticulocyte Count and Blood Specimen Collection

Reticulocytes are produced to either **replace aging RBCs** or in **response to an inadequate supply of RBCs** (i.e., blood loss, etc.). Reticulocyte cell counts are typically reported as a percentage of the total number of RBCs, as derived from an original count of NMB stain-reactive cells per 1000 red cells. The veterinarian will apply this count in an attempt to assess potential disease states. In most animals, reticulocytes should constitute less than 1% of all RBCs. However, situations such as blood loss, disease-shortened RBC life, general anemia, and low oxygen intake can all cause the reticulocyte count to rise (reticulocytosis).

The reticulocyte count can sometimes be **artificially inflated**. In situations of anemia (low RBC count) reticulocytes, as a percentage, can appear artificially high. To correct for this, the **Reticulocyte Production Index** (RPI, or "corrected reticulocyte count") was created: Reticulocyte Count X (hematocrit / normal hematocrit) — with "normal" usually defined as 30 to 45, depending on animal type. If the count is 100,000 mm^3 or higher, the anemia is likely of the hyperproliferative type (i.e., hemolytic anemia or anemia from blood loss, etc.). If it is under 100,000 mm^3, the anemia may be hypoproliferative (iron, B12, or folic deficiency, suppressed bone marrow, etc.). It should be noted that this assessment may not be valid in a horse, as horses do not discharge reticulocytes into the circulation directly from the bone marrow except in cases of severe chronic anemia.

Additional Procedures Applied for Blood Collection with Gaining a Reticulocyte Count

A modest amount of blood should be sufficient to run this a **reticulocyte cell count**. However, supplemental tests may be needed to verify the results. Thus, the technician should fill a tube to

90% capacity. A tube containing an anticoagulant such as ethylene-diamine-tetra-acetic acid or EDTA will be needed. When blood is drawn, the veterinarian should avoid any unnecessary voids or vacuums which may cause the cells to be harmed. Voids or vacuums are caused during the aspiration of the syringe when fluids are withdrawn from the body with suction. The veterinarian should not take a second sample too close to the original extraction site in the same time period, as this may cause harm to the patient.

The veterinarian may observe a **lipemic condition** in the blood sample. This can be attributed to patients that have recently eaten prior to the sample collection. In addition, the veterinarian should note any vaccinations that were given recently. These vaccinations may play havoc with the readings of certain tests. The veterinarian should be aware that EDTA is solely an anticoagulant and that it has no preservative qualities. Therefore, the sample should be analyzed as quickly as possible. As always, the veterinarian should be aware of the patient's emotional state during a clinical exam, especially when inflicting pain such as when drawing blood. This state may be described as afraid, keyed up, harassed, anxious, or inhibited. Remaining aware can help both the veterinarian and the patient avoid injury during the exam and specimen collection processes.

Erythrocytes

Characterizing the Size of Mature Erythrocytes in a Blood Film

Mature erythrocytes come in many sizes. Typically, the size can be attributed to the type of animal from which the erythrocyte was taken. Unusually large RBCs can be referred to using the term **macrocytic**. This characteristic is also common to immature RBCs. Well developed, mature erythrocytes generally have a uniform, average size referred to as **normocytic**. Cells that are smaller than average are referred to as **microcytic**. These smaller erythrocytes may be caused by vitamin or mineral deficiencies, genetic traits, or certain iatrogenic conditions. They also are associated with a diminished MCV (mean corpuscular volume) and MCHC (mean corpuscular hemoglobin concentration), causing them to be hypochromic (paler than normal). Substantial discrepancies in RBC size (often referred to as "red blood cell distribution width" or RDW) may be referred to using the term anisocytosis. The size of the RBCs observed should be compared with the size of RBCs normally found in the animal's species. This comparison should allow the veterinarian to judge the average RBC size for that species. The veterinarian will note the presence of larger, normal, or smaller sizes using the terms mild, moderate, or marked to indicate observed severity.

Acanthocyte, Crenation, and Echinocyte Cell Shapes in a Stained Erythrocyte Film

Spiculated cells include acanthocytes and echinocytes. **Acanthocyte** refers to cells exhibiting obvious blunt protrusions extending out from the cell wall. These types of cells have an inconsistent shape. Acanthocyte cells are also called "spur cells." Acanthocytosis is caused when RBC membranes contain excess cholesterol as compared to phospholipids. It may be caused by high blood cholesterol and/or abnormal plasma lipoproteins.

The term **crenation** describes the process where **cells contract due to a lack of water**. Crenated cells, with their characteristic notched or scalloped edges, can be seen when RBCs are allowed to dry on a blood film (smear). This slow drying process will produce visible barbs on the film.

Echinocytes (or "burr cells") have copious amounts of little spicules (micro-spikes) protruding from a roughly spherical surface. Burr cells are found in animals with renal disease. However, the blood cells of a horse may exhibit these characteristics after vigorous exercise. Canines with lymphosarcoma and renal disease may also exhibit burr cells. Other causes of echinocytosis include: uremia, pyruvate kinase deficiency, liver disease, low potassium or low ATP in red cells, hypomagnesemia, hypophosphatemia, high calcium in RBCs, the absence of a spleen, hyperlipidemia, myeloproliferative disorders, and heparin therapy. Also, specimen handling errors such as procuring a blood smear immediately after a transfusion, or artifact due to improper drying, may cause the condition.

Color in a Stained Erythrocyte Film

Fully developed cells with a normal amount of hemoglobin are known as **normochromic** cells. Cells with an inadequate concentration of hemoglobin are called **hypochromic** cells. Normochromic cells will turn a pinkish color when a stain has been applied; hypochromic cells will be a much paler shade of pink. A mammal's normochromic erythrocyte cell has a whitish, innermost area, due its biconcave formation and lack of a nucleus and cell organelles. However, reptiles, birds, and amphibians have nucleated red blood cells. These reticulocytes turn a light blue when a stain has been applied. The color originates from the **residual organelles** found in the cytoplasm that have not yet disintegrated. The presence of these cells in a stained peripheral blood smear is referred to as polychromasia. The veterinarian can observe this condition in a regular blood film (slide smear). However, whenever special staining is applied, as in the case of NMB, then the ribosomal RNA organelles will be visible as reticulum. Thus, the cells in this application will be referred to as reticulocytes. **Hypochromic** is the term used whenever there has been a reduction in the stain's concentration. This reduction is caused by the hemoglobin (or Hb) in the cell, often from a lack of iron. Macrocytic erythrocytes may be mistaken for hypochromic cells. Both are characterized by large widths. However, the distinction can be evident when hypochromia and microcytosis are both found in the same sample. This is further confirmed by MCV results.

Target, Leptocyte, and Stomatocyte Cell Shapes in a Stained Erythrocyte Film

A **leptocyte** is described as an abnormally thin, flattened cell. It is sometimes referred to as a Mexican hat cell, due to a central rounded area of pigmented material, a clear unpigmented mid-zone, and an outer pigmented cell rim. This form may be attributed to a reduction in hemoglobin volume or to an inordinate increase in the surface area of the cell membrane. Leptocytes are found in cases of regenerative anemia.

Codocytes are sometimes referred to as "target cells" for their dark circular "target" appearance. As an erythrocyte it has hemoglobin, but potentially not in adequate amounts. The target-like appearance may be due to cell membrane collapse secondary to minimal hemoglobin content. Other suspected causes include increased cholesterol and lecithin content, bile insufficiency, liver disease, splenectomy, or anemia.

Stomatocytes present with an abnormal-appearing center. Rather than the circular pale center of a normal erythrocyte, the pale center of a stomatocyte is rod-shaped, or even smile-shaped, in appearance. An inherited disorder has been linked to the presence of stomatocyte cells in dogs, and liver disease may also predispose the condition.

Leptocytes, codocytes, and stomatocytes are all in same family.

Vocabulary Terms

Spherocytes, Schistocytes, and Poikilocytosis

Spherocytes: Red blood cells having a round, spherical form instead of the biconcave disk shape of a normal RBC. Although typically involved in immune-related hemolytic anemias, other causes include defective membrane assembly and traumatic or toxic injury to the erythrocytes. Spherocytes are two-thirds the diameter of a normal RBC, with a decreased surface area. Their hemoglobin is denser and stains a deeper red, and the cell lacks a central pallor. They are more readily seen in dogs than many other animals that already have smaller erythrocytes with less central pallor (cats, horses, etc.). However, in thick areas of a dog's blood smear all the RBCs may resemble spherocytes. Therefore, clinicians must focus on the monolayer areas of the blood film.

Schistocytes: Fragmented RBCs of varying shapes — some with horn-like keratocytes, triangle-shaped triangulocytes, and helmet-shaped cells. Typically the fragmentation occurs when erythrocytes are cut by fibrin strands lining microvessels. True schistocytes are not the softer-edged "bite cells" which occur when the spleen ingests abnormal hemoglobin (i.e., a Heinz body), leaving a bitten-apple appearance (although they are often lumped together). Schistocytes are seen in burns, uremia, various hemolytic anemias, and in disseminated intravascular coagulation (DIC) disorders.

Poikilocytosis: A condition in which there is a 10% or more increase in the amount of unusually shaped RBCs in the body.

Ghost Cell, Eccentrocytes, and Torocyte

Ghost cell: Refers to a red blood cell that has lysed or ruptured in a hypotonic solution, spilling out its hemoglobin contents. Over time it will resume its normal disk shape, and will likely have retained at least some of its prior hemoglobin contents. Thus, when stained it appears as a very pale, ghost-like cell.

Eccentrocytes: RBCs that have been subject to the harmful effects of oxidation, resulting in adhesion of the cell membranes from opposing sides of the cell. The hemoglobin is thus forced to one side of the cell. These effects can cause the RBC to appear semi-circular in form. Eccentrocytes are associated with fragmented anemia, keratocytes, and schistocytes. Often presented as synonymous with blister cells (with both undergoing oxidative damage, etc.), it appears they differ in the membranous adhesions as opposed to the blister-like vacuole development. Causes include onion and garlic ingestion (in dogs, cats, etc.), and the administration of oxidant drugs.

Torocyte: A red blood cell with an abrupt transition from pale center to the red hemoglobin-rich ring of the outer cell circumference. It is sometimes referred to as a "punched out" cell due to this appearance. This presentation is typically induced by poor slide smear technique. However, it should be noted that horses, cattle, and some other animals have naturally low central pallor, making observation of this condition more difficult.

Rouleaux, Agglutination, Blister Cells, and Ovalocytes

Rouleaux: Erythrocytes that are gathered in chains or stacks — not unlike stacks of coins. In such formations, the cells are not free to readily absorb and carry oxygen. It is a precursor to many serious diseases, including inflammatory or plasma protein transformations. However, a certain degree of rouleaux is expected in horses.

Agglutination: This term refers to erythrocytes that are clustered together without any clear structural constriction. This type of cell formation can be detected by noticing a grainy appearance on the slide. The veterinarian will not be able to continue with an automated RBC counting or sizing when agglutination has been detected. This phenomenon can be associated with the presence of an antibody or in situations of immune disease.

Blister cell (Pyknocyte, Hemighost): This term refers to an RBC where a blister or a vacuole has formed, and is absent of any hemoglobin content. This is often a result of oxidation damage on the cell's surface potentially due to iron deficiency anemia. Later rupture or removal of the blister by the spleen may result in a keratocyte, or "horn cell." However, if the cell forms only one slim horn-like protrusion, it is sometimes called an "apple stem" cell.

Ovalocytes: This term is used to describe elliptocytes — cigar- or egg-shaped erythrocytes. These cells have an elliptical form which can be attributed to a flaw in the membrane. They can be found in animals that have any of a number of types of anemia. The center of the cell has the typical erythrocytic light or pale color.

Inclusions

Basophilic Stippling and Nucleated RBC

Basophilic stippling is the granulated appearance of ribosomal RNA clusters found in certain erythrocytes. They can be easily observed through the use of **New Methylene Blue stain**, which makes the RNA appear as tiny, blue-colored granules inside the red blood cells or erythrocytes. This basophilic stippling is a result of ineffective heme formation, often due to various pathologies, including some anemias found in cattle, sheep, and felines, and lead poisoning in certain animals. However, it is also characteristic of active erythropoiesis in sheep and cattle.

A **nucleated RBC** (abbreviated as NRBC) is a less developed and slightly smaller RBC that has retained its nucleus. The cytoplasm in this cell has the capability of staining a dark color. NRBCs are not normally found in mammalian peripheral blood films, and tend to indicate serious bone marrow stress, from hemolytic anemia to metastatic cancer. However, NRBCs are normal in animals that are not mammals. For instance, birds, reptiles, fish, and amphibians have well developed NRBCs. These mature cells have an elliptical shape.

Howell-Jolly Bodies and Heinz Bodies

Howell-Jolly bodies are defined as erythrocytes that did not entirely expel their nuclear DNA, now visible as purple-blue basophilic inclusions upon staining. These inoperative, basophilic DNA fragments are stored in the cell. The veterinarian will notice the dark staining qualities. The inclusion shape will be circular. In addition, non-refractive qualities are apparent when the microscope is out of focus. The presence of these Howell-Jolly bodies can be found in cases associated with splenectomy, regenerative anemia, or spleen disorders. It should be noted, however, that most cats and horses will have about 1% of all their RBCs defined as Howell-Jolly bodies.

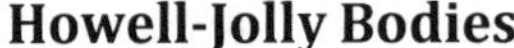

Howell-Jolly Bodies

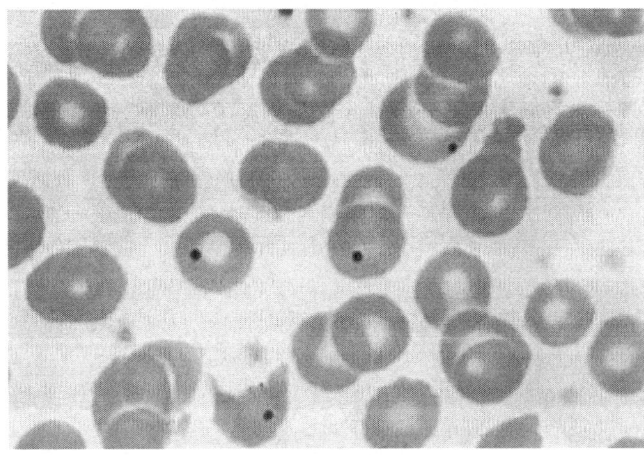

Heinz bodies (or Heinz-Ehrlich bodies) are small inclusions of **denatured hemoglobin** found within RBCs. The veterinarian can view Heinz bodies with Wright's or Diff-Quick stains. However, an easier observation can be made with New Methylene Blue (NMB) stain. Heinz bodies are associated with the use of oxidant drugs, lymphosarcoma, and hyperthyroidism, as well as with the consumption of onions by dogs, cats, and certain primates. Heinz bodies are frequently found in felines. An abrupt rise in the number of Heinz bodies in a feline can indicate diabetes mellitus.

VOCABULARY TERMS

BABESIA SSP AND ANAPLASMA MARGINALE

Babesia spp (spp, for multiple subspecies; sp for a single subspecies): This term refers to a blood-borne parasitic protozoan of the genus Babesia. It causes the disease referred to as **Babesiosis**. Transmitted by ticks, it affects many domestic animals including cattle, horses, sheep, goats, pigs, and dogs. The particular type that is associated with the infection of dogs is known as Babesia canis, and the type found in horses is known as Babesia caballi.

These blood parasites can be found inside the RBC. The presence of a pairing of large-sized, pear- or droplet-shaped blood cells can be observed in blood films from infected animals. The cells typically amass together under the buffy coat. Thus, the buffy coat (i.e., smears, etc.) may also be used for identification.

The **Babesia blood parasite** can be carried by the **Ixodes tick**. The veterinarian will be able to detect the presence of this parasite through serology antibody testing. Serology is the study of the animal's blood serum. The veterinarian may also lyse or disrupt the bonding of the cells. Then, a Giemsa stain will be applied to assist in the observation and analysis of the chromosomes.

Anaplasma marginale: This term refers to a blood parasite found within a host's RBCs. This parasite looks like a tiny circle within the cell. The parasite will turn a dark color when the RBCs are stained. This dark stain occurs in the RBCs of cattle and wild ruminants. They may be mistaken for Howell-Jolly bodies, due to their similar appearance and roughly equivalent size.

HEMOBARTONELLA FELIS, HEMOBARTONELLA CANIS, AND CYTAUXZOON FELIS

Hemobartonella felis (recently renamed Mycoplasma haemophilus; also called feline infectious anemia): This is the name of the tiny, flea-borne blood parasites that appear as cocci or rods. However, as a true mycoplasmic organism, it has no cell wall and cannot survive independently. It is easily stained with Wright's stain. The stain will produce a dark purple color. These parasites are observed on the boundaries of feline RBCs, and are routinely treated with tetracycline and transfusions.

Hemobartonella canis: This term refers to the blood parasites located on the surface of canine RBCs. These parasites look like extended chains of cocci or rods, and may be stained a dark purple color with Wright's stain. This parasite is most commonly found in dogs that have had a splenectomy or that have compromised immune systems. This type of blood parasite is comparable to the Eperythrozoon found in pigs, cattle, and llamas.

Cytauxzoon felis: This term refers to tiny, tick-borne parasites that live within erythrocytes. The erythrocytes contain "piroplasms" that may appear as round or oval "signet rings," or in "safety pin" forms, tetrad forms, or as round "dots". The dotted form may appear in linked cell chains. The nucleus stains dark red to purple with a light blue cytoplasm. These parasites are also located inside the feline's lymphocytes and macrophages. However, this type of blood parasite is not at all common.

NEUBAUER HEMACYTOMETER METHOD

The **Neubauer hemacytometer method** is a manual means of determining the number of red blood cells (among other cells). The veterinarian will normally apply the **Unopette system** in the preparation of the sample to be tested. This system requires that the calibrated blood sample be diluted or weakened with acetic acid. The dilution ratio for this mixture is 1:100. This is necessary to reduce the amount of cells that require counting. The red blood cells or RBCs require a 10-minute period to hemolyze following the dilution process. Next, the hemolyzed RBCs are placed into the hemocytometer chamber. This chamber has 9 compartments which have been separated by a counting mechanism. Each compartment is occupied by a specified amount of cells. These cells can be measured under a microscope at 10x objective magnification to determine the exact quantity present.

COLLECTING CELLS FOR MICROSCOPIC EXAMINATION BY FINE NEEDLE ASPIRATION

Collecting various blood and tissue cells for examination is often necessary. The veterinarian will use a **fine needle aspiration** to gather the cell samples from the skin, lymph nodes, and internal organs. The appropriate size includes a 22 to 25 gauge needle with a 3 to 12 mL syringe. Smaller gauge needles and smaller syringes should be employed with softer or more pliable tissues or cell accumulations. However, **larger-bore syringes and larger gauge needles should be employed in gathering cells that are compact and solid when pressed**. The veterinarian should release the suction pressure on the syringe before moving the syringe to another area. This allows multiple samples to be gathered from a wide variety of distances from the top to the bottom of a given mass or area of diagnostic concern. This also allows the veterinarian to take samples from different locations. The veterinarian will place the samples on a sterilized microscope slide. Next, the veterinarian will apply a staining solution. This will increase the ability of the veterinarian to carry out a thorough inspection of the cells.

EVALUATING AND DIFFERENTIATING LEUKOCYTES

There are many kinds of **Leukocytes can be differentiated by staining**. The best methods employ the largest occupied section of the film. Thus, the veterinarian will pay attention to patterns of blood dispersion across the stained region. A monolayer arrangement of the cells will yield the best results. Feathered edges are not useful in detection. The form and structure of the leukocyte must be examined. There are 5 types of leukocytes, in 2 main groups: polymorphonuclear leukocytes (also granulocytes — characterized by stain-revealed granules in the cytoplasm), including neutrophils, eosinophils, and basophils; and mononuclear leukocytes (non-granular), including monocytes and lymphocytes. "Banded" cells refers to granulocytes in an immature state. They may be elongated and narrow, with non-segmented nuclei. Neutrophils may be referred to as "toxic" when they undergo morphologic changes (shape, color, etc.). The degree (based on numbers of cells affected and changes incurred) is noted as mild, moderate, or marked. Severe toxic change is indicated when toxic granulation, diffuse cytoplasmic basophilia, or cytoplasmic vacuolation are present.

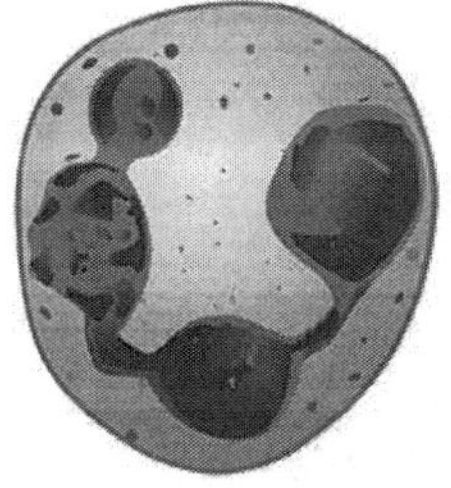
Neutrophil

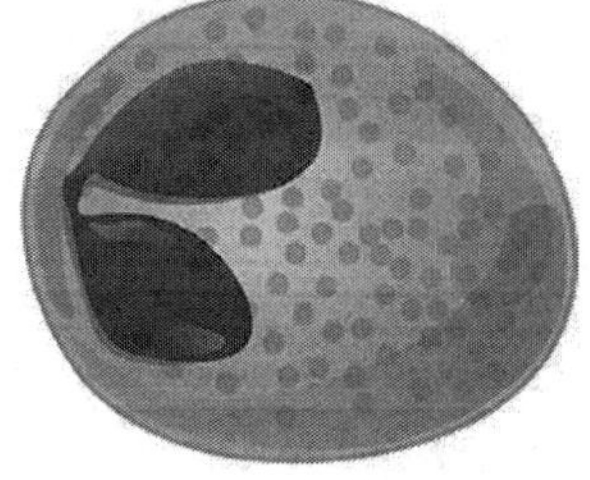
Eosinophil

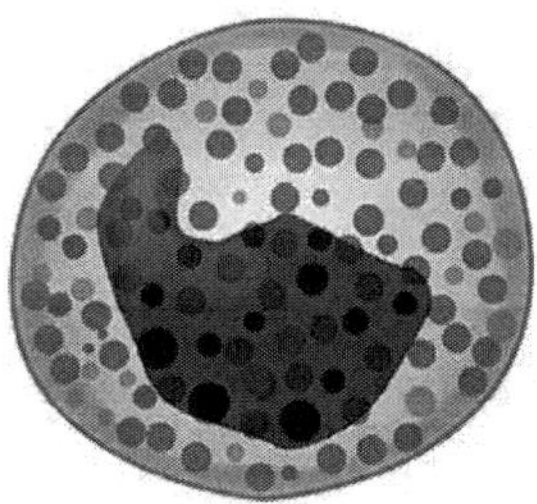
Basophil

Neutrophils and **lymphocytes** are the **most common leukocytes**. The largest WBCs are monocytes, staining with a gray-blue cytoplasm. Monocytes are found in peripheral blood. Eosinophils are granular cells with cytoplasm of a unique red-purple stain. Basophils are almost never found in peripheral blood. Their cytoplasm is distinguished with a blue or blue-black stain.

EXFOLIATIVE CYTOLOGY

NEUTROPHILS AND NECROTIC PROCESSES REVEALED

Exfoliative cytology (cells shed from body surfaces) may reveal neutrophiles that are comparable in appearance to the neutrophiles located in peripheral blood. The veterinarian may notice **degenerative characteristics or structural changes**. These observances can be found by scrutinizing the neutrophile underneath a microscope. **Hypersegmented neutrophils** may have 5 or 6 sections or lobes. Other neutrophils may be undergoing pyknosis, which is the inexorable degeneration of chromatin in a cell nucleus when undergoing cellular death or apoptosis. Still other neutrophils may be undergoing **karyolysis** which is defined as the **digestion of chromatin** in the nucleus by way of the enzyme DNAse. This digested material is known as karyorrhexis. **Karyorrhexis** is defined as the fragmented particles of the cell's nucleus undergoing necrosis. **Necrosis** is defined as the death and decay of parts of cells or whole cells in a patient's tissues or organs. The detection of necrosis can lead the veterinarian to diagnose an injury. Necrosis may also be indicative of a disease (such as cancer or other decay-inducing processes) associated with the patient's condition.

TYPES OF STAINS THAT ARE AVAILABLE FOR STAINING CYTOLOGY SAMPLES

There are 3 types of **Romanowsky stains**. The types include: **Wright's**, **Giemsa** and **Diff-Quik.** These stains are employed in the examination of cytology samples. There is a noticeable variation in the staining quality of these products. Therefore, the veterinarian should employ one type of stain on a consistent basis to reduce the likelihood of misinterpretations due to the stain style and quality variations.

The new **methylene blue stain** is abbreviated as NMB. This stain is used to examine cell nuclei, mast cell granules and most infectious organisms and agents. However, there are limitations associated with its use. NMB should only be applied to the examination of nucleated cells, bacteria, fungi, and mast cells. The veterinarian may apply this stain directly to a slide that has been allowed to dry in the air.

The veterinarian may classify bacterial agents by the employment of a gram staining solution. The veterinarian will note the pink coloration for cells and bacteria that are gram-negative, in contrast to the purple color that indicates a gram-positive result.

The veterinarian may employ a hematoxylin/eosin stain in the examination of histological studies. In particular, the veterinarian will employ the use of stains that can expose the nuclear detail of the sample. These solutions are known as Papanicolaou stains.

Field Stain

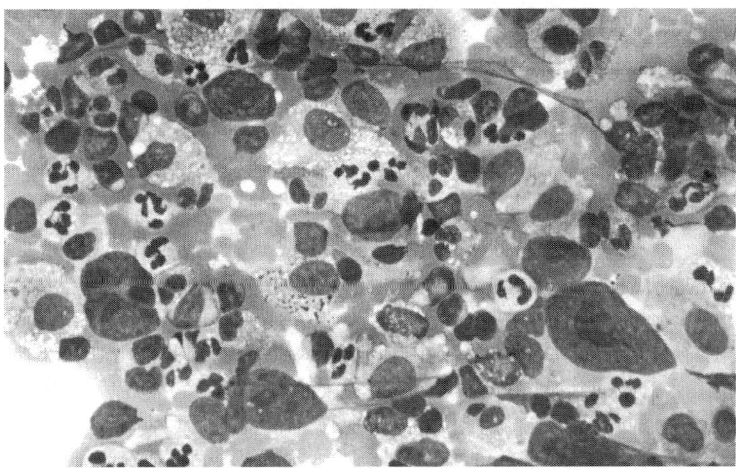

Mesothelial Cells and Mast Cells Found

Mesothelial cells form **mesodermal tissue**, which provides the interior lining of a body cavity or the covering of an embryo. This lining is specifically found on pleural, peritoneal, and visceral surfaces within the body. Mesothelial cells generally have a circular shape and a single nucleus. However, some mesothelial cells are known to be multinucleated. In addition, these cells contain a network structure of nuclear chromatin and slightly basophilic cytoplasm. The basophilic descriptor indicates that the cytoplasm has little difficulty in being stained with ordinary dyes.

Some cells function to **remove unwanted or phagocytic debris**. They can be identified by looking at the cells with cytoplasm, nucleoli, or a corona.

Mast cells have a distinctive shape and color. These cells have either round or elliptically formed nuclei. In addition, there is a bluish-purple coloration found in a majority of the cytoplasmic granules.

Lymphocytes, Plasma Cells, Erythrocytes, and Eosinophils Found

Exfoliative cytology (cells shed or gathered from body surfaces, as opposed to body fluids) can reveal cells and changes not always available via peripheral vascular fluids. **Lymphocytes** and **eosinophiles** present similarly, as when found in peripheral blood. However, plasma cells will be visible as **elliptical cells**. These elliptical cells have an abnormal nucleus. In addition, these cells also have a basophilic cytoplasm and perinuclear clear zone. **Erythrocytes** can sometimes be observed in the interior of phagocytic cells. This is especially true in macrophages found in the exfoliative sample. **Macrophages** are large cells that are critical in the protection against infections in the body. These sizeable cells come from the monocytes found in peripheral blood. The nucleus in the macrophages will have an elliptical shape. These cells are pleomorphic. **Pleomorphic** is defined as the presentation of 2 different forms arising within its overall life cycle. **Exfoliative cell chromatin** will form chromosomes that have the appearance of lace. The chromatin may also form denser or more condensed molecules. The veterinarian will also apply a stain. If the stain turns the cytoplasm blue, then the veterinarian should check to see if the compartment in the cytoplasm of the cell or vacuole is filled with phagocytic debris. This is indicative of a macrophage. Macrophages can have one or more nuclei. Macrophages can also range from normal sizes to overly large sizes.

Vocabulary Terms for Malignant Neoplasia

Coarse Chromatin Pattern, Nuclear Molding, Multinucleation, and Nucleoli

The veterinarian will use cytological samples to explore and confirm or reject the presence of a **malignancy**. Specifically, the veterinarian will note the **presence or absence of changes in the cell nucleus** to determine if a malignancy is present. For example, the coarse chromatin pattern in a cell nucleus bears distinctive markings. This pattern appears to resemble a cord or rope. Changes in this expected pattern may well be problematic.

A particularly concerning pattern of nucleus deformity is called nuclear molding. **Nuclear molding** occurs when the nucleus in one cell spontaneously changes to a deformed state in response to other deformed nuclei in the same cell, or to match the deformed nuclei of neighboring cells. If a cell contains 2 or more nuclei, it is known as multinucleation.

The veterinarian will also make note of the **size, shape, and number of nucleoli** in the cells when looking for precursors pointing to the presence of a malignancy. **Anisonucleolosis** is the term used to describe an inconsistency found in the size and profile of the nucleoli. In addition, the veterinarian will take special care to examine any deviation within the same nucleus.

The veterinarian will find that round or oval nuclei shapes are usually normal. However, pointed shapes indicate angular nucleoli. **Macronucleoli** is the name given for the larger nuclei which may point to a malignancy. The existence of a multitude of nucleoli also suggests that a malignancy is present.

Anisokaryosis, "N:C" Ratio, and Mitotic Activity

Malignancy is a term given to describe a cancerous growth. **Metastasis** describes a cancer that spreads to other parts of the body. This growth can be detected through changes that occur in the nucleus of a cell in a cytological sample. For example, a sizeable variation can be found in the measurement of a cancerous cell's nucleus. This difference can be beyond that which is normally anticipated for the tissue type involved. **Nucleus size variation** is a condition known as anisokaryosis. The **normal cellular N:C**, or nucleus to cell cytoplasm ratio, is typically in the range of 1:3 to 1:8. However, cancerous tissue types may not display these same N:C ratios. Thus, the veterinarian may suspect that a malignancy is present whenever the N:C ratio is on the rise. This rise is such that it cannot be explained by normal operations with a tissue. The process for mitosis may also signal an unusual occurrence. Normally, cells will divide and split evenly into 2 cells. Therefore, when cells do not split evenly, the veterinarian may suspect the presence of malignant cells. Again, it is a rare and concerning occurrence when mitotic figures or cells have not split evenly.

Collecting and Evaluating of Lung Tissue Lesions

The veterinarian can also identify masses of growth through **radiographic technology**. However, this is just one early step in a potentially lengthy evaluation process. The next step in the process is to **take samples of the cells by using fine needle aspiration**. The animal may respond with complications such as pneumothorax and hemorrhage during a fine needle aspiration; thus, caution and careful post-aspiration follow-up is important. The other technique involves a scraping and/or impression taken of any suspicious looking tissue. The tissue is often collected during a procedure for biopsy.

The veterinarian may also examine normal cells in a comparison with cells taken in a tracheal wash. The cancerous cells associated with the lung include **carcinoma** and **adenocarcinoma**. Inflammation found in the lungs can be a result of the following: a) Bacteria known as Mycobacterium sp, b) fungi known as Cryptococcus sp, Blastomyces sp, c) parasites known as Toxoplasma sp, Pneumocystis sp, and d) viral diseases. The veterinarian may apply an aspiration technique known as nasal flushing to gather further samples of nasal exudates and masses. The veterinarian may further observe inflammations caused by trauma or foreign bodies. In addition, the veterinarian may observe any bacterial or fungal organisms obtained. The presence of a neoplasm or a tumor within the naval cavities strongly suggests a malignant tumor.

Collecting and Evaluating Cutaneous and Subcutaneous Tissue Lesions

The veterinarian will use 4 techniques to examine tissue samples. The 4 techniques include: **swabbing**, **scraping**, **imprinting**, and/or **fine needle aspiration**. These 4 techniques can be applied in gathering samples of both cutaneous and subcutaneous tissues. The veterinarian should take a sample of the lesion region before and after the lesion is cleaned. In addition, care should be used in the removal of all scabs or healed-over areas.

The veterinarian will apply the **scraping technique** along a variety of different surfaces associated with the lesion. Inflammatory lesions are a common occurrence in response to bacterial, fungicidal, and parasitic infections.

Phagocytic cells found in such lesions are laden with infectious agents. These agents include gram-positive cocci, gram-negative bacilli, fungi and parasites. This debris may offer further diagnostic information upon further evaluation.

The veterinarian should carefully examine the skin of cats and dogs. The skin in these animals is a common site for the growth of **neoplasias** or the **formation of tumors**. The animal may be suffering with a number of neoplastic lesions. The more common types include the following:

lipomas, mast cell tumors, histiocytomas, squamous cell carcinomas, fibromas, and hemangiosarcomas.

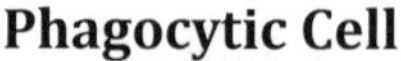

Phagocytic Cell

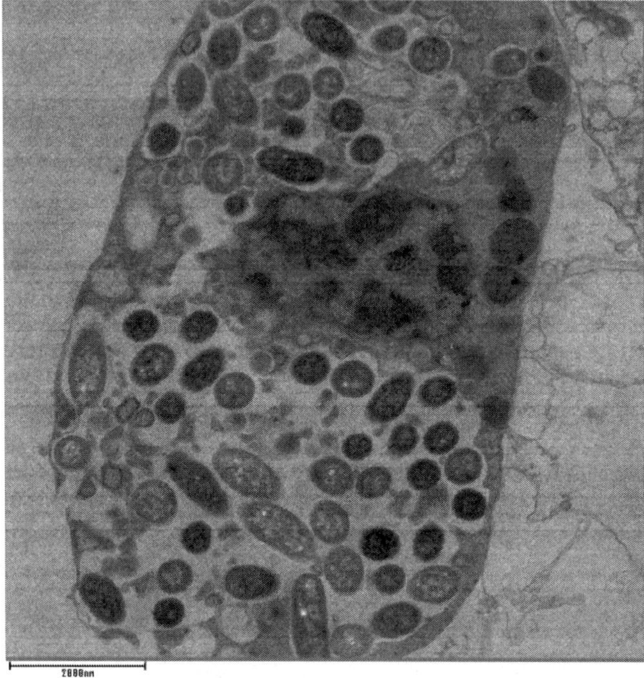

Collecting and Evaluating of Spleen Tissue Specimens

The veterinarian may apply fine needle aspiration or biopsy collection techniques in gathering cells from the spleen. **Spleen samples** are needed for analysis when certain other signs of ill health are present. However, the **splenic tissue is frail**. Therefore, the fine needle aspiration technique must not be approached carelessly. The veterinarian should proceed painstakingly to prevent the occurrence of any tears or undue bleeding in the tissue.

The veterinarian must employ a **cytology evaluation** to derive an appropriate identification of the results. The veterinarian will also compare these results with other clinical signs that will assist in obtaining an accurate diagnosis.

Hyperplasia is defined as an enlargement which is a result of an abnormal multiplication of cells. Hyperplasia may be the result of a variety of infectious or immune-mediated conditions. In addition, hyperplasia can be a result of parasites or fungi infiltration. Further, splenic hyperplasia can sometimes be attributed to a condition known as extramedullary hematopoiesis involving the spleen. Many tumors are associated with the spleen. Two common types are known as hemangiosarcoma and fibrosarcoma.

Collecting and Evaluating of Tissue Lesions on the Sensory Organs

The veterinarian will apply a scraping or fine needle aspiration technique when collecting cells from the **eyelids**. This is a common site for the growth of tumors. These tumors also frequently occur in the **sebaceous glands** around the eyes (although skin-oil-producing sebaceous glands are all over an animal, and any such gland can become tumorous). The **conjunctiva** is the membrane located under the eyelid and covering the eye. The tool often used to collect a sample from this region is a smooth, circular shaped spatula. This spatula is used to scrape the conjunctiva in order to obtain a greater number of cells than can be obtained by sterile cotton swabbing alone. The scraping may then reveal the cause of a chronic conjunctivitis, following a thorough analysis of the conjunctival tissue specimens. The veterinarian will spread a layer of topical anesthetic before gathering samples from corneal lesions.

The veterinarian will use cotton swabs to collect secretions or discharges located within the ear canals. These secretions are used as cultures and slide samples. During an exam, the veterinarian may detect a neoplasm in the ear canal. Tumors in the ear canal are frequently found, but most are not malignant. However, the ear canal is frequently troubled with infections caused by microorganisms in the body. These microorganisms are normally of the bacterial or fungal family. However, some infections are caused by parasites. Parasites that are commonly located in the ear canal include Otobius sp and Otodectes sp.

Cellophane Tape Method

The **cellophane tape method** is beneficial in the **identification of intestinal pinworms and skin mites.** Pinworms are threadlike nematode worms that invade the intestines. Parasitic pinworms can be found in and around the perianal area, while mites can be found on the hair and on the surface of the skin. The cellophane tape method requires the following: cellophane tape, mineral oil, and a microscope slide.

The cellophane tape method involves applying tape to the outside of the skin. The tape is used to pull off the outer epidermis and related debris from the skin's surface. This sample is left on the tape. Then, a single drop of mineral oil is applied to the surface of a glass microscope slide. The tape is then positioned on top of the oil on the microscope slide. Finally, the sample is examined closely under a microscope set at a 10-power objective. In this way it can be determined if there are pinworms or mites on the sample.

Elevation of Nucleated Red Blood Cells (nRBCs)

In most animals, **nucleated red blood cells** (nRBCs) are young red blood cells. If there is an increase in nRBCs in the blood, that means the body is making RBCs too quickly and is not allowing them to mature before they are released into the bloodstream, which can be a result of anemia. The nRBCs have a dark staining nucleus and a bluish-red cytoplasm and are of significance if there are more than 5 in a 100 WBC count.

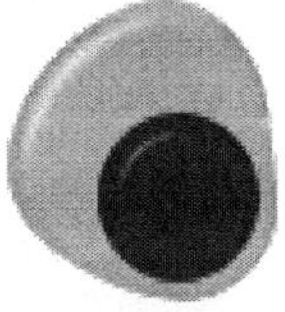

Immune-Mediated Hemolytic Anemia (IMHA)

Immune-mediated hemolytic anemia (IMHA) results when the body's immune system attacks and removes its own RBCs. The majority of IMHA cases are primary (there is no underlying cause), whereas some cases are secondary to an infectious or neoplastic disorder. A normal RBC lives 120 days, and then the liver and spleen remove aged RBCs in a process called extravascular hemolysis. The iron from the RBC is delivered to the liver in the form of bilirubin, the proteins from inside the RBC are used for building new proteins, and the spleen decides which cells are taken out of circulation. When the immune system removes too many RBCs, the spleen enlarges because it is taking in an increased number of damaged RBCs, and the liver becomes overworked by large amounts of bilirubin. There eventually will not be enough RBCs circulating to transmit enough oxygen to the body's tissues and to remove waste gases, causing patients to become weak. There is a 25%–50% mortality rate of patients with IMHA. In cats, IMHA results from either the feline leukemia virus or from infection with *Mycoplasma haemofelis* (an RBC parasite).

RBCs, WBCs, and Epithelial Cells That May Be Seen in a Urine Sediment

Red blood cells (RBCs) appear pale yellow and are smaller in comparison to **white blood cells (WBCs).** More than five RBCs per high-power field (hpf) is abnormal. WBCs in a urine sediment appear 1.5 times larger than RBCs and are mostly neutrophils that are spherical and granulated. More than five WBCs/hpf indicates inflammation and infection. Three types of **epithelial cells** may be present, including squamous, transitional, and renal. Squamous epithelial cells come from the urethra, vagina, vulva, and prepuce, and they resemble potato chips with a small nucleus and a large, flat, irregular shape. Transitional epithelial cells derive from the bladder, ureters, and renal pelvis, and more than one/hpf is a significant finding indicating inflammation and cystitis. Transitional cells vary in diameter, have an eccentric nucleus and are pear shaped with a granular cytoplasm. Renal epithelial cells come from the renal tubules and appear larger than WBCs with a large nucleus and granular cytoplasm; more than one/hpf indicates renal tubular disease.

Types of Casts That May Be Seen in a Urine Sediment

Casts that may be seen in a urine sediment include RBC casts, WBC casts, hyaline casts, fatty casts, and granular casts. Casts are formed in the distal tubules or distal nephron and are tube shaped because they are formed in the kidneys' tubules. They appear cylindrical with parallel sides and have rounded or blunt ends. Any structure that may be present at the time that the cast is formed will embed itself into the cast (RBCs, WBCs, or renal cells) and can indicate renal degeneration, irritation, and chronic nephritis. RBC casts indicate bleeding from within the nephron, and WBC casts indicate inflammation of the renal tubules. Hyaline casts are protein precipitants and may appear in large numbers with fever or renal disease. Granular casts could mean renal disease if they are found in large numbers. Fatty casts are uncommon, but they are found in cases of diabetes mellitus.

Animal Care and Nursing

Initial and Ongoing Evaluations

Clinical Signs That Should be Noted for the Skin and Coat During a Physical Examination

There are a number of potential issues associated with the condition of an animal's skin and coat. Therefore, the technician should be careful to note whether or not the animal's skin and/or coat has a healthy shine to it. A **dull coat** may indicate that the skin is dry, and may ultimately contribute to a condition known as alopecia. Alopecia is the loss of hair or the persistent absence of hair from the body. In some animals, this can be aggravated by excessive scratching and ultimate injury to itchy, dry skin.

The skin's **elasticity** or **turgor** (i.e., hydrated plumpness) should also be examined. This evaluation can help detect problems associated with dehydration. Skin that is poorly hydrated usually does not exhibit proper flexibility, and thus will not snap back into place when pulled outward. Instead, the skin is slow to go back into place. The skin at the thoracolumbar region in particular should be pulled upon to determine if the skin can be described as properly or poorly turgid or pliable. However, turgor must be evaluated in relation to the degree of dehydration. Thus, specific documentation may describe skin turgor as: good or normal, decreased, poor, or doughy. Briskly responsive, pliable skin is diagnosed as normal.

Basic Physical Examinations

A veterinarian is responsible for supervising the veterinary technician. This includes overseeing the technician's collection of information regarding a patient's anesthesia risk factors. This information will be used to promote a comprehensive anesthesia plan. The **anesthesia plan** should be strictly adhered to during the performance of any procedure. Further, it should be used to check the status of a patient's recovery following the administration of anesthesia. **Medical record documentation** should bear out adherence to the anesthesia plan. To this end, there should be an authentication process applied for all medical record entries.

The technician is responsible for consulting with and **keeping the veterinarian informed** of any irregularities or unexpected situations and occurrences. The physical exam of the patient is beneficial in obtaining information about any health concerns that have not previously been addressed by a medical professional. This physical examination is the first step in assessing the patient's overall health. The technician should adhere to a **preset, standard routine** regarding the physical examination. This will help ensure a more complete and **uniform examination**. The routine also prompts the technician to adhere to important portions of the exam which may easily be overlooked when a less consistent routine is used. Each body system requires a thorough perusal in a comprehensive examination.

Clinical Signs That Should be Noted for the Eyes, Ears, and Nares

The animal should also be examined for **proper reflexes** and **appropriate responses to visual stimuli**. This is essential in determining problems associated with the eyes. Likewise, the technician should record any leakage or matter that is released from the eyes. The color of this leakage may be clear or purulent. **Purulent** describes an exudate that contains pus or a similar yellowish or greenish fluid. This may indicate an infection in the animal.

The examination should note any **irregularities in the cornea**. Likewise, the **clarity of the conjunctiva** (the membrane covering the eye's surface) and the **color of the sclera** (the whites of the eyes) are both noted. The technician will manipulate the ear in checking its health. The technician will note any auditory stimuli response, abnormal or disproportionate odor, and the presence or absence of matter in the ear canal.

The technician will note the quality of any movements involving the patient's head. Any favoring of one side, disequilibrium, poor coordination, etc., should be recorded. The technician will check the nares or nostrils. The **color and consistency of mucus released in the nasal region** should be noted. This includes any sneezing or congestion observed. The nostrils should also be checked for any obstructions that may be causing a congested response.

Clinical Signs That Should be Noted Regarding the Skin and Coat

The presence of **poor or doughy skin turgor** should produce a closer examination for other signs of **dehydration**. Ideally, the degree of dehydration should be determined. Dehydration is classified as follows: mild= (6% to 8% fluid loss), moderate= (10% to 12% fluid loss), and severe= (12% to 15% fluid loss). Regions of the body that have an excessive amount of skin are not good candidates to test for turgor. Therefore, the cervical area will not produce valuable information.

A complete physical examination should also **include the detection of any fleas, lice, mites, ticks, or lesions**. The technician should examine the animal by **palpation** — described as a gentle pressure applied by the fingers over the animal's body. This should be useful in **detecting lumps, swellings, and in producing reactions to painful points** that the patient may be experiencing. Any unusual masses or changes in organ size, or other tissue enlargements, should be recorded. These observations will be used to further determine the patient's overall health. Indeed, all available information should be used to diagnose and treat the patient fully and properly.

Clinical Signs That Should Be Noted for the Respiratory System

The technician will need to listen to the patient's internal organs with a **stethoscope**. This is referred to as **auscultation**. For **pulmonary auscultatio**n the stethoscope should be placed on the back or the side of the thorax. The **thorax** is located between the neck and the abdomen. Moving the stethoscope to various points throughout the thoracic area can aid in obtaining a complete **evaluation of the upper and lower lobes of the lungs and the trachea**. This may be particularly important with larger animals. The technician should listen closely for any sounds that are irregular. This can involve **crackling, wheezing, stridor, rhonchi, or rales**. **Stridor** refers to a severe, struggling, high-pitched gasping for air, arising from an obstructed or highly constricted airway. **Rhonchi** are wet, mucus-laden wheezing or snoring sounds. **Rales** refer to a crackling, bubbling sound that emanates from the chest region. Some sounds may present only at the time of inspiration or expiration, with others present during both inspiration and expiration.

Clinical Signs That Should Be Noted in Finalizing the Check of the Respiratory System

Sounds coming from the animal's upper airway and trachea should be checked further, particularly if an obstruction appears to be involved. Likewise, any problematic breathing should be noted. The **animal's respiratory pattern, rate, and depth**, and any changes noted with exertion may be important. The animal may exhibit hyperventilation or hypoventilation, panting or shallow breathing, and dyspnea.

Hyperventilation refers to a deep, quick-paced breathing that may be induced by anxiety or by an organic disease process. In particular, the disease of an organ may contribute to problems associated with carbon dioxide levels in the blood. The animal may then experience dizziness or weakness.

Hypoventilation refers to a shallow breathing that that allows carbon dioxide to build up in the bloodstream. **Dyspnea** refers to difficult or labored breathing, often associated with heart disease coupled with overexertion. These problematic symptoms should be recorded. Felines that exhibit quick, shallow breaths or open-mouth breathing may be in physiological distress. This observation should be carefully noted to further promote the proper diagnosis of the animal.

Clinical Signs That Should be Noted for the Gastrointestinal System

The technician will appraise the gastrointestinal system by checking the animal's mouth, teeth, and gums. The technician should make a note of all **fractured, missing, or discolored teeth** found in the animal's mouth. The **animal's gums** should be inspected for periodontal disease. Likewise, the presence of halitosis (bad breath) should be recorded. The technician will also make notes regarding any signs of malocclusion or unusual alignment of the teeth. The technician will seek to determine the age of the animal as related to dental status and overall health.

The **animal's tonsils** should be examined for any growth or excess size. In addition, the technician should document any **disproportionate salivation** or **problems associated with swallowing**. The technician will record any greenish- or yellowish-colored mucus. The mucous membranes should be pale pink in color to be considered normal. Any irregularities should be recorded. The gingival tissue should be checked for capillary refill time (abbreviated as CRT). This can be examined by applying gentle pressure on the gums and then quickly releasing in order to determine how long the gum tissue takes to return to a normal color. The refill process should be brisk and uniform in its re-saturation.

Maintaining a Normal Fluid Balance and Abnormal Fluid Loss

The body is uniquely designed to maintain a **proper balance of fluids** and other biochemistries. This design incorporates a body makeup of about 60% water. The amount of water is divided between intracellular and extracellular components within the body. However, this constant need to maintain a fluid balance must be met by metabolic functions and by the restoration of lost fluid through oral means. The act of drinking restores fluid by oral means. Then, the body's metabolism plays a part in how that fluid is allocated, maintained, and utilized. Some metabolic functions include losing fluids through respiration, excretion, and episodic routines such as sweating and milk production.

Furthermore, fluid can be lost by atypical adverse conditions. These adverse conditions may include the following: vomiting, diarrhea, and/or abnormally excessive urination. Some diseases induce polyuria (excessive urination). Available fluids may also be reduced due to the patient's state of health. For example, chronic disease or severe injury can negatively impact the patient's ability to take in fluids. Ill dogs that have rapid respiration or excessive panting may also suffer from further fluid loss.

Signs to Estimate Mild-To Moderate Dehydration

The animal must also be carefully checked to determine the degree of dehydration. The following factors should be considered in that determination: **weight** (especially recent rapid changes likely due to fluid loss), **skin turgor**, **moistness of mucous membranes, heart rate, and CRT** (capillary refill time). These factors must be evaluated through a physical inspection of the animal. Animals with a rate of dehydration under 5% of total normal fluid status do not typically show obvious signs or symptoms. However, animals with rates of 5% to 6% dehydration will usually exhibit a mild degree of skin turgor evidenced by a lack of pliability to the skin. Animals with 8% dehydration will exhibit a more moderate rate of skin turgor, a minor rise in CRT, and some dryness in the mucous membranes. The CRT can be examined by applying gentle pressure on the gums and then quickly releasing in order to determine how long the gum tissue takes to return to a normal color. The refill process should normally be brisk and uniform in its resaturation of the gum tissue.

Signs to Estimate Severe Dehydration

Animals with dehydration rates of 10% to 12% total body fluid loss will exhibit **moderate to severe skin turgor, hollow-looking eyes, a marked rise in CRT** (capillary refill time), **dry mucous membranes, rapid heart and respiratory rates, cold limbs, and perhaps signs of shock**. The CRT can be examined by applying gentle pressure on the gums and then quickly releasing in order to determine how long the gum tissue takes to return to a normal color. The refill process should normally be brisk and uniform in its resaturation of the gum tissue.

The animal exhibiting 12% to 15% dehydration will be extremely **metabolically depressed**. In addition, the animal will likely already be in shock. This animal is in danger of dying from the severe level of dehydration and shock.

Tests can be given to come to a determination about the degree of dehydration present. A dehydration test measures the packed cell volume or PCV, total plasma protein or TPP levels, urine-specific gravity, and a lower rate of urine production. The degree of dehydration should be classified as follows: mild (6% to 8%), moderate (10% to 12%), and severe (12% to 15%).

Electrical Impulses That Lead to the Contractions of the Muscles of the Heart

The **heart** organ is motivated by an **electrical impulse** which works to cause the tightening and the relaxing of the heart muscle. This tightening or contraction is referred to as **cardiac systole**, or the **systolic phase**. The relaxation or loosening of the muscle is known as **diastole**, or the **diastolic phase**. These phases describe the heartbeat or continuous pulsation of the heart muscle that is responsible for the circulation of blood throughout the body. The contraction of the myocardium (systole) is immediately preceded by (and thus is sometimes referred to as) depolarization. In like manner, the relaxation of the myocardium may be referred to as repolarization. The electrical impulse is transmitted through the regions of the heart in a systematic, recurring pattern. Electrical activity begins at the point known as the sinoatrial node. Another term for the sinoatrial node is the cardiac pacemaker. It consists of a small mass of fibers positioned in the heart's right atrium. The heart's cells are all closely linked. This linkage allows the depolarization and repolarization to move along at a rapid pace.

Electrocardiography, Electrocardiograph, and Electrocardiogram

Non-invasive electrocardiography can be accomplished through the use of bioelectrical leads placed in such a way as to externally sense the heart's electrical conduction activity. The device is used in making a profile of the electrical impulses that govern and regulate the function of the heart. Each impulse is given immediately prior to various areas of the heart experiencing muscle contraction or movement.

The **electrocardiograph** gathers signals through the use of a voltmeter that has the capacity to gauge the amount of electricity that radiates through electrodes positioned on the outside of the person's chest. The signal is recorded ("traced") on a continuous roll of thermograph paper, which provides a permanent record of the electrocardiogram. The abbreviation for electrocardiogram is ECG (or EKG, to differentiate it from the ultrasonographic abbreviation for an echocardiogram). ECG tracings are visible when drawn by a heated stylus on heat-sensitive graph paper, or as transiently displayed on a monitor screen. The ECG is capable of measuring the amplitude or strength of electrical activity, and the duration or length of time associated with each electrical impulse. Normal heart contractions are recorded and viewed as normal rhythms on the ECG.

ECG Waveform

The **electrocardiogram** may be described as a graph-based display and recording of the heart's electrical functions. This graphic display is produced by way of an electrocardiograph instrument. The electrical activity induces motion in a tracing stylus that then produces a line drawing of a continuous wave tracing of electrical activity. The continuous line drawing of linked sequences of electrical impulses transmitted across the heart constitutes the electrocardiogram or ECG.

The series of electrical events that begin and end a single heartbeat is referred to as **waves**, **complexes**, and **intervals**. For purposes of evaluation, the electrical activities of a heartbeat are broken into 4 parts. These 4 parts are known as the P wave, the PR interval, the QRS complex, and the T wave. The P wave is a result of the depolarization that takes place in the right and left atrium. The P wave lasts for about 0.12 seconds or less. The section of the ECG that begins with the atrial depolarization (the P wave), to the point known as the ventricular depolarization (the QRS complex), is referred to as the PR interval. The PR interval is described as a breadth of time that can range from 0.12 to 0.20 seconds. The QRS complex is a result of the ventricular depolarization (contraction).

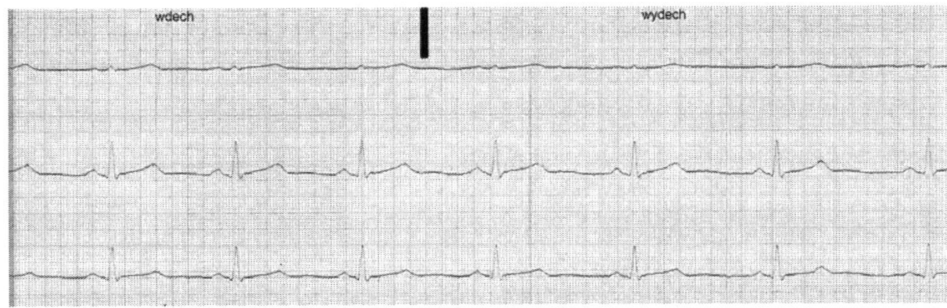

Movements Which the Electrical Impulses of the Heart

The electrical activity is carried by various **nerve fiber bundles** from the sinoatrial node to the right and left atria and then toward the ventricles. The electrical activity continues until it reaches the atrioventricular (AV) node. The **AV node** is the junction where the atria and the ventricles are interconnected. The AV node produces a brief transmission delay once activated. This allows the ventricles a momentary period of time to fill with blood prior to a contraction. The ventricles are the lower, larger chambers of the heart. The **atria** are the upper, smaller chambers of the heart that serve solely to fill the ventricles in preparation for significant blood movement through the lungs or body. **Depolarization** spreads through the interventricular system between heartbeats. It moves through the left and right bundle branches. At the **apex** or tip of the heart, the **Purkinje Fibers** or neuroelectrical conduction branches finally end. The impulse transmission then radiates upward and outward through the ventricles, producing a smooth, upward rippling, milking-like contraction. Effective cardiac contraction is vital, as it causes the blood to be pumped into the arteries on its way to the lungs or throughout the entire body.

ECG Waveform and the Supplies Needed for Electrocardiography

The **QRS complex** typically lasts between 0.04 to 0.12 seconds. **Repolarization** of the ventricular myocardium can be viewed in a segment of the graph-based tracing of the ECG. This segment is known as the T wave. **Atrial repolarization** activity is overshadowed by the QRS complex. Thus, it cannot be viewed on the tracings represented in an ECG.

When performing an ECG the patient should be given a protective coverlet, and cushion or mat to reduce the harmful effects associated with a steel table's ability to conduct electricity. The patient should be swabbed with alcohol, conducting gel, or paste. These substances give a boost to skin where contact is made. Some machines designed for taking human ECGs can be adapted for use with animals. Necessary modifications include the use of a filed or bent alligator clip. This modification inhibits the pinching or bruising that is often associated with the use of strong alligator clips applied directly to the skin. In addition, the continuous monitoring offered by pads (applied to shaved skin) or even subcutaneous wires can also be employed.

Normal Electrocardiographic Interpretation

The wave segments denoted as P, Q, R, S, and T are considered the key features of a normal heartbeat. Each QRS complex is associated with a P wave. The **P wave** has a **positive deflection** in lead II. However, either a positive or a negative deflection can be associated with the T segment. The PR interval is relatively normal. In most domestic animals, a normal cardiac rhythm can also be referred to as a sinus rhythm. The measured values should be examined for similarities and differences in association with the normal values as denoted by each species of animal. This comparison should take place at the end of a complete ECG. The complexes should be evaluated by the veterinarian or a trained technician. The number of complexes in a 3 second period should be counted. This will allow the professional to also determine the heart rate of the animal examined.

Procedures Followed When Taking an Electrocardiogram

Keeping each limb from touching the other body parts will **reduce the contact of skin upon skin**. This is important for an accurate ECG reading. Leads are fastened at the center point or proximal left and right of the elbow bone or olecranon processes. Leads can also be fastened to the center point or proximal left and right stifles of the hind leg and the chest. This includes the dorsal or the back of the thorax near the seventh thoracic vertebra in the chest region. A sedative should help an animal that is overly anxious or unruly.

It is usually best to take a standard recording with the paper speed set at 25 mm/sec. Typically, 30 cm or 12 inches for each lead is recorded for an ECG that incorporates all the necessary information for proper evaluation. The paper speed is often set at 50 cm/sec for small dogs and cats. Various animals with faster or slower heart rates may require different paper speeds to provide adequate tracing differentiation and clarity. The ECG tracing should also incorporate pertinent patient identification and procedural information including: the date of the ECG, patient name and species, client name, and any other relevant information.

Adult Horse Examinations

Normal Temperature and Pulse

A mature, fully grown horse has a normal body temperature between 37 to 38.5 °C (between 98.6 to 101.3 °F). The normal pulse rate is in the range of 28 to 45 beats per minute. The veterinarian can auscultate, or listen to, the horse's heart with a stethoscope. When doing so, the veterinarian may well hear only 2-3 specific heart sounds. However, there are times that more than 3 are heard. The full array of 4 can be notated according to the phases of the cardiac cycle, as depicted by the symbols S1, S2, S3, and S4. The most prominent sound is normally associated with ventricular contraction. This sound is depicted by the symbol S1. The second sound that the animal will display is associated with the semilunar valves closing. This second sound is depicted by the symbol S2. The third sound that the animal will display is associated with the blood rushing into the ventricles. This faint sound is depicted by the symbol S3. The fourth sound, rarely heard, is associated with atrial contraction. This fourth sound is depicted by the symbol S4.

Atrioventricular Blocks

The term **atrioventricular block** is abbreviated as AV block. This condition occurs when the atrial depolarization is not relayed to the ventricles, or when there is an unduly prolonged delay between atrial depolarization and ventricular depolarization. There are 3 recognized degrees of AV block. First-degree AV block is characterized by a lengthened PR interval, arising from dysfunction of the AV node. There are few symptoms or problems associated with this degree of AV block. In second-degree AV block, one or more (but not all) of the atrial impulses fail to communicate on to the ventricles. While few patients show symptoms, those who do may experience fainting and dizziness. In third-degree AV block (sometimes referred to as "complete" heart block), no atrial impulses (sometimes called supraventricular impulses) are relayed to the ventricles. This leaves the ventricles to generate a rhythm from alternate conduction sites (often septally derived). In an electrocardiograph, the P wave and the QRS complex can be seen to function independently from each other. These factors will be used to establish the presence of a complete heart block. Some horses with second-degree heart block may be in poor health. However, a horse with second-degree heart block may or may not be diagnosed with a heart disease.

Normal Cardiac Rhythm

The mature horse has a number of heart rhythms that can fall within the normal range. A **thorough examination** should be completed and all of the following cardiac performance indices and measures should be recorded: heart rate, rhythm, intensity, any deficiency or absence of standard sounds, and any unusual sounds — all of which can be classified as cardiac arrhythmias (sometimes referred to as dysrhythmias). Two of the more common and prominent abnormal rhythms in the heart are tachycardia and bradycardia. **Tachycardia** is a sustained overly-rapid heart rate. This is defined (in a horse) as a heart rate of more than 50 beats per minute. Bradycardia is an unusually slow heart rate. This is defined (in a horse) as a heart rate that is lower than 20 beats per minute. Irregular beats, skipped beats, incomplete beats, etc., are often associated with both of these forms of arrhythmias. The condition known as hypocalcemia can result in brachycardia. Hypocalcemia is a condition where the animal has an extremely low level of calcium present in the blood.

Normal Respiration

The **normal respiration** or **breathing rhythm** for a mature horse is 8 to 20 breaths per minute. The veterinarian will make a careful observation of the horse's flanks and nostrils in observing respiratory function. In addition, the veterinarian will use a stethoscope positioned on the trachea and in the left and right lung fields to listen to the passage of air during inspiration and expiration. In this process the veterinarian is trying to find evidence of sounds associated with abnormal respiration.

The normal respiration rhythm of the horse has a **consistent pattern**: 1) a **pause**; 2) followed by **inspiration** or breathing inwards; and 3) **expiration** or breathing out. Horses that are in an excited condition can exhibit deeper inspiratory breaths than expiratory breaths (i.e., gasping, etc.). This can be seen in an abnormal respiration rhythm. Further, strenuous exercise may bring on the following: coughing, nasal discharge, epistaxis (nose bleeds), hyperpnea (abnormally deep or rapid breathing), and dyspnea (difficult or labored breathing). These symptoms can indicate that the animal has a respiratory condition. The horse should next receive an endoscopy. This test will be beneficial in helping the veterinarian to determine the condition of the horse's pharynx and trachea.

Common Clinical Signs of Gastrointestinal Ailments

Gastrointestinal ailments in horses can be attributed to a number of possible problems. These problems include overfeeding, parasites, twisted intestines, defective feed, an irregular feeding schedule, and sudden changes in feed. The animal exhibiting the following clinical signs could be suffering from a gastrointestinal ailment: restlessness, getting up and down frequently, agitation, hoof pawing, persistently pacing the stall or confinement area, rolling, biting at, or persistently watching their flank, and kicking at the abdominal region. Other bodily symptoms include: a distended abdomen, sweating, grinding teeth, increased heart and respiration rates, increased CRT (capillary refill time, usually in the gingival area), and diminished appetite. The animal's mucous membranes and gums should be checked. The gums can have a visible red or blue toxic line located right above the horse's teeth. The mucous membranes can change to a pale, bright brick red or bluish color. **Cyanosis** is indicated by a bluish color, and means there is not enough oxygen in the horse's bloodstream. The following conditions may also be present: hypermotility, hypomotility, or the entire absence of gastrointestinal motility. The horse may even sit in a stance like a dog or with its legs extended out in a sawhorse-like posture.

Physical Examination for Ruminants

A veterinarian can glean considerable useful information by taking a few moments to observe an animal from outside its enclosure. The veterinarian should take stock of the condition of the animal's **eyes**, **stance** and **carriage**, **the body tone, movement and gait**, as well as urine and manure output. In addition, the veterinarian should ascertain and document how much food and water is being consumed by the animal.

There should be a specific set of procedures applied to every physical examination to ensure that it is thorough and complete. These procedures will produce consistent results for each patient examined. Typically, the procedures flow forward from the originating point of the examination, which should begin at the animal's nose. The examination should then move from the head of the animal down to the tail, with attention paid to intervening areas of the patient. The veterinarian should use a stethoscope to listen to the sounds coming from the animal's heart, lungs, and abdomen. The condition of the animal's skin, coat, mane, tail, and hooves should also be observed and recorded.

Final Procedures to a Physical Examination and an Oral Dosage Instrument

Thorough documentation is important. A complete recording should include all **abrasions**, **swellings**, and **discharges** emanating from the patient. The veterinarian should record the animal's **temperature**, **pulse**, and **respiration** (or TPR). The stethoscope is applied to the left paralumbar fossa to pick up any sounds emanating from rumen contractions. The ribs, vertebral column, and pelvis should be palpated (i.e., examined by touch) with a gentle pressure. This helps the veterinarian determine if the animal is suffering from **areas of sensitivity**, and to check for malnourishment by detecting the musculature and adipose layers of the animal.

The **balling gun** is a plastic or metal instrument used to give a ruminant animal an **oral medication** or **vitamin dosage**. The animal's head should be immobile when the balling gun is applied. The animal will be forced to open its mouth when the bridge of its nose is held. Stress should be directed to the hard palate. The balling gun is then inserted into the opening. The oral dosage is directed to the base of the patient's tongue. The jaws of a swine are held ajar with a bar speculum. The boluses or capsules can then be inserted at the base of the tongue by utilizing the balling gun.

Nuclear Scintigraphy

Nuclear scintigraphy is an imaging technique used to evaluate the kidneys, bones, thyroid gland, and brain. It requires that **technetium** (a radionuclide or radioactive isotope) be infused into the body with a syringe. The infusion is given to the horse by intravenous means. The animal will then be scanned to locate and track the radioactive isotope. The isotope appears as a radiographic "hot spot" approximately 2 hours after the injection has been given to the animal. The lower limbs of the animal should be scanned about 20 minutes after infusion of the isotope. The horse will be in a radioactive state for a period of 24 to 36 hours following the procedure. During this time the animal should be left alone except for feeding and watering. However, water should not be given to the animal whenever the pelvis is being examined, as the full bladder will obscure certain views of the pelvis. The veterinarian may give the horse a diuretic to reduce the size of the bladder. One example of a diuretic is Lasix, which may be administered parenterally.

Nuclear scintigraphy is an appropriate examination for tendon injuries, suspected suspensory injuries, and horses with a crippling injury or lameness. Of particular benefit is the ability to detect tibial stress fractures, condylar fractures, and pelvis, carpus, and hock injuries.

Conducting a Radiographic Examination

The procedures surrounding a radiographic examination primarily involve appropriate measures for the **safe use of radiation**. One standard view taken is with the horse standing with its leg directly underneath the plate. The technician will hold the plate parallel to the leg to obtain a proper radiographic view approximation. Other standard radiographs involve the following views: lateral, medial oblique, lateral oblique, anterior-posterior, flexed for the fetlock and carpus, and skyline of the carpus. Additional radiograph views may be obtained with the horse standing on a cassette enclosed in a sturdy Plexiglas shield. This technique provides extra views of the feet. A portable unit is best applied in obtaining views of the feet, fetlocks, carpus, and hocks. The larger units (stationary and immobile due to size) are more efficient for obtaining views of the shoulder, stifle, and head regions. Radiographs of the pelvis are taken when the horse is in a dorsal recumbent position. However, the horse will need to be sedated with an anesthetic for this procedure to be carried out.

Disease Referred to as Navicular Syndrome

Navicular syndrome is not fully understood. The origin of the disease remains a mystery. However, the disease does produce a lameness and specific deterioration of the navicular bone (a small bone in a horse's foot). Horses suffering with navicular syndrome may display a variety of symptoms. These symptoms include stumbling, shorter strides, and periods where the horse goes lame. The horse's aversion to hoof testing may be attributed to the extreme amount of pain the horse is experiencing in the hoof region. **Mechanical hoof testers cause considerable pain when pressure is applied to the sole of the foot of a horse with this disease**. The horse that exhibits this reluctance should also be given the following tests: flexion tests, nerve blocking, and radiographs.

The horse can be treated with the following: anti-inflammatory medication, vasodilators, and corrective foot trimming and shoeing. One vasodilator often used for this condition is isoxsuprine hydrochloride. Some horses require a **surgical neurectomy**. This procedure is conducted along the nerve to the foot. The nerve is cut above the fetlock. However, this procedure should only be used when all other alternatives have been exhausted.

Parts of the Abdomen That Must Be Palpated Upon Examination and What to Look/Feel For

When examining a patient, the **abdomen** must be examined for signs of distension or any lesions or bruising. The abdomen must also be palpated beginning at the spine, moving around and down toward the belly. Palpate with one or both hands to feel for any masses, fluid, or even fetuses if pregnancy is suspected. By palpating the abdomen, the veterinarian may find an enlarged organ, a mass, an obstruction in the small intestine, or even an extremely full bladder, which could mean an obstruction. The patient may show pain upon palpation, which may need to be investigated further. The stomach, liver, spleen, and pancreas lie in the cranial abdomen; the kidneys and part of the spleen are located in the middle of the abdomen; and the bladder, prostate, uterus, and colon are in the caudal part of the abdomen. The small intestine is found throughout the entire abdomen.

Organs in the Abdomen and Their Function

The stomach breaks down food, and gastric acid in the stomach helps digest the food.

The digested food leaves the stomach and enters the small intestine, which is a tube-like structure extending from the stomach to the large intestine and is 2.5 times the animal's body length. The small intestine has three parts: The first is the **duodenum**, the **jejunum** is the middle, and the **ileum** is the smallest part that connects to the large intestine. The gallbladder and the pancreas attach to the duodenum. Enzymes and other secretions important for digestion are produced by the liver and pancreas and pass through the pancreas to mix with food in the duodenum. The jejunum contains tiny fingerlike projections (villi) that absorb nutrients. The large intestine connects the small intestine to the anus and absorbs water from feces to keep the animal at an adequate hydration status, as well as holds feces. The large intestine is divided into three parts: the ascending colon, transverse colon, and the descending colon where fecal matter exits the anus.

Complete Physical Examination of the Patient's Chest, and the Organs in the Chest Cavity

Part of the physical examination is to examine the **chest cavity** of the patient. The veterinary technician or veterinarian will locate the heart by placing the stethoscope over the side of the chest between the fifth and sixth intercostal space. Once the heartbeat is heard with the stethoscope, you can record the heart rate and listen for any murmurs or abnormalities. Also, while listening to the heart, you will listen to lung sounds to make sure they sound clear with no crackling. The anatomy of the thoracic cavity begins with the diaphragm, which separates the abdominal cavity from the thoracic cavity. The heart is located in the thoracic cavity and is responsible for pumping and carrying blood rich with oxygen and nutrients to the rest of the body providing the cells with energy. The lungs are located in the thoracic cavity as well and are a main part of the respiratory system with the important function of delivering oxygen to the blood and removing carbon dioxide from the blood through an exchange that occurs in the alveoli.

Dogs Becoming Socialized and What to Look for in Puppy Exams

Dogs build relationships with people as a result of handling in the early stages of life, **socialization**, **genetics**, as well as **learning**. In the first 3 weeks of a puppy's life, **maternal care** and handling are crucial. Attentive maternal care leads to a dog that can better handle stress as well as a more mature nervous system, so puppies that are bottle fed may have a harder time socializing. The transition period is when interactions with litter mates are crucial to social skills. Puppies do not make social attachments as easily after the **socialization phase**; therefore, it is crucial for puppies to have adequate socialization during the first **4–12 weeks**, or it can lead to an increased response to stimuli through fear and aggression, as well as an inability to communicate. When an owner comes in with a new puppy for an exam, it is important for the veterinary technician to discuss how to introduce the puppy to other dogs, children, and other adults. Telling the owners to handle the puppy constantly and to play with its paws, ears, and mouth is crucial because this will get the puppy used to being handled and not to be fearful.

Body Condition Score (BCS) Chart of Dogs and Cats

A **body condition score (BCS) chart** is designed to evaluate the patient's **nutritional status**. The chart ranges from 1 to 5 with 1 indicating emaciation, 3 being a healthy weight, and 5 being obese.

With a BCS of 1, the ribs and pelvic bones are visibly noticeable and the patient has no body fat or muscle mass. A BCS of 2 means that the patient is underweight and the ribs can be felt easily, as well as no obvious waistline or abdominal tuck to the patient. A BCS of 3 means that the patient is at a healthy weight and the ribs can be felt with no obvious amount of fat covering and the abdomen is tucked nicely. A BCS of 4 means that the patient is overweight, the ribs are palpable with difficulty, the waist is absent or barely visible, and an abdominal tuck may be present. A BCS of 5 means that the patient is obese, has large fat deposits over its chest and back, and the abdomen appears distended. This score chart is important because it is a visual to show the owner where the pet's weight should be and what they should look like. After they recognize that their pet may be overweight, the feeding plan can be set, and the pet would need to be weighed regularly to monitor progress.

Maintaining a Hospitalization Form for a Hospitalized Patient

If a patient is presenting with an illness that requires hospitalization, then routine monitoring of the patient must be recorded. Hospitals will commonly have a **hospitalization form** on the patient's kennel for the duration of the stay. The form will have the patient's name, client's name, breed, sex, weight, date, and the illness or injury. Any medications given or that will need to be given will be recorded on the form including the strength, dose, and how many times per day it is to be administered. If IV fluids are being administered, that will be recorded on the form as well, along with the rate and type of fluids. Routine temperature, pulse, and respiration (TPR) measurements will be taken throughout the day and will be recorded on the hospitalization form also, along with the patient's temperature. The attending veterinarian will record how often the patient should be examined and if certain tests need to be run such as a CBC on the form. Once the requested treatments and exams are done, the person should initial the form so other staff members will know what has been done. Hospitalization forms are an effective form of communication.

Mentation Status in a Patient

Mentation refers to the mental activity or level of consciousness of the patient. Mentation status should be documented for each patient and can be labeled as normal, dull, obtunded, stuporous, and unresponsive. **Normal** means the patient is bright, alert, and responsive to stimuli and its surroundings. **Dull** means that the patient is interactive by nudging or walking up and seeming interested in people but seems depressed. **Obtunded** means the patient is reacting to stimuli but not necessarily interested and is slower moving and more depressed. **Stuporous** mean the patient is disconnected and only responds to painful stimuli, whereas unresponsive means the patient is disconnected and does not respond to any sort of stimuli.

Blood Pressure Values and Normal Reference Ranges for the Dog and Cat

Systolic arterial pressure (SAP) is created when the left ventricle contracts and blood is pushed into the aorta. Then, that left ventricle empties and relaxes, and it begins to fill again while the aortic pressure decreases, giving the diastolic arterial pressure (DAP). The mean arterial pressure (MAP) is measured through a calculation from both the systolic and diastolic values. The actual calculation is MAP = DAP + 1/3 (SAP – DAP). **Blood pressure** can be monitored directly using an arterial catheter (a catheter inserted into an artery) giving continuous monitoring or indirectly by use of a Doppler or automated blood pressure cuff to detect the arterial blood flow in a peripheral artery. Normal blood pressure values for a dog's SAP range from 90-140 mm Hg, and MAP in dogs ranges from 60-100 mm Hg. Normal systolic values for cats range from 80-140 mm Hg, and normal mean pressures in cats range from 60-100 mm Hg.

Pulse Oximetry Monitor

Pulse oximetry measures the percentage of hemoglobin in the blood that is oxygen saturated by passing light through the tissues using two wavelengths, red and infrared. Well-oxygenated hemoglobin will absorb more infrared light and allows more red light to pass through, whereas deoxygenated hemoglobin absorbs more red light, allowing more infrared light to pass through. The difference in this light absorption is calculated and gives a final percentage, which is the SpO_2. There are a few areas to place the pulse oximeter probe, such as the ear, tongue, lip, in between the toes, prepuce, or vulva. Normal SpO_2 values are between 95 and 100 when the patient is getting 100% oxygen. Patients that are hypothermic or in shock will have a very low SpO_2 value due to vasoconstriction.

Capnography

Capnography works by measuring the amount of carbon dioxide by the use of infrared waves in the breath at the end of expiration, also known as the end tidal CO_2. Capnometry gives us a way of estimating ventilation and how well the lungs are removing CO_2 from the body. A normal range is between 35 and 45 mmHg. An elevated end-tidal CO_2 occurs with hypoventilation, whereas a lowered end-tidal CO_2 occurs with hyperventilation. The end-tidal CO_2 number gives information about cardiac output as well. If there is a decreased cardiac output to bring CO_2 to the lungs, then the amount exhaled will decrease. Capnography machines provide a waveform in which the height corresponds to the amount of carbon dioxide exhaled and the length of the waveform represents time. If the waveform is tall, that represents an increase in exhaled CO_2, and if the waveform is short, that indicates a fast respiratory rate.

Indirect Oscillometric Blood Pressure (BP) Reading

To perform an accurate **oscillometric blood pressure (BP) reading**, the cuff size needs to be accurate for the patient. An appropriate cuff size will measure 40% of the limb circumference in dogs and 30% in cats. The cuff can be measured by laying it lengthwise along the limb, making sure that the edges measure 25-50% of the circumference of the limb. The limb chosen should be level with the heart. Common placements are the midradius on the front leg, midtarsus on the rear leg, or the tail base. The tubing from the cuff should run along the artery at whichever limb is chosen and leading toward the BP monitor not the patient. The cuff should be placed around the limb securely but not too tight, and it should never be taped in place because this would result in inaccurate readings. This BP monitoring is done with a machine that will inflate and deflate the cuff and display the systolic, diastolic, and mean arterial pressure on a screen.

Doppler BP Measurement

The **Doppler measurement of BP** uses a crystal instead of a stethoscope to detect blood flow. The equipment needed to perform a Doppler BP reading includes a tape measure, a sphygmomanometer, ultrasound gel, inflatable cuff, and the Doppler unit. An appropriately sized cuff is chosen and placed on the patient's front limb (just below the elbow) or the hind limb, and then the cuff tubing is connected to the sphygmomanometer. A small area is shaved distal to the cuff over the artery (if it is the front limb, shave between the carpal and metacarpal pads). Apply ultrasound gel to the Doppler crystal, and then place the crystal on the shaved area to find an audible pulse. Inflate the cuff using the sphygmomanometer until you cannot hear the pulse anymore, and then slowly release the pressure while listening for the pulse to return. Record the number that the sphygmomanometer reads when the pulse is heard again. The reading mostly relates to the systolic BP in dogs, whereas in cats it is more closely related to the mean arterial pressure.

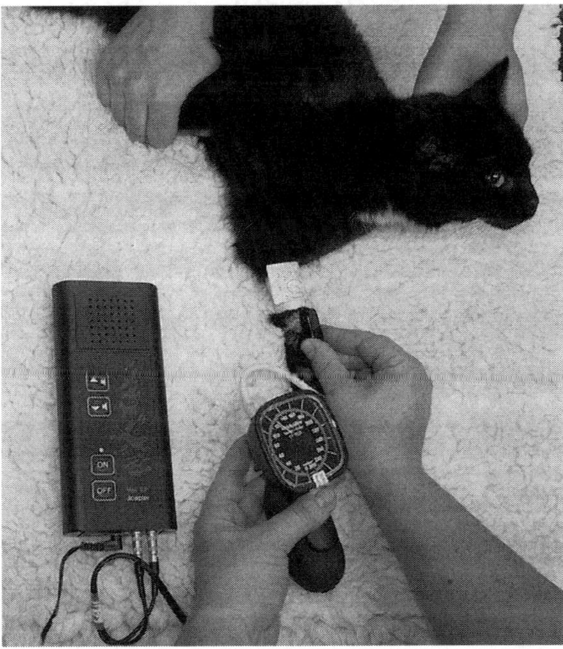

Obtaining an SpO_2 Reading

The first step to obtaining an accurate **SpO_2 reading** is to find a hairless area on the body with not a lot of pigment to place the **pulse oximetry probe**. The probe must be placed on an area where a pulse can be detected; common areas used include the ear, lip, tongue, prepuce, vulva, or in between the toes. The machine will either show a waveform that will represent pulse quality, or the machine will show just the pulse rate along with the SpO_2 reading. If the SpO_2 reading is low, there may be other factors affecting that such as patient movement, skin pigment, or the tissue being too thin. It is best to evaluate the location and probe placement, as well as the patient's other vital signs, before determining if the low SpO_2 reading is legitimate.

Common Conditions and Treatment

Sinus Bradycardia

A particularly slow but regular ventricular heart rate can be described as **sinus bradycardia**. This term is generally used when the heart rate is less than 70 beats per minute for dogs that weigh under 20 kg or 45 lb. This rate is also given for dogs that have a heart rate less than 60 beats per minute when weighing over 20 kg or 45 lb. Heart rates measured at 100 beats per minute or less are indicative of sinus bradycardia in cats. Animals experiencing profound bradycardia can exhibit **symptoms such as weakness, hypotension, and syncope.** Both excessive and reduced parasympathetic tone may result in sinus bradycardia. Sinus bradycardia can sometimes also be attributed to respiratory disease. The disease can cause the animal to experience a number of problems, including struggling to draw in air, gastric irritation, increased cerebrospinal fluid pressure, hypothyroidism, hypothermia, hyperkalemia, and hypoglycemia. Certain drug therapies may also induce the condition.

Sinus Arrhythmia as Related to Respiratory Rate

Sinus arrhythmia (also called respiratory sinus arrhythmia or RSA) is refers to a normal variation in heartbeat, as influenced by respiratory patterns. Both **inspiratory** and **expiratory respirations** can alter the heart's sinus rhythm. Typically, the heart rate increases during inspiration and decreases during expiration. Theorists suggest that this maximizes cardiac output during more effective ventilatory periods. Variations are more pronounced in younger animals and moderate with age. The "sinus" term refers to the sinus node (or the sinoatrial node), which is the heart's natural pacemaker. It is important to know of respiratory sinus arrhythmia, as these changes will be apparent during an ECG. Neurologically induced cardiac variations (as seen in altered vagal tone and parasympathetic system responses, including emotions) can also contribute to the magnitude of sinus arrhythmia experienced. Finally, any respiratory disease in an animal may also bring about an altered sinus arrhythmia.

Benign and Malignant

A **growth** may be described as either **benign** (non-cancerous) or **malignant** (cancerous). Cancer is often defined in terms of the **tumor site**, the **severity**, and the **type of tissue** in which the growth is located. Other terms often used to describe a growth include **mass**, **lump**, **lesion**, **neoplasm**, **tumor**, and **malignancy**. The least severe cancerous tumor is one that is described as "localized". Localized tumors have not spread to other parts of the body. These tumors are often fairly simple to remove if they are also encapsulated (i.e., a lump with clear margins), but may be more difficult if they are diffuse (fuzzy, or tentacle-like). Normally, the primary danger associated with a benign tumor is derived from the place it occupies inside the body. A tumor can obstruct or prevent the body from performing normally, and thus can be dangerous or even life-threatening. More serious tumors are those described as both cancerous and metastatic. These types of tumors are invasive and malignant. These cancer cells often break free and move into a secondary region of the body. The regions frequently involved include the lymph nodes, bones, lungs, and other internal organs. This spreading of cells from the primary site to the secondary position is known as metastasis. These locations need not have any relative connection. The terms primary and secondary are used only to designate the original tumor as opposed to any that later emerge if the cancer spreads.

Types of Therapy to Treat Tumors

It is often possible to entirely remove a tumor through a surgical procedure, particularly when it is both localized and encapsulated. It is important to note that malignant tumors should be removed along with approximately 2 to 3 cm or 1 to 2 inches of healthy tissue bordering the tumor. One type of surgery known as **cryosurgery** is done by freezing tiny external epithelial lesions with liquid nitrogen or N_2O. The cancerous tissue is thereby frozen, following which it dies and can be sloughed off, débrided, or otherwise removed.

Another procedure, known as **chemotherapy**, applies cytotoxic agents to the cancerous regions. Chemotherapy cannot be described as a cure-all for cancer, as it is toxic not only to cancer cells but to healthy cells as well. However, chemotherapy has been able to create a state of remission in some patients. The types of cancers which best respond to this type of treatment are known as systemic and metastatic cancers.

Another procedure known as **radiotherapy** applies a dose of ionizing radiation to the cancerous region. Radiography interrupts the cell's DNA replication, which results in its death. Yet another technique is known as cauterization. This technique uses various methods to burn away tiny epithelial tumors.

Classification of Tumors

Tumors can be described as either benign or malignant and are often classified according to origination site, severity, and tissue type involved. Sarcomas are classified as a malignancy that grows in muscle, tendon, bone, fat, or cartilage, along with various other soft tissues. Sarcomas originate in mesenchymal connective tissues or the embryonic mesodermal tissues found in muscle, bone, fat, or cartilage.

The formation of the term has specific meaning. The prefix (sarco-) comes from the Greek word "sarkos," meaning "flesh." The suffix (-oma) also comes from the Greek and means "swelling" or "tumor." The suffix, (-oma), is typically used to refer to a benign tumor. Thus, the term fibroma refers to a benign tumor that has its starting point in the fibers of muscle or nerves. Unfortunately, however, some tumorous growths that are cancerous also use the suffix (-oma). Therefore, a chondrosarcoma refers to a malignant tumor that originates in the cartilage, and sarcoma refers more generally to any cancer of connective tissue. Other malignant tumors ending in the suffix (-oma) include melanoma, insulinoma, seminoma, and thymoma.

Characteristics of Melanoma

Melanoma is a malignant tumor or cancer that may or may not be accompanied by a dark pigmentation (if pigmented, it is usually black). This type of cancer is more commonly found in dogs than in cats. Melanoma can be unrelenting, and it often **grows quickly**. The tumor can **metastasize** or spread within the body quite rapidly. The spreading of this cancer occurs when the original tumor is **transported by the lymphatic system** to the lymph nodes or via the vascular system in blood cells. Dogs have a 1 in 20 chance of having any tumor diagnosed as malignant melanoma. The most common sites for development of melanoma are on the skin, on the animal's digits, and in the mouth (more particularly found on the face, trunk, feet, and scrotum). Animals with malignant melanoma are generally older, frequently 9 to 12 years of age. The tumor may have produced ulcers or bleeding. This form of cancer responds best to early detection and treatments. The chances for metastatic spread are increased with late detection of the cancer. Often, late detection will have given the cancer time to spread to various bodily organs.

Later Staged Melanoma, and Squamous Cell Carcinoma

The late diagnosis of malignant melanoma may preclude successful treatment. Certainly the prognosis is never as good as it could have been with earlier detection. **Late-staged melanoma** is **not treatable with chemotherapy or radiation**. The animal can be expected to survive for 2 to 3 months when the cancer reaches its most advanced stages.

Both cats and dogs can be diagnosed with **squamous cell carcinoma**. This is the most common type of malignant tumor that can develop in the epithelial layer of the skin, but it can also develop in the mucous membranes. This type of cancer is primarily found in cats, but it can also occur in dogs. It attacks the adjacent tissue and can spread to destroy bone in the animal's skeletal structure. The tumor appears grayish white or pink. It has an abnormally shaped mass. It is most often located in the gingiva, tonsils, and nose. Ulceration is associated with this cancer. Squamous cell carcinoma is aggressive but treatable. The veterinarian may apply surgery, radiation, or hyperthermia in the removal of the tumor.

Epulis and Gingival Hyperplasia

Epulis is a **non-malignant cancer** that begins along the **periodontal ligament**. It will attack the adjacent tissue and spread to the bone. There are 3 kinds of epulides: fibromatous, ossifying, and acanthomatous. **Fibromatous epulides** are fashioned from a resilient tissue fiber. **Ossifying**

epulides are fashioned from bone cells and fibrous tissue. The Ossifying tumor can develop into cancer.

Acanthomatous epulides are detrimental to the bone structure. They are extensively intrusive and will infiltrate (grow into) normal bone. Once it has engulfed the bone it will destroy it. The animal may exhibit drooling, loss of appetite, difficulty eating, and bad breath. The tumor may also be of a size and located in such a way as to cause the animal difficulty in breathing.

Gingival hyperplasia is a condition which occurs in animals that produces an excessive growth of gum tissue. This can be a genetically inherited condition, or it can be drug induced.

Complications of Chemotherapy

Cytotoxic agents are capable of destroying neoplastic cells, primarily by disrupting nucleic acid and protein synthesis. Cytotoxic agents (often referred to as chemotherapy medications) are toxic to all cells, but tend to be taken up faster by cells that are rapidly dividing — a characteristic common to cancer cells. Because bone marrow cells also divide rapidly, patients often become immunosuppressed when cytotoxic agents delay the production of crucial blood and immunological cells.

Common side effects of chemotherapy include alopecia, cardiotoxicity, vomiting, diarrhea, pancreatitis, hepatosis, neutropenia, thrombocytopenia, anemia, neurotoxicity, and renal toxicity.

Staff should wear protective garments to reduce harmful side effects induced by even incidental contact with powerful cytotoxic agents. Recommended garments include latex gloves, long-sleeved lab coats or long-sleeved surgical gowns, and safety goggles. The sleeves on the garments should have close-fitting cuffs. In addition, the waste products must be discarded according to specific biomedical waste guidelines. This waste includes syringes, IV administration sets, gauze, and gloves. The waste should be discarded in a plastic bag that has been securely closed.

Health Issues in Horses

Causes and Management of Colic

Colic can cause a horse to experience **considerable pain in the abdominal region**, and is the number one cause of premature equine fatality. This common problem can be a result of the following: poor feed or feeding and hydration patterns; intestinal tears, displacements, torsions, or hernias; disproportionate gas; sporadic cramps; ileus; parasitic infections; volvulus; intussusception; impactions; obstructions; displacement; inguinal hernias; or ulcers. The colic's degree of severity may not be readily evident depending upon the disposition of the horse. Therefore, careful observation is recommended. In addition, the horse can be placed on a treatment regimen involving the following: fluid therapy, anti-inflammatory drugs, mineral oil, anti-flatulence medication, and anti-ulcer medication. Intestinal injuries (tears, torsions, hernias, etc.) typically require corrective surgery. The horse will need the following checked: vital signs, motility, and fecal output. The horse's state of hydration may be observed when a nasogastric tube is passed and gastrointestinal reflux is achieved. The horse will require regular moderate exercise, typically by being walked. The animal should be reintroduced to food slowly and gradually to reduce upset in the animal's digestive system.

Fluid Therapy Management of Colitis

A horse with **colitis** should be treated with **fluid therapy**. This should reduce the inflammation and spasms experienced by the horse in the colon and abdominal region. The fluid therapy should consist of a **balanced electrolyte solution**. Sometimes adequate amounts of potassium, chloride, and calcium are missing from the animal's diet. This can be corrected via supplementation during fluid therapy. Fluid therapy can also be used for the correction of **metabolic acidosis**. Metabolic acidosis is caused by an increase in the acidity of the blood. The result is a low blood pH level. The correction is made by adding sodium bicarbonate or anti-inflammatory drugs to the fluid therapy administered to the animal. However, a plasma transfusion is required when the total protein is low.

A **vasodilator** is an agent that opens and expands the blood vessels. This agent can be effective in combating the natural tendency toward vasoconstriction found in the equine medial and lateral digital arteries (located between the hoof wall and the distal phalanx). One commonly used vasodilator is known as nitroglycerin.

Causes, Symptoms, and Management of Colitis

Acute colitis is a condition that has yet to be fully understood. The exact cause of the disease is still a mystery. However, it appears some animals may develop colitis due to the following: dietary changes, excessive consumption of carbohydrates, Clostridium perfringens or colitis X, Clostridium difficile, Potomac horse fever, antibiotic therapy, and the overuse of NSAIDs. Acute colitis may be present in the horse that exhibits the following signs and symptoms: inappetence, listlessness, depression, abdominal pain, hyper- or hypomotile gastric motility, increased heart and respiration rates, discolored mucous membranes, increased CRT (capillary refill time), diarrhea, dehydration, hypoproteinemia, imbalance of electrolytes, metabolic acidosis, and shock. Shock, in this situation, can often be attributed to endotoxemia (caused by endotoxin molecules released during the rapid growth or death of gram-negative bacteria).

Mucous membranes that have a **brick or dark red color,** or else a muddy or bluish or cyanotic coloration, can be associated with acute colitis. The animal should be treated with fluid therapy, consisting of a balanced electrolyte solution.

Causes, Symptoms, and Management of Salmonellosis

Many horses with diarrhea are diagnosed with **salmonellosis**. Salmonellosis is the number one cause of infectious diarrhea in horses for at least 2 reasons. First, salmonella is a **zoonotic organism** (can be passed from animals to humans) that is essentially ubiquitous in the equine environment (up to 20% of all horses may "shed" the organism, as it is present in their natural intestinal flora). Second, it is **extremely contagious** to other equines. Therefore, this contagious disease must be managed very carefully.

Salmonellosis can also be triggered by stress in the animal. Some causes for a significant degree of stress are evident in the following: animals transported in a trailer, sudden changes in feeding, use of antibiotics, sickness, surgery, or immunosuppression. It is important for signs of the disease not to be mistaken for similar signs displayed in animals with colitis. The animal can also have an acute case of diarrhea. Notably, the consistency and categorization of the diarrhea is profuse, watery, and foul-smelling. The animal may have pyrexia (a fever), and may also show signs of anorexia.

Concerns Regarding the Management of Salmonellosis and Intestinal Clostridial Infections

In the event infectious **Salmonellosis** is discovered, the animal should be isolated and only one handler should treat the animal to **reduce cross-contamination risks**. The handler should wear a gown, gloves, and protective boot covers. Hand washing with a bactericidal solution is essential. Boots worn in the isolated horse's stall must be washed in a foot bath. Fluid therapy is given using a balanced electrolyte solution to reduce chances for dehydration and electrolyte disorders.

Animals with hypoproteinemia may well need a plasma transfusion. The animal's vital signs must be taken at regular intervals to ensure that the body is functioning adequately. The horse can be fed as often as its appetite allows. However, grain is not included in the diet during this time.

Intestinal clostridial infections cause severe inflammation of the intestines. Colitis X, a widespread form of this disease, is usually discovered only after the death of the animal (during a postmortem examination). It is similar to colitis. Diarrhea is not observed in its early stages. Chronic pain is generated in the abdominal region within hours of contracting the disease. Hypermotility is typically seen. It is treated with an oral dose of antibiotics such as bacitracin. This disease should be treated in largely the same manner as that of colitis or salmonellosis.

Management of Anterior Enteritis

Horses are **unable to expel excess stomach** contents by way of emesis (vomiting). Thus, the treatment of anterior enteritis involves insertion of a nasogastric tube (NG tube). This tube is used to collect any gastric reflux fluids and to relieve gastric and intestinal fluid distension. Without placement of this tube, outright gastric rupture may occur from fluid overload. If the patient exhibits a lessening in symptoms after the NG tube is placed, then it is highly probable that the patient does not have an intestinal obstruction and it is more likely that the patient has anterior enteritis. Anterior enteritis often is mistaken for an obstructed bowel. A rectal exam is needed for verification purposes and to make a more conclusive (albeit not always definitive) diagnosis. Fluid therapy provides replacement of essential fluids, as oral fluid intake is trapped by the enteritis. A jugular vein access is usually needed, as the animal may require as much as 60 to 100 liters (16 to 26 gallons) of replacement fluids daily. The horse requires the monitoring of these vital signs: temperature, color of mucous membranes, CRT (capillary refill time) in the gingival area, and digital pulses. Toxemia can occur as a result of the bacterial toxins present in the horse's bloodstream. This poisonous condition can be a direct result of the severe intestinal upset that accompanies anterior enteritis.

Causes, Symptoms, and Management of Potomac Forse Fever and Anterior Enteritis

Potomac horse fever is abbreviated as PHF. It is also known as **monocytic ehrlichiosis**. One common vector implicated in spreading the infective organism, Ehrlichia risticii, is through snails. In the northeastern United States a peak season exists for the spreading of this disease, largely between the months of June through August. Signs of the disease include depression, anorexia, and pyrexia; a decrease in sounds in the gut; abdominal pain; and diarrhea. Treatments involve: a) isolation of the animal; b) oxytetracycline; c) fluid therapy consisting of a balanced electrolytic solution; and d) frequent monitoring of vital signs. Laminitis is a serious concern. Vaccines preventing PHF have a high rate of effectiveness, but are not totally foolproof.

Anterior enteritis can be linked to Clostridium spp (i.e., including multiple subspecies). However, this disease is normally thought of as idiopathic, with no apparent or known source. Clinical symptoms of this disease involve the following: severe colic, higher heart and respiration rates, and a probability of pyrexia (fever).

Causes, Symptoms, and Treatment of Tetanus

The bacteria known as **Clostridium tetani** can be found in some soils. This bacterium is responsible for the infection known as **tetanus** or "**lockjaw**." The bacterium typically enters the body through a **puncture wound**. The neurotoxins created by the clostridium tetani are able to severely impact the nervous system. The horse shows the following symptoms: a) muscle stiffness as evidenced in a sawhorse stance; b) a decrease in water and feed consumption; c) hypersensitivity to light and noise; and d) muscle fasciculations. The horse that has tetanus should receive a tetanus antitoxin booster. This booster is beneficial in binding the circulating tetanus toxins to the antitoxin in the vaccine. The **puncture wound** requires cleansing. In addition, any excess fluids around the site should be drained off. Topical penicillin is rubbed onto the injury. The animal should be given an IV infusion with penicillin and other fluids. It is recommended that horses receive an annual tetanus vaccination. This cuts down on the likelihood that an animal will contract the infection at a later date.

Causes, Symptoms, and Management of Hyperkalemic Periodic Paralysis

Genetic mutations can cause some diseases to occur in animals. Some Quarter Horse sires have a particular genetic mutation that brings about the disease known as hyperkalemic periodic paralysis. **Hyperkalemic periodic paralysis** can be abbreviated as HYPP. This disease has the following clinical symptoms: muscle fasciculations; incidences of colic, sweating, respiratory distress, and a prolapsed third eyelid (the nictitating membrane which lies on the inside corner of the eye and closes diagonally over it); loose feces; and ataxia (unsteady gait). A blood test can be used to reveal if the horse is a homozygous affected animal, with 2 identical genes. Or, the test may reveal that the horse is a heterozygous carrier with genetic variants. Ideally, however, the test will reveal that the horse has a normal genetic makeup. Breeding is not recommended for horses that have a positive blood test. In addition, horses that have HYPP should not be ridden, as gait and balance issues can present a danger to both the animal and the rider. The horse should be given a low potassium diet, and lots of fresh water. It is best not to give the horse alfalfa hay, feeding grass, or oat hay. In addition, stress should be reduced as much as possible.

Causes, Symptoms, and Management of Rabies

Rabies is a result of a virus known as rhabdovirus. This virus works to damage the central nervous system. The bite of an infected animal allows the transmission of the disease to another animal. The infected animal's saliva is an infective source of the rhabdovirus. This virus can also be transmitted through any open wound or through the mucous membranes. Some infected animals will exhibit high levels of aggression. Other symptoms include dysphagia, hydrophobia, and self-inflicted wounds. If the handler suspects that a horse has rabies, the horse should be immediately isolated. The handler should protect himself by wearing the appropriate clothing, including gloves and other protective gear. Rabies can be transmitted to the handler, as it is a virus with **zoonotic** (animal to human transmission) **potential**. This high potential, in conjunction with the lack of a cure for rabies, results in a rabid horse's euthanasia. Since rabies can only be positively identified through a postmortem examination, it becomes necessary to also euthanize animals that are suspected of having rabies. The best medical advice is to make sure that the animal receives its annual vaccination.

Causes, Symptoms, and Management of Strangles

The bacteria **Streptococcus equi** (S. equi subsp. equi) is a gram-positive coccus that can harm the infected horse's upper respiratory system. The bacteria produce the condition known as Strangles. This condition causes the horse to experience a number of problems associated with breathing and swallowing. This is a highly contagious disease that requires the animal to be placed in isolation. The horse suffering with Strangles will have significant swelling in the lymph nodes, particularly those located underneath the mandible, the guttural pouches, and in the throat. Over time, the lymph nodes develop into empyema abscesses (pus-filled lesions). The horse should receive hot packs on these swellings. The hot packs facilitate the abscesses opening and draining. In addition, many of the abscesses may require lancing to allow the excess fluid to drain. During this time the infected horse may experience dysphagia, finding it difficult to swallow. If this happens, the horse should be given additional fluids. The infected horse should also be fed slurries, which are a liquified mixture of water and feed.

Additional Concerns Regarding Strangles

The animal infected with **Strangles** requires liberal, readily available amounts of fresh water. The infected horse should be kept warm and dry. The horse should also be given antipyretics and antibiotics.

An **antipyretic** is a drug to reduce the animal's fever. **Antibiotics** are beneficial in destroying the virulent bacteria in the body. However, this highly contagious disease must still be carefully monitored. All materials that come into contact with the sick animal should be disposed of by fire or disinfected thoroughly.

This disease does not have a vaccination that can entirely halt its progression. However, the vaccine that is available has been proven to reduce the seriousness of the symptoms associated with the disease. Vaccines should be given to the horse by way of an intranasal administration (through the nose of the animal).

Symptoms and Management of Equine Herpes Virus 1 (EHV-1)

The acronym for **Equine Herpes Virus 1 is EHV-1**. This viral rhinopneumonitis is an organism that primarily infects the respiratory system and endothelial tissues, but which is capable of attacking the nervous system as well. Typical infective symptoms include: fever, depression, inappetence, nasal discharge, and a cough. However, if neurologically afflicted, the horse can exhibit the following symptoms: ungainly movements, incontinence, posterior ataxia (lack of muscle control in the hind limbs), and an absence of tail tone. The horse may be found sitting as a dog or in a recumbent position. This is attributed to the paralytic state of the animal's hind legs. The infected expectant mother may spontaneously abort an unborn fetus.

To reduce fetal risks, the animal should be given a vaccination in the 5th, 7th, and 9th month of the pregnancy. The vaccine is Pneumabort K +1b. Abortion does not necessarily have to occur if the animal is infected during later gestational periods. Harm to the foal in utero is evident when a stillbirth foal is delivered. A live foal may also die shortly after delivery. The horse may be given antibiotics, anti-inflammatory drugs, or corticosteroids. It is recommended that horses receive a preventive vaccination. However, abortions or neurological diseases can still occur if the vaccination does not provide enough protection.

Causes, Symptoms, and Management of Equine Herpes Virus (EHV)

The acronym for **Equine Herpes Virus 4** is EHV-4. This virus produces a rhinopneumonitis, and is common throughout the globe. However, its infectious patterns differ significantly from those common to EHV-1. Although EHV-1 also affects the respiratory tract and lymph nodes, it is predisposed to infecting endothelial tissue in the nose, lungs, adrenal glands, thyroid, and central nervous system. Thus, neurological problems and spontaneous abortions in gravid horses may also occur. By contrast, EHV-4 infections are largely localized to the respiratory tract and associated lymph glands, without these neurological and pregnancy issues.

EHV-4 is spread through close contact or through aerosolized body fluids (i.e., droplets scattered when sneezing, etc.). This viral disease targets the horse's upper respiratory system, and causes increased respiratory symptoms such as wheezing, rhonchi, rales, and stridor. In addition, the lymph nodes will swell from the infection. It is highly recommended that the horse be placed in isolation, as there is a significant danger of cross-contamination. The horse's environment should be protected against undue cold and be well ventilated. The horse should be placed in a stall that is quiet, and should not be placed under stress. The animal will require brief periods of exercise, as this is beneficial to blood circulation and lymph systems. This disease cannot be totally prevented by preemptive vaccination, but post-infection vaccination is thought to reduce the seriousness of the associated symptoms.

Symptoms and Management of Equine Infectious Anemia (EIA)

The acronym for the **Equine Infectious Anemia virus** is EIA. Another name for this condition is **Swamp Fever**. This virus can be found in an animal's blood and semen. Transmission of the disease occurs primarily through blood, spread by biting flies (arthropods) and other blood-feeding insects. However, the animal can also contract this virus through blood transfusions and unsanitary needles used in various medical treatments. Finally, the disease can also be spread through semen, infecting mares and (because it can penetrate the placental barrier) their young. Infection is for life, with periods of remission and exacerbation recurring in due course. Infected horses will have the following symptoms: pyrexia (fever), depression, weight loss, anorexia, and anemia. All infected horses are carriers of this disease even when they display no symptoms. The animal with this disease should be euthanized. In each state or province, local, state, provincial, and federal regulations should be consulted regarding the laws concerning euthanasia. Horses that are not put to sleep should be placed in isolation to prevent further contamination of other animals. This isolation must last the length of the horse's lifespan, as there is no known cure for Swamp Fever or EIA. Total isolation (including insect-free isolation) is the only way to keep other horses from contracting the disease.

Laminitis

The disease known as **laminitis** impacts a horse's feet. This disease causes the laminae or protective plate inside the horse's hoof to become swollen and irritated. This inflammation is usually experienced more in the front hoofs of a horse than in the hind hoofs. However, there are occasions when the hoofs in the hind quarters will also become inflamed. Laminitis can result from the following: overconsumption of grain, ingesting too much cold water, endotoxemia, concussion, hormonal influences, aftermath of a viral respiratory disease, aftermath of a drug treatment, and overeating in lavish pastures. Horses with this condition display a lack of motivation and energy. Some horses display apprehension. Other symptoms include pyrexia, depression, lack of appetite, and sensitivity when hoof testing is conducted (typically by way of a manually operated device that tests for pressure-sensitive points on a horse's feet). Horses with laminitis will exhibit an irregular gait characterized by toe pointing and rocking onto the heel. This gait relieves pressure on the tender area of the toe. The hoof wall will also be hotter to the touch than is normally experienced.

Treatment for Laminitis

With the **hoof disease laminitis**, the heat felt in the hoof wall is the result of increased in blood flow in that area. The digital pulses will also be out of the normal range. In acute cases, the coffin bone will rotate and penetrate the sole of the horse's foot. A radiograph can detect the extent of the rotation. Treatment includes anti-inflammatory drugs, acepromazine, fluids such as LRS (lactated Ringer's solution), and trimming the hoof in a restorative fashion.

Vasodilators known as isoxsuprine hydrochloride and nitroglycerine can be applied to the horse's medial and lateral digital arteries. Vasodilators are medicines that can expand the blood vessels to lower blood pressure and ease the flow of blood. The horse should be given grass and hay to eat. Grains are not recommended. Cold hosing and icing the feet are treatments that have been applied by some veterinarians. However, others strongly disapprove of this practice.

Estrous Cycle

The **phases of the estrous cycle** circumscribe the duration of time that a female mammal can exhibit signs of sexual receptivity that may attract a mate. During this period of time the female has reoccurring physiological changes that can be attributed to the effects of reproductive hormones. There are 4 estrous phases: proestrus, estrus, diestrus, and anestrus. Some schema include a fifth phase called metestrus, which is very brief (1-5 days) immediately following the estrus phase.

Proestrus is the time period just before onset the estrus cycle. The proestrus period is designed to prepare the uterus to receive an embryo. **Follicle Stimulating Hormone** or FSH induces ovarian follicles to develop and give off estrogen. **Estrogen** is a steroid hormone produced by the ovaries, which builds up in the uterus and uterine horns. During proestrus, estrogen induces endothelium to grow and form an inner layer in the uterus. This inside layer develops in preparation for a potentially fertilized egg to implant.

Additional Phases of the Estrous Cycle

With the **onset of estrus**, the female is able to function in the reproductive process and ovulation occurs. The female's uterus and uterine horns are **fully prepared to accept an embryo**. Canines also experience a surge in **luteinizing hormone** (LH), which comes from the pituitary gland. The luteinizing hormone is responsible for ovulation, and indicates that the egg or eggs from the ovaries are ready for fertilization. Ovulation in cats and rabbits occurs through the breeding process, as they are nonspontaneous or induced ovulators.

A third phase called **metestrus** begins as luteinizing hormone levels begin to drop. In this post-ovulatory phase, each egg-containing follicle changes, bursts, and grows into a corpus luteum. A corpus luteum is a yellow mass that produces progesterone to continue thickening the lining of the uterus. The corpus luteum is needed to begin and to maintain a pregnancy, and functions to produce hormones during the next phase of the estrus cycle (diestrus). Finally, all sexual hormonal activity ceases during the concluding phase called anestrus (the resting phase).

Estrous cycle, Placenta, and Umbilical Cord During Pregnancy

Pregnancy exists when a female animal carries an unborn offspring inside her body. A healthy pregnancy lasts from the time of fertilization to the birthing process. During the estrus cycle, the corpus luteum will work to consistently produce essential pregnancy- related hormones throughout most or all of a pregnancy. The duration of the production of hormone will vary in accordance with the type of species. Some types of animals will require the hormones to be produced throughout the entire period of the pregnancy. Other types of animals will only require the hormones until the placenta is formed.

The **placenta** is a transient organ inside the uterus that pregnant female mammals produce to supply oxygen and food to a fetus. Nutrition, oxygen, and other substances are delivered to the fetus through the umbilical cord. The umbilical cord is a flexible tube that links the abdomen of the fetus to the mother's placenta. This tube is also used to expel waste. The intrauterine corpus luteum will break down or decompose if a pregnancy does not actualize (i.e., if a fertilized egg does not implant there).

Female Reproductive System

The female reproductive system consists of many interrelated organs and anatomical features. The ovaries are a pair of organs necessary for female reproduction. The oval-shaped ovaries are located in the female's abdomen. **Ovaries** are responsible for the production of ova and hormones. The ova are female reproductive cells. **Ova** is a Latin word for "eggs," and the words may be used interchangeably. In most species, the ova will pass from the ovary to the uterine horn or uterus, down to the uterine tubes (or Fallopian tubes or oviduct). The **uterus** has the following parts: uterine horns, body, and cervix, leading to the opening of the uterus. **Uterine** horns are the projections from the uterus that extend toward the uterine or fallopian tubes. Some animals do not have uterine horns.

Some animals are **polytocous** or **multiparous** (which means that the animal is able to have more than one baby at a given time), and will typically have longer uterine horns in order to carry several offspring. The species that have only 1 baby are known as monotocous or uniparous. Their fetuses will grow & develop in the uterus itself. There are 3 layers within the uterus and uterine horns. These 3 layers are: endometrium, myometrium, and perimetrium. During the birthing process, the fetus will pass out of the uterus to the exterior environment. The vehicle for this passage is known as the vagina or birth canal. The vulva is the name given to the external female genitalia, which consists of the labia and opening to the urethra and internal sex organs.

Educating Clients and the Public

Zoonosis

Zoonosis is any disease that can be transmitted from animals to humans, or any disease that normally is in an animal but can infect humans. There are three routes of transmission including contact, aerosol, and vector-borne. Contact may be direct, for example, ingestion or puncture wounds, or it may be indirect by exposure to fomites by handling the dirty laundry, dishes, or housing of an animal. There are certain zoonotic parasites such as hookworms that can be transmitted from dogs and cats to humans through the feces. Roundworms are also zoonotic parasites that can be transmitted to humans through feces, and they can cause visceral and ocular larva migrans (where larvae settle in the eye). Rabies, which is fatal, is also a zoonotic disease transmitted through saliva, bites, or scratches from infected animals.

Types of Heartworm Prevention for Dogs or Cats

Heartworm preventatives, including ivermectin, moxidectin, milbemycin oxime, and selamectin, are effective against heartworm disease. Heartworm preventatives work by killing the infective larvae that have infected the patient within the previous month. **Ivermectin** (Heartgard, Iverhart Plus, and Tri-Heart) is an antiparasitic drug that is administered as a chewable oral tablet monthly at a very low dose as a heartworm preventative. Medications include **pyrantel pamoate**, which also will kill hookworms and roundworms (Heartgard Plus). **Milbemycin oxime** (Trifexis and Sentinel) is an antiparasitic drug given as a monthly oral tablet that will also kill roundworms, hookworms, and whipworms. **Selamectin** (Revolution) is a topical monthly application that is an antiparasitic drug that kills heartworm infective larvae as well as fleas, hookworms, roundworms, and ear mites. **Moxidectin** (ProHeart 6 and Advantage Multi) is an antiparasitic drug that kills heartworm infective larvae and hookworms. Advantage Multi is a topical drug applied once monthly, and ProHeart 6 is an injectable given SQ once every 6 months.

Tick-Borne Illnesses and the Clinical Signs

Anaplasmosis is transmitted by deer ticks and black-legged ticks. Dogs and cats can acquire *Anaplasmosis,* and clinical signs include joint pain leading to lameness, fever, vomiting, and diarrhea. **Ehrlichiosis** is transmitted to dogs by the brown dog tick and the lone star tick. Clinical signs of ehrlichiosis include depression, anorexia, fever, joint pain, and bruising. **Rocky Mountain spotted fever** (RMSF) is transmitted by the American dog tick and the RMSF tick and can infect dogs and cats, but the tick must be attached for at least 5 hours to transmit RMSF. Signs of RMSF are anorexia, joint pain, fever, vomiting, and diarrhea, pneumonia, kidney and liver failure, and neurological signs. **Lyme disease** (borreliosis) is caused by the bacteria *Borrelia burgdorferi* and is transmitted by deer ticks. Clinical signs for Lyme disease include fever, swollen lymph nodes, and anorexia; in more severe cases, kidney disease and heart conditions may develop. There is a vaccine given for Lyme disease for dogs. All of these diseases are commonly treated with a course of antibiotics.

Lone Star Tick

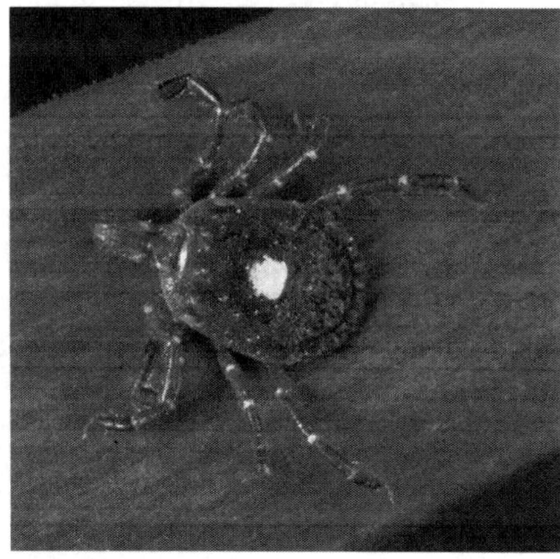

Canine Distemper Combination Vaccine

The **canine distemper vaccine** is a combination vaccine that protects against more than just the distemper virus. The canine distemper vaccine protects against **distemper**, **canine adenovirus-2** and **-1 infection** (hepatitis and respiratory), **parvovirus**, and **parainfluenza**. The abbreviated vaccines are labeled DA2PP or DA2PPV. The D is for canine distemper, which is a virus that affects the respiratory system, digestive system, and the brain and nervous system of canines. The distemper virus is highly contagious and can be fatal. A2 refers to the canine adenovirus-2, which can cause respiratory disease. P stands for parvovirus, which is an incredibly contagious and potentially fatal disease that attacks the immune and digestive systems causing diarrhea and vomiting. P refers to parainfluenza, which is a viral respiratory disease in dogs, with the V referring to virus.

Bordetella Bronchiseptica

Bordetella bronchiseptica is a strain of bacteria associated with respiratory disease in canines, but it may also affect cats, rabbits, and very rarely humans. It is the most common bacterial cause of tracheobronchitis in canines, also referred to as kennel cough. *Bordetella* is very contagious and is transmitted through direct contact or even through the air. In young puppies or older dogs with a compromised immune system, *Bordetella* can cause major illness and even death. Mostly, in healthy adult canines, *Bordetella* causes mild illness. The *Bordetella* vaccine is a noncore vaccine; therefore, it is not administered to all dogs or cats and is typically used for those likely to come in contact with the bacterial organism in kennel situations, such as at the groomer or boarding facility. Puppies may receive the intranasal *Bordetella* vaccine as early as 3–4 weeks of age, and they can receive the injectable vaccine at around 6–8 weeks of age, with a booster between 10 and 12 weeks of age. Dogs should then receive a booster *Bordetella* vaccine every 6–12 months.

Leptospirosis

Leptospirosis is caused by the *Leptospira* bacteria that are found in water and in soil, and there are numerous strains that can cause disease. Leptospirosis is zoonotic, where infection in humans can cause flu symptoms and could cause kidney and liver disease. Leptospirosis is very common in dogs and is rare in cats. Dogs are exposed to the *Leptospira* bacteria by drinking out of contaminated rivers, ponds, streams, or from living in areas where infected wildlife mammals may be present. If the dog's mucous membranes or open wounds come in contact with the infected urine of wildlife mammals, the dog can become infected. Dogs may also become infected if they eat an infected animal or get bit by an infected animal. *Leptospira* bacteria can be transmitted through the placenta to puppies as well.

Booster Vaccines

Young puppies and kittens are at risk for acquiring infectious diseases because of their **immature immune systems**. Antibodies from the mother's milk provides protection but does not last long, and there can be gaps in protection because the antibodies in the milk decrease and the pet's immune system matures. The first vaccine given is to jump-start the puppy or kitten's immune system against the virus or bacteria, and then **booster vaccines** are needed to further stimulate their immune system to produce antibodies to protect the animal. Vaccines for puppies and kittens are given 3–4 weeks apart, starting at 8 weeks, with the final booster given at around 4 months of age. The rabies vaccine will be given after 12 weeks of age and is given as a booster in one year. An incomplete or missed vaccine in a puppy or kitten series leads to incomplete protection and leaves the pet vulnerable to infection.

Ctenocephalides Felis

Ctenocephalides felis is a common cat flea. The fleas lay their eggs in the fur of the host (dog or cat), and the eggs will fall onto the carpet or outside onto the dirt where they hatch about 1–6 days later. The flea larvae that just hatched will feed on organic debris in the environment and the feces of adult fleas. In order for the larvae to develop, the environment must be warm, shaded, and moist. Fleas inside of a house will dig deep into carpet fibers or floor cracks and damp basements. Mature larvae produce a cocoon where it pupates, and once the pupa is mature, it emerges from the cocoon when stimulated by physical pressure or heat. If not stimulated, the adult flea may remain in the cocoon for a few weeks up to a year if conditions allow. Adult fleas normally do not leave their host unless forced off, and they begin feeding immediately once on the host. Fleas mate in a couple of days after feeding and can produce up to 50 eggs a day, and they continue producing eggs for up to 100 days.

Feline Leukemia Virus (FeLV)

Feline leukemia virus (FeLV) is a retrovirus that is spread through saliva, nasal secretions, feces, urine, as well as through nursing mothers to their kittens. FeLV is defined as a retrovirus because the virus invades the body's cells and inserts a copy of its personal genetic material into the cells through an enzyme produced by the retrovirus called reverse transcriptase. Cats that live primarily outdoors are at a higher risk of contracting FeLV, but exposure does not always mean that the cat will become infected because the virus may not replicate. There are three specific groups of FeLV, including FeLV-A, FeLV-B, and FeLV-C. FeLV-A affects all cats infected with FeLV and causes severe immunosuppression, is easily transmitted, and is the group used in making the FeLV vaccines. FeLV-B occurs in about half of the cats infected with FeLV and causes neoplastic disease. FeLV-C affects less than 1% of infected cats and causes severe anemia. There is no treatment for FeLV; therefore, vaccinating is crucial.

Rabies Virus

Rabies is an acute viral encephalomyelitis caused by lyssaviruses that affects mammals, primarily carnivores and bats. Rabies is **mainly transmitted through saliva** to the tissues by a bite of an infected animal, and it may also be contracted through salivary glands and the brain coming in contact with fresh wounds or mucous membranes of the body, but this is rare. Once clinical signs appear, the virus is considered contagious, but in cats and dogs, the virus is contagious a few days prior to noticeable clinical signs. After an animal is bitten by an infected animal, the virus remains at the inoculation site for the duration of the incubation period. The virus then migrates through the peripheral nerves to the spinal cord and up to the brain, and then it travels through the peripheral nerves to the salivary glands and is shed intermittently. After the virus replicates in the CNS, every organ will become affected.

Feline Calicivirus (FCV)

One of the most common causes of feline upper respiratory infection and oral disease is **feline calicivirus (FCV)**. There are more than 40 different strains of the calicivirus, and the severity varies greatly between strains. FCV is **transmitted through saliva as well as eye and nasal secretions and is highly contagious.** The calicivirus can survive for up to a week in optimal environmental conditions. Cats can become infected by being exposed to contaminated objects in an environment contaminated with FCV, and humans can transmit the virus by touching infectious secretions on objects or other cats and transmit it to susceptible cats. Once the cat becomes infected with FCV, the virus goes through a 2- to 6-day incubation period before symptoms develop, and the infection can last up to 21 days. Cats that are infected can shed the virus for up to 3 weeks, and after recovering, many cats develop a carrier state in which they continue to shed viral particles occasionally or consistently. The carrier state can last a few months or even a lifetime; therefore, those cats are contagious.

Feline Panleukopenia Virus (FPV)

Feline panleukopenia virus (FPV), also known as feline distemper, is a highly contagious and often fatal disease in cats. FPV is transmitted oronasally through feces, urine, blood, and fomites such as shoes or clothing. FPV can also be transmitted in utero as well as through the breast milk of an infected mother. Stray cats are usually exposed to FPV before they reach 1 year of age, and those that survive an acute FPV infection will build a strong immune response. FPV infects and kills the rapidly dividing cells of the bone marrow, intestines, and lymph nodes. Usually if kittens are infected transplacentally, they will be stillborn, but if they become infected immediately after birth from nursing, it could cause cerebellar hypoplasia as a result of the virus damaging the part of the brain responsible for muscle activity.

Ringworm

Ringworm (dermatophytosis) is a **fungal disease that infects the skin, hair, and claws of patients**. The ringworm fungus feed on the keratin found in the layers of these areas. Most ringworm is caused by the *Microsporum canis* species in dogs, although some cases are caused by the *M. gypseum* or *Trichophyton mentagrophytes* species. Once infected, dogs will develop lesions of alopecia and crusts, as well as bumps on the skin (mainly on the face, ears, tail, and feet). Ringworm is zoonotic and is spread very easily by contact with contaminated objects or infected animals; however, some humans and animals can be asymptomatic carriers, which means that they have ringworm but show no symptoms. Coming in contact with an infected animal does not necessarily mean that it will cause infection, which depends on the species of fungus and the age, health condition, and other factors of the host.

Macroconidia of *Microsporum Canis*

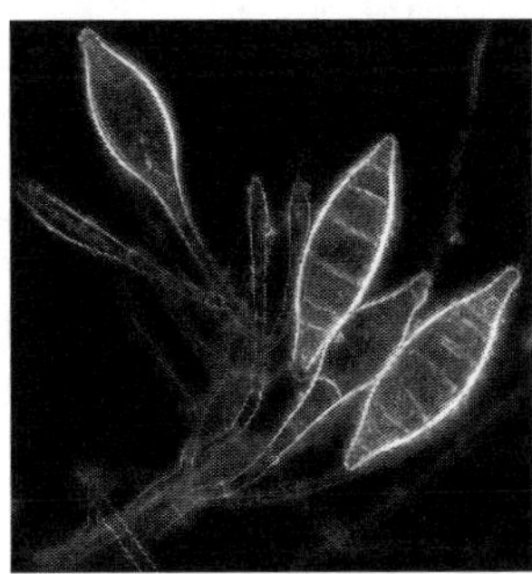

Obesity and Its Effects

Obesity can cause irreversible damage to the pet's organs, bones, and joints. Obese pets are more prone to diabetes because the extra fat leads to insulin resistance in cats. Obese cats also run the risk of developing hepatic lipidosis, which can result if the cat gets stressed and stops eating and the body starts metabolizing body fat for calories. The liver in a cat is not meant to process such a large amount of fat, so it becomes overwhelmed and eventually fails, which can be life threatening. Pets can develop arthritis because there is an excess of weight being put on the joints leading to pain and discomfort caused by the degeneration of the joints. Obesity, especially in brachycephalic breeds, can cause trouble breathing because of the extra fat constricting the chest, making it harder for the pet to take deep breaths, and also causing the pet to cough because the lungs cannot inflate fully. To maintain a healthy weight for a pet, be sure to use an actual measuring cup to measure the amount of food per serving, limit treats, only give healthy table food such as fruits and veggies, and give the pet daily exercise whether it is walking a dog or using a laser pointer for a cat to chase. There may be an underlying medical issue contributing to the pet's obesity such as Cushing's syndrome or hypothyroidism, and testing should be done to rule out suspected disease.

Spaying or Neutering a Pet

Spaying or neutering a pet is important for the pet's health. Spaying a female animal eliminates the potential to develop uterine or ovarian cancer, and it also eliminates the risk of pyometra (infection of the uterus). Spaying a female also **lowers the risk of mammary cancer**. Neutering a male animal **eliminates the risk of testicular cancer** and greatly **reduces the risk of prostate** and **perianal cancer**. Spaying and neutering pets also helps with the overpopulation issue. Humane societies and shelters are constantly overpopulated with dogs and cats, and there are not enough staff members or funds to provide help to all of the stray or abandoned animals so that many are euthanized. Altering a pet will also benefit the owner, because the females will not go into heat and it significantly lowers the need for males to mount, urine marking, aggression, and their desire to seek out a female in heat, therefore decreasing the urge to roam away from the home, resulting in less of a risk of getting hit by a car or fighting with other animals.

Food Allergies in Dogs

A dog's immune system will overreact to a certain protein in the dog's food, and this is called a **food allergy**. Certain meats as well as grains and vegetables are sources of proteins in dog foods, but the most **common food allergens are beef, dairy, chicken, and wheat**. When the dog ingests the food, stomach acid helps break down the food into smaller pieces, and then the enzymes and stomach acid break down complex proteins. The food is digested until the proteins are broken into their smallest forms called amino acids, which are absorbed by the body. Enterocyte cells are the cells that allow the body to absorb the amino acid, but they also turn away amino acids. Sometimes an entire protein will be digested into the intestine before being broken down; this causes an immune reaction because it is identified as a threat, resulting in clinical signs of a food allergy in the dog.

Preventing the Spread of Canine Parvovirus (CPV)

To prevent environmental contamination and the **spread of canine parvovirus** (CPV) to other dogs, infected patients must be kept in an isolation ward in the hospital away from other patients. When personnel handle dogs with CPV, they must be wearing gloves and a gown (specified for that infected patient), and they must also step through **a diluted bleach foot bath** with their shoes before entering or leaving the isolation room. Every surface should be cleaned with a diluted bleach or an accelerated hydrogen peroxide disinfectant. **Vaccinations for canine parvovirus** should be administered to puppies at 8 weeks, 12 weeks, and 16 weeks of age; there is a booster a year later and then every 3 years to prevent and control this deadly virus. CPV can remain viable in the environment for long periods of time; therefore, in kennels, shelters, and hospitals, every surface needs to be cleaned, disinfected, and dried twice before reuse.

Cleaning a Kennel

The first step to **cleaning a kennel** is to remove the animal and any bedding, bowls, and toys. Next, wipe away any feces, urine, or vomit from the kennel. Use a bristle brush to scrub the kennel with the disinfectant starting at the top with the ceiling of the kennel, all sides, door, and floor of the kennel. All hinges and latches need to be scrubbed as well. The disinfectant solution must sit for 5–10 minutes to be effective, and then it should be rinsed with water. All dishes should be soaked in the dilute disinfectant after being cleaned with soap and water. All blankets should be washed.

Maintaining Diagnostic Equipment and Supplies

Electrocardiogram

Electrical signals from the heart can be conveyed to the **electrocardiograph** in many ways, including: 1) by wireless ECG devices positioned near the animal; 2) by use of adhesive ECG pads; 3) by rubber straps holding small metal plates to the skin; or 4) by the subcutaneous placement of ECG wires. Each method has advantages and disadvantages. If pads are used, the pad is placed directly on the animal's bare skin. The animal's fur is clipped to allow complete contact. If alligator skin clips are used, they may be clipped directly to the animal's skin. However, this technique can be painful. Other techniques may provide the animal with a less traumatic experience. Where necessary (particularly for long-term monitoring) ECG wires can be placed subcutaneously. The placement of surgical wire can be accomplished after cleaning the area. The wire is cleansed with alcohol. Then, a 20 gauge needle is used to introduce the wire under the skin. The ends of the wire are bent along one end and adhesive tape is applied. This is done to prevent harm in long-haired animals. In addition, this method allows easy removal of the wire following the procedure.

During the **ECG recording process** the animal can be placed into a right lateral recumbent position. Some larger sized animals may remain in an upright position on their feet. Cats are normally more comfortable in a crouch position on the table. Regardless, the animal requires manual restraints.

Running Quality Controls on Laboratory Instruments

Running **quality controls** on lab equipment should be done at each shift ideally. There should be a log book in which the results of the control are logged and tracked to look for trends. Each quality control should be assessed for accuracy according to the reference ranges before patient samples are run. Quality control results are accurate when they fall into the **average reference ranges**. Differences in quality control results must be evaluated; for example, if one day the reading is at the high end of the reference range and the very next day it reads at the low end of the reference range, then something may be wrong with the instrument because this could reflect the difference between a normal and an abnormal value in a patient. Proper handling and storage techniques must be used with quality control material: Some may need to be refrigerated, some may need to be reconstituted with distilled water (not tap water), and certain products have a short shelf life after being opened, so carefully reading instructions is vital.

Proper Disposal of Sharps

Used sharps need to be disposed of into a sharps container directly after use. **Sharps containers** are sealed and made of a material that is resistant to punctures. After the container is full, the lid is closed, and it is nearly impossible to open again. Once sealed, sharps containers are water resistant. The sharps container should be labeled as a biohazard. Items categorized as sharps include an item with rigid corners or edges that could cut an individual. Sharps include **needles, blades, broken glass,** and **slides**. After using a syringe, the needle should not be removed or bent in any way and you should not recap the needle. A medical waste disposal company will pick up and dispose of the sharps.

Nursing Tasks and Administration of Medications

Oral and Topical Routes of Drug Administration

The patient should be given medication by mouth in an oral dosage that is liquid, semisolid, or in a pill or capsule form. **Liquid medication** can be injected in the pocket of the cheek via a dropper or syringe. The **pill** or **capsules** should be positioned towards the back of the animal's tongue. This is accomplished with one hand, while the other hand works to keep the animal's mouth open. Once the pill has been positioned, then the animal's mouth is held closed until the animal has swallowed noticeably.

The animal cannot be given an oral medication if there are certain adverse conditions present. Contraindicating adverse conditions include **vomiting, injury in the oral cavity or esophagus**, or **problematic swallowing**. In these situations the use of oral medication is contraindicated and highly inadvisable.

Other medications may be applied **topically**. These medications can be placed on or rubbed into the skin. The animal's skin must be sanitized and clipped of any hair in any region to be used for medication application.

Parenteral Administration of Drugs

IM injections are given with a 22 to 25-gauge needle. The injection is administered into the lumbar muscles or bicep femoris muscle. This injection is delivered in a volume that is no more than about 2 mL in any one location. Therefore, a number of sites may be needed to obtain the desired effect. IV administrations can be given in the cephalic, femoral, saphenous, or jugular veins. The IV is the quickest route to produce the desired effect. This also is an ideal method when a large dose of medication or fluid must be given. The cephalic region refers to the area within or on the head. The femoral region refers to the area of the thigh or the femur. The saphenous vein is found in the leg and refers to 2 major veins which travel from the foot to the thigh. The jugular vein refers to one of the 4 main pairs of veins found in the neck.

Topical and Parenteral Administration of Drugs

Topical medications are placed upon the skin. The animal's skin must be sanitized and clipped of any hair in any region to be used for medication application. This must be done before any medication is applied to the area. However, it is perfectly acceptable to place appropriate topical medications directly on any lesions or wounds. The directions accompanying each medication will provide specific information regarding the amounts recommended to be applied at any given time. In addition, the directions should note the time it takes for the medication to be absorbed. The technician that applies the medication should wear gloves to prevent accidental absorption into the skin.

Some drugs are best delivered through an **injection**. All drugs taken by any means other than via the digestive system (i.e., by way of skin absorption, inhalation, injections, etc.) are referred to as parenteral medications. However, the term is most often used in reference to injectable drugs (whether administered by syringe, IV, or other infusion method). Medications by injection typically take effect much more quickly, will not be regurgitated or expectorated, and are more completely absorbed into the system than drugs administered orally.

Routes of Drug Injection and Sites of Injectable Drug Administration

There are 3 ways that an injectable drug can be administered by parenteral means. These 3 routes are subcutaneous, intramuscular, and intravenous. **Subcutaneous** is abbreviated as SC or SQ. Intramuscular is abbreviated as IM. **Intravenous** is abbreviated as IV. However, there are additional distinctions which may be involved, including intradermal, intraperitoneal, intracardiac, intratracheal, intramedullary or intraosseous, intranasal, intrathecal, and intra-arterial. **Intradermal** (between skin layers) is abbreviated as ID. **Intraperitoneal** (into the abdominal cavity) is abbreviated as IP. **Intracardiac** (into the heart) is abbreviated as IC. Intratracheal (into the trachea) is abbreviated as IT. **Intramedullary** or intraosseous (into a bone) is abbreviated as IO. Intranasal (into the nose) is abbreviated as IN. **Intrathecal** (into the space around the spinal cord) is also abbreviated as IT, and thus is context specific. Intra-arterial (into an artery) is abbreviated as IA.

In most cases, SC injections are given with a 22 to 25 gauge needle. SC injections are often administered in the back of the hips or neck of an animal. This is an ideal location due to the excess skin found in these regions. Vaccinations are normally given in subcutaneous injections under the skin.

Fluid Therapy

Contraindications

There are times when an animal's immediate condition may make it inadvisable to pursue rapid fluid replacement. For example, pulmonary edema may make rehydration problematic. **Pulmonary edema** is an excess of fluid accumulating in the lungs. This is a concern that requires regular and frequent observations until all troubling fluid dynamics can be adequately addressed and resolved. Other problems that may make rapid fluid replacement therapy inadvisable include: pulmonary contusions, brain injury, severe ascites, cerebral edema from any cause, and congestive heart failure. If the animal shows signs of over-hydration, then fluid therapy must be halted. **Over-hydration symptoms** include: restlessness, an elevated respiratory rate, wheezing or other sounds of respiratory compromise emanating from the lungs, an abnormal rise in blood pressure, chemosis, and pitting edema. **Chemosis** is demonstrated by an enlargement or swelling of the eye whites. **Pitting edema** is a sign of fluid overload in the extremities, seen when the tissues are firmly pressed and do not rebound (leaving a "pit" or dent where previously pressed). At the conclusion of fluid replacement therapy the animal is again evaluated. The weight of the animal should be taken. The specific gravity and amount of any recent urine voiding should also be noted. The recorded amounts, patient reactions, and veterinarian's instructions are applied in making any changes needed for further fluid therapy.

Routes

Fluids can be given to a patient in a number of ways. **Fluids can be given through oral, subcutaneous, percutaneous, intravenous, or intramedullary routes** into the body. A syringe or a feeding tube is often used in the administration of fluids by oral means. However, an oral administration route is not advisable in animals displaying certain adverse conditions. These include: vomiting, esophageal injury, and/or pancreatitis. Pancreatitis exists when the digestive and endocrine gland known as the pancreas becomes inflamed and swollen.

A subcutaneous fluid replacement route is often used in cases that exhibit symptoms of mild dehydration. However, the subcutaneous fluid route cannot be applied if the patient is in shock or in cases of severe dehydration. This is due to the relatively slow rate of absorption associated with poor peripheral circulation, which is a symptom of shock. Therefore, it is best to administer intravenous fluids to patients in shock accompanied by moderate to severe dehydration. Younger animals, or those that are very small, should be given fluids by intramedullary infusion. This method allows the fluid to be absorbed quickly, since it is delivered directly into the highly vascularized bone marrow.

Calculating the Fluid Replacement Volume

Fluid levels must be promptly replaced in patients that are suffering from hypovolemic shock, or severely dehydrated conditions. These patients should receive 60 to 90 mL/kg/hr of fluids to replace the lost volume. The replacement fluids should be given to the patient over a 12- to 24-hour time frame in order to avoid inducing other problems. The total fluid amount needing to be replaced can be calculated by determining the daily fluid requirements. The calculation for the amount of replacement fluids required is the percent dehydration (as a decimal point figure) multiplied by the animal's body weight in kg, multiplied by 1000 to obtain the replacement amount in milliliters.

The quantity of maintenance fluid needed is approximately 40 to 60 mL/kg/day. A measurement must be taken to determine the volume of urine excreted on a daily basis. In addition, diarrhea, vomitus, and other concurrently lost fluids should be measured. This includes any fluid that drains from an injury. This provides an estimated amount of the total fluid needed to provide rehydration, maintenance, and replacement fluid for that which is continuously excreted in one form or another.

Replacement solutions include Normosol R and lactated Ringer's solution or LRS. Maintenance solutions are known as: Normosol M and normal saline with KCl.

Canine Blood Donor Requirements

There are 2 kinds of dog blood types: Type A- (A negative) or Type A+ (A positive). The A- blood type is regarded as the universal blood donor type for dogs. This is because all dogs, whether they are A- or A+, can tolerate receiving this blood type via transfusion, while A+ blood is only well tolerated by dogs that are also A+ in blood type. A blood donor gives blood to another patient in need. The ideal donor can be found among any breed of dog. Further, the ideal donor can be either male or female. However, the animal should have been neutered or spayed, to reduce blood hormone levels. Neutering is defined as the surgical removal of the animal's testicles or ovaries. In addition, the animal's weight is a factor. It should be larger than 25 kg or 55 lb. Age is also a factor. It should be between the age of 1 and 7 years old. The animal should have received all of its vaccinations. The donor's blood type should already have been determined. The animal should have the following additional tests on a yearly basis: blood chemistry, CBC, and urinalysis. The ideal donor should receive a normal result from these 3 tests before the blood is extracted.

Additional Requirements with Canine Blood Donors

A **blood donor animal** requires regular checkups and tests to allow the doctor the opportunity to gauge whether or not the donor animal remains a suitable candidate. These checkups should be scheduled at 6-month intervals. The checkups should be used to detect parasites in the animal, among other health conditions. Of particular importance is an evaluation regarding the presence of heartworms or intestinal parasites. The presence of any infectious diseases will rule out the donor's suitability for giving blood. Infectious diseases include the blood parasites, and other parasites responsible for rickettsial diseases. The primary blood parasites are Babesia canis and Hemobartonella canis. The parasites responsible for rickettsial diseases include Ehrlichia canis, Ehrlichia platus, Borrelia burgdorferi and Rickettsia rickettsii. The rickettsial parasites are primarily transmitted through ticks. Ticks are defined as blood-sucking insects that burrow into the skin. These insects have the ability to attach themselves to humans and animals. Therefore, it is important to check the animal's skin thoroughly for any signs of ticks after being outdoors. The canine blood donor should fast before giving blood to reduce the likelihood of producing a lipemic (fat or lipid laden) blood specimen.

Feline Blood Donor Requirements

There are 3 kinds of **feline blood types**. The 3 types are known as Type A, Type B, and Type AB. Type A is the most common type found in domesticated cats. This is true of both longhair and shorthair species. However, purebreds most often have the blood type known as Type B. It is not necessary to determine the type of blood in the feline before the blood withdrawal procedure. The ideal feline blood donor will be under 8 years of age. The cat will be neutered or spayed. The cat will have received all of its vaccinations. In addition, the cat will not be overweight or underweight. The ideal weight for the cat is a lean body mass of not lower than 4.5 kg or 10 lb. The cat with a good disposition and that has been accustomed to living indoors will usually find the procedure to be less traumatic.

Fresh Whole Blood, Packed Red Blood Cells, and Plasma

Fresh whole blood is given when an animal exhibits one or more of the following: hemorrhagic shock, anemia, excessive surgical hemorrhage, clotting disorders, non-immune-mediated hemolytic anemia, and sometimes immune-mediated hemolytic anemia.

Crystalloid (an isotonic or hypertonic fluid, such as Lactated Ringer's solution, used as a blood volume expander) is given in combination with packed red blood cells (RBCs) when it becomes necessary to maintain the animal's fluid balance and osmotic pressure. Packed RBCs can be given to the animal that has suffered from hemolytic and nonregenerative anemias. RBCs may be maintained in an "extender" solution such as ADSOL (adenine, glucose, mannitol, and sodium chloride). Packed RBCs stored in ADSOL will naturally have a greater total volume than packed RBCs stored alone. Further, the unit volume of RBCs packed in other preservatives (i.e., Optisol or Nutricel, etc.) may vary from that of ADSOL. However, the cell count per unit should be the same regardless of the solution used. When mixing packed RBCs with ADSOL, add the solution to the cells rather than the cells to the solution. This reduces the degree of hemolysis during and after mixing. The shock and burn patient can benefit from a plasma transfusion. This type of transfusion will supply volume replacement when tissue-based fluids are lost in the absence of skin. In addition, other medical conditions such as hypoproteinemia, pancreatitis, and sepsis can benefit from this type of transfusion.

Orogastric Intubation

Orogastric intubation is described as a method employed to purge the stomach of its contents. This method can also be employed to dispense food or nutrients to animals that have been orphaned at a young age. In particular this may include neonate animals, usually less than one month of age. In addition, orogastric intubation can be employed to flush out stomach contents with a flow of water in a gastric lavage. Finally, it can also be used to distribute medications or radiographic contrast agents, such as barium, into the abdominal and gastrointestinal regions.

The veterinarian will need to use a variety of supplies when performing an orogastric intubation. The supplies include a stomach tube, speculum, adhesive tape, and a lubricant. Smaller animals such as puppies and kittens will require a 12 F to 18 F infant feeding tube. Larger dogs, ranging over 10 kg or 22.2 lb, will require an 18 F foal stomach tube.

Equipment Needed for an Orogastric Intubation

The animal's jaws should be held tightly shut against the speculum by the staff member assigned to the job of restraining the animal. The lubricated tube should be inserted into the mouth opening through the speculum and down to the pre-marked location on the tube. Proper placement should be verified before any fluids or other materials are inserted (typically by withdrawing stomach contents using gentle suction, or by putting 1 mL of sterile water into the tube to cause coughing if pulmonary intubation has occurred). If the tube is found to be located in the trachea, then the tube must be promptly taken out to avoid respiratory compromise and introducing fluids into the lungs. The procedure will have to be repeated until the location is verified as accurate. Once an accurate location has been reached, then necessary fluids and substances can be inserted into the tube. This is followed by a flushing with water, using approximately 6 mL. The tube should not produce any seepage. If this occurs, the seepage can be stopped by placing a thumb over the tube. If this still does not work, then it should be kinked or bent over to stop the flow.

Additional Equipment Needed

When performing an **orogastric intubation**, larger dogs will require a foal stomach tube. To facilitate the intubation process, the medical instrument known as a speculum can be employed. The veterinarian can use a canine speculum to hold the mouth open, or a roll of adhesive tape measuring 1-2 inches wide can be placed crosswise in the mouth to serve as an open speculum when the tube is inserted. The following is also required: an appropriately sized orogastric tube, sterile saline solution in a syringe, tape or a permanent marker for depth marking on the tube, and an appropriate sedative (if needed). If the animal requires any other drugs or substances, these are given via a syringe or a funnel.

Usually, an orogastric intubation does not require sedation. However, in some cases a light tranquilizer can be employed. The animal can remain standing or be positioned in a sternal recumbent position. The tube should be measured against the length of the animal (typically from the mouth to the ninth intercostal space). This will give an approximate length needed to gain access into the stomach of the animal. The oral tip of the tube (i.e., that which will remain immediately outside the mouth) should be designated with tape. Then, the speculum should be introduced into the animal's mouth.

Nasogastric Intubation

A **nasogastric intubation** is described as procedure in which a tube is inserted through the external nares, the nasal cavity, pharynx, and the esophagus, into the stomach region. The veterinarian will typically employ this particular procedure in an effort to supply nutrition in a liquid form to the animal. In addition, this method is suitable for supplying water and other liquids to the animal. A nasogastric tube can be left in place over a long period of time, whereas an orogastric tube cannot. Animals that are anorexic may require lengthy nasogastric feedings if they are extremely thin or unhealthy. Thus, placement of a nasogastric tube can be used to provide the animal with proper nutrition. This may be particularly effective for an anxious animal that is a poor candidate for forced feedings. This procedure also allows the veterinarian a method to introduce medication or a contrast medium into the animal's stomach. One contrast medium that may be used is barium, which is applied in radiology in evaluating the gastrointestinal tract for certain lesions, obstructions, and other problems.

Procedure for a Nasogastric Intubation

Nasogastric intubation should only be administered to alert patients. Sedation is usually not necessary. The tube is measured first. The tube's measurement consists of the length estimated by assessing the distance between the ninth to thirteenth rib and the nares or nostrils. A topical anesthesia is given at 4 to 5 drops in one nostril. This is followed by the addition of more drops in the same nostril once a period of 2-3 minutes has elapsed. The lubrication of the nasogastric tube is completed at this juncture. The animal's head is then held in one hand. The other hand should be applied to introduce the tube into the anesthetized nostril. The animal must be checked to find out if the tube is properly positioned (stomach versus lungs). This is accomplished by inserting 1 mL of sterile saline into the tube. The animal will cough if the insertion is incorrect. Optionally, gentle suction may be applied until frank stomach contents are aspirated and visualized. Prompt extubation and reinsertion of the tube is necessary if pulmonary intubation has occurred.

Equipment Needed

The **equipment needed for nasogastric intubation** includes a nasogastric feeding tube, a topical ophthalmic anesthetic, lubricating jelly, a syringe, sterile saline solution, injection cap, and any medications or substances needing to be introduced into the patient's stomach. The tube that is employed in the procedure can be of various sizes and materials. For instance, an infant feeding tube can be made from either red rubber or polyurethane. However, the critical elements of this tube are its small diameter and its composition from a flexible material that is soft. Animals that are under 5 kg or 12 pounds require a size 5 F feeding tube. Animals that range in size from 5 to 12 kg or 12-33 pounds require a size 8 F feeding tube. The insertion of the nasogastric intubation also requires a topical ophthalmic anesthetic (to reduce nasal insertion discomfort), lubricating jelly, a syringe containing sterile saline (1 mL), an injection cap, and any medication or liquid to be introduced into the animal's stomach. In some cases, the need for the tube to remain in place for an extended time necessitates that securing dressings be used.

Insertion of the Nasogastric Tube

The onset of coughing in the animal will be a decisive factor in determining that the tube has been placed in the wrong location. The location is tested by inserting 1mL of sterile saline into the tube. The animal will cough if the tube is in the trachea. This requires that the tube be removed and reinserted. For long-standing tube utilization, the tube should be fastened along the side of the patient's neck with a binding. The tube requires a cap. The cap is essential in keeping the animal from aspirating air into the stomach. Each feeding necessitates that the location of the tube be rechecked. In addition, the tube should be aspirated or suctioned at that time. A finger can be placed over the top of the tube when the tube must be extracted. This keeps any seepage from occurring in the pharynx or throat while the tube is being withdrawn.

Canine Male and Female Urinary Catheterization

A urine sample that is free from infective organisms and other contaminants can be used for analysis and cultures. The urine discharge collected in a catheterization tube from the patient should be measured. The urine is most sterile when it is extracted directly from the urinary bladder. A **catheterization tube** can be used to bring relief to the patient experiencing a ur**ethral obstruction.** The catheterization tube can also be used for dispensing medication or contrast media. Contrast media are used in radiology examinations.

A pneumocystography is an example of a test that necessitates a urinary catheterization. The veterinarian should carry out a urinary catheterization on the patient personally. The supplies needed for this procedure include a gentle soap, a sterile urethral catheter, sterile lubricant, and sterile syringes or other sterile collection containers. In addition, female patients require the following: a vaginal speculum, sterile gloves, viscous Xylocaine or 0.5% lidocaine jelly, and possibly a steel catheter. Normally, the catheter is made from polyethylene, vinyl, or rubber. Less flexible and larger catheters can result in a traumatic experience for the patient. Catheters are available in sizes 3.5 F, 5 F, 8 F, and 10 F.

Manual Compression of the Urinary Bladder

Manual compression of the urinary bladder can also be used to expel the contents for collection purposes. However, this procedure must not be used if a urinary obstruction is suspected. The urine is collected for inspection of solute concentration, physical properties, and chemical constituents. This unsterile urine sample should not be used for urine cultures. The bladder on the animal can be found by palpating or applying a gentle pressure along the abdomen. This pressure should begin at the site where the very last rib is located. The examination should be carried out by moving from the front to the rear portion of the body in a caudal direction. Another technique used in locating the bladder consists of palpating along the upper portion of the rear legs. The movement starts at the back of the body and continues along towards the front lower portion of the body. Once located, pressure should be applied lightly over the bladder in a sustained or continuous manner to allow the urine to be expelled from the bladder. The expelled urine is then promptly transferred into a sterile container. Following this the urine sample can be analyzed.

Cystocentesis

Cystocentesis is a **needle aspiration technique** used to collect a urine sample from a patient. This technique can be applied to cats or dogs. The animal may be in a state of sleepiness or under sedation. The animal should be placed in a dorsal or lateral recumbent position. The bladder should be examined medically and palpated using gentle pressure to detect the fullness of the bladder. Alcohol is wiped over the site where the needle is to be inserted. The veterinarian should prevent any shifting of the bladder with one hand. The other hand is needed to insert the sterile needle and syringe in a caudodorsal direction into the bladder site. It is important to prevent any squeezing pressure from being applied to the bladder during this procedure so as to prevent urine leakage into the peritoneal cavity. The urine is extracted through the syringe with a negative pressure applied on the plunger device. The needle and syringe should then be pulled out of the body as soon as the plunger is released. It is recommended that the sample be immediately transferred to a sanitized, marked container.

Injections in Horses

Intravenous Injections

The animal receiving an **intravenous injection** should have the injection site cleansed to prevent infection and to destroy disease-carrying microorganisms. This can be accomplished by using a cotton ball doused in alcohol and firmly swabbing the injection site.

The horse's jugular vein is a prominent vessel that meets the criteria for an injection site. However, there are times when other sites may be more appropriate. Alternate sites include the thoracic, cephalic, and saphenous veins.

An IV injection is an effective way to administer a **fast-acting drug**. An IV route can also be used to introduce sizeable quantities of fluid into the animal's body. In addition, an IV site can be used when blood is collected from the animal. The veterinarian can be assured that an injection has been correctly administered into the vein when blood can be drawn back through the needle or catheter.

The aspiration or suction of fluids or gases from the body can be accomplished with a syringe. An indwelling catheter used for these purposes can be fastened into place with a sewing technique or glue. The site should be further protected with an overlay of tape and Elastoplast for added hygienic protection and security.

Intramuscular Injection

The animal receiving an **intramuscular (IM) injection** should have the injection site cleansed to prevent infection from occurring. This is accomplished by using a cotton ball doused in alcohol and firmly swabbing the injection site. Some likely places for an intramuscular injection are in the muscles of the neck, the semitendinosus muscle (in the thigh), the gluteus muscle (in the flank), and the pectoralis descendens (a chest muscle). The medical staff should be careful to avoid injections near joints, blood vessels, or large fat deposits. The effectiveness (in duration) of some drugs can be extended with the application of an IM injection.

It is also important to note that some drugs require administration into the body through intramuscular injections alone. For instance, an injection of procaine penicillin directly into the bloodstream will result in a harmful reaction in the patient. The severity of the reaction is usually directly related to the time that it takes for the reaction to take place. Acute reactions can be produced instantaneously. However, a longer period of time may elapse before evidence of a milder reaction appears. The medical staff should be on the alert for the following reactions: restlessness, agitation, head tossing, snorting, eye rolling, violent thrashing, or a state of collapse.

Administering Drugs and Taking Samples in Cattle

The **jugular vein** is the ideal spot to **administer large amounts of fluids and/or medications** to an animal. This spot can also be utilized to take venous blood samples from the animal. The animal's head is held immobile through the use of a head catch device. The device should be pulled in an upward direction towards the opposite side of the animal. The syringe must be of adequate size (measured in mL or cc) for the liquid being injected. The needle used usually ranges from 16 to 18 gauge (the smaller the number the larger the bore) and 1 to 3 inches in length.

The **vein in the tail** is ideal for **smaller quantities of fluid**. Smaller animals should be held securely in place by bending the tail straight forward from its base. The animal will not be able to make a movement to the left or to the right when this hold is firmly applied. The syringe must be of adequate size for the liquid being injected, with a needle that ranges in bore diameter from 18 to 20 gauge and about 1 to 1.5 inches in length. A smaller size syringe is applicable for the administration of more modest amounts of fluid.

Another spot that can be employed for injections is the milk vein. However, this vein does have a tendency to form hematomas when stress is applied. The needle used with this vein is frequently 14 gauge and 2 to 3 inches in length.

Intramuscular Injections in Cattle

Cattle can receive intramuscular injections through the lateral cervical muscles of the body. Mature cattle will receive injections with a 16, 18, or 20 gauge needle that is 1.5 to 2 inches in length. It is comparable to a 3.75 to 5 cm needle. Only 15 to 20 mL of medication can be administered at each specific intramuscular (IM) injection site. Smaller-sized calves may require smaller-sized needles. The smaller-sized needles can be used to administer 10 to 15 mL of medication into an animal.

The area should be desensitized with a couple of modest taps from the flat side of the hand in a balled up position with fingers closed (i.e., a half-fist). This will also give the animal an opportunity to steady itself before the needle is inserted. The best way to apply the intramuscular injection is to align the needle in the proper position before attaching the syringe. The medication can then be introduced into the patient with this intramuscular injection.

Administering Drugs and Taking Samples in Pigs

Swine should be given large quantities of intravenous liquid through the cranial vena cava. The mature swine requires use of an 18 to 20 gauge needle, 3 to 4 inches in length. This is comparable in length to a 7.5 to 10 cm needle. The jugular fossa closest to the manubrium sterni of the pig can be employed as a guide to ensure proper placement or alignment into the cranial vena cava. The needle must be inserted in a perpendicular direction towards the neck facing the left shoulder.

The ear artery is known as the caudal auricular artery. This artery is ideal for giving the pig smaller quantities of liquid. The syringe should be inserted with gentle pressure. The syringe must be of adequate size for the liquid being injected. The needle used usually ranges from 18 to 22 gauge and 1 to 1.5 inches in length. This needle is comparable to a 2.5 to 3.75 cm needle length. Intravenous administrations within the vein typically require the use of a 19 to 21 gauge butterfly needle.

Subcutaneous Injections in Cattle, Small Ruminants, and Pigs

Subcutaneous injections for cattle are administered in site regions from the cranial area to the shoulder and lateral to the animal's neckline. The ideal needle bore will range from 16 to 18 gauges, with a 1.5 inch or 3.75 cm needle length. The veterinarian can use his or her discretion to establish the volume of the injection. However, it is best that adult cattle only receive about 250 mL/site, at most. Younger cattle should receive a maximum of about 50 mL/site.

Smaller ruminants will be given an injection along the cranial to the shoulder region. This injection is given in a lateral direction from the neck. The animal should only receive about 5 mL of fluid per site. The recommended needle bore ranges from 18 to 20 gauge, with a 1 inch or 2.5 cm needle length.

The injection is given at the lateral side of the neck near the base of the pig's ear, with 1 to 3 mL injected per site. The maximum amount is dependent upon the size of the pig. The recommended needle bore ranges from 16 to 18 gauge with a 1 to 1.5 inch needle. This is comparable to a 2.5 to 3.75 cm needle.

Intramuscular Injections in Sheep, Goats, and Pigs

Sheep and goats can receive an intramuscular injection through the lateral cervical muscles. Mature sheep and goats will receive injections with a needle ranging from 18 to 20 gauge and 1.5 inches in length (comparable to a 3.75 cm needle). Smaller sized animals will need a 20 to 22 gauge needle. The maximum capacity of medication intramuscularly given to an adult-sized animal is 15 mL. The normal quantity typically measures about 5 to 10 mL.

Swine are given the injection through the dorsolateral neck muscles. This site is deemed to be the most appropriate for pigs. The pig will require an 18 to 20 gauge needle that is about 1.5 inches in length (comparable to a 3.75 cm needle). This is an appropriate size for a mature pig. The maximum amount of fluids appropriately given intramuscularly is 1 to 15 mL, depending upon the size of the animal and the area injected.

Administering an SQ Injection

Certain medications such as antibiotic or pain control injections and even vaccines will need to be administered **subcutaneously** (SQ, or under the skin). To administer an injection SQ, first find an area of loose skin — between the shoulder blades generally works well — and gently pinch the loose skin between your thumb and forefinger. Pull the skin up to create a tent, and the area pinched between your fingers creates a small indentation. Take the cap off of the needle, and insert the sterile needle into the skin tent indentation parallel to the skin's surface. Once inserted, pull back on the syringe plunger to be sure no blood is drawn back, and you are in the SQ layer. If no blood is seen, push the plunger and medication forward into the skin. Remove the needle once the syringe is empty.

Administering Oral Medications to Cats and Dogs

To properly **administer oral** tablets or capsules to a dog, have a restrainer hold the dog in a standing restraint and quickly yet gently lift the top jaw with one hand and place the pill at the back of the dog's throat with the other hand. Quickly close the dog's mouth, and hold its head upward. Wait for the dog to swallow before letting go; sometimes, gently rubbing the dog's neck will initiate swallowing. A pill popper device may also be used. A pill popper is a long plastic handle with a rubber end with a slit to hold the pill, and once the popper is placed in the dog's mouth, the plunger is pushed from the opposite end forcing the pill out and into the dog's throat. Tablets and capsules can also be hidden inside of soft treats or canned food and be fed to the dog. In order to administer a tablet or capsule to a cat orally, there should be somebody holding the cat while the other person quickly lifts up the top jaw and places the pill at the back of the cat's tongue so that it is swallowed.

Routes of Administration of Medications

The **oral route of administration** is used for tablets, capsules, solutions, and suspensions. Oral dosing is generally used for systemic effects after drug absorption from the GI tract; however, the disadvantage of the oral administration route is the slow onset of action for the drug as well as irregular absorption. Parenteral routes of administration include intravenous (IV), intramuscular (IM), and subcutaneous (SQ). Injectable medications or fluid therapy via a needle are used for these administration routes. IV administration has a quick onset of action, usually within seconds, and the onset of action for the IM and SQ routes is within minutes. The topical route of administration is used for parasitic control, local skin treatments, and therapeutic agents. Drugs applied to the skin (topical) for a local effect include antifungals, anti-inflammatory agents, and antiseptics. Topical drugs come in different forms including powders, creams, liquids, and sprays.

Importance of Understanding If Other Medications Have Been Taken

It is important to ask owners if their pet is taking any **medications** or supplements, or if they have treated the illness or injury the pet is presenting for. Certain medications should not be administered to dogs. Aspirin and ibuprofen, for example, are human NSAIDs, but they can be dangerous if given to dogs even if it is the correct dose due to sensitivity. They can also cause stomach ulcers and kidney failure. If an owner gives their dog Tylenol (acetaminophen) at the incorrect dose, this can cause liver and kidney damage, and it converts hemoglobin to methemoglobin, which results in decreased oxygen delivery to the tissues. If the owner has been giving their pet NSAIDs, then the veterinarian cannot prescribe an NSAID designed for dogs because they cannot be taken together. Any of these medications should be avoided at all costs in cats because even one dose of Tylenol given to a cat could cause death.

Monitoring Giving Lifelong Medications

If a patient is on a **lifelong medication** such as a **thyroid medication**, it is necessary to **recheck the pet's thyroid level regularly** to ensure that they are on the right dosage and determine that the patient's health status is normal while on the medication. If an animal is **diabetic**, then you will want to be sure that the client is administering the correct dose of insulin to the patient, because there can be serious complications if the pet is given an incorrect dosage, such as hypoglycemia if the pet is given too much insulin. If the patient is taking **phenobarbital** to help control seizure activity, it is crucial to ask the owners if the pet has had any seizures while on the medication and how they are doing in case the dosage needs to be adjusted. Also, if the patient is taking phenobarbital regularly, a phenobarbital level blood test will need to be run once a year to make sure that the dosage is accurate.

Collecting Specimens

Collecting Blood from a Donor

The procedure for **preparing a blood donor** begins with a sedative. The animal is given a sedative suitable for the canine species. The animal is then placed in a lateral recumbent position with its neck stretched out for the procedure. This position allows easy access to the jugular vein. The jugular vein is ideal for withdrawing the blood from the patient. The cephalic vein is also concurrently used to give the animal needed replacement fluids. Both the cephalic vein and the jugular vein are in need of preparation before commencing the blood withdrawal. The preparation includes clipping the hair in the area of venipuncture. A catheter is a thin tube that is used to inject fluid into the cephalic vein. The blood is drawn out of the jugular vein by means of a 16 gauge needle. The blood is collected in a bag that holds an anticoagulant. A full collection of blood is measured at 450 mL.

Additional Procedures Used in Collecting Blood from a Donor

A **scale** is applied to gain an exact measurement of the blood collected. This exact measurement is used to ensure that the collection bag is not filled too much or too little. A full collection of blood is measured at 450 mL. There is a risk to the animal of developing a **hematoma** (a clotted mass of blood) at the jugular venipuncture site. This risk can be diminished by placing a firm, but gentle force directly on the jugular vein for 2 minutes following the closing stages of blood withdrawal. In addition, it is advisable to only take a maximum of 10 to 20 mL/kg at an interval of at least 3 weeks. The veterinarian should make every effort to replace the blood extracted with fluids given at rates measuring 3x the volume of blood lost. The replacement fluids should be administered to the patient via a catheter through the cephalic vein in the region of the patient's head.

Vaccinations Given to Horses in the United States and Canada

There are routine **sets of vaccinations** that should be administered to horse based upon **geographical location**. The prevalence of a particular disease can relate directly to the region in which the animal resides. Animals in the United States should be given the following vaccinations: Eastern and Western encephalomyelitis, tetanus, and influenza. Young horses should also receive the vaccination known as rhinopneumonitis. Some locations also recommend the administration of the vaccination known as the Strangles vaccine. Use of this vaccination is becoming more widespread. In addition, the intranasal administration of many vaccines is also increasing. It is a common occurrence to vaccinate an animal for rabies regardless of the geographic location.

Revised vaccination protocols have increased the prevalence of the West Nile virus and Potomac horse fever vaccines. These vaccinations should now be given to horses in areas that are both high and low risk.

Horses located in the Ontario, Canada region should be given the following vaccinations: rabies, tetanus, Rhinopneumonitis or EHV-4/1, and West Nile virus. Horses that travel outside of the region will be given the following vaccinations: Eastern and Western encephalomyelitis, Strangles, and Potomac horse fever or equine monocytic ehrlichiosis.

Feline Blood Collection

The first step in preparing the cat is to clip the hair away from the jugular and the cephalic vein regions. The next step involves providing an aseptic cleansing to the regions involved. The animal should next be given a sedative. The cat is then placed in a lateral recumbent or sternal recumbent position. A 19 gauge butterfly needle is inserted into the jugular vein. To diminish the movement associated with the needle in the jugular vein, the staff should utilize a 60 mL syringe with 8.5 mL of anticoagulant joined with a flexible phlebotomy tube to the butterfly needle. In addition, the staff should maintain a focus on the animal's vital signs, including its pulse, respiration, and blood pressure throughout the procedure. Partway through, the cat should be given replacement fluids. The blood and anticoagulant should be mixed often. The withdrawal should be finalized at the time that the 60 mL syringe is measured in its fullness. This is followed by the removal of the butterfly needle. Then, the staff places pressure on the jugular vein to prevent a hematoma or blood clot from developing. The replacement fluid is completed at 180 mL, or 3 times the amount of blood extracted.

Collecting a Milk Sample for Bacterial Culture

The identification and treatment of mastitis is critical to an animal's good physical condition. **Mastitis** is inflammation of the animal's udder. This condition can have particularly detrimental effects upon a dairy herd. The dairy herd will have a sample of its milk taken for a culture. The samples are first tested for a simple positive or negative result, as this screening reduces the costs associated with more detailed laboratory testing. Any positive test result will indicate the need for further, more definitive testing. The samples should be collected from the animals before the milking process begins. However, samples may also be collected from an animal after milking has been completed, during the 6 or more hours that follow the prior milking episode.

In taking a sample, the udder should be thoroughly cleansed. Each teat should be wiped with alcohol beginning from the farthest point to the nearest in proximity. Then the teat should air dry. The initial milk stream must be thrown out. The midstream milk is collected and saved for the sample. The milk stream is aimed in a straight line towards the sample vial.

Collecting Urine Samples to Be Used for a Urine Culture and Sensitivity Test

The ideal urine **sample for a culture and sensitivity** test would be obtained via cystocentesis. To obtain a urine sample via cystocentesis from a dog, the dog will be placed on its back with a restrainer holding the front half and a restrainer holding the back half. The person collecting the sample will use an ultrasound probe to probe over the area of the bladder until it is seen on the ultrasound to guide it in the right direction. Depending on how large the dog is, a 3 ml syringe with either a 22-gauge ¾-inch needle or a 22-gauge 1 ½-inch needle will be used to insert perpendicular to the skin above the bladder and down into the abdominal cavity. Once inserted, pull the plunger back slightly to see if urine is drawn into the syringe, and if not then let go of the plunger and redirect the needle to try again using the ultrasound as a guide. It is easier to hold cats in a lateral restraint and palpate and isolate the bladder, then insert the needle once the bladder is isolated.

DIFFERENT WAYS TO COLLECT A URINE SAMPLE

One option for **obtaining a urine sample** is to get a voided sample. A **voided sample** can be obtained by simply following the dog outside while the dog is on a leash and once the dog urinates, place a small tray or container underneath it so the urine flows into the tray. Another technique used for male dogs is to **catheterize** them to obtain a urine sample. You will need sterile gloves, sterile lubricant, scrub, a catheter sized for the dog, and a syringe (commonly a 3 ml syringe Luer slip). The dog will be placed in a lateral restraint while the restrainer extrudes the penis. The penis will be scrubbed with a chlorhexidine solution, and then the lubed catheter is placed into the lumen of the penis and advanced until it is inside the bladder. Once the catheter is in the bladder, the syringe is attached to the opposite end of the catheter and urine is drawn into it by pulling back on the plunger. Once the urine is collected, the catheter is pulled directly out of the penis.

Patient Information

GENERAL INFORMATION (SIGNALMENT) NEEDED FOR THE PATIENT

The **patient's signalment** includes their age, breed, and sex. If the patient is geriatric, then a comprehensive blood work panel is recommended and the veterinary technician will want to ask the owners probing questions on how well the patient is getting around to see if there are any signs of osteoarthritis. Age is also an important factor when dealing with puppies or kittens to determine which vaccines they are due for. The breed is an important factor because certain breeds of dogs are predisposed to certain diseases. For example, boxers can be genetically predisposed to cardiomyopathy, so annual ECG monitoring may be necessary. The sex of the patient is important, as well as if the patient is neutered or spayed. If a female is not spayed, then watching for signs of pyometra and mammary cancer is crucial.

Managing Hospitalized Patients

MAINTAINING AN IV CATHETER FOR A PATIENT

An **IV catheter** may be in place for up to 72 hours in a hospitalized patient. During hospitalization, the IV catheter must be monitored to make sure that proper placement is maintained and that the catheter is still patent. The patient may move around and twist the IV line or even pull on the IV catheter, which could pull it out of the vein. The patient could also attempt to bite or pull at the catheter with its teeth to try and remove it. To make sure the catheter is patent, a syringe of flush (lactated Ringer's or sodium chloride) can be administered through the catheter to feel if it is moving through the vein or pull back on the plunger to see if blood pulls into the syringe from the vein. The patient must be monitored to ensure that the foot doesn't get swollen if the tape for the catheter becomes too tight.

OBTAINING A TPR ON A PATIENT

TPR stands for temperature, pulse, and respirations. A normal rectal temperature in a dog is 99-102.5 °F. A cat's normal body temperature can be 100.5-102.5 °F. A temperature greater than 103.5 °F in a cat or dog is considered to be pyrexia (fever). A normal heart rate for a dog is 90-120 beats per minute (bpm) for small breeds, 70-110 bpm for medium breeds, and 60-90 bpm for large breeds such as Great Danes or mastiffs. In cats, a normal heart rate is between 150-200 bpm. To get an accurate heart rate on the patient, place the stethoscope over the animal's chest and find the heartbeat. Count the beats for 6 seconds, and then multiply that by 10 to get the beats per minute. A normal respiration rate for a dog is 18-24 respirations per minute (rpm) and 20-30 rpm for cats. To obtain a respiration rate, palpate or watch the patient's inspiration/expiration and count for 15 seconds, and then multiply by 4 to get the rpm.

Getting a Hospitalized Patient to Eat

If the patient has **not been eating enough** food to meet its **resting energy requirement** (RER), then a feeding plan must be in place to provide nutrients. In order to create a feeding plan, the patient's ability to eat should to be evaluated. **Enticing** the patient to eat by placing a small amount of canned food in the mouth may be just enough to get the patient to eat. **Syringe feeding** is another method that is done with a liquid mixture of canned food and water in a feeding syringe. To syringe feed a dog, the tip of the syringe is placed inside of the cheek, emptying small amounts at a time while waiting for the dog to swallow. Another method is to place a **feeding tube** and administering either a liquid or blended food product through the tube. While in the hospital, the patient should be fed on a schedule according to their caloric requirements. To calculate the patient's RER, use the formula of 15 kcal/lb for the dog and 20 kcal/lb for the cat. The feeding schedule will be decided by how well the patient tolerates being fed, and feeding the amount close to the patient's RER is recommended.

Wound Care and Physical Rehabilitation

Wounds

Basic Steps of Wound Treatment

Appropriate wound treatment involves protective measures, evaluation, and treatment. The initial protective measure requires that the wound be covered with a dressing and/or a splint of some sort. The second step involves an evaluation of the wound's degree of severity. The most severe cases are those that require control of hemorrhaging. Once any hemorrhaging is under control, the wound should be checked to lessen further contamination and infection risks. Hair or other debris should be cleaned and clipped away from the area. The border surrounding the wound should be thoroughly cleansed with an antimicrobial/detergent scrub. This step also involves washing out any hollow body parts or organs. Getting rid of necrotic tissue is the step known as débridement. This is necessary so that new tissue can grow over the wound. Necrotic tissue would hinder this process. In addition, it may be necessary to place a drainage tube to allow excess air and fluid to exit the wound site.

Types of Open and Closed Wounds

Open wound refers to an injury that has an external break in the tissue. An abrasion is an open wound that involves a loss of the epidermis plus some of the dermis layer. An avulsion is an open wound that is a result of the tissues being torn from their attachments. An incision is an open wound caused by a sharp tool (surgery). A laceration is an open wound caused by tearing, which creates superficial and deeper tissue damage. A puncture is an open wound created by a sharp object (e.g., tooth) that could cause severe tissue damage and are at a high risk for infection. **Closed wounds** are the result of damage beneath the skin's surface. Closed wounds consist of contusions defined as blunt force trauma that does not break the skin but does damage to it and the tissues underneath. Crushing injuries are closed wounds caused by force placed upon an area of the body over any length of time.

4 Phases of Wound Healing

There are 4 phases associated with **wound healing**: inflammatory, débridement, repair, and maturation. The **inflammatory phase** is the initial phase that follows an injury. This phase is associated with the appearance of scabs. Scabs are a crust over the injured area. This dried substance can be formed from blood, serum, and pus. This crust protects the wound so that healing can begin. The **débridement phase** commences about 6 hours after the injury takes place. Neutrophils and monocytes work to remove foreign material, bacteria, and necrotic tissue from the wound. Both neutrophils and monocytes can be described as white blood cells. In most cases, the **repair phase** starts within approximately 3 to 5 days after the initial wound. However, the time associated with this phase is contingent upon foreign substances being adequately extracted from the infected area. The final phase is known as maturation. **Maturation** can extend for a number of years (i.e., to include scar lightening, etc.). Refashioning the collagen fibers and other fibrous tissue promotes complete wound recovery. Multiple phases may sometimes operate simultaneously, accomplished by a series of overlapping actions.

Bandages

3 Major Layers of a Bandage

The 3 principal layers of bandages are the non-adhesive primary layer, the secondary layer, and the tertiary layer. The **non-adhesive primary layer** is used without anything in between it and the wound. The type of tissue that forms over a wound, known as granulated tissue, should be treated with a non-adhesive primary layer. This bandage layer prevents further trauma to the injury site.

Exuded substances are soaked up by the cushioned, secondary layer. Common name brands include Kling or Sof-Kling.

Finally, the exterior layer is known as the **tertiary layer.** This layer gives the 2 bottom layers more reinforcement. This reinforcement is due to the type of bandage used, including adhesive tapes, elastic bandages, Vet Wrap (3M), and conforming stretch gauze. The adhesive tape gives the bandage the ability to bond to the other layers. The elastic bandage and stretch gauze is expandable and flexible over the layers covering the wound.

Types of Absorptions Used in a Bandage Application

There are 3 types of bandages used on a wound. These include: dry-to-dry bandages, wet-to-dry bandages, and wet-to-wet bandages.

Loose necrotic tissue should be addressed with a **dry-to-dry bandage**. The dry gauze stays in place with the follow-up application of a dry, absorbent wrap. The patient will experience pain whenever the bandage is removed, but dead and dying tissue is naturally débrided and removed with it.

It is best to use a **wet-to-dry bandage** on any infected or open wounds. If an exuded substance is present then the wound may require a wet, saline-moistened or medicated bandage placed inside and dry bandage coverings outside. This type of bandage is advantageous as it is able to treat infection and still absorb exudates that emanate from the wound. This type of bandage can also reduce pain associated with the removal of exuded substances attached to the binding. The bandages soak up excess fluid from the wound. The bindings are not taken off of the patient when wet. **Wet-to-wet dressings** can sometimes be useful for chronic wounds or for larger, ulcerated wounds that require internal tissue regrowth before epidermal tissue can grow and provide protective coverage. Deep pressure sores are one possible example. This form of bandage is removed while still wet.

Reasons and Precautions for Bandaging the Limbs

A patient's limbs may require bandaging for a variety of reasons. These reasons include: to **reduce or stop movement** (i.e., in bone fractures), to keep a wound **safe from infection** or further contaminants, and to maintain the **positioning and stability of a limb** for purposes of **fluid therapy** (i.e., a subcutaneous infusion or IV line, etc.).

The best bandage application provides an **even distribution of pressure** throughout the bandaged area of the limb. Equally distributed pressure ensures reasonably unimpeded circulation in the limb. In addition, the entire limb requires a bandage whenever the upper sector of the appendage has been injured. Otherwise, continued movement in the lower area of the appendage may impair healing in the upper area. Whenever an extremity bandage has been placed, it is necessary to carefully ensure adequate circulation. Symptoms of impaired circulation include: swelling around the toes, coldness to touch, and paleness around the nail beds. This requires prompt readjustment and loosening of the bandage. Ideally, when sufficiently loose, 2 fingers can be inserted beneath the binding.

The animal's bandage should be covered with a protective bag such as an ordinary plastic bag, a rubber glove, or unfilled fluid bag whenever the animal is up and about. This covering should help keep the binding unsoiled and dry. This covering can be secured for a short time by affixing one end of the protective bag to the proximal end of the appendage.

Reasons and Precautions for Bandaging the Head and Neck

The patient's head and neck may require a protective bandage after certain surgeries. The following surgeries are associated with this need: postocular surgery, aural hematoma repair, and ear surgery. In addition, a bandage of this type may be needed to firmly secure a jugular catheter or a nasogastric or pharyngostomy tube into place.

Wound edema is a condition in which serous fluid builds up in excessive amounts in the patient. In the head and neck area, this condition can endanger the patient's life. Therefore, the condition of the wound and surrounding swelling should be checked often. This may require removal of the bandage to allow an inspection of the site. The patient's respiration, skin color, and involved mucous membranes should be carefully checked. The bandage should be slack enough to allow the insertion of 2 fingers underneath the bindings. Patients with respiratory concerns should have their bindings loosened. It may be necessary to reapply a different bandage. Animals that are opposed to wearing a head or neck bandage may need to be given an Elizabethan collar. The Elizabethan collar is used to prevent the animal's access to the bandaging material.

Reasons and Precautions for Bandaging a Tail

There may be occasions when an animal's tail may also require a bandage. This bandage should incorporate and be able to cover the animal's wound. An animal that has had a tumor removed or a partial tail amputation will also benefit from the application of a bandage.

An animal experiencing a period of **persistent diarrhea** may also benefit from the application of a **tail bandage**. This bandage can bundle up both the appendage and any associated hair, and thereby better help in securing and maintaining the cleanliness of the animal at this difficult time.

An **amputation** can involve **persistent bleeding**. This bleeding can be induced, exacerbated, and/or perpetuated by excessive tail wagging or by bringing the intact portion of the tail in contact with a hard object. Tail wagging movements can be reduced by sedating the animal. However, this is only a temporizing intervention and one of last resort, due to the negative effects of such medication. An optional way to lessen tail movement is to slide a tube-shaped item over the bottom of the remaining portion of the tail. This should reduce the momentum of the tail wagging, and provide some additional protection to the animal's tail. Analgesics or painkillers can also be given to the patient to reduce the animal's distress and painful symptoms.

Layers of the Skin

Skin is composed of three layers: the epidermis, dermis, and hypodermis. The epidermis is the outer layer, which provides protection from sources of infection. The epidermis is made up of cells that have certain responsibilities such as keratinization, producing the skin's color, producing an immune response to foreign substances, and to provide sensory signals to the animal. The basement membrane zone is the protective layer connecting the epidermis to the dermis. The dermis contains protein collagen, elastic tissue, and fibers that gives skin its strength and support. The dermis contains sensory nerves that respond to painful stimuli, touch, and hot or cold temperatures. Finally, beneath the dermis is the hypodermis, which attaches the skin to the muscle and consists of connective tissue, providing insulation and protection to the body.

Placing an IV Catheter

Depending on the size of the patient, **IV catheters** range in size with a 24 gauge being smaller and used in the critical, smaller patient such as a cat to a 20 gauge being larger and used in large-breed dogs. In surgery or emergency treatment, it is best to use a larger catheter in the patient to allow a larger port of access to the vein. First, shave the area where the catheter will be placed, vacuum excess hair, and scrub the area rotating between chlorhexidine solution and alcohol approximately three times. The person restraining the pet will hold off the vein, and the person placing the catheter will locate the vein. Start low on the vein in case the catheter does not advance and you need to try again; that way, you can try again higher on the same vein. Insert the needle/catheter into the vein, and blood should flash into the hub of the end of the needle you are holding. Once blood is flowing back and the catheter is in the vein, swiftly advance the catheter over the needle into the vein as you are pulling the needle out of the vein. Place an injection plug into the end of the catheter to stop blood from flowing out. Last, tape in the catheter so it is secure to the leg.

Underwater Treadmill

The **underwater treadmill** works to improve the dog's range of motion, increase muscle strength, and increase endurance. The underwater treadmill also helps patients with soft-tissue injuries, weak muscles, and postsurgical care such as an amputation or orthopedic surgery. The temperature of the water is kept at around 95 °F, which helps with flexibility and allows for an improved range of motion for affected joints. Depending on the patient's size and progress, the water is level, and the speed of the treadmill is adjusted accordingly. A water level right above the feet is helpful to patients with reduced flexion in the carpus and hock. A water level at the elbows is great for athletic dogs to improve their endurance because there is a lot of resistance and not a lot of buoyancy. Water levels at the shoulder benefit patients with osteoarthritis or surgical recovery because this provides the most buoyancy with little weight on the joints.

Euthanasia

Euthanasia

Euthanasia is when death is induced without pain or distress put upon the animal. A drug is administered intravenously to cause loss of consciousness immediately followed by cardiac and respiratory arrest resulting in lost brain function and death. The drug used for euthanasia is pentobarbital, which is a barbiturate and has a depressive effect on the CNS. Pentobarbital is actually a seizure medication, but when given in large doses, it leads to complete loss of heart and brain function in less than 2 minutes. When a pet is brought into the hospital for euthanasia, an IV catheter is placed and the animal is sedated first. After the patient is fully sedated, the euthanasia solution is administered via the catheter at the appropriate dose for the patient's weight and the patient is checked for a heartbeat. Once no heartbeat is detected, the animal is pronounced deceased.

Role of the Veterinary Technician

When an owner comes in with their pet to be euthanized, the hospital staff must have a protocol in place to ensure that the process goes smoothly. Once the owner arrives with their pet, it is best to get them into a room quickly so they do not have to sit in the waiting area very long. The **veterinary technician** or receptionist will have the owner sign a euthanasia consent form documenting that they provide consent to put their pet "to sleep." The veterinary technician will explain the process that an IV catheter will be placed and a sedative will be administered first so that their pet is under no stress. The patient is commonly taken into the treatment area for the IV catheter to be placed and the sedative to be given. The veterinary technician will make sure that there is a soft blanket in the room for the patient to lay on and plenty of tissues for the owners. The veterinary technician usually is the shoulder to cry on and can give support to the owner, which may mean giving them a call a few days later to see how they are doing or creating a clay pawprint for them.

Proper Handling of the Deceased Patient Post Euthanasia

Normally, there are two options for pet owners for **cremation services**. They can choose from general cremation or private cremation. **Private cremation** means that their pet is cremated alone and they will receive the ashes back in an urn of their choice. With **general cremation**, the owner does not get the remains back because the pet will be cremated along with other pets that are to be generally cremated. Cremation services are normally done at an outside service. The body of the deceased pet is kept in a freezer in the hospital until the cremation servicer picks up the body. The body is placed into a bag, and the bag is labeled with the patient's name, client's name, and the hospital name. The proper form filled out with the patient name, breed, weight, and color will be needed for identification purposes as well.

Restraining Animals

Restraint Techniques for Dogs

One commonly used **restraint technique** for dogs is to have the dog stand and the holder faces the dog's side placing one arm underneath its abdomen and the other arm under the dog's neck holding the dog close. Another method is done while the dog is sitting and the holder places one arm around the hind end of the dog and the other arm underneath the neck holding the dog close. Lateral restraint is holding the dog on its side with the holder standing or sitting along the dog's back. While the dog is in lateral restraint, hold the dog's head down by applying firm pressure with the arm over the neck, then hold the front limbs with that hand and a finger in between the two legs to secure the grasp, and the holder's other arm will lay across the dog's lower half and grasp the rear limbs with that hand.

Tools Used for Restraining a Dog

A common tool used to **restrain a dog** is a leash. The **leash** is either looped around the dog's neck or clipped to their collar. A **muzzle** is a device that is wrapped around the dog's nose and mouth and clipped behind the ears to prevent the dog from biting. The muzzle also helps to distract the dog from what the veterinary technician is doing for a short period of time. A **rabies pole**, otherwise known as a **head snare**, can be used if the dog is attempting to attack and there is no other way to get a hold of the dog. The rabies pole is a long metal handle in the shape of a tube with a thick wire that retracts inside of it. The wire inside of the tube is long and is pushed out in a loop.

When pushing the wire out, make sure the loop is wide enough to go around the dog's head while the handle allows the restrainer to stand at a safe distance, and once the loop is around the dog's head, it is pulled tight.

Restraint Methods for Cats

A common **restraint technique** for drawing blood from the back leg is the lateral method. To hold a cat in lateral recumbency, one hand will hold the cat by the scruff while stretching the cat on its side with its back against the holder's body. The back leg that is closest to the table is left down while the restrainer's other hand is holding the leg on top while occluding the vein of the leg on the table. The technique used for jugular blood draws on cats is the kitty stretch. To perform the kitty stretch technique, the restrainer will stand on one side of the cat and wrap the arm closest to the cat around its body and grasp the front paws with that hand and stretch the paws off of the table as the other hand is lifting the cat's head up so its nose is pointing up. The kitty stretch technique should only be performed on cats that will tolerate it.

Tools Used for Restraining a Cat

There are muzzles made just for cats, and they slip over the nose, cover the eyes, and Velcro behind the ears. There is a small hole where the nose and mouth are so the cat can breathe, but the eyes are covered, which helps to calm a feline patient. Sometimes a combination of a cat muzzle and wrapping the cat in a towel will help calm the cat even further by making them feel secure with the towel swaddled around them and calm because they cannot see what is happening around them. There are cat bags that the cat's body is placed in and the head is left out while the bag is zipped up along the cat's back. There is a hole in the front of the bag to extend a front leg through either to place an IV catheter or draw blood from if needed. Again, the cat bag and cat muzzle will work well together. If the cat is extremely fractious, it may be necessary to use sedatives.

Restraint Methods for Cattle

The **tail restraint technique** is done to distract the cow from kicking, as well as from paying attention to a part on its body being worked on. Tail restraint is performed by lifting the tail straight over the back with both hands at the base firmly until resistance is felt. Rope halters are placed on a cow by holding the slip lead and the top of the nose piece in the left hand and the head stall in the right, then placing the nose piece over the cow's nose from the left side and the slip lead under the chin with half of the stall over the top of the cow's head and behind its ears. Mechanical restraint, such as a squeeze chute may also be used. A squeeze chute is designed with a headgate, tailgate, and sides that move to change the width of the chute. As the cow moves its head through the headgate, a handler will close the head gate while the second handler puts in the tailgate bar and slowly squeezes the cow with the sides of the chute to prevent it from moving too fast and injuring itself. Applying enough pressure in the squeeze chute allows the cow to stand up and balance while also calming the animal. Once the cow is properly in the chute, a halter can be used to restrain the head.

Restraint Techniques Different Personality Traits of Cattle

Dairy bulls may seem gentle and calm, but they are actually very unpredictable and untrustworthy. Dairy bulls should always be restrained for any sort of procedure or handling. Beef bulls should be dealt with carefully and should be restrained in squeeze chutes because ropes are not strong enough to hold them. Dairy cows, such as Holstein and Jersey cows, need little restraint because they are very excitable and fearful, so restraints will only upset them, but simple handling will usually calm them enough to submit. **Restraint techniques** must be appropriate for the size and temperament of the cow that is being handled, as well as they must be appropriate for the procedure being performed. For example, if a blood draw is needed on a beef bull, then tight and secure mechanical restraint must be used such as a squeeze chute, but if a dairy cow needs to be examined, a simple halter restraint can be used.

Restraint Methods for Horses

A common **restraint technique for the horse** is a chain over its nose that is ideal for veterinary visits, but this method must be used with caution because excessive pulling on the lead rope with the chain can cause damage to the horse's nose bone. A **lip chain** puts pressure on the gums and under the upper lip and should be used cautiously with a slow and steady pressure because yanking on the lead will cause injury to the horse. The **lip twitch** comes in three forms with the chain being the safest because the links on the chain will not twist too tight on the horse. A skin twitch is used as a distraction from what the handler is trying to work on with the horse that is easily done by pinching the skin between the thumb and forefinger. The **skin twitch** works by releasing endorphins, which calms the horse and decreases the sensation of pain. If you need to work on one of the horse's legs and they won't stand still, then having another person pick up an opposite leg can help you finish the job.

Types of Aggression That Dogs May Display

Fearful aggression is often displayed when the dog feels threatened. Sometimes being on a leash or being confined in a cage will bring out fearful aggression if the dog is trying to escape but can't get away. Also, if a dog realizes that being aggressive helps to remove the threat, then they will continue that behavior. **Territorial aggression** is when the dog becomes aggressive toward someone or another animal coming onto its property but does not seem bothered by the same interaction outside of its territory. **Predatory aggression** is an attack with the intent to kill prey with no warning. **Food** or **possessive aggression** is displayed when the dog becomes aggressive when someone or another pet comes up to the dog when it is eating or has a possession such as a toy.

Diagnostic Imaging

Radiographic Concepts

Amplitude, Time Period, Attenuation, and Acoustic Impedance

Amplitude: The intensity or height of a wave.

Time period: The equivalent of one cycle of the wave. This is given the symbol (T).

Attenuation: A loss of vitality, amplitude, or power. With sound, this occurs when intensity is lost as an ultrasound beam passes through tissue. The loss can be attributed to the way the beam is absorbed into the tissue as it makes its way through. The absorption process creates heat and results in a loss of energy. Tissue that has sound refractory characteristics can scatter the sound in a multitude of directions.

Acoustic impedance: The capability of something to withstand or resist sound conduction. The density of tissue may be reflected in its degree of impedance. However, both air (not dense) and bone (very dense) will significantly obstruct the passage of sound. Thus, both bone and air have a high rate of acoustic impedance, despite their widely differing density. On the whole, however, tissues respond favorably to the passage of sound waves. Therefore, most bodily tissues have a low rate of acoustic impedance.

Basics of Sound Waves

A wavelength is defined as the span of distance that a wave travels in one repeating cycle. Wavelength is written in an abbreviated international symbolic or notation form as: λ (i.e., the lowercase Greek letter lambda).

Audible sound has a wavelength that spans a lengthier distance than the wavelength displayed by an ultrasound.

A transducer is a device that converts one form of energy into another form. The defining features of the transducer may influence the wavelength.

A second is defined as a unit of time measured in a given cycle. This measurement is applied to number the times a cycle is replicated.

The frequency is how many times the cycle occurred. Frequency is given the following symbol: (f). The wavelength will extend for a longer distance or increase as the frequency decreases. The frequency range for ultrasonic waves is measured at 2 to 10 MHz. The frequency range for human auditory perception is approximately 20 Hz–20 kHz.

Velocity is given the following symbol: (v). Sound velocity is defined as the speed at which a sound wave travels through a medium. The formula for velocity is given as the frequency multiplied by the wavelength.

Ultrasonography

Ultrasonography is noninvasive and records reflections of ultrasonic waves to allow internal organs to be seen in real time. A narrow beam with high-frequency ultrasound waves is directed into the area on the body that is of interest through the use of a probe and is transmitted through the tissues, or the waves may be reflected or absorbed. The waves that are reflected from the tissues come back to the probe and are called "echoes" that transfer to an image displayed on the monitor as a 2D image. Ultrasound waves do not pass through organs that contain air, such as the lungs, and they stop at bone, so bones are not seen in an ultrasound. B-mode ultrasonography produces a 2D image and is used to diagnose pregnancy, examine the organs in the abdomen, and evaluate the function of the heart. M-mode ultrasonography produces a tracing of the structure in motion, and, combined with B-mode, it is a good diagnostic tool to examine the chambers and valves of the heart. The speed and direction of the blood flow in the vessels and heart can be viewed by Doppler ultrasound.

Magnetic Resonance Imaging (MRI)

Magnetic Resonance Imaging (MRI) uses a powerful magnet that surrounds the body of the patient that is laying on a table. All soft tissues of the body can be viewed with MRI, but bone and air are difficult to produce. As the soft tissues respond to the magnet, signals are produced and converted to a cross-sectional image. An MRI produces high-contrast, detailed images using electromagnetic signals from protons in the tissues. All tissues have protons that have a charge and spin on their axis, naturally creating an electromagnetic field. During the MRI, the region of the body being imaged is inside of the large and powerful magnet that causes all of the protons to align with the magnetic field.

CT Scan Machine

CT stands for **Computed Tomography**. The patient must be still and lay on a table for this scan, so they must be under general anesthesia, while the veterinary technician and veterinarian are separated by a large window where they can monitor the pet. The table that the patient is laying on is slowly directed into the machine for the scan (this table is called a gantry). The large X-ray tube that the patient is now in rotates 360° around the entire patient recording the X-rays from different angles, and every scan takes less than 30 seconds. Once a scan is finished, the table advances further and the next scan is taken. The computer processes the information, creating a cross-sectional image of the body part of interest, and then the image is displayed on the monitor.

What a Computed Tomography (CT Scan) Will Show

A **CT scan** is used mainly for looking into parts of the brain or spine of the patient. A CT scan works as X-ray beams move through the body, and then the transmitted energy from the X-rays is recorded by detectors on the opposite side of the patient. This energy from the x-rays sent as an electrical signal to the computer to produce an image. A gray scale is images of tissue that appear white, black, and gray. The amount of gray reflects the tissue's ability to absorb the X-ray beams, helping to compare abnormal tissue to normal tissue. Some CT scan machines produce a 3D image and display the tissue's height and width. A CT scan only looks at a slice of the body at a time, and thinner slices produce better quality images. CT scans show the different levels in density of the tissues to produce a highly detailed image.

Echocardiography

Echocardiography is a noninvasive ultrasound used to evaluate the heart's anatomy and function. A narrow sound beam is projected into the heart, and the echo pattern and strength are shown on the screen. The M-mode format provides the ability to evaluate fast-moving structures such as the heart's valves as well as the pattern of the heart chamber's wall movement due to its high resolution. M-mode is combined with B-mode to further evaluate the shape of the heart's chambers because it will help improve the beam's placement. Doppler echocardiography looks specifically at the heart's blood flow and will help to identify valve leaks or abnormal blood flow movement between the right and left sides of the heart. Doppler echocardiography can also detect any obstructions to blood flow to and from the heart.

Fluoroscopy

Fluoroscopy is an ongoing series of **low-dose X-ray images** that allow the veterinarian to see the internal organs in motion. The images produced are similar to that of an X-ray image, but because the images are continuously produced, it creates motion in real time similar to a movie. To perform a fluoroscopy, the patient is placed in a plastic box whether sitting or standing and a continuous X-ray beam is generated at the patient. The C-arm of the fluoroscopy machine has two sides with the patient in between, and the body of the machine along with the C-arm can move together if needed to be adjusted with the patient's height and position.

Producing Diagnostic Imagery

Safety Practices When Taking Radiographs

Radiation treatments cannot be conducted when a pregnant person is present in the room. When conducting radiological procedures it is best to use nonmanual restraints on the patient, even if the state allows manual restraints, to avoid unnecessary x-ray exposure.

Persons in the room should wear the following: protective gloves, thyroid protectors, and aprons.

The x-ray machine itself should not be handled without protection. It is necessary to use a 2.5 mm aluminum filter to eradicate the lower-energy portion of the x-ray beam. The x-ray machine requires routine maintenance and calibration. It is important to keep body parts out of the path of the primary beam. This is necessary because of the primary beam's ability to transmit 25% of its radiation through a body shield. The technician should wear a dosimeter next to the outside collar of the apron. Ideally, diagnostic radiographs will be achieved with the fastest (i.e., lowest dosing) film-screen systems employed by the attending technician.

Radiation Dosage and Hazards

Radiation exposure standards are set to ensure patient and staff safety. The maximum radiation exposure allowed is defined in terms of dose rates and exposure time (dose = dose rate × exposure time). Thus, the maximum exposure time permitted is a function of the environmental and occupational dose rate. In clinical settings, the criteria are set according to guidelines issued by the **National Committee on Radiation Protection and Measurements** (the NCRP). These are derived from the recommendations produced by the **International Commission on Radiological Protection** (the ICRP).

The NCRP, and almost every province and state, has established radiological protection guidelines. These guidelines specify acceptable rates of exposure when, for example, one is holding an animal for an x-ray (some states, however, prohibit any type of manual animal restraint). To provide an extra measure of protection, staff will wear an individual dosimeter at the work site. It provides a cumulative record of radiation exposure over time, and is evaluated by a federally approved laboratory on a routine basis.

Contrast Radiography

Contrast radiography allows hollow areas of the body (vessels, intestines, etc.) to be more meaningfully viewed. Two variations of the contrast medium include positive and negative contrasts. The **positive contrast agents** are known as radiopaque agents. These agents are found in products like barium and iodine. Radiopaque agents have the capacity to absorb x-rays more thoroughly than the absorption rate found in bones. This causes the structure filled with the radiopaque agent to appear whiter on the film than any other structure in view. Barium is typically employed when examining areas of the gastrointestinal tract. This is an insoluble positive contrast agent.

Soluble contrast agents are found in products with iodine. These products are appropriate for the examination of the renal, articular, vascular, myelographic, and gastrointestinal systems. It should be noted that some patients can exhibit toxic reactions to these agents, although these reactions rarely occur. Soluble iodinated contrast agents can be attributed to a hyperosmotic condition.

Negative contrast agents include air and carbon dioxide, and are known as radiolucents. Radiolucent media will show up as black (indicating a void) in radiographs. This is because it is entirely unable to absorb x-rays. Both positive and negative contrast agents are employed by professionals using double-contrast studies.

Diagnostic Radiographs

Non-manual restraint of an animal is always recommended because of its minimization of radiation exposure for staff.

Calipers are measuring instruments used to determine the number of centimeters involved in an area to be radiologically exposed.

The recommended views are taken from **two right angles**. However, this is not true for thoracic views, contrast studies, equine radiography, and injuries that present only one view option. It is best to achieve a close up shot with the film nearest to the subject as is workable. The beam should be centered over the specified portion of the body. The film is positioned in a parallel direction. The x-ray beam is set perpendicular to the portion of the body to be shot. Some accommodation may be necessary for certain anatomy parts. This accommodation may be in the form of collimating (bringing into a direct line) the machine to use the smallest field available. Extremities are shot with the proximal and distal joints of long bones included in the image. The patient may need to be repositioned to get the best view. It is best to take the time necessary for repositioning so that retakes will not be required.

Sonographic Appearances

Liver, Gallbladder, and Kidneys

The largest part of the **spleen** is hyperechoic. It has a standard granular profile. It is also surrounded by an illuminated capsule. The patient's spleen should be ultrasonographically imaged from the left side. This side provides the best option for examining the spleen, with the least amount of surrounding tissue interference. The spleen lies just below the skin and facia, behind the stomach and under the diaphragm.

Viewing the spleen from the trailing edge of the liver provides important imaging advantages. The liver's outer layer has a thick surface which presents an echogenic disparity that should be avoided.

The **gallbladder** (or cholecyst) is located under the liver. The liver has a multitude of vessels and bile channels. Sonographic images of the gallbladder are displayed as anechoic, as it is largely fluid (bile) filled. Thus, it presents itself as an illuminated wall. Sludge or solid deposits can occasionally be found and visualized in the gallbladder. Animals that have not eaten before a sonogram often have large (i.e., dilated) gallbladder sonographic images.

The **kidney** will present as ovoid or egg-shaped. It will be enclosed by an illuminated capsule, as the cortex of the kidney is hyperechoic. The medulla of the kidney presents itself as anechoic. The pelvic fat will be displayed as an illuminated central zone. The sagittal view should be measured to determine the size.

Heart and Spleen

Sonography is an imaging system used to produce a visual likeness of organs found in the body. The heart is visualized using 2 types of sonographic imagery: M-mode or two-dimensional B-mode imaging. Sonograms of the heart require that 2 separate directional views be taken along both the long- and short-axis of the organ. The Doppler imaging technique can then be applied to determine the turbulence and velocity of red blood cells within the heart.

For an **echocardiogram** (cardiac sonogram), the animal should be placed in a lateral recumbent position. The heart is normally ultrasonographically examined by aiming the ultrasound transducer between the fourth and fifth ribs. In this way, it is possible for the transducer beam to reach the heart from the underside of the animal.

A hyperechoic appearance is seen in the walls and valves of the heart. A hyperechoic condition results when the tissue or an organ (or parts thereof) are highly reflective of an ultrasound beam, thus producing a brighter or whiter appearance on the ultrasound image than the surrounding tissue.

Stomach, Bowel, Pancreas, and Adrenal Gland

The presence of **gas or flatus in the abdomen and intestines** presents a routine obstacle in ultrasonography. This is because air is hyperechoic and thus intestinal flatus limits the imaging of anything in the far field behind it. Even so, the intestinal walls on a sonographic image will look white or dark gray on the screen.

Depending upon its contents, the stomach may be hypoechoic. However, the rugal folds of the stomach are usually visible in the image created.

The **pancreas** is sandwiched between the spleen and the stomach. It is adjacent to the duodenum. The pancreas is a digestive and endocrine gland found in the body.

The **adrenal gland** appears as a standard (isoechoic) gray color. The adrenal gland is responsible for the secretion of hormones in the body. The adrenal gland itself is hypoechoic.

As reference points, the cranial pole of the kidney is situated toward the middle of the adrenal gland. The renal artery is next to the caudal pole found in the adrenal gland. The renal artery connects to the aorta.

Bladder, Prostate, and Uterus

A sonographic image of the **urinary bladder** is typically dark, as it is fluid filled and thus is relatively anechoic. However, the bladder has a wall that presents itself as hyperechoic, and it is not unusual to find debris in the bladder that aids in visualization.

In the male, the **prostate** can be ultrasonographically located by following the urethra to the pelvic inlet. The **urethra** is encircled by the prostate. The prostate is composed of 2 lobes. The prostate has an illuminated capsule in its ultrasonographic image.

In the female, the **uterus** is evident as the organ adjacent to an enlarged bladder. The wall of the uterus is hypoechoic.

The optimum time to discover an early uterine pregnancy in small animals is at about 30 days into gestation. In horses, the optimum early confirmation time is around 11-14 days into the gestation period. At these junctures, the sonographic equipment should be able to detect viable embryos in their gestational sacs. However, it can often be hard to distinguish the exact number of fetuses inside the sac. This is due to the problem of superimposition and the usual presence of gas in the intestines.

Nuclear Scintigraphy

In **nuclear scintigraphy imaging**, the patient can be given gamma emissions from radioactive material or radionuclides applied by a variety of methods. These methods include intravenous injections, transcolonic applications, or aerosol insufflation (i.e., blown into or onto the body). The radioactive material is picked up by sensors found in the gamma scintillation camera. The organ is then pictured on x-ray film, formatted in black and white shades of varying contrast.

Clinical nuclear scintigraphy is typically performed on the thyroid, bone, and liver. The results derived from this technique provide physiological, pharmacological, and kinetic data.

Nuclear scintigraphy is beneficial in many treatments provided to horses. However, the handler and persons coming into contact with the horse having this procedure should use the recommended safety equipment. This equipment should prevent undue exposure to the harmful effects of radioactive material. The animal will expel the radiopharmaceutical elements in its bodily waste. The contaminated urine and feces is normally expelled within 24 to 72 hours after the procedure was completed.

Computerized Axial Tomography

Computerized Axial Tomography (i.e., a "CAT" scan) is primarily employed as a diagnostic test to determine the health of the central and peripheral nervous system, although it is also used for many other kinds of evaluations. This imaging technique can detect numerous forms of disease in a variety of animals. However, it is also one of the costliest examinations used by veterinarians. The animal having this procedure will require general anesthesia to limit movement. The equipment used in computerized tomography requires that the patient be moved slowly through a circular gantry while remaining virtually motionless. This circular segment of the machine holds the x-ray tube and detectors. The equipment has the capability of moving completely around the patient, encompassing 360 degrees in total.

Each movement of the scanner produces a recording of a single cross-sectional slice of data. This recording is created when x-rays are picked up by the scanner. The x-rays are transformed into electronic signals with a wide range of intensity levels. These varying levels are produced through radiant attenuation. The image is then computed and shown in a re-creation produced by the computer.

Magnetic Resonance Imaging

Magnetic Resonance Imaging (MRI) produces cross-sectional images of anatomy. This technique has some shared characteristics with those found in computerized axial tomography. However, magnetic resonance imaging does not employ the use of ionizing radiation to create a likeness of the tissues or organs. Instead, it incorporates a magnetic field to produce the desired image being scanned. Enclosed coils in the device are able to transmit and receive magnetic field signals. Then the computer organizes those signals into an image. Magnetic resonance imaging provides an image resolution that has a better quality than other techniques used. Indeed, this device is sensitive enough to display detailed portions of an animal's anatomy and tissue makeup. Magnetic resonance imaging particularly lends itself to head and spine appraisals that require more intricate images to be produced.

Common Radiographic Positioning Techniques

To describe **radiographic positioning**, the terms used when the X-ray beam enters or exits the body or head are ventrodorsal or dorsoventral. To describe how the X-ray beam enters or exits a limb, caudocranial or craniocaudal is used. A lateral (side) view is when the patient is placed with its side on the X-ray table and is defined as where the X-ray beam exits the body; for example, left lateral positioning is when the patient's left side is on the X-ray table. Ventrodorsal views are taken as the patient is on its back and are defined by where the beam enters through the ventral surface of the body and exits out of the dorsal surface. Dorsoventral is when the patient is sitting sternal and is defined as where the beam enters the body through the dorsal surface and exits through the ventral surface. Craniocaudal positioning is defined as where the beam enters the front side of the limb (cranial) and exits out of the back of the limb (caudal), whereas caudocranial is defined as where the beam enters the back side of the limb and exits out the front.

Positive and Negative Contrast Media

Contrast media are used to allow the veterinarian to assess the size and shape of a specific organ. Positive contrast media, such as barium, are radiopaque making it possible to identify minor defects in the walls of an organ, and they will help identify a lesion or organ from the surrounding tissues. Taking multiple radiographs throughout the day after administering positive contrast media will show how the organ in question is functioning; for example, if the barium is not passing through the intestines, there may be a foreign body present. Negative contrast media appear radiolucent (transparent to X-rays) compared to the surrounding tissues, allowing the veterinarian to assess the size and thickness, as well as the location, of a specific organ. Negative contrast media will also help in identifying masses and foreign bodies.

Diagnostic Imaging on a Patient

After collecting a patient history and presenting complaint as to why the patient is in the hospital, the veterinarian may need to take an inside look to gather more information on where the issue lies. For example, if the owner thinks that the pet has eaten an inanimate object and now will not eat or when the patient eats followed by vomiting, abdominal radiographs may be necessary to look for an obstruction. An ultrasound may be used as well to provide more detail of the organs. Another example is if the patient presents with limping, radiographs of the limb may be necessary to look for any fractures.

Positioning for Radiographic Views

Thoracic Radiographic Views for the Small Animal

Dorsoventral (DV), ventrodorsal (VD), and lateral views are commonly taken for **thoracic radiographs**. If the animal is having trouble breathing, then a DV view may be taken instead of a VD, in which the animal is placed on its back. To place the animal in right lateral recumbency, the animal will be laid on its right side with its front legs extended forward (cranially) and the head should not be extended too much because this can create a false image of a narrow airway. Center the beam over the caudal dorsal aspect of the scapula, collimating the entire chest with the edge of the collimation being right in front of the scapula. To position for a VD view, the patient will lay on its back (dorsal) with the front legs extended and the head laying straight between the front legs. The other restrainer will hold the rear legs and extend them back so the patient is straight on its back. Collimate only to include the chest cavity, centering over the heart. Take both images upon inspiration. To perform DV positioning, the patient is sternal with the front legs extended out and the head is straight between the front legs. Collimate over the area of the chest, centering over the heart, and take the image at inspiration.

Cervical Spine Radiographic Views for the Small Animal

When taking radiographs of the patient's spine, it is best to have the pet sedated because these images require specific positioning. Routine positions for **spinal radiographs** are lateral, including flexion and extension, and VD. For cervical lateral spine radiographs, place the patient on its side with the spine parallel to the table and the forelimbs will be pulled back toward the abdomen (caudally). An extension lateral view of the cervical spine is taken with the patient on its side, front legs pulled toward the abdomen and the head moved dorsally. The flexion lateral view of the cervical spine is taken with the patient on its side, with the front legs pulled caudally toward the abdomen and the head pulled toward the thorax. For a VD view of the cervical spine, the patient is on its back (dorsal) with the nose pointing up, the front legs are extended caudally and can be secured with a loop tie or tape. The base of the skull and the second vertebra of the thorax should be included in the VD view.

Pelvic Radiographic Views for the Small Animal

Common views requested for **pelvic radiographs** include extended-leg VD, lateral, and frog-leg VD. For lateral positioning of the pelvis, the patient will be laying on the side that is affected. The femur on the bottom will be pulled cranial with the stifle flexed, and the leg on top will be extended caudally. The beam should be centered on the greater trochanter, collimating for the pelvis. To position for the VD view of the pelvis, the patient needs to be in dorsal recumbency with the front legs extended with the head laying between. The other person restraining will extend the rear legs while rotating the stifles in so that the legs are straight and the sternum and spine are superimposed. Collimate for the crest of the ilium of the pelvis and down to the stifle joints. To position the patient for a VD frog-leg position, place the patient in the dorsal recumbent position making sure that the sternum and spin are superimposed and the rear legs are left to fall into a normal flexed position with the femurs at a 45-degree angle to the spine. Collimate for the VD frog-leg position starting at the crest of the ilium of the pelvis, including the stifle joints, and centering on the greater trochanter.

Dosimetry Badges

Dosimetry badges are worn to monitor the amount of exposure to scatter radiation for each individual. These badges have a radiation-sensitive film inside of a plastic holder with a clip to attach to the area on a person's body most at risk, such as the collar (thyroid). The badges are checked quarterly to evaluate each individual's radiation dose for that period of time, and the amount of exposure should not exceed 5 Roentgen equivalent man (rem) per year. A laboratory develops the film inside these badges and measures the level of radiation exposure. A control dosimetry badge is the same as the personnel dosimetry badges, but it is used to monitor the background radiation from shipment and storage at the location. The control dosimetry badge should be kept away from the radiology suite and is shipped back with the other personnel badges for dose readings in which the control normally reads low and that reading is subtracted from the other badges to obtain the occupational dose.

Personal Protective Equipment (PPE) Used for Taking Radiographs

Personal protective equipment (PPE) includes items that are worn to protect the person from health hazards. PPE used for personnel obtaining radiographs include lead aprons, lead gloves, lead thyroid collars, and lead-rimmed glasses. Lead is an extremely dense material and serves as a barrier against scatter radiation. Lead aprons, gloves, and thyroid collars should be made of at least 0.25–0.5 mm of lead. Lead aprons should fit correctly, there should be various sizes available, and they need to have enough shielding from the neck to the middle of the thighs and wrap around the sides. Thyroid collars wrap around the neck, and lead gloves should be used during each exposure.

Producing Images with a Swallow Study with the Use of Fluoroscopy

Swallow tests may be performed on a pet if they are having trouble swallowing their food, an esophageal disorder is suspected, or they are having issues with regurgitation. The patient is put into the plastic box, and a variety of different types and consistencies of food is prepared. The consistencies of the food should range from liquid to slightly formed, up to dry kibbles, and each type of food will have a contrast media added to it. As the continuous X-rays are produced, the veterinarian can easily watch the food travel through the esophagus and watch for any abnormalities.

Echocardiograms

Most of the time, the patient will not need to be sedated to perform an **echocardiogram**. The patient will lay on a padded tray, and using the ultrasound transducer probe, the veterinarian will place it over the area of the heart. There are specialized trays available to lay the patient in allowing the heart and lungs to be viewed from underneath the patient so there are fewer reflections from sound waves. The hair can be shaved if needed and must be wet to allow the transducer access to the skin. Ultrasound gel is placed on the transducer probe liberally and may be repeatedly applied throughout the analysis. The images in real time show on the screen, and the doctor can identify leaks in the valves of the heart as well as evaluate the movement of blood between the left and right sides of the heart. Echocardiography is commonly used to diagnose different forms of heart disease including valve abnormalities, dilated cardiomyopathy (dilation of the heart), and tumors in the heart.

Methods Used for Identifying External Parasitic Mites

Superficial or Light Skin Scraping Method

Parasites are those organisms which live on or in a host organism. **Ectoparasites** live on the surface of the host, and include fleas, ticks, lice, and mites. Endoparasites live inside the animal, and include heartworms, roundworms, hookworms, lungworms, whipworms, and tapeworms. Parasites can cause harm to the host, and thus appropriate examinations should take place. While fleas, ticks, and lice are usually easily seen and identified, mites are too small, and thus require microscopic examination.

Scraping the skin for external parasite identification requires a number 10 scalpel, mineral oil in a dropper bottle, microscope slides, and a microscope. The scalpel blade is first moistened on a slide laden with mineral oil. It is then ready to obtain a scraping. The blade of the scalpel should be held in a perpendicular position towards the skin to ensure that an incision in the skin is not accidentally made. Grasp the skin gently between the thumb and index finger of one hand. The other hand should be used to make contact with the skin as the scraping motion is performed. Some parasites require deeper scrapes than other parasites. Therefore, a tentative determination should be made to classify the presenting case according to potential types: sarcoptes (burrowing mites), Demodex (hair follicle mites), Chorioptes, and Cheyletiella (both surface, non-burrowing skin mites). The burrowing mites require a deep scrape or rub to be collected.

Deep Skin Scraping Method

Non-burrowing mites such as Demodex, Chorioptes, and Cheyletiella require only **superficial skin scraping** or **rubbing** for specimen collection. This should be sufficient to dislodge the loose scales and skin crusts in which they live. Scales are flaky pieces of skin. **Crusts** are dry, hardened outer layers of blood, pus, or other bodily secretion that forms over a cut or sore on the skin.

Cheyletiella is sometimes referred to as "walking dandruff" due to the mites' habit of carrying dermal scales (i.e., dandruff) over the surface of the host. Burrowing mites (Sarcoptes) are more difficult to collect. To ensure adequate material collection, the skin in an affected area should be taken down just deep enough to produce a slow leak of blood.

The material that is collected through either scraping method should be placed on a prepared slide laden with mineral oil. The slide should then be covered with a coverslip. The slide is scrutinized under a microscope at 10 power magnification. At least 10 slides should be inspected to ensure accuracy in making the external parasite identification.

Initial Stages of the Baermann Technique

There are 4 categories of **endoparasites**, often classified according to the part of the body they infect: **blood**, **digestive system, organs,** and **sinus cavities**. Many parasites have a life cycle that results in the presence of eggs (oocytes), larva, or the parasites themselves in excreted feces. The **Baermann Technique** is one test used to examine fecal matter for parasites and parasitic ova and larva.

One of the parasites found in the feces is lungworm, living in the larval stage. The **lungworm** is a form of roundworm that lives in the pulmonary tissues of mammals and birds. Lungworm is introduced into the body through the ingestion of a contaminated food source. This worm can cause the host to have a number of respiratory problems. One indication of lungworm infestation is a severe cough.

The external identification of this parasite is accomplished via the **Baermann Technique**. It requires the use of a paper cup, disposable cellulose tissue or Kimwipe, elastic band, sedimentation jar, long Pasteur pipette with a bulb, and a dissecting microscope. A small amount of feces is examined for the presence of the lungworm. The feces sample is collected in the paper cup. A Kimwipe or a disposable cellulose tissue is placed on the cup as a cover. This cover is held in place with an elastic band.

Final Stages of the Baermann Technique

The **Baermann Technique** for fecal examination requires a small hole to be made in the underside of the cup containing a fecal specimen. The cup must be covered with a Kimwipe or disposable cellulose tissue, which is secured with an elastic band. Warm water is used to fill a sedimentation jar halfway. Then, the cup should be submerged with the Kimwipe or cellulose tissue-end placed facedown in the water. All of the tissue should be in the water. The sample requires submersion in this manner for 12 to 18 hours.

After ample time has elapsed, a sample of water should be collected from the underside of the sedimentation jar. The sample is collected using a long Pasteur pipette with bulb. This is a small glass tube that allows liquid to be drawn into it by use of an attached suction bulb. At least 3 or 4 samples should be collected. The samples should be inspected under a dissecting microscope. The examination should show movement by any living larvae. Diligent perusal of the feces sample should allow ample opportunity for the external parasite to be identified. Lungworm can produce death in the host animal, and thus prompt treatment is essential.

Feces Examination

Direct Smear Method

Fecal matter may also be examined for parasitic infestation by way of a glass slide smear. The **direct smear method** is also used to discover the existence of protozoa in feces. Protozoa are single cell organisms that feed on organic compounds. The direct smear method can aid in a rough calculation of the number of parasites present within the body. The direct smear method requires the following: microscope slides, coverslips, and applicator sticks. Lugol's iodine or methylene blue stain may be used, but neither is required. Fresh fecal matter is also required (at or near body temperature and ideally less than an hour old). **Trophozoites** in older specimens will lose motility, degenerate, and become very difficult if not impossible to recognize.

A single drop of saline solution (not water, which may rupture trophozoites) should be placed alongside an equal amount of feces on the surface of the slide. If stain is to be applied, then it should be added at this juncture. The blending of the feces and saline solution is accomplished with an applicator stick. This blend is thinly spread across the flat surface of the glass plate or slide. The larger pieces of feces are removed for uniform magnification and ease in slide viewing. Parasite eggs can be viewed with a 10-power magnification objective. Protozoal organisms can be viewed using a 40-power magnification objective.

Initial Stages of the Standard Vial Gravitation Flotation Technique

The **standard vial gravitation flotation technique** is used to find **parasitic eggs in fecal matter**. The principles and processes involved are not difficult. Further, the cost of this test is fairly low, which is an added benefit. However, this test may also be inaccurate, with false negative results not uncommon. The accuracy can be jeopardized by numerous variables in the testing process. The primary variable is the relative specific gravity of the flotation solution chosen. With the density of water as the reference point, a solution of higher specific gravity should cause parasite eggs or oocytes to float to the surface as the eggs have a lower specific gravity than the floating solution. However, different parasites have oocysts of varying specific gravity, and thus flotation may not always occur. Further, old fecal samples may experience egg degradation and altered flotation patterns, and poor straining strategies may trap eggs and remove them from the flotation solution.

The standard vial gravitation technique requires a paper cup filled with about 60 mL of floating solution. Then, 2 to 4 grams of feces is placed into the solution. The feces are handled with a tongue depressor. The solution and the feces are blended thoroughly. The blended solution is filtered through a strainer and poured into a second cup. This results in the reduction of extraneous waste material. This strained or filtered mixture is gently churned to disperse the eggs.

Final Stages of the Standard Vial Gravitation Flotation Technique

The final stages of the **standard vial gravitation flotation technique** require that this churned mixture be poured into a glass vial. The vial is filled to the top until a **positive meniscus** (upward curving solution surface) is formed. A coverslip or cover glass is positioned on top of the vial at this juncture, making contact with the meniscus. Then, the eggs are permitted to float to the surface of the vial. The parasite eggs or oocysts should float since they have a lower specific gravity than the flotation solution.

Once this has been accomplished, the cover glass can be removed. The cover glass should be carefully lifted off in a straight, upward direction. The cover glass is placed on top of the glass slide. The slide is now ready to be systematically and painstakingly examined. A cautious inspection should reveal the parasite oocysts present in the waste material, and allow for proper parasite identification.

OVC Puddle Technique to Observe Cryptosporidium Oocysts

The **OVC Puddle Technique** is utilized to detect and **monitor Cryptosporidium oocysts or eggs** in feces. This technique requires the use of a microscope, glass slide, and coverslip; applicator stick;

and a saturated sugar solution, such as corn syrup. A very small measure of feces is blended with a bit of the sugar solution. This blended solution is placed on a slide. The cover glass is placed on the slide at this juncture. The sample should be examined under a microscope using a 40-power objective.

The coloration of the Cryptosporidium Oocysts is a light pinkish color. These oocysts are not to be confused with fungal spores that can also be present in the waste material. Fungal spores can be similar in shape and size as the oocysts or eggs. However, the fungal spores will start to bud after a period of time has elapsed, while the eggs will not.

Buffy Coat Method

The **buffy coat method** is used to examine a blood specimen for blood parasites. When blood is placed in a centrifuge and spun at a high rate, the 3 primary components of blood are separated from each other. The top layer is clear plasma; the bottom layer is red blood cells. In between is the "buffy coat" – a thin, creamy-yellowish (sometimes greenish) layer of white blood cells. If the buffy coat is placed on glass slides and examined under a microscope, the presence of parasites in the blood can often be revealed. The method requires the following: microhematocrit tubes and sealer, centrifuge, microscope slides and coverslips, saline solution, methylene blue stain, and a small file or glass cutter.

A microhematocrit tube is filled with blood. This tube of blood goes through centrifuge process for 3 minutes. The packed cell volume (PCV) is then read (it is an important overall indicator of hematological health). Next, the tube is scored at the level of the buffy coat. Then the tube is cautiously snapped before lightly tapping the buffy coat onto a slide. The buffy coat layer is inspected under a microscope. One drop of saline solution and one drop of methylene blue stain are placed on the slide. A coverslip is then positioned over the sample. The slide is then inspected for the presence of microfilariae. Finally, the plasma is retrieved from the microhematocrit tube's residue to be evaluated for total protein. Total protein is a good indicator of overall animal health.

Skin Digestion Technique for the Identification of External Parasites

The **skin digestion technique** is useful for the identification of external parasites. **Skin scraping** samples which have a significant amount of scurf (scales, epidermal shards) and skin debris is ideal for the skin digestion technique. The following is required for this technique: 15 mL conical centrifuge tube, 4% NaOH solution, hot plate, beaker, and centrifuge. The scalpel is used to place the sample in the centrifuge tube. Then, about 10 mL of NaOH solution is applied to the sample within the centrifuge tube. Next, the tube is positioned in a glass beaker water bath and boiled for 5 to 10 minutes.

The centrifuge tube is then placed in the centrifuge for 5 minutes at 1000 rpm. Upon removal of the tube, the supernatant should be poured off from the top of the tube. Then, a drop of the sediment should be placed on a microscope slide and covered with a coverslip. Finally, the slide should be inspected for parasites using a microscope which has been set at a 10-power objective.

Enzyme-Linked Immunosorbent Assay or ELISA Parasite Antibody Test

Parasitic blood infestations will cause the body to develop antibodies to the presence of these foreign bodies. The **enzyme-linked immunosorbent assay** (ELISA) kits detect these antigens in the blood. While this test can reveal a host's antibody response to parasites, it cannot detect the microfilariae themselves. ELISA tests are particularly beneficial in the detection of occult heartworm (Dirofilaria immitis).

Commercial kits available for this use include Dirochek from Synbiotics, PetChek/Snap from Idexx, and Witness from Binax. The tests are performed on a tray with an indented surface. The kit supplies a membrane or wand that has parasite-specific monoclonal antibodies bound to its surface. Blood samples containing this particular antigen can thus become bound to the antibody. Next, an additional antibody is labeled with an enzyme and applied to the sample. This will also bind to the antigen. A color-producing agent is then applied.

If **parasite-specific antibodies** are present after the introduction of this agent, then an antibody-enzyme complex will be formed, producing a specific color. The specific color is an indicator that the antigen (i.e., the parasite) is present. If there is no parasite-specific antigen in the sample, the enzyme-labeled antibody will wash away without any color-change result.

Equipment and Related Materials

X-Ray Tube

An **x-ray tube** consists of the following components: a cathode filament, an anode plate, a focusing cup, a target, a glass envelope (within which a vacuum is created), an aluminum filter, and a beryllium window. The x-ray tube generates the photons carrying the electromagnetic charge, and directs them along a targeted pathway. The cathode filament is usually made from tungsten. The tungsten filament is a coiled wire that releases electrons when heat is applied to its surface. The cathode filament is situated across from the focusing cup and the anode plate. The filament maintains a negative potential throughout the heating process. The electrons are drawn to the positively charged anode at great speed. The anode can be immobile or it can be put into a rotation. The target is described as tungsten with a copper stem. The target is fastened to the face of the anode. The entire x-ray device is encased within a tube-shaped Pyrex capsule that creates a vacuum. This is essential for x-ray generation. The x-rays are sent out through a small window fashioned from a thin section of glass. This glass absorbs a small quantity of x-rays or electromagnetic radiation.

X-Rays

X-rays are derived from the energy produced by electrons or negatively charged particles within an atom. This energy is converted to **electromagnetic radiation**. The radiation produces energy particles known as **photons**. Photons do not have any mass or electrical charge, but they can carry **electromagnetic (EM) energy**. When EM-carrying photons crash into and pass through matter, the x-ray picture is created. An x-ray tube has filters that are able to direct the source of electrons at the object toward which it is aimed. The x-ray tube must have the following components: a source of electrons, a method to accelerate the electrons, a defined path, a target, and an encompassing envelope in which to create a vacuum. The electrode pair (a heated cathode and an anode carrying a powerful voltage charge) is the source from which the EM-charged photons are derived. The cathode is capable of releasing electrons when subjected to heat. The electrons are sped up when drawn toward the charged anode, and their collision with the anode produces EM-charged photons, which are aimed to produce a collision with the intended target. Approximately 99% of the energy created is heat and 1% is x-rays (photons carrying EM energy). EM energy is measured as a kilovoltage peak or potential kVp. This energy can be harnessed and adjusted in accordance with the specifications of the particular x-ray machine. The kVp of the electrons establishes the penetration strength of the x-rays.

Screens and Screen Speeds Used in X-Ray Film

The x-ray machine incorporates an **intensifying screen** made from a synthetic base covered in sheets of small **luminescent phosphor crystals.** These crystals function as a protective covering.

Two intensifying screens are located on the interior fabric of the x-ray cassette. The film is packed in between these 2 screens. Visible light exposes the light-sensitive emulsion of the x-ray film when **radiation connects with and illuminates the surface of the phosphor crystals**. This is referred to as indirect imaging, and is responsible for more than 95% of the film's exposure to light. The screen functions to decrease the exposure time necessary to create a diagnostic image on film. Differences in intensifying screen speeds refer to the amount of exposure time required for the production of a diagnostic film. Screen speeds are measured as slow, medium, and fast. The best quality image is gained when slower speeds are used. Further, slower screen speeds do not have any significant problems relating to exposure times. Gradually, computerized x-ray machines are moving into the field. Relying on digital media, they are much more versatile to use, and they bypass the film development step altogether. Further, they have greater file-sharing and archival capacities. Thus, they are slowly replacing the older film and intensifying screen-based processes. In the interim, however, familiarity with traditional x-ray equipment remains important.

X-Ray Machine

The x-ray machine must also include the following components: electrical circuits to control the x-ray tube, a control panel, and a tube stand. It has filters, collimators, and grids as part of its framework. The electrical circuits utilize high-voltage electricity to generate energy and speed. This speed allows the electrons to develop a high electromagnetic potential. The electrical circuits also supply a low-voltage electric current used for heating the cathode filament. A timer switch operates to measure exposure time in seconds. The rectification circuit is used to change the current supplied to the tube from alternating to direct current.

The control panel is utilized to manage and regulate the kilovoltage peak, milliampere, milliampere-seconds, and/or seconds. This regulation is dependent upon the capacity of the x-ray machine. The kVp potential establishes the class of energy. The mA (milliampere) and involved time establishes the intensity of the x-rays. Kilovoltage peak is abbreviated as kVp. Milliampere is abbreviated as mA. Milliampere-seconds are abbreviated as mAs. The x-ray tube is set up on a foundation known as the tube stand.

X-Ray Film

Nonscreen Film and Appropriate Darkroom Conditions

Nonscreen x-ray film does not utilize intensifying screens. It has improved sensitivity to direct ionizing radiation. However, the nonscreen film will require a longer exposure time to work. Even so, it has the advantage of producing an image that has better detail-revealing resolution than that of an image gained via an intensifying screen. The film is packaged in a heavy envelope that does not allow light to pass through. This film is often used in dental offices, where the bulkiness of radiographic film coupled with an intensifying screen is prohibitive. The film speed is depicted by the label D or E. The faster nonscreen film speed is the E label.

Proper darkroom conditions must also be maintained in clean, well- ventilated, temperature-controlled facilities. The correct wattage should be used for a safelight. A filter for the safelight that matches the sensitivity of the film being developed should also be utilized. The light should be positioned at least 4 feet away from the work space.

Screen Speeds and Characteristics of Screen Film

Fair to good resolutions can be obtained with **medium-speed x-ray films**. These require relatively low exposure times. **Fast- speed films** allow a shorter exposure time and provide superior patient x-ray penetration. However, they trade speed for image quality. The poorer quality image is caused by the larger crystals and thicker layers applied in fast-speed screens. These blurred images show less detail than images taken with a medium or slow speed screen.

Film made with **silver halide crystals** or grains has a superior rate of sensitivity to the waves of light produced from the intensifying screens. This increased sensitivity allows a diagnostic radiograph to be created using a **shorter exposure time**. Greater resolution is obtained because of the finer image resolution grains on the film. This greater resolution is accomplished through longer exposure times. Shorter exposure times can only be achieved with larger grains on the films. The veterinarian will find that x-rays performed on animals usually require only a medium-grain film. This medium- grain film is a concession made to obtain a reasonably good image resolution without an extended exposure time.

Pointers for Manually Processing Film

Processing of film involves the following steps: developing, rinsing (in a stop bath), fixing, washing, and drying. The chemicals must be diluted and mixed according to the manufacturer's directions. The chemical solutions are mixed at a temperature of 20 °C or 68 °F. The manufacturer lists detailed information about the time-temperature development of each chemical. The film should be shaken at regular intervals to prevent any air bubbles from forming while in the developing fluid. The oxidation of developing chemicals can be reduced by keeping lids securely fastened on the tanks. As the developer solution is used, the exposed silver halide crystals are changed to black metallic silver.

If the expected density or contrast does not appear, then the solution has weakened and should not be used. The fixer solution is used to remove unexposed, undeveloped silver halide from the image. It also hardens the film. It should be discarded if it takes longer than 2 or 3 minutes for this step to be completed. The process is finished when the image goes from a hazy, cloudy image to a clear image.

Appropriate Darkroom Conditions as Related to Safelight Illumination

A **darkroom light switch** should have a delay to minimize any accidental light exposures. Wet and dark areas should be separated to prevent unintended exposures. The images should be processed by technicians wearing appropriate safety equipment. This includes proper gloves and protective eye wear. An eyewash bottle should be kept in the vicinity, in compliance with state, province, and/or federal regulations regarding timely treatment following an accident.

Light leakage is defined as an event which leads to fogging of the images in the radiographs. A check for fogging can be accomplished by placing an open, unprocessed film cassette in the darkroom. Three quarters of the film should be covered with a lightweight paper board for a period of 1 minute. The other portion of the cardboard should be covered for the second minute. The first section should be uncovered during this time. Continue in like manner, until the entire board has had 1 minute of covered exposure. This takes a total of 3 minutes time. On the fourth minute, the film is left uncovered in its entirety so that the film can be totally exposed. After development, any darkened areas on the film will indicate conditions which permit film fogging to occur.

Factors That Influence Radiographic Density

Radiographic density ultimately relates to the degree of darkness or blackness present on the developed film's surface. The density level is directly correlated with the number of photons that have affected the film. The density can vary according to the total number of x-rays that come into contact with the intensifying screen, transferring the image to the film. It can also be altered by the penetration strength of the x-rays. Density can be further influenced by the development time and temperature. **Focusing filters and grids** can make the beam weaker. In addition, tissue density and patient coverings and support pads can lessen the strength of the beam. The beam strength and exposure duration is measured in milliampere-seconds of x-rays that come into contact with the intensifying screen. The more x-rays that come into contact with the intensifying screen (a function of both strength and time), the more densely activated (darkened) is the film. The strength of penetration is determined by the measurement of kVp (kilovoltage peak). The higher kVp settings produce higher energy x-rays. These higher energy x-rays have higher levels of penetration strength. This results in an improved film density. Thicker or denser tissue causes a reduced film density (lighter film). In like manner, thinner tissue causes an increase in film density (darker film).

Automatic Film Processing

Mechanized film processors can be employed to provide **automated film processing**. The film is routed through the chemical solutions and out to a dryer on a roller assembly. The temperature ranges from 20 to 35 °C (77 to 96 °F). Mechanized film processing can take as little as 90 seconds or as long as 8 minutes. The procedures and chemicals are much like those used in the manual processing methods. However, these mechanical chemicals are mixed in a much more concentrated manner. The hardener is mixed directly into the developer solution. There is no rinsing step between the developing and fixing steps in this method. The mechanical process can only be accomplished by maintaining very clean equipment. The rollers, roller racks, and crossover rollers cannot be dirty. Chemicals should be replaced at recommended intervals to give optimum performance in the mechanized film development process.

Responsibilities and Hazards Involved in Radiation Safety

The practice owner should be responsible for applying the appropriate **radiological safety procedures** in accordance with state or province requirements. These guidelines involve the use of **dosimeter devices**, efficient **radiation detection devices**, **equipment registration**, **staff certification**, and **radiologically appropriate room design**. The health department is normally responsible for regulating these devices and safeguards. Trained personnel are necessary to apply the appropriate radiation safety guidelines. Personnel must be able to use the devices correctly, according to instructions received. Every cell in an organism can be affected by ionizing radiation. Ionizing radiation generates charged particles that are able to modify or disintegrate a molecule. Modified molecules may not perform their intended functions appropriately. This can dangerously interrupt the normal functioning of tissues. This harm may not be immediately apparent. Some effects do not become evident for hours, days, months, years, or even generations. Intergenerational delays may occur when damage presents itself only in the genetic makeup of reproductive cells. Other alterations may not be readily apparent because of concurrent tissue restoration. Even so, somatic cell damage may take place throughout the body. The region of the cell most susceptible to the effects of ionizing radiation is the nucleus, and those aspects central to cellular reproduction.

Factors That Influence Radiographic Contrast and Subject Contrast

Black and white can be combined to produce a variety of different shades of gray and degrees of intensity. The degree of difference between the shades is defined as the radiographic contrast. Radiographic contrast can be impacted by the following: kilovoltage, scatter radiation, processing features, and physical aspects. Some examples of physical aspects include beam attenuation and fogging effects.

Kilovoltage or kVp has the strongest impact on radiographic contrast. The x-ray beam is polychromatic, with many wavelengths. Lower kVp ratings offer wider ranges of energy levels. Higher kVp ratings produce more consistent penetration and fewer disparities. Objects along the pathway of the beam scatter the effect. This creates a reduction in the film's contrast and is displayed by overcast shades of gray on the film.

Subject contrast distinguishes between the density and mass of 2 adjacent structures. A high subject contrast will produce a more prominent radiographic contrast. The thickness and density of the anatomic structures being imaged will also impact subject density. Higher tissue density is translated into higher subject density. Bones are an example of an object with high subject density, as bones are more opaque to x-rays, and will thus image as white or light gray on a radiographic image.

Transducers

Types of Transducer Crystals, and the Function of the Linear Array Transducer

Natural crystals are often utilized as **transducer crystals**. These crystals include: quartz, tourmaline, and Rochelle salts. Some synthetic crystals are also utilized as transducer crystals. **Synthetic crystals** include the following: lead zirconate titanate, barium titanate, and lithium sulfate. Sound vibrations are promoted via a piezoelectric electric effect. A dampener is applied to terminate the vibrations after they have been received. Then new echoes received come into contact with the crystals and initiate the vibration again. These vibrating movements back and forth are subsequently transformed into electrical energy.

One version of transducer is known as the **linear array transducer**. The linear array transducer has a tiny row of crystals that operates in a regular rhythm. The linear array transducer produces a composite image from many parallel lines. These lines form an image in a rectangular shape. Thus, the linear array transducer is often best applied to imaging a wide, near field such as transrectals and equine tendons.

Purpose of a Transducer and the Function of the Transducer Crystal

A transducer is a device that transforms one form of energy into another form. The transducer probe is the principal transforming component of the ultrasound machine. This device will transform sound waves into electrical energy, from which an image can be obtained.

The sound waves produce echoes that can be received as they bounce back in return. The pulsed-wave transducer is a device that emits a short pulse of sound, and works to send and receive these signals in a patterned sequence.

An additional form of a transducer probe is known as a continuous-wave transducer. This device actually utilizes 2 transducers. The first transducer sends out a constant sound wave, while the second transducer continuously receives sound waves as they echo back.

Ultrasound devices function with transducer crystals to enhance the electrical energy conversion process. However, a transducer crystal cannot send and receive sound waves simultaneously. Thus, the transducer must perform these functions in an alternating pattern (unless a dual-crystal [continuous] wave transducer is used).

Types of Transducers

Another kind of transducer is known as the **mechanical multiple angle** or **sector scanning transducers**. The mechanical sector transducer utilizes one or more crystals in its operations. The device will create an image that has the form of a pie wedge or circle segment. It is often a better choice when deep tissue penetration and a large, far-field view is needed.

Another version of a transducer is the phased array sector scanner. This computerized device has the ability to guide ultrasound pulses from about 20 crystals through a particular area. Providing images of time-motion (TM) activity, the phased array sector scanner is best applied to echocardiography. However, this compact device can be an expensive purchase.

Another version of a transducer is the broad bandwidth transducer. This version utilizes a piezoelectric ceramic and epoxy material in the probe. It is a lightweight device with a minimum of acoustic impedance. Importantly, these transducers can operate on a variety of frequencies. These frequencies or short-duration pulses are available because of the transducer's ability to transmit over a wide range of bandwidths.

Resolution, Lateral Resolution, Axial Resolution, and Sound Beam Zones in Ultrasonography

A properly resolved (clearly seen) image on an ultrasound is defined as 2 small objects in close proximity which can be individually recognized. The frequency of the transducer is critical to the resolution quality of the image. Resolution is increased when higher frequencies are applied. This is due to the shorter wavelength used to gain the image. Lateral resolution refers to the ability to properly resolve 2 objects that are both side-by-side and perpendicular to the beam. The beam functions to visually separate the 2 objects from each other. The degree of lateral resolution is also a function of the beam's width. Objects in parallel position to each other are best able to be identified when they are spaced farther apart than the diameter of the beam. Axial resolution is the ability to resolve 2 objects are located one above another in the beam's pathway. In this situation, greater resolution and differentiation is obtained at lower frequencies. The size and design of the transducer controls the ultrasound beam zones. The near field (also called Fresnel zone) refers to the entire area of the ultrasound beam that precedes the focal point and is most proximal (nearest) the crystal. It is characterized by a narrowing, gradually converging beam shape.

Sound Beam Zones and Display Formats Used for Ultrasound Images

The **near field** is that portion of the ultrasound beam that is closest to the crystal. The narrowest position or spot that is reached is known as the beam's focal point. The shifting of the focal point closer to the image can produce a better resolution of the image. The transducer can be brought into focus by "shaping" (manipulating) the crystal. The focus can also be improved by adding a lens to the transducer. The section of the beam that gets broader, and less intense, as it moves away from the focal point is known as the far field (also called the Fraunhofer zone).

The different display formats for ultrasound images include: amplitude mode, brightness mode, and motion mode. The amplitude mode is abbreviated as A-mode. It can provide the depth and dimensions of a target. A-mode is demonstrated as a one-dimensional graph with a succession of rising points. Each rising point stands for a returning echo. A point that is higher on the graph is indicative of a larger, more intense echo coming back.

Additional Display Formats Used for Ultrasound Images

The **brightness mode** (B-mode) produces a two-dimensional map of data represented by dots or small marks on a graph. The dots represent the returning echo. The deepness of the mirrored image is indicated by the location of the dot on the graph's baseline. The baseline is used to reference the results found.

The **motion mode** (M-mode) is represented by a one-dimensional wave graph. Its vertical axis indicates the immediate position of the moving reflector. The horizontal axis represents the time. Objects in motion are represented by wavy lines on the graph. Stationary or immobile objects are represented by straight lines on the graph. The M-mode is best applied for cardiac examinations on a patient. The M-mode provides a beneficial evaluation of the condition of cardiac valves, walls, and chamber sizes.

These display formats are essential to the ultrasound's ability to provide a display that meets the criterion for each particular purpose sought by the technician obtaining the image.

Propagation Artifacts and Attenuation Artifacts

Propagation artifacts: Reverberations, refraction, and mirror images. Reverberations are exhibited as linear echoes. Reverberations are a result of sounds reflected between a strong reflector and the transducer in a continuous pattern. An example of a strong reflective (i.e., reverberation-prone) surface is illustrated by bones.

Refractions are a result of sound beams changing directions as they are bounced off one medium and strike another medium's surface. Refractions are to blame for the manifestation of organs in unusual positions. An example of this is when an image is duplicated and appears as if it exists on both sides of a reflecting axis. This phenomenon is often due to the close proximity of strongly reflective organ to the reflector. This is a typical occurrence in ultrasound images taken of the liver and of the diaphragm.

Attenuation artifacts: Include acoustic shadowing and acoustic enhancement. *Acoustic shadowing* is found when an object reflects a sound wave in its entirety, producing an acoustic shadow of the actual structure. *Acoustic enhancement* occurs when a propagated wave passes largely unimpeded through an anechoic structure, resulting in an artificially strong wave and echo from otherwise deeper tissues.

Echogenic, Sonolucent, Anechoic, Hyperechoic, Hypoechoic, and Isoechoic

Echogenic: Tissues with the capacity to produce return echoes. These echoes are singled out by the transducer, and displayed in a black and white image (with varying gray tones) that represents these tissues. Organs in proximity to each other will produce a larger echo reflection, indicating the gap between each organ.

Sonolucent (also called echolucent): Something that does not reflect sound, and thus produces no echo.

Anechoic: An absence of echoes. A condition sometimes characteristic of chambers, spaces, or fluid-filled areas, where the sounds pass deeper into the tissue without producing returning echoes from that area. This produces a black image on the viewing screen, which sometimes represents tissue saturated with fluid.

Hyperechoic: Strong echo reflection. Also, a greater amplitude wave return. The result is a whiter image appearance from the high degree of sound that is transmitted back to the transducer. Examples of hyperechoic tissues include bone, tendons, and ligaments when perpendicular to the beam.

Hypocholic: Giving back few echoes. A condition where less sound echoes back to the transducer, as compared with adjacent tissue. This less reflective tissue creates a darker ultrasound image.

Examples include: muscle as compared to tendon fiber, soft atherosclerotic plaque, and some tumor tissue.

Isoechoic: Similar amplitude wave returns. Areas of similar echogenicity are considered to be isoechoic to each other.

Doppler Imaging

Doppler imaging is beneficial in examining aspects of the body that remain in constant motion. One such part of the body is blood. Doppler imaging uses differences between sound wave frequencies received at a remote point as opposed to the frequency found at the sound's origin to analyze certain characteristics about motion. The difference is most pronounced when there is activity between the original sound and the receiver. Specifically, the sound wave frequency can increase when the receiver is moving towards the originating location of the sound, and it can decrease when the receiver moves away. Thus, the frequency will increase or decrease in relationship to any movement between the receiver and the originating source. The position-dependent wave amplitude changes between a stationary object and one in motion are referred to as a "Doppler shift." In Doppler imaging, a continuous-wave ultrasonic beam is sent to and received back from a part of the body in motion. Using the sound wave frequency data obtained from movement such as blood flow, the blood's velocity can be calculated. Doppler imaging is beneficial in determining whether or not a lesion or a mass exists in a vessel. Doppler imaging can also help in locating portal systemic shunts and in assessing cardiac function and effectiveness in the body, etc.

Attenuation Artifacts That Can Occur in Ultrasound Images

Posterior shadowing occurs when an object blocks sound waves from passing deeper into the body. This type of shadowing can be a result of calculi and/or gas in the intestines. Calculi are defined as stones or hard fragments that are formed in the kidney, gallbladder, or urinary bladder.

Objects located on the backside of organs filled with fluid may present with **enhanced echoes**, when compared to adjacent objects or tissues. This enhancement is a result of a fluid's anechoic nature, allowing sound waves to more readily pass through, and thus resulting in acoustic enhancement.

Attenuation artifact occurs when tissues in the near field reduce the intensity of the ultrasound beam, leaving tissues in the focal region and far field poorly imaged. Attenuation artifact may cause a lesion itself to be perceived as a hypoechoic mass or cyst.

Hypoechoic conditions exist when certain tissues direct less sound back to the transducer than adjacent tissues. This less reflective tissue creates a darker appearance than the neighboring tissue. Examples include muscle compared to tendon fiber, soft atherosclerotic plaque, and some tumor tissues.

Parts of the Ultrasound Machine

The **transducer probe** is a handheld probe that sends and receives sound waves by using the piezoelectric effect. The transducer probe consists of many crystals that rapidly change shape when an electrical current is applied. The rapid shape changes produce sound waves that travel outward. There are a few different sizes and shapes of transducer probes, which will determine the viewing field. The transducer pulse control changes the frequency and length of the sound waves. The central processing center is the computer that performs the calculations and holds the electrical power for the transducer probes and the central station itself. The display screen will present the image received from the ultrasound data that the central processing unit has processed.

Radiographic Image

X-rays are forms of electromagnetic energy carried by photons with **high energy and a short wavelength**. Mineralized tissues of the body such as bones and teeth absorb the most X-rays, soft tissues like the spleen and kidneys absorb some X-rays, and air doesn't absorb any X-rays. The X-ray machine has a narrow beam of photons that aims at a specific area of the body with a cassette underneath that obtains the X-rays as they pass through to it. The areas that absorb the x-ray photons appear white, whereas areas that allow more photons to pass through will appear black. Areas that are fluid filled appear black or dark gray because those areas do not absorb many X-ray photons. For example, when taking a radiograph of a dog's front leg, the bones will appear white and the muscles and tendons will appear gray.

Proper Maintenance of Lead Aprons and Gloves

Lead aprons and gloves should be checked at least every 6 months to ensure there are no holes or tears. Lead gowns and gloves are inspected by using a fluoroscopy or radiographic machine set at 80 kVp and 5 milliampere seconds (mAs) to check for any cracks, which would appear dense. If there are any signs of cracks or radiation leakage, the item must be replaced. There should be a rack, normally on the wall in the radiology suite, that the gowns and gloves can hang on so they do not get folded or stacked on top of one another. Hanging them will also keep them from accidentally getting punctured or cut by any sharp object. The gowns and gloves can be washed with mild detergent and warm water, but chemicals and machine washing are not recommended.

Maintaining and Caring for the Ultrasound Machine

The **transducer probes** must be wiped down and cleaned with a specific ultrasound cleaner to rid them of any excess ultrasound gel. All wires and connections must be inspected regularly, and any wires that are frayed or not working properly must be replaced. The central processing center must be regularly assessed to be sure that all buttons work correctly and that the image produced is of good quality. If the ultrasound machine contains a printer, it must be filled regularly with the correct paper to print the ultrasound images. The **ultrasound machine** itself must be stored in an area with low traffic that is dry so nothing leaks onto the machine. Some hospitals may even cover their machines to prevent dust and debris from accumulating.

Anesthesia

Classifications of Anesthetic Drugs

Indications for Benzodiazepines

Patients that have **epileptic fits** or **convulsions** may find treatment with **benzodiazepines** beneficial. Others who may benefit are patients that require emotionally traumatic cerebrospinal fluid tap or myelograms. Benzodiazepines are used as tranquilizers. Drugs containing benzodiazepines include the following: diazepam or Valium, zolazepam, midazolam or Versed, and lorazepam or Ativan. All of these variations of the drug may result in depression of the cardiovascular or respiratory systems. However, the remote risk has been determined to be acceptable for both geriatric and pediatric patients. Candidates found to derive the greatest benefits from the drug are elderly, depressed, and/or nervous patients. Benzodiazepines used in conjunction with ketamine may serve as an effective general anesthetic induction agent.

Diazepam is soluble when placed in oil. However, water does not dissolve diazepam. Diazepam may work faster when it is used in conjunction with other drugs. Opioids like butorphanol and oxymorphone easily mix with the midazolam. Midazolam is a medication that is known to be water-soluble.

Indications, Contraindications, and Side Effects of Phenothiazines

Occasionally, healthy animals will be scheduled for an **elective surgery**. These animals can be given phenothiazine, which provides a sedation effect. Phenothiazines include acepromazine and chlorpromazine. Phenothiazines are also given to patients in need of an antiemetic to stop nausea and vomiting.

Acepromazine is contraindicated for any patient with a history of convulsions, epilepsy, or head injuries. Acepromazine is known to decrease the threshold level for seizure activity.

Phenothiazine-induced peripheral vasodilation in patients with symptoms of shock or hypothermia may cause hypotension (i.e., low blood pressure). Patients with depression or liver or kidney diseases should not be prescribed phenothiazines. These drugs should only be given to the very young or old with careful observation. A lower dose or alternate medications such as benzodiazepines may be given instead.

Unexpected antihistamine effects can occur when animals are not given a medication-specific allergy test beforehand. Some animals experience adverse effects from taking phenothiazines. These effects include abnormal heartbeat, an unexpected reaction of excitability replacing the desired effect of sedation, and personality changes. These side effects normally subside within 48 hours of taking the medication.

Contraindications and Side Effects of A_2-Agonists

Ignoring the contraindications associated with α_2-agonists can produce serious risks for a patient. These risks include cardiac disease, respiratory disease, and liver or kidney disease. Dogs in a state of shock should not be given this medication. In addition, dogs in a state of incapacitation should not be treated with this class of drug. Other concurrent conditions such as extreme heat or fatigue can produce stress in the animal that can be harmful in conjunction with this medication. Intravenous administration of this medication may produce serious side effects. The animal may experience temporary behavioral and personality changes. Patients given this medication when suffering from dehydration may suffer from reduced pancreatic secretions, resulting in transient hyperglycemia. Opioids may exaggerate these side effects. The effects of xylazine can be reversed by Yohimbine or tolazoline. Another name for Yohimbine is Yobine. Atipamezole is a reversal agent used to counteract medetomidine. Another name for Atipamezole is Antisedan.

Indications for A2-Agonists

Medications that are α_2-agonists (alpha-2 agonists) provide sedation, analgesia, muscle relaxation, and anxiolysis. Some α_2-agonists include xylazine, romifidine, detomidine, and medetomidine. Xylazine is also known as Rompun and Anased. Detomidine is also known as Dormosedan. Medetomidine is also known as Domitor.

α_2-agonists are not to be used as preanesthetic medications. Instead, this medication is more suitable for general sedation purposes. The potential for side effects exceeds its benefits as a preanesthetic medication.

A vicious animal destined to be euthanized can be given α_2-agonists to produce a sedative effect. This medication is also beneficial when given as an analgesic or pain reliever. However, the relief will only last for about 16 to 20 minutes. There is a 50% chance that dogs will become nauseated to the point of vomiting when given this drug. This chance increases to 90% when the medication is given to cats. There are 2 α_2-agonists employed for treatments in horses. These are xylazine and detomidine. Ruminants may be given a significantly lower dose of xylazine.

Indications and Contraindications for Use of the Phencyclidines

Phencyclidines are available under the following names: Ketamine or Ketaset, Ketalean, Vetalar, and tiletamine hydrochloride. Tiletamine hydrochloride is a combination of zolazepam and Telazol. Another name for phencyclidines is cycloheximide. Patients that need to remain immobile will benefit from the application of this drug in their treatment. This drug is a beneficial preanesthetic when applied to the mucous membranes in the mouth or oral cavity.

Felines are the only animals that can take phencyclidines as a solitary form of medication. Other animals should never have this medication in solitary form. Dogs do not respond well to phencyclidine as a preanesthetic medication. It is best to avoid its use in patients with a history of seizure activity. It is best to avoid use for patients with suspected brain herniation or suspected perforation of the eye chamber. Visceral analgesia (pain relief for pain arising in the internal organs) is inadequate. However, the response is much better when given for the purpose of peripheral analgesia. It should be noted that the animal's recovery period after being given this drug may be extensive and unpredictable.

Opioids

The following medications are opioids: morphine, oxymorphone or Numorphan, butorphanol or Torbugesic and Torbutrol, hydromorphone, meperidine or Demerol, Pethidine, and fentanyl. Opioids have the following effects on the body: analgesia, sedation, dysphoria, euphoria, and excitability. These effects are precipitated by the drug's interaction between one or more dedicated receptors in the brain and spinal cord in various reversible combinations.

Opioids can act as an agonist or antagonist against each dedicated receptor. Preanalgesia medication is given to the patient as an induction agent or for a more balanced anesthesia transition. It also aids in controlling pain after the surgery. The effects of this medication can be reversed by giving the patient a pure antagonist agent. Opioids are categorized as narcotics in Canada and as Schedule II drugs in the United States. Neither country allows the dispensing of these medications without a prescription from a licensed physician or veterinarian.

Benefits and Harmful Effects of Barbiturates, Phenobarbital, and Pentobarbital in Treatment

Two common barbiturates are phenobarbital and pentobarbital. Barbiturates are considered sedative-hypnotic medications. This category of drugs can also be applied to depress respiration and the cardiovascular system in general. The effects of barbiturates are not reversible and no other medication can fully counterbalance their effects. Barbiturates bind to proteins in the body. Thus, the rate and amount of absorption can change when the level of plasma protein is altered.

The most widespread use of phenobarbital in veterinarian medicine is as a sedative for dogs. This drug can be used to calm animals that have reached a level of high excitement. It is also beneficial when used as an anticonvulsant. Varying the dosage may cause the drug to last for shorter or longer periods of time. When given in a high dose, it may have sedative effects for a period ranging up to 24 hours.

Pentobarbital has been replaced with ultra-short acting barbiturates. In the past it was often employed for the purpose of anesthesia inductions.

Indications and Contraindications for Neuroleptanalgesics and Barbiturates

Neuroleptanalgesics are combinations of analgesics with a neuroleptic tranquilizer. Versions of this drug include oxymorphone and acepromazine. Neuroleptanalgesics are employed when it is necessary to produce a deep sedative effect. The dose can be reduced for less extensive procedures, resulting in shorter durations. These shorter time frames may include treatments involving the suturing of an injury or the removal of porcupine quills. Neuroleptanalgesics are beneficial in the treatment of patients with conditions resulting in cardiac distress or shock. Naloxone or nalbuphine are reversal agents for neuroleptanalgesics.

Some side effects include hyperactivity, auditory stimuli, defecating, vomiting, panting, and in some cases, bradycardia.

Barbiturates can be used for sedation, as anticonvulsants, and for general anesthesia. This drug can serve as an induction agent prior to endotracheal intubation. The drug may be given as an inhalant anesthetic for maintenance purposes. In some cases the drug will produce unconsciousness in the patient.

Phenobarbital and Pentobarbital, and Propofol in Treatment

Phenobarbital is also used for seizure control. Sedation is achieved when the drug is given to the patient by intramuscular means. It has no negative effects upon tissue. The drug will reach its optimum effect about 5 minutes following the injection. Intravenous administration works more quickly, and the patient may respond after only 1 minute following administration. The patient should exhibit a strong effect from the medication. Sheep take longer to recover from this medication than any other type of animal. The majority of animal species will respond quickly and have an easier recovery period when given this drug. Pentobarbital may also be given with phenobarbital. While it is not an anticonvulsant, its sedative properties can reduce symptoms while waiting for the phenobarbital to take effect.

Propofol is also known as Diprivan or Rapinovet. This drug is useful in veterinary medicine for the following purposes: sedation, anesthesia induction, and anesthesia maintenance. It is also effective as an anticonvulsant. Propofol usually results in an induction procedure that is relatively easy and stress free.

Other Characteristics Associated with the Use of Propofol

The drug known as propofol is a short-acting sedative that is rapidly dispersed throughout the body, including the brain. Although it is oil-soluble, the medication is not retained in the muscle or fat and is metabolized out of the body very quickly by the liver. Metabolic clearance of this drug is faster than required for barbiturates. This is also the preferred preanesthetic induction medication for the sight hound breeds (i.e., whippets, greyhounds, Deerhounds, Irish Wolfhounds, Pharaoh Hounds, Afghan Hounds, Salukis, Borzois, Ibizan Hounds, Basenjis, Rhodesian Ridgebacks, and a select few others). It is also preferred for low body mass index (skinny) patients. Further, it is useful as an injectable maintenance anesthesia due to its fast-acting properties. It should be noted that propofol may cause tachycardia, bradycardia, temporary arterial and venous dilation, and depressed cardiac contractility. Typically, however, this medication has no effect on the cardiovascular system.

Characteristics of Guaifenesin and Fentanyl

Guaifenesin is also known as glycerol guaiacolate. This drug is described as a decongestant and antitussive. Guaifenesin works on the central nervous system and skeletal muscles as a relaxant. It is most often used for treatment in large animals. This medication can serve well for anesthesia induction and recovery. The animal will experience only mild effects on the respiratory and cardiac systems. While the drug is able to cross the placental barrier, the fetus should not experience any harmful effects.

Fentanyl is most often used as an analgesic (pain reliever). Unconsciousness can result from the use of fentanyl. Mainly, this drug is employed in conjunction with a tranquilizer, sedative, or benzodiazepine. It is considered to be an injectable induction agent. This drug does not cause problems with apnea. While it can cause contractility or cardiac output changes, it is not contraindicated for most high-risk patients. Fentanyl is usually classified as a neuroleptanalgesic.

Use of Etomidate for Anesthesia Induction

Etomidate is also known by the name Amidate. This drug is used as an anesthesia induction agent. It is considered to be safe and fast acting. It is dispersed rapidly throughout the body and does not build up in any tissues or organs. An animal is administered the drug through a repeated bolus or continuous infusion. During this time the animal may suffer from vomiting, diarrhea, and excitement. This can be attributed to the drug, the induction process, and/or postanesthesia effects. The animal may show brief signs of apnea (a pause in breathing), and thus should be monitored carefully.

Etomidate is a medication that can cross the placental barrier. However, it is usually harmless due to the liver's ability to metabolize the drug quickly. Etomidate is able to mildly depress the respiratory system. It can also have a rare side effect that results in extreme muscle rigidity and seizures in horses and cattle.

An animal may experience a great deal of pain when given an IV injection of etomidate. Thus, some veterinarians also administer lidocaine for pain control. The injection can also result in phlebitis or inflammation of the veins. However, inflammation more often occurs in smaller-sized veins.

Advantages of Inhalation Anesthesia Over Injectable Anesthesia

Inhalation anesthesia has certain advantages over injectable medications. These advantages include the anesthetic depths achieved and the ease in regulation. The patient's recovery is also considered to be more rapid. Further, inhalation anesthesia provides a drug that is metabolized at a nominal rate. This is a result of the body's ability to easily expel the excess medication through the respiration process.

A patient's airway is used when an endotracheal tube is applied. The patient will require assisted breathing at this juncture. Inhalation anesthesia should be delivered in an initial dose that is considered a fully safe concentration, and then increased as needed. This will allow the induction of anesthesia without undue depression of the respiratory and cardiovascular systems. Inhalation anesthesia typically has both analgesic and muscle relaxant properties, and both will benefit the patient. Patient recovery is considered to be more rapid due to the capacity of these medications to be quickly eliminated from the body. Inhalation medications do not persist or accumulate within the body's tissues or systems.

General Considerations When Using Inhalation Anesthetic Medication

There are certain factors that should be recognized when using inhalation anesthetic medications. First, the lungs absorb inhalation anesthesia as either gases or vapors. The medication is rapidly carried from the alveoli or air sacs in the lungs to the brain and body. During initial dispersal, this medication remains in the same chemical form (it has not yet been changed by the liver or other metabolic events). The amount ultimately delivered to the patient can be impacted by variables such as vapor pressure, boiling point, and the anesthetic delivery system used. The medication has to be carried through the lungs subject to alveolar partial pressure, the inspired concentration, and the alveolar concentration. To be effective, the tissues must be able to readily absorb the medication. Delivery from the lungs to the brain is contingent upon the drug's solubility, the relative rate of blood flow in the arteries and tissues, the strength of the anesthetic, the tissue type, and the blood saturation of the tissues.

MAC is the acronym for minimal alveolar concentration. This abbreviation stands for the level of anesthetic vapor concentration in the lungs needed to prevent a motor response to surgical pain in 50% of all patients. The potency level rises as the MAC number is reduced.

Advantages and Disadvantages of Isoflurane

MAC is the acronym for Isoflurane is known to induce only insignificant metabolic changes in the liver. Isoflurane is also considered to be a prudent treatment as related to the cardiovascular system. Indeed, this drug exhibits low arrhythmogenicity even while simultaneously enhancing cardiac productivity. Isoflurane is a medication that rapidly induces anesthesia, and with a shorter recovery period than many other medications. The dosage of this drug can be also be adjusted easily, given the drug's low solubility characteristics. In fact, it offers a much quicker dosage adjustment and response time than that available through the drug halothane.

Even so, there are some problems associated with isoflurane. These issues pertain to respiratory depression, difficult recovery periods, and rising costs, as both halothane and isoflurane require an out-of-circle precision vaporizer to raise vapor pressures. Isoflurane produces blood pressures associated with normal rates when linked with vasodilation.

The minimal alveolar concentration (MAC) of isoflurane for canines is 1.2%. The MAC of isoflurane in cats is at 1.6%. This refers to the level of anesthetic vapor concentration in the lungs needed to prevent a motor response to surgical pain in 50% of all patients. The potency level rises when the MAC is reduced.

Advantages and Disadvantages of Halothane

MAC is the acronym for minimal alveolar concentration. One of the benefits of halothane involves its modest respiratory depression effects. Further, it is not considered to be nephrotoxic, and can be mask induced.

Some drawbacks of halothane anesthesia are found in the risk to the patient of cardiac arrhythmias, hypotension from cardiac depression, minimal analgesic or pain-relieving impact, and hepatotoxic effects. The patient should be given an out-of-circle precision vaporizer to maintain the required elevated vapor pressure. This practice provides the patient with the safest exposure to Halothane.

Methoxyflurane has a lower solubility factor than halothane. This creates a faster rate of anesthesia induction and recovery level for the patient. The veterinarian can thus respond to adjustments needed in the concentration levels at a faster pace.

The minimal alveolar concentration (MAC) of halothane is 0.8%. This refers to the level of anesthetic vapor concentration in the lungs needed to prevent a motor response to surgical pain in 50% of all patients. The potency level rises when the MAC is reduced.

Advantages and Disadvantages of Desflurane

The MAC rating for Desflurane is 7.2%. MAC is the acronym for minimal alveolar concentration. This refers to the level Desflurane promotes rapid anesthesia induction and recovery. This can be attributed to the drug's low solubility and consequent rapid dispersion. It does not display a tendency for either hepatotoxicity or nephrotoxicity.

Desflurane requires the use of a unique, electrically heated vaporizer in its administration. This type of vaporizer can be extremely costly to purchase. Further, Desflurane has a pungent odor that can irritate the respiratory tract. Thus, patients tend to cough and hold their breath when being administered this drug. Some animal species will experience a malignant hyperthermia from the use of this drug. Other patients may recover before treatment is finished. Patients that experience a premature recovery will need more sedation given immediately.

The MAC rating for Desflurane is 7.2%. MAC is the acronym for minimal alveolar concentration. This refers to the level of anesthetic vapor concentration in the lungs needed to prevent a motor response to surgical pain in 50% of all patients. The potency level rises when the MAC number is reduced.

Advantages and Disadvantages of Sevoflurane

Sevoflurane is considered to have a very low solubility, and therefore provides speedy anesthesia induction and recovery periods. Further, it does not readily induce cardiac arrhythmias. The animal should also respond with a superior rate of muscle relaxation. The drug has an analgesic quality used to bring pain relief to the patient.

Sevoflurane is considered to be a particularly appropriate analgesic inhalant for the majority of avian or bird species. Sevoflurane is considered to be less overpowering than other inhalants. Thus, it leaves the patient with no symptoms resembling a hangover, as might otherwise be expected from the use of a psychoactive drug.

Sevoflurane and isoflurane both produce respiratory depression in the patient. Sevoflurane can also cross the placental barrier. This can result in concurrent fetal depression. Finally, this drug is typically more costly than either halothane or isoflurane.

Sevoflurane is MAC rated at 2.4%. MAC is the acronym for minimal alveolar concentration. This refers to the level of anesthetic vapor concentration in the lungs needed to prevent a motor response to surgical pain in 50% of all patients. The potency level rises when the MAC number is reduced.

Pre-Procedural

Preanesthetic Blood Work

Before a patient undergoes a surgical procedure, it is important to run **preanesthetic blood work.** Preanesthetic blood work may include a CBC, chemistry panel, and electrolytes. The major reasons that these tests are important is because a CBC can detect clotting disorders or an abnormally high WBC count indicating infection, which would put the patient at risk for an anesthetic procedure and surgery. Certain anesthetic agents will metabolize through the liver and be excreted via the urine, and a chemistry panel will indicate the kidney (blood urea nitrogen, creatinine, phosphorus) and liver (alanine transaminase, alkaline phosphatase, and bilirubin) function. If the chemistry panel shows an abnormal level of kidney and liver enzymes, this can mean that the patient could have a slower, abnormal recovery from anesthesia and the anesthetic plan may need to be altered. Electrolytes, including potassium, sodium, and chloride, will indicate signs of dehydration as well.

Fasting Before Anesthetic Procedures

The patient will need to be fasted (**no food or water**) commonly after 10 p.m. the night prior to the anesthetic event. The reason for fasting the patient is because most anesthetic drugs cause vomiting. While the patient is under general anesthesia, the larynx relaxes, which is the part of the body that prevents matter from going down into the trachea. If the patient were to vomit while anesthetized, the vomited material could risk going down into the trachea to the lungs (aspiration) rather than into the esophagus to the stomach. If the patient does aspirate, this can lead to pneumonia.

Explaining Anesthetic Procedures to Alleviate a Client's Concerns

When the patient arrives for an **anesthetic procedure**, the veterinary technician and the veterinarian will perform a full physical exam and evaluate the patient's medical history. Based on the patient's health status, species, and weight, a premedication protocol will be implemented. The patient will be premedicated prior to the surgery to sedate and provide analgesia preemptively. Once the patient is adequately sedated, they are induced to put them under general anesthesia, commonly with an IV drug agent. Once induced, the patient is intubated and maintained on a low level of anesthetic inhalant. From the moment of induction, the patient is continuously monitored by a licensed veterinary technician who will be adjusting the vaporizer and oxygen settings as needed and manually assessing vital signs including the heart rate, respiration rate, mucous membrane color, and capillary refill time, pulse quality and strength, and temperature. Monitoring equipment will also be used, including blood pressure monitoring, ECG, capnography, and pulse oximetry. After the surgery is completed, the patient will be extubated once they show signs of waking up (swallowing). During the recovery phase, the veterinary technician will keep a close eye on the patient and continue to monitor vital signs until the patient is alert and standing.

Placing an ET in the Patient

First, the patient must be sternal with the head and neck extended in a straight line so you can see the larynx. The restrainer can hold the patient's head and place their thumb and forefinger behind the canines on the maxilla and pull the head up and out straight. The person who will be intubating will pull the tongue out of the mouth over the lower incisors and open the mouth wide. A laryngoscope should be used because it has a light to better see as well as free up the epiglottis if it is hidden behind the soft palate. Once the correct **ET** is chosen, it is inserted into the trachea and not advanced past the thoracic inlet. Use a tie (either gauze string or an IV line) to tie around the ET tube and then up behind the canines and tie behind the patient's ears or on top of their nose. To determine if the ET tube is placed correctly, you can watch for the reservoir bag to inflate and deflate with respirations, watch for fog to appear in the ET tube from respirations, or confirm with capnography because the presence of CO_2 means that the ET tube is placed correctly.

Inflating an ET Cuff Correctly on an Anesthetized Patient

In order to correctly **inflate an ET cuff**, you will need two people. The cuff is inflated with air from a syringe that attaches to the cuff. A 3 ml syringe should be used for cats, and a 10 ml syringe can be used for dogs with larger ET tubes. Once the patient is intubated, one person will close the pop-off valve and squeeze the reservoir bag up to 20 cm H_2O while the anesthetist listens close to the patient's mouth for leaks. If a leak is heard while squeezing the reservoir bag, then a little more air may be needed to inflate the cuff. Open the pop-off valve when reinflating the cuff and after no leaks are heard. The person squeezing the reservoir bag should say "breathing" when they squeeze and "release" when the bag relaxes because a leak will only be detected on inspiration and the bag would empty when squeezed as the air goes past the tube into the oral cavity.

Benefits of Preoxygenation

Preoxygenation can be done around 5 minutes prior to induction by delivering pure oxygen to the patient through a mask via the anesthetic machine. Preoxygenation aids to replace nitrogen in the patient's lungs with oxygen, reducing the risk of possible hypoxemia that can result from induction agents. Hypoxemia is the insufficient oxygenation of arterial blood in the body resulting in poorly oxygenated vital organs in the body, causing cyanosis in the patient. Brachycephalic breeds will benefit from being preoxygenated especially given the fact that intubation may take longer to accomplish. Obese and pregnant patients will also require preoxygenation because they are at risk for oxygen desaturation.

Advantages and Disadvantages of Preanesthetic Medication

Pre-anesthetic medication lowers the stress level of an animal, when it is given before a procedure. This medication produces a state that supports a smooth induction and effective recovery period. The patient that receives a preanesthetic may well benefit from a reduced need for anesthesia induction and maintenance medications. Preanesthetic medication may also produce some intraoperative and postoperative analgesic effects. These medications have also been known to lower certain secretion levels and to reduce certain autonomic reflexes. This effect gives the handler a more manageable animal that is easier and safer to handle.

However, the application of preanesthetic medication can come with some drawbacks. Specifically, time and medication cost factors are involved. However, some of these costs can be counterbalanced though the reduced need for subsequent induction and maintenance agents. Most preanesthetic medications will reach maximum effectiveness levels approximately 20 minutes after an intramuscular injection.

Additional Advantages and Disadvantages of Preanesthetic Medication

Pre-anesthetic medication can remain effective for a period of up to 2 hours, and can be given to the patient by a variety of means. The most common administration is through an intramuscular (or IM) injection. An intravenous (or IV) injection works faster than other methods. However, an IV injection should be given with careful consideration, as administration via this route may induce certain temporary behavior and personality changes. Various side effects from preanesthetic drugs are associated with xylazine, acepromazine, opioids, and diazepam.

Anticholinergic medications may be used to block nerve impulses from reaching the vagus nerve. Examples of anticholinergics include atropine and glycopyrrolate. Pharmacologically blocking this nerve with a vagolytic medication is necessary when the veterinarian is treating bradycardia in a patient. Anticholinergics and opioids can be used in conjunction with each other.

The synergistic effects of these drugs can produce lower levels of salivary and tear secretions. Anticholinergics can also diminish bronchodilation. Contraindications associated with anticholinergics include administration to patients at high risk for tachycardia (often geriatric patients), those with a history of congestive heart failure, and patients with constipation or ileus.

Anesthetic Process

Stages and Planes of Anesthesia

The first **stage of anesthesia** is the voluntary excitement stage, which begins at induction. The patient is conscious and may display the fight-or-flight response. Stage two is labeled involuntary excitement, and it starts when the patient goes unconscious up until breathing is established. Surgical anesthesia is the third stage, consisting of three planes. Plane one is light anesthesia in which the patient is able to be intubated and short exams and surgical procedures can take place. Plane two is medium anesthesia in which most surgical procedures can take place. Finally, plane three is deep anesthesia and is not normally necessary for most surgical procedures. The fourth stage of anesthesia is excessively deep, and if the patient gets to this stage, you must react quickly because this can lead to cardiovascular and respiratory depression and can lead to death.

Reflexes That Are Used to Determine Anesthetic Depth

There are **reflexes** that the technician can assess on the patient to determine anesthetic depth. The palpebral reflex is determined by lightly touching the medial canthus of the eye to stimulate blinking. If the patient still displays the palpebral reflex, the patient may be too lightly sedated for certain procedures. With the pupillary light reflex, the pupils respond to light by constricting. The pupillary light reflex disappears during medium anesthesia, which is stage 3 and plane 2. The pedal reflex is when the patient pulls its leg back in response to pinching between the toes, and it may be too light for certain procedures. Jaw tone is resistance given when opening the patient's mouth, and it means that the patient is too light to intubate. The pharyngeal reflex enables swallowing, and the laryngeal reflex enables coughing and closing of the larynx.

Hypothermia Effects on the Body Under Anesthesia

Hypothermia is a drop in body temperature below the normal range: Hypothermia is considered to be mild until the core temperature drops below 98 °F. Moderate hypothermia is 95-98 °F, severe is 92-95 °F, and critical is below 92 °F. Hypothermia affects several different areas of the body, including the cardiovascular, respiratory, and metabolic systems, as well as decreasing immune function, which in turn increases the risk of infection. While under anesthesia, if the patient becomes hypothermic, their metabolic rate decreases causing slower drug metabolism and elimination, leading to longer recovery times. When the body temperature gets as low as 95 °F, vasodilation occurs and leads to hypotension (low blood pressure); at temperatures any lower than this, the body can't regulate its own body temperature. When a patient is hypothermic, the blood thickness and PCV increase, which increases the work for the myocardium (the muscular tissue of the heart).

Interpreting the Mucous Membrane Status and Capillary Refill Time

Check the patient's **mucous membranes** easily by lifting the lip and looking at the gums. The mucous membrane color represents the blood flow to the tissues. If the patient's mucous membranes appear pale, this could mean that the patient is anemic, and it represents poor perfusion. Mucous membranes that appear blue or purple (cyanosis) mean that there is a decreased amount of oxygen in the tissues; this is a medical emergency. If mucous membranes are yellow, this commonly indicates a liver problem, when the bile is not being excreted by the liver but is instead accumulating in the tissues, giving them a yellow color. The **capillary refill time (CRT)** is determined by applying pressure with a finger onto a spot on the gums, stopping blood flow to that area; then lift the finger pressure off and allow the blood to return to the area, counting the number of seconds it takes for the color in the area to return. A normal CRT is <2 seconds, and if the CRT is more than 2 seconds, the patient could be experiencing hypotension, vasodilation, or hypothermia.

IV Induction Agents vs. Gas Anesthetic

Delivering gas anesthetic to induce a patient via a mask or chamber should be avoided because even though using a lower dose of inhalant gas during maintenance anesthesia is safe, using a high dose to induce the patient is not. Inhalant drugs used as the only anesthetic agent cause extreme dose-dependent hypotension, low body temperature, and hypoventilation. The patient will go through the excitement phase and release catecholamines, which causes secondary effects such as hypertension and tachycardia that can cause complications to the patient and even result in cardiac arrest. **Induction** takes longer and requires more gas anesthetic to get the patient asleep due to catecholamine release, and when the patient does actually reach the end of induction and is asleep, it is too deeply anesthetized. Maintenance is also dangerous if only inhalant gas has been used because the patient has no analgesia to alleviate responses to surgical stimuli so high inhalant concentrations are needed to keep the patient under anesthesia. Along with being dangerous to the patient, masking down the patient exposes the staff to dangerous anesthetic gas, which can cause irritability, headaches, and other health issues.

Anesthetic Plan Developed for the Geriatric Patient

A complete blood panel is recommended for **geriatric patients** to evaluate kidney and liver function, as well as a complete blood cell count and electrolyte panel. Lowered drug dosing will be used to lower cardiovascular effects and lower the amount of work on specific organs for elimination of these drugs. The geriatric patient should be placed on a warming device such as a heating pad with a blanket between the pad and the patient's body, IV fluid warmer, and foot covers to prevent heat loss because these patients are more susceptible to hypothermia because of less body fat. Geriatric patients need to have their temperature monitored closely during the procedure as well as during recovery. Hypothermia leads to hypotension and arrhythmias, and the vital signs must be watched closely because they will greatly affect the geriatric patient.

Anesthetic Plan for the Brachycephalic Breed

A complete physical exam must be done for the **brachycephalic breed** prior to administration of pre-medications, including full panel blood work, auscultation of the heart and lungs, as well as an evaluation of the degree of upper airway obstruction. Any abnormal upper airway sounds or heart murmurs should be noted because this will affect the drugs used as well as the monitoring of the patient. An SpO_2 reading should be taken in room air on the patient to get a baseline reading of the patient's normal reading because brachycephalic breeds normally have a lower SpO_2 reading (93%–95%) than other breeds. Premedication should include an anticholinergic, which will prevent bradycardia and will dry the patient's oral secretions, along with a sedative that provides analgesia and buprenorphine or morphine. The brachycephalic breed must be preoxygenated for 5 minutes prior to induction, and a laryngoscope must be used to intubate because it will be difficult to visualize the back of the throat. It is necessary to wait until they are alert and swallowing to extubate, and they must be closely monitored during recovery until they are standing and bright, alert, and responsive (BAR).

Anticholinergics in Anesthesia and Their Contraindications

Anticholinergics such as atropine or glycopyrrolate are used as part of the premedication protocol as a way to avoid the effects of the parasympathetic reflexes. These drugs block the vagal reflexes, preventing cardiac arrhythmias, drying out secretions, and reducing gastric reflux while under anesthesia. Dosing must be accurate because if given at a higher dose, these drugs can cause tachycardia and low dosing can cause an AV block. They are contraindicated in patients that have a preexisting tachycardia, any cardiac disease, and patients that have GI stasis. Anticholinergics are recommended in pediatric patients (patients younger than 6 months of age) due to the fact that they rely on the heart rate to maintain CO, any airway surgery because this can stimulate a vagal reflex, as well as patients who are brachycephalic breeds because they commonly have a high vagal tone. Anticholinergics are also used in emergency situations administered IV with a rapid onset of action.

Analgesics in Anesthesia

Analgesia will give the patient pain relief by inhibiting pain stimuli from connecting with the pain pathway so that the patient has no perception of the pain. Analgesia should begin prior to the surgical procedure as part of the premedication protocol. Every patient will have its own analgesic protocol after a full physical exam, blood work, and evaluation of medical history. Certain drugs may not be suitable for some patients; for example, Rimadyl (an NSAID) should not be given if the patient is taking prednisone because it is contraindicated. Alpha 2 agonists should not be used in patients with heart disease, and some drugs will need to be used in conjunction with other drugs to provide appropriate pain relief. A multimodal approach to analgesia is most effective, in which different classes of drugs are used or combined to block different areas of the pain pathway to provide adequate analgesia to the patient.

Difference Between a Rebreathing and Nonrebreathing System

The two main anesthetic circuits are **rebreathing and nonrebreathing** systems, and their main function is to deliver oxygen and anesthetic gas to the patient while eliminating carbon dioxide. Rebreathing circuits are recommended for patients weighing more than 10 pounds; they work to push the expired gas through the soda lime canister, which absorbs the carbon dioxide, and then it is rebreathed by the patient. A rebreathing system forces the patient to open the one-way valves, which provide slight resistance, so the patient must work to overcome that. In a nonrebreathing circuit, the oxygen flows through the flow meter and into the vaporizer, and then the gases leaving the vaporizer flow through the hose straight to the patient. Exhaled gases in a nonrebreathing circuit pass through another hose and flow to the reservoir bag but not a CO_2 absorber, and then this gas is released into the scavenger system. Because the gas flows in and out in the nonrebreathing circuit, there is no resistance for the patient to overcome. A higher fresh gas flow is required with the nonrebreathing circuit because the fresh gas has to push the expired gas away from the patient so that it is not rebreathed.

Implementing an Anesthetic Plan Specific for the Pediatric or Neonatal Patient

Neonatal refers to patients younger than 4 months of age, and **pediatric** refers to those patients 6 months of age and younger. Pediatric and neonatal patients' cardiac output and blood pressure maintenance solely rely on the heart rate and stroke volume, so if the heart rate decreases (bradycardia), then the cardiac output decreases and so does blood pressure. Pediatric patients have a higher chance of hypoxia during apnea due to their reduced pulmonary reserve. Pediatric and neonate patients have a more pliable rib cage and weak intercostal muscles; therefore, they use more energy and effort for breathing, which could lead to airway collapse and respiratory fatigue. Pediatric patients are prone to hypoglycemia because of their minimal glycogen stores, so their blood glucose should be monitored, and they should only fast for a few hours before an anesthetic procedure as well as be fed a couple of hours after recovery. Pediatric and neonatal patients are prone to hypothermia due to their immature thermoregulatory system, so monitoring temperature pre, peri, and post anesthesia is vital.

Implement Monitoring of Vital Signs in the Anesthetized Patient

Once the patient is induced, the technician hooks the patient up to the anesthetic machine with the gas and oxygen flow and immediately checks the patient's heart rate and respiratory rate. Adjust the vaporizer setting as needed. The **monitoring** equipment used will include blood pressure, ECG, capnography, and pulse oximetry. Every 5 minutes, the technician should be manually checking the patient's vital signs, including listening to the heart rate, respiration rate, and lung sounds using a stethoscope. The technician should be assessing the mucous membrane color and the capillary refill time, along with the patient's pulse strength and quality every 5 minutes. The oxygen and vaporizer settings should also be checked every 5 minutes and adjusted according to the patient's depth and status. The patient's temperature should be measured every 5 minutes as well, and as soon as there is a decrease, steps should be taken to stabilize the temperature. The technician will also be assessing the patient's ECG reading to look for any abnormalities.

Classes of Sedative and Tranquilizer Drugs Used in the Premedication Protocol

Tranquilizers such as acepromazine or midazolam or **sedatives** such as medetomidine can also be added to the premedication protocol, remembering that tranquilizers and sedatives will sedate the patient but sedatives provide analgesia as well. Acepromazine causes vasodilation leading to hypotension, as well as decreases the patient's seizure threshold, but it also is an antiemetic and an antihistamine. Medetomidine is an α_2 agonist sedative and muscle relaxant that also provides analgesia and can be reversed with atipamezole (Antisedan). Medetomidine use will lower the amount of other anesthetic agents needed for the patient such as inhalants and induction agents. Medetomidine is contraindicated for use in sick patients because it has adverse effects on the cardiovascular system. Benzodiazepines such as midazolam are used for sedation, they are anticonvulsants, and they inhibit anxiety, but they do not provide analgesia so they should be combined with a drug that does. Benzodiazepines are contraindicated in patients with kidney or liver disease because the drug is metabolized mainly through the liver and eliminated via the urine.

Two Classes of Opioids Used in the Premedication Protocol

Opioids consist of two classes: pure mu agonists including morphine, hydromorphone, and fentanyl and partial mu agonists including buprenorphine. Because morphine and hydromorphone cause vomiting in most patients, they should not be used with patients who have obstructions of the esophagus or GI tract, and they also should not be used in patients with eye issues because vomiting causes an increase in cranial pressure. Opioid agonists such as morphine are highly addictive with the potential for abuse and are classified as a Schedule II drug. Buprenorphine has a long duration of action and provides less analgesia than pure mu agonists, but it will provide less respiratory and cardiovascular depression. Butorphanol is an agonist-antagonist, meaning it is an antagonist at the mu receptor, preventing activation. Butorphanol is also an agonist at the kappa receptor meaning it activates these receptors. Therefore, because butorphanol is an agonist-antagonist, it partially reverses the effects of full agonists. Naloxone is used to reverse the effects of other opioids because it is an opioid antagonist.

Routes of Administration for Pre-Medications and Postoperative Medications

The most common **routes of administration** for premedication drugs are IV, IM, and SQ. The first factor to consider when choosing a route of administration is which route the specific drug is labeled for because some drugs may not be given IV and others may not be given SQ or IM. For example, diazepam should only be given IV because of its solubility. Another factor to consider is how long do you want the onset of action to be, because the IV route is the fastest whereas SQ would be the slowest. An antibiotic injection may be given perioperatively if needed, such as in an orthopedic surgery. You may be required to administer cefazolin, which is given IV slowly over the course of 10 minutes. An injection for pain is often required after any painful procedure, for example, carprofen (an NSAID) is given SQ and oral medications will be given by the owner at home starting the next day for continued pain relief.

Calculating for the Correct-Sized Reservoir Bag for the Patient

To choose the correct-size **reservoir bag,** you take the patient's tidal volume and multiply that by six. The patient's tidal volume, which is the amount of inhaled and exhaled air with each breath, is normally around 20 ml/kg. For example, for a dog that weighs 10 kg: 10 kg × 20 ml/kg = 200 ml × 6 = 1,200 ml. Then, to convert milliliters to liters, because rebreathing bags are weighed in liters: 1,200 ml ÷ 1000 = 1.2 liters. So a 1 liter bag would be used for that patient.

Importance of a Reservoir Bag (Rebreathing Bag) in the Breathing System

The **rebreathing bag** permits fresh and exhaled gas to accumulate and be available for the patient's next breath. It is important to have the correct-sized rebreathing bag for the patient because if the bag is too small the patient won't be able to make a full breath before using up the gas in the bag and deflating it first. If the rebreathing bag is too big for the patient, then the anesthetic system's volume increases, which prolongs the time to change the inspired anesthetic concentration. The rebreathing bag is also used to manually breathe for the patient that is not adequately breathing on its own under anesthesia or in emergency situations when the patient must be intubated and manually ventilated.

Importance of an IV Catheter

An **IV catheter** provides direct access to the vein. It is important to place an IV catheter in every patient going under anesthesia as well as hospitalized patients. An emergency could happen at any time while the patient is under anesthesia, when emergency medications such as epinephrine or atropine must be administered intravenously. Placing an IV catheter prior to surgery is more efficient than having to place one during an emergency when circulatory collapse occurs most of the time, leading to low blood pressure and making it harder to place an IV catheter. An IV catheter is also useful when administering fluids to a patient under anesthesia to maintain blood pressure by allowing the movement of blood to the body's vital organs. While patients are hospitalized, it is ideal to have an IV catheter placed for fluid therapy and to ease administration of IV medications.

Manual Monitoring While the Patient Is Under Anesthesia

Certain vital signs must be **manually monitored** and recorded every 5 minutes while the patient is under anesthesia, including heart rate, respiratory rate, pulse strength and quality, mucous membrane evaluation, capillary refill time, temperature, vaporizer setting, and oxygen levels. If the patient is experiencing a sinus arrhythmia under anesthesia, the ECG monitor may not be able to catch every beat, so taking a heart rate using a stethoscope is important. The respiratory rate given on the monitor may pick up inaccurate movements, so manually measuring the patient's respiratory rate is important as well as listening to lung sounds with a stethoscope to make sure that they are clear. The mucous membrane color and capillary refill time can only be evaluated by the technician because a machine cannot observe this. Taking the patient's temperature every 5 minutes during a procedure will help you to notice a decrease early so warming techniques can be applied such as warm blankets, etc., to prevent hypothermia.

Perioperative Sinus Bradycardia

When the patient's heart rate decreases to fewer than 60 bpm in large dogs, less than 80 bpm in medium to small dogs, and less than 100 bpm in cats, this is **sinus bradycardia**. Heart abnormalities, hypothyroidism, and hyperkalemia can all cause sinus bradycardia. Common causes of sinus bradycardia are a result of low body temperature and the patient being too deep under anesthesia, which is why vital sign monitoring is important. A patient with sinus bradycardia can exhibit hypotension and poor tissue perfusion. If sinus bradycardia is not treated with atropine, which can be given to increase the heart rate, it can lead to a longer recovery time due to decreased drug metabolism through the kidneys.

Perioperative Sinus Tachycardia

Sinus tachycardia is defined as an abnormally high heart rate, which would be more than 200 bpm in cats and more than 160 bpm in medium-sized dogs. The ventricles need to dilate and fill in between heart beats, but when the heart rate is too fast, there is not enough time so the stroke volume decreases, causing hypotension. If the heart cannot compensate for the decreased stroke volume caused by sinus tachycardia, then the oxygen demand increases. Certain drugs, such as anticholinergics, can cause sinus tachycardia, as well as the patient becoming stimulated during a surgical procedure due to inadequate anesthetic depth. Constant monitoring of the patient's anesthetic depth is vital, and the vaporizer setting may need to be adjusted accordingly if the patient is not under a correct anesthetic depth. Adequate pain control will need to be administered as well to prevent the patient from having an increased heart rate in response to a painful stimulus.

Managing a Patient with Cardiac Disease Under Anesthesia

Stress-reducing techniques prior to surgery should be implemented because stress activates the sympathetic nervous system, which in turn causes the heart to work harder. If the patient is under stress during induction, this can cause increased blood pressure, tachycardia, and an increased oxygen demand on the heart. If the patient is struggling during induction, this causes a release of catecholamines (hormones including epinephrine, norepinephrine, and dopamine) and can lead to arrhythmias. Providing stress-free techniques in the hospital as well as preop analgesia will benefit the patient by decreasing the amount of induction agent needed and lowering the percentage of inhalant. Patients with **cardiac disease** should be preoxygenated before induction to increase oxygen saturation during. Patients with cardiac disease will need their IV fluid therapy given to effect, and it should be given carefully to avoid fluid overload, which can cause congestive heart failure. Monitoring the patient's blood pressure, oxygenation, and lung sounds will need to be done to determine if fluid therapy should be stopped or slowed.

Fluid Therapy During Anesthesia

The decision to have a patient receive **fluid therapy** during anesthesia depends on the patient's age, physical condition, as well as the length and type of anesthetic procedure. Fluid therapy during an anesthetic procedure makes up for the ongoing fluid loss as well as provides cardiac support and allows the body to maintain fluid volume for longer procedures. While the patient is under anesthesia, the anesthetic gases and premedications can lower blood pressure, whereas if the patient receives IV fluid therapy, it will offset this decrease. Low blood pressure can result in kidney damage, so IV fluids are critical in keeping blood pressure up so the vital organs are properly oxygenated. IV fluids also help to protect the kidneys and hydrate the patient because fasting for surgical procedures can lead to dehydration as well as blood loss from certain procedures.

Sometimes the patient's body temperature will decrease while under anesthesia, and administering warm IV fluids can keep the patient at an ideal body temperature. IV fluids also aid in the excretion of anesthetic from the kidneys and liver, which leads to a smooth recovery.

Medical History for Develop an Anesthetic Plan

A complete patient physical exam and **medical history** are necessary to be able to provide an appropriate anesthetic plan. Any chronic diseases that the patient may have, such as kidney or liver disease, must be noted. Some anesthetic drugs are metabolized through the liver and excreted via the urine, so these drugs should be avoided. If the patient has a history of cardiovascular disease, certain premedications such as dexmedetomidine should not be used. Any medications that the patient is currently taking are necessary to know because some medications may not be taken together, for example, steroids and NSAIDs. If the patient has a history of seizures, then certain anticonvulsant drugs may be added to the premedications.

Responseif the Patient Will Not Remain Anesthetized

If a patient will **not remain anesthetized**, you must check their respirations. If they exhibit shallow respirations, this could lead to the patient being under a light stage of anesthesia possibly due to the gas anesthetic not entering the lungs. The patient may need to be given manual breaths with oxygen and gas anesthetic until adequate anesthetic depth is reached. The ET may too short, or the cuff may not be properly inflated. Vaporizer settings and oxygen settings must be checked. If the gas anesthetic is too low, the patient could be too lightly under anesthesia and painful stimuli such as an incision could easily arouse the patient.

Response If the Patient Is Dyspneic and/or Cyanotic Under Anesthesia

Dyspnea is when the body is not able to obtain enough oxygen using a normal respiratory effort, and **cyanosis** is inadequate tissue oxygenation (the patient's tissues will appear blue/purple). Common causes of respiratory distress while under anesthesia could be an empty oxygen tank, the oxygen flowmeter may be turned all the way down, or it could be a damaged circuit. An airway obstruction or respiratory disease such as pulmonary edema may be a cause as well. The anesthetic depth must be evaluated as well: If the patient is inhaling an excessive amount of gas anesthetic, they may be too deep. If respiratory distress is noticed, the first step is to deliver 100% oxygen to the patient and turn the vaporizer off. Ventilate with oxygen until the patient has a normal mucous membrane color (pink/moist) and the SpO_2 reading is within normal limits (> 95%). Always alert the attending veterinarian in this emergency situation.

Cardiac Arrest on a Patient Under Anesthesia

If the patient under anesthesia has no heart rate and is not breathing, the first thing to do is turn off the vaporizer and alert the veterinarian. Signs that could indicate oncoming cardiac arrest include low blood pressure and weak or irregular pulse, cyanosis, and a trend in a decreasing respiratory rate that is noticed during 5-minute-interval monitoring. **Cardiac arrest** is when there is no pulse or heartbeat, apnea, and a loss of certain reflexes such as the palpebral reflex. The patient's eyes will appear fixed and wide open with dilated pupils that are unresponsive to light. In order to respond quickly to this emergency, it is critical that the person monitoring take manual heart rates, respiratory rates, and check the mucous membrane color and capillary refill time as well as feel pulses for the duration of anesthesia to notice trends such as a slow decrease in respirations. Monitoring equipment is helpful, but can be unreliable; for example, an ECG will appear normal even if the heart is not contracting.

Ventricular Premature Contraction (VPC)

Ventricular premature contractions (VPCs) happen before the heart has time to fill making it harder for the heart to pump blood effectively. VPCs occur in the ventricles of the heart, and when more than three happen in a row this causes ventricular tachycardia. Less blood is pumped to the body as a result of ventricular tachycardia because of the VPCs making it harder to pump effectively; therefore, the heart can stop if the abnormal beat happens at the wrong time. Cats are normally treated for an underlying issue rather than treating the VPCs because they are rarely life threatening in cats. Dogs that present with a serious arrhythmia are normally hospitalized and given IV lidocaine to stabilize the arrhythmia. Once the underlying disease is treated (if it is curable), then the VPCs will go away, but with a chronic disease, the prognosis will depend on how well the arrhythmia can be controlled. Oral drugs used to control arrhythmias in dogs include sotalol and mexiletine, and cats may be prescribed atenolol or sotalol.

Response If the Patient's Blood Pressure Drops While Under Anesthesia

The main focus is the mean arterial **blood pressure** while the patient is under anesthesia, which should range from 80 to 100 mm Hg. If the MAP is less than 60 mm Hg, this can lead to delayed recovery from anesthesia, decreased metabolism of drugs via the kidneys, renal failure, and CNS abnormalities. Severe untreated hypotension can lead to cardiac and respiratory arrest. The first step is identifying the cause of hypotension in the anesthetized patient. Many anesthetic drugs affect blood pressure, so if the patient is otherwise healthy with normal vital signs other than BP, then anesthetic drugs are the likely culprit. If the drug has a reversal agent, then it should be administered or the anesthetic depth should be lowered. IV fluids are to be administered at 10 ml/kg/hr for the anesthetized patient in order to compensate for vasodilation and replace the patient's ongoing losses. If hypovolemia is the cause, then a bolus of IV fluids should be administered and the patient's BP should be reevaluated. If the patient is experiencing blood loss, this should be replaced at 3 ml crystalloid fluids to 1 ml of blood loss, whereas Hetastarch may be required for an extreme blood loss.

Adjusting the Vaporizer Setting for the Anesthetized Patient

Directly after the patient is induced, the **vaporizer** will be set at or higher than (~3%) for a few minutes to reach an adequate anesthetic plane. However, if certain drugs such as dexmedetomidine were given as a premedication, then the vaporizer setting may be lower (1.5%) right after induction because dexmedetomidine causes cardiovascular and respiratory depression. Every 5 minutes or more frequently, the vaporizer setting should be checked along with the patient's vital signs and adjusted accordingly. If the patient is under a light plane of anesthesia showing signs of an increased heart rate or is responding to the palpebral reflex, the vaporizer setting should be increased and the patient should be reevaluated after a couple of minutes. If the patient appears to be too deep under anesthesia showing signs of a decreasing heart rate or lower respiratory rate, then the vaporizer setting should be turned down accordingly and the patient should be reevaluated continuously until the patient is at the appropriate depth.

Regulating the Patient's Body Temperature Under Anesthesia

Using large amounts of scrubbing solutions or using alcohol for ECG lead contact can cool a patient, so limiting scrub solutions and using gel instead of alcohol for ECG lead contact will help keep the **patient's body temperature** from decreasing. The patient should be placed on top of a towel, warming blanket, or a forced-air warming device such as a Bair Hugger, and should not be placed directly onto the cold surgery table. If the patient is undergoing a dental procedure, their face must be kept as dry as possible by placing towels under the neck and switching out damp towels often because this can quickly lower their body temperature. Always wrap the patient's feet with socks, towels, or warming blankets because the feet are a source of heat loss. To warm the body from the inside, IV fluid warmers are necessary and they must be placed as close to the patient's IV catheter as possible or else the fluids will cool by the time they reach the patient.

Administering Anesthesia to Domestic Small Animals

Monitoring the Corneal Reflex and Pupil Size

The small animal placed under anesthesia should be very carefully touched along the lateral aspect of the cornea to stimulate the corneal reflex. If reflex closure of the eye does not occur with this stimulation, then the patient is moving into a deep plane 2 state, and may be over-anesthetized. Minimize use of this reflex test to avoid injury to the cornea. Other monitoring devices should be more frequently relied on.

The patient can be determined to be in a light, nonsurgical plane of anesthesia when the patient's pupils do not dilate. The patient's pupils will spontaneously constrict when a light, surgical plane has been reached. It is in the deeper, more intense plane of anesthesia (i.e., plane 3) that the patient's pupils again dilate. However, there are other factors that can induce dilation of the patient's pupils. These include the early "excitement" phase response to a preanesthetic medication or anesthesia, sympathetic responses to pain, or other drug-induced responses.

Monitoring the Eye Position and Palpebral Reflex

Patients that are in stage III, plane 2 of anesthesia will not exhibit eyeball movement, and the pupils will begin to dilate and the eye will rotate to a ventral medial (central) position. In dogs and cats, the eyeball rotates down when under halothane, isoflurane, barbiturate, and propofol anesthesia, and does not revert to a central position until deeper in plane 3. Patients that exhibit any eye movement or blinking are not sedated heavily enough for surgery to commence. The veterinarian can gently touch the medial or lateral canthus of the eyelid to stimulate the palpebral (i.e., pertaining to the eyelid) reflex or blinking reflex in the eyes. The patient's medial palpebral reflex will fade away after the lateral reflex becomes more intense. In stage III, plane 2 of anesthesia the medication causes the patient's reflex to grow slower and weaker until it ebbs to nothing. The only acceptable reflex is found in that of a mild medial palpebral reflex that can be viewed after an analgesic has been given to the patient. This reflex is also present when an injectable anesthesia is used as a solitary medication. It may also be present when methoxyflurane is used. The corneal reflex disappears at the deeper end of plane 2. Gentle palpation of the lateral aspect of the cornea will produce eyelid closure if the reflex is still intact. If not, sedation may need to be lightened. This reflex is more difficult to determine if the eyeball is significantly rotated downward, as occurs with dogs and cats.

Monitoring the Heart Rate, Pulse Rate, and Rhythm

The heart rate should be carefully monitored during general anesthetic procedures. It is best to use a stethoscope to obtain an accurate assessment. Mechanical monitoring equipment with a digital readout can also be employed. Canines given anesthesia should have a heart rate ranging from 70 to 140 beats per minute. Felines given anesthesia should have a heart rate ranging from 100 to 140 beats per minute. The animal's heart rate may slow down when the anesthetic plane deepens in the patient. However, sometimes this may not be the case. Bradycardia can be caused by a number of drugs, as well as end-stage hypoxia and vagal nerve stimulation. In such situations the heart may still maintain a constant rate even when the patient falls into a dangerously deep state of anesthesia. Bradycardia can also be caused by hypotension.

The pulse rate can be obtained by feeling the pulse along its artery. Pulse deficits are defined as diversions between the actual heartbeat and a palpable pulse response. These pulse response deficits must be recorded on the patient's chart.

Arterial palpation and electrocardiograms should be used together to monitor the patient for arrhythmias. The electrocardiogram is the most precise device used.

MONITORING THE PEDAL REFLEX AND JAW TONE

Another way to evaluate the depth of anesthesia is to check for the pedal reflex. This requires the technician to firmly squeeze (i.e., modestly pinch) the patient's skin— specifically, between the toes in dogs and cats, squeezing together the claws in cattle and swine, or applying firm pressure on the pastern of a horse. This action stimulates the animal's pedal reflex. The usual reaction is for the animal to pull the leg away. However, if properly anesthetized, the anesthetic plane greatly reduces the animal's response and reaction time. There are times when this response will disappear entirely. Patients considered to be within a surgical plane will not be able to respond to the stimulus at all.

The jaw tone or muscle tone of the animal can also be tested to determine the animal's depth of sedation. The test is conducted by grasping the lower jaw of the animal and attempting to open the animal's mouth widely, up to 3 times. This test is given to the animal prior to endotracheal intubation. The animal will usually resist the mouth-opening efforts. However, the anesthetic puts the patient into a very deep sleep, sufficient for the resistance response to dwindle. This response fades away to nothing when the animal reaches a light surgical plane. However, there are occasions when the addition of a strong analgesic or methoxyflurane can produce some signs of response. This does not indicate that a suitable plane of anesthesia has not been reached.

MONITORING THE CAPILLARY REFILL AND MUCOUS MEMBRANE COLOR TIME

The capillary refill time is abbreviated as CRT. It is calculated as the amount of time it takes for blood flow to come back to an area after digital compression has been applied to an unpigmented mucous membrane (gingival tissue is a common site). The normal CRT is measured at less than 2 seconds. During general anesthesia, the CRT levels also require observation. In addition, the patient's blood pressure should be monitored concurrently. Blood pressure and CRT levels are both indicative of the quality of peripheral perfusion arising from cardiac output. CRT indices are expected to become more protracted as the anesthetic plane deepens and if hypovolemia (blood loss) ensues in the patient.

Unpigmented areas of mucous membrane are seen as pink when in a normal state. The discoloration of these tissues can be attributed to lower O_2 levels. At such times the mucous membranes may change to the gray or blue coloration common to cyanosis. This transformation can be rapid or it may be delayed. A brilliant pink coloration can be attributed to the condition known as hypoventilation. This vasodilated color is the result of high CO_2 levels within the body caused by incomplete respiration and/or CO_2 retention.

MONITORING THE BLOOD PRESSURE AND RESPIRATORY SYSTEM

The peripheral pulse should be palpated with a gentle pressure to determine any increases or decreases in the beats. However, palpation cannot be used to come up with the actual cardiac and vascular performance values associated with the peripheral pulse. Commercially purchased, indirect or direct arterial blood pressure monitoring systems will give a more accurate measurement of blood pressure.

Normal readings for blood pressure are: 100 to 160 mm Hg for the systolic, 80 to 120 mm Hg for the mean arterial, and 60 to 100 mm Hg for the diastolic. In most cases, the animal will be in deeper anesthetic planes when exhibiting a drop in blood pressure. Canines generally maintain a minimum level of 60 mm Hg for their mean blood pressures.

Blood pressure can rise with hypercapnia (high levels of blood carbon dioxide, usually due to hypoventilation). However, blood pressure may sometimes be reduced with hypercapnia. Thus, the animal's rate and depth of the ventilation must be carefully monitored.

Monitoring the Temperature

When the patient's metabolism slows down, the demand for anesthesia sufficient to maintain the surgical plane lessens as well. This is also true when the body temperature is reduced. Thus, the vital signs and body temperature should be carefully watched to prevent any complications from occurring during the procedure. The patient may require additional body temperature support when the anesthesia is first introduced into the body. This support may also be required during the recovery period. A digital thermometer can be used to monitor the axilla, peripheral, or rectal temperature of the animal. An esophageal temperature probe can be employed to find the animal's core temperature. Patients suffering with hypothermia require a warming treatment. This treatment is given to warm the body to 37.5 °C or 99 °F. Hyperthermia is avoided by terminating the heating support when the body reaches the correct temperature. The body can be warmed with hot water bottles or by way of BAIR hugger machines.

Stages I, II, and IV of Anesthesia

Stage I of anesthesia encompasses initial anesthetic administration up to the point of the loss of consciousness. This is known as the stage of induction, early analgesia, and altered state of consciousness. The patient may experience the following: dulled sensations, pain loss, blood pressure elevation, vomiting, inspiratory struggling, and coughing. The patient's pupils will begin to dilate as Stage II approaches. The patient's breathing rate is usually high and irregular at this time.

Stage II commences with the loss of consciousness. In Stage II, the patient may experience the following: delirious activity and sounds, symptoms of involuntary struggling, and physiological agitation and excitement. During this time it is expected that the patient's eyes will remain closed and its jaw will be set. The patient's point reflexes may be amplified. The patient's pupils will be dilated and respond to light. Stage II does not last long.

Patients experiencing fairly uncomplicated inductions can move from stage I to stage III (the "surgical" stage) without incidence. Should the patient experience prolonged apnea, cardiac arrest, and/or brainstem or medullary paralysis, the "overdose" or fourth stage of the anesthesia will have been encountered and prompt remedial steps must immediately be taken.

Stage III of Anesthesia

The third stage of anesthesia is maintained during the actual surgery. During this stage the patient's pupils will constrict further and the patient will gradually lose its palpebral (blink) reflex. However, the patient's breathing will be full and regular.

There are 4 planes associated with Stage III anesthesia. In plane 1 of Stage III, the patient retains its capacity to blink its eyes. The patient also retains its swallowing reflexes, and should be able to produce regular respirations with a respectable measure of chest activity.

The patient will no longer be able to blink in plane 2 of Stage III, but will demonstrate a fixed pupil response. Respirations will continue to be regular and the chest and muscles in the diaphragm will continue to exhibit a good amount of movement. Plane 2, stage III is appropriate for the surgery executed by veterinarians.

In plane 3 of stage III, the patient's breathing becomes shallow. This is due to a partial intercostal paralysis, limiting the patient's ability to breathe with its chest and abdominal muscles.

In plane 4 of stage III, the patient enters an unstable and potentially life-threatening stage that should be avoided. This stage is formally reached when the patient ceases to breathe.

Analgesics During Surgery or Painful Procedures

Analgesics given for anesthetic purposes require attention to the following factors: the timing of administration, the length of analgesia required, and the route of administration. A patient in pain can have some of its symptoms reduced with the application of an analgesic. This medication should not only reduce the animal's pain, but its anxiety as well. This can provide an easier preanesthetic and induction period for the pain-racked patient and for those laboring to render treatment.

The amount of induction or maintenance agents needed may be lessened when analgesics are given to the patient preoperatively.

The patient that is in the recovery period should continue to be given analgesics following a surgical procedure. The goal of the medication is to reduce the patient's stress and postoperative pain. Carefully administered analgesics are beneficial in reducing the patient's pain without rendering the patient unconscious. In this way the patient will remain in a more relaxed, responsive, and recovery-conducive state, where appropriate medications continue to alleviate the pain.

Muscle Relaxants While the Patient Is Under Anesthesia

Neuromuscular blocking agents are employed during a surgical procedure to bring the patient into a state of more complete relaxation. The muscle relaxants have a number of beneficial effects. The positive effects include the following: an increase in the ability to manipulate the joints and bones, an improved contact and observation of the region being operated on, greater ease in regulating ventilation, easier endotracheal intubation, and the elimination of any residual eye movement in ocular surgical procedures.

Muscle relaxants are particularly beneficial for those occasions when the patient cannot be subjected to a substantial amount of a deep anesthetic. In these cases, the patient experiences a reduction in the quantity of anesthetic agent required in the patient's treatment, and muscle relaxant adjuvants will enhance the surgical outcome and experience.

A muscle relaxant–assisted surgical procedure should be conducted with the patient receiving constant ventilation. The patient should continue to be checked to determine the depth of anesthesia the patient is experiencing, with adjustments made accordingly.

Nonsteroidal Anti-Inflammatory Drugs

Nonsteroidal anti-inflammatory drugs are abbreviated as NSAIDs. These drugs include the following: aspirin, acetaminophen, carprofen, ketoprofen, and meloxicam. These drugs are not dangerous to use in combination with opioids. NSAIDs are appropriate for the treatment of musculoskeletal pain. They are frequently applied in the treatment of patients with arthritis and other joint diseases. However, long-term NSAID therapy should not be used by patients with chronic kidney problems. The use of NSAIDs by this population can result in nephrotoxicity. It is best to use meloxicam in long-term therapy for renal-compromised patients, as has a lower risk for nephrotoxic results.

It is never appropriate to administer acetaminophen to a cat. Dogs should only be given acetaminophen on atypical occasions. Analgesics that are considered strong and safe can be given in direct postoperative orthopedic procedures. Pain medications are also particularly beneficial in the treatment of painful degloving injuries (where a large section of skin is severed from its underlying blood supply). Alternative medications include ketoprofen and carprofen.

Concerns When Ventilating a Patient Under Anesthesia

The use of assisted ventilation predisposes the delivery of additional anesthetic to the patient. Thus, the patient will require a reduction in the percentage of delivered inhalant anesthetic at this juncture. The patient that demonstrates spontaneous breathing while receiving IPPV is being underventilated. Overventilation is not advisable, as it can cause the pulmonary alveoli to be harmed.

The patient in an underventilated state will have a reduced cardiac output. Respiratory alkalosis can be a result of unwarranted levels of CO_2. The patient with pneumothorax requires careful treatment. The danger of a collapsed lung is a strong possibility.

The patient should receive continued ventilatory support for a few minutes after the inhalant anesthetic is turned off. This additional ventilatory support will be essential to the patient's speedy recovery. This directly assists in ridding the body of residual inhalant anesthetic.

Checking the Depth of Anesthesia and Ventilation for Patients Under Sedation

A muscle relaxant–assisted surgery will mask some of the usual signs used to monitor depth of anesthesia. Thus, regularly checking the depth of anesthesia takes on additional importance. Further, the patient will need another type of analgesic to reduce the pain. There are a multitude of neuromuscular blocking agents (muscle relaxants) that can be employed in patient care, including succinylcholine, gallamine, pancuronium, atracurium, and vecuronium. When such agents are employed, ventilation must be regulated by manual or mechanical means. One form of mechanical ventilation is referred to as intermittent positive pressure ventilation or IPPV. It involves establishing a preset respiratory rate.

Successful ventilation can help preserve normal acid-base levels by oxygenating the patient and reducing CO_2 retention. Assisted ventilation is usually necessary for overweight patients, patients in head-down recumbency, and patients with hypothermia or pulmonary disease. Ventilation is controlled with patients that receive neuromuscular blocking agents. In addition, patients with thoracic surgery, diaphragmatic hernia, gastric torsion, or hypoventilation should receive this same care. The veterinarian should note the respiratory rate, inspiration-to-expiration ratio, tidal volume, and inspiratory pressure. These outcomes should be reassessed continuously throughout the surgery. Ventilation is further checked by looking at the animal's chest motions arising from the breathing process.

Respiratory Acidosis

Respiratory acidosis is a result of CO_2 excretion that is lower than the CO_2 produced. An escalation of CO_2 levels in the blood gases can be attributed to this situation. Conditions that contribute to hypoventilation include: a state of deep anesthesia, pulmonary disease, or respiratory obstruction. Reduced ventilation is also responsible for CO_2 retention.

These circumstances can bring about respiratory acidosis. Patients that have a more concentrated level of CO_2 will more than likely have a lower pH level. Thus, the patient's acid levels will rise as the CO_2 builds. Cardiac outputs will also rise in patients with hypertension. This condition points to respiratory acidosis. In addition, vasodilatation or ventricular arrhythmias can also suggest respiratory acidosis.

The body is able to compensate for this circumstance with time. Initially, the body releases acid buffers. In 3-5 days, kidney excretion of carbonic acid rises as does bicarbonate reabsorption. Respiratory acidosis can be treated by ventilatory volume and by treating the underlying disease that caused the higher levels of carbon dioxide.

Replacement Fluids for Stable Anesthetic Cases

The sedated and stable patient can be given IV fluid replacement crystalloids like Normosol R or Plasmalyte 148. Maintenance crystalloids include Normosol M or Plasmalyte 56. Replacement crystalloids are comparable to plasma because they have high sodium and chloride levels with a reduced potassium concentration. These medications can be administered according to the following general formula: 5 to 10 mL/kg/hr. Longer applications will require that the first hour be run at 10 mL/kg/hr, with additional hours reduced to 5 mL/kg/hr. The patient that loses fluids should receive supplemental fluids. This includes patients that have need for replacement of blood lost. The medical staff should be prepared to act in case of an emergency when a patient receives IV fluids. The medical staff will adhere to patent IV standards in this administration of IV fluids.

Metabolic Acidosis and the Interpretation of Blood Gases

Metabolic acidosis can be attributed to a low adjusted base excess. The low adjusted base excess can be written as ABE. Metabolic acidosis can also be a result of low HCO_3^- — as confirmed by blood gas analysis. Metabolic acidosis can also be brought on by lactic acid gain, renal failure, and losing and not reabsorbing HCO_3^- rich body secretions. Diarrhea can also lead to this problematic condition. Higher levels of H^+ can be detected when HCO_3^- is lost.

Hyperventilation can produce a natural relief to this problem. An alkalinizing IV solution can also be administered to the patient to correct a minor imbalance. Sodium bicarbonate can be administered to patients to restore more acute imbalances.

However, this can be a deadly approach for patients suffering from dehydration. In this situation the patient would be suffering from 2 disorders. However, one is considered the primary disorder. The other is a secondary disorder which contributes to the primary problem. The blood gas results should be noted and interpreted according to the factors associated with both the primary and secondary disorders.

Respiratory Alkalosis

Respiratory alkalosis is a result of a patient's excreting more CO_2 than is produced. Lower levels of CO_2 in blood gas analyses point to this condition This may occur as a result of mechanical respiratory hyperventilation. It can also be caused by spontaneous hyperventilation in patients suffering from extreme pain or some other source of overstimulation. Lower levels of CO_2 will produce lower quantities of acids and drive an increase in basic pH. The patient suffering from respiratory alkalosis may exhibit tachycardia and other electrocardiographic anomalies. The kidneys may be able to counteract the effects, if given enough time. Further, a mechanically ventilated patient can be given a lower minute volume of ventilation to reduce the effects of respiratory alkalosis. Hyperventilation should be addressed by the medical staff.

Common Oxygenation and Anesthetic Equipment Problems

Some problems associated with anesthetic delivery can be traced to mechanical dysfunction. The problem can be as simple as a disconnected endotracheal tube, rebreathing bag, or breathing hose. The problem may also be found in leaking or blocked equipment. These issues can contribute to the poor oxygenation of a patient.

Sometimes such a problem will lead directly to medication overdosing or under-dosing. For example, anesthesia under-administration may be traced to an empty vaporizer. A broken or ineffective setting on a vaporizer can also cause this problem. In addition, sometimes the problem is found in hoses that are not securely fastened, poorly connecting the patient to the device.

Too much carbon dioxide can be the result of an exhausted CO_2 absorbant or a stuck unidirectional valve. Sometimes, the mixture of anesthesia administered to a patient may be in a hypoxic form. This happens when the nitrous oxide levels are too high when matched with the O_2 flow. The higher settings on the vaporizer can result in a patient that has been over-anesthetized. The patient may then suffer from acute hypercapnia or hypoxia. Consequently, all mechanical equipment must be examined prior to use, and maintained regularly.

Interpretation of Blood Gases

The veterinarian should always monitor a patient's pH levels. These levels should range from 7.35 to 7.45. Lower rates of pH are indicative of acidosis. Higher rates are indicative of alkalosis. The PCO_2 can also be used to determine the patient's respiratory condition. The ABE (adjusted base excess) levels can be used to determine the patient's metabolic condition. The primary disorder will be the one that produces the most change in the patient. The patient's pH can be indicative of the direction in which the changes are taking place. The metabolic state is determined by the ABE levels, despite the presence of irregular levels of CO_2. This can be attributed to the changes in PCO_2 that are assessed along with the ABE level. Normal levels of CO_2 suggest that the metabolic state can be determined through analysis of the HCO_3^-. Metabolic acidosis can be detected when HCO_3^- is less than 20. However, levels over 26 imply metabolic alkalosis exists.

Properly Recovering a Patient from Anesthesia

Patients must be monitored closely during the **recovery phase** of the anesthetic procedure. Once the patient has swallowed twice, the ET can be removed (extubation) while the patient is in sternal recumbency (in case of vomiting). The patient's vital signs must be monitored during the recovery phase including the heart rate, respiratory rate, mucous membrane color, and capillary refill time. The patient's temperature should be monitored every 15 minutes until it is within normal range. To promote circulation during the recovery phase, the patient may be walked around or moved around to provide stimulation. If the patient becomes hypothermic (lower than a 98-degree body temperature) during recovery, place a heating pad covered with a towel under the patient and place towels on top of the patient; also make sure a reversal agent was given if needed. Check the patient's temperature frequently and remove heat sources as necessary to prevent the patient from becoming hyperthermic.

Maintaining, Cleaning, and Preparing Equipment

Parts of an Anesthesia Machine

An anesthesia machine is fashioned from the following: medical gas cylinders, a regulator, flowmeter, vaporizer, inhalation or exhalation flutter valves, check valves, y-connector, a rebreathing bag or reservoir bag, carbon dioxide absorber, soda lime canister, exhaust valve, manometer, oxygen flush valve, scavenger system, and a negative pressure relief valve.

The gas cylinders hold compressed gas which is subjected to extreme pressures. Full containers of oxygen are pressurized at around 2000-2200 psi. (pounds per square inch). Full containers of nitrous oxide are pressurized from 750-770 psi. A regulator can reduce the pressure of the gas exiting to around 50 psi. The flowmeter sets the gas delivery at a certain rate. The flowmeter can further reduce the pressure to approximately 15 psi.

The liquid anesthetic is changed to a vapor with the vaporizer. It regulates the quantity of anesthesia combined with the carrier gas. The circle system utilizes a check valve to ensure and control the unidirectional flow of gas.

Other Parts of an Anesthesia Machine

The circle system's inspiration and expiration tubes are linked to the endotracheal tube with a y-connector. The reservoir bag achieves an improved form of breathing with its gas reservoir. Animal size is a crucial variable that must be accounted for in the gas flow rate. Thus, minimum gas volume requirements are around 60 mL/kg of patient weight. The circle system's carbon dioxide absorber removes the carbon dioxide from the expired gas. The tanks must be replaced every 6 to 8 hours when in use.

The exhaust valve is utilized in extracting the exhaust gas from the machine into the scavenger system. The manometer can detect the amount of pressure of gas in the lungs and airway of the patient. It measures the pressure using the following increments: mm of Hg or cm of H_2O. The system can be cleansed with pure oxygen by releasing the oxygen flush valve. The waste gas is accumulated and directed out of the building. A second alternative allows the waste anesthesia to be extracted by a charcoal canister in the scavenger system. The negative relief valve is described as a safety valve that releases to allow room air in when a negative pressure is formed.

Advantages and Disadvantages of Nitrous Oxide

Nitrous oxide (chemical symbol: N_2O) is a very weak general anesthetic with a MAC rating of 105%. However, it is very effective as a "carrier gas" for other more powerful anesthetics. Mixed in a 2:1 ratio with oxygen, it serves to increase the rate of inhalation induction in the patient. At the start of anesthesia induction, large quantities of nitrous oxide are distributed from the alveoli into the bloodstream. For some animals (depending upon the procedure), N_2O alone may provide sufficient anesthesia. Other animals may require further analgesics to be administered. Nitrous oxide has an immediate effect due to the body's inability to metabolize the medication (less than 0.004% of this gas is metabolized). The body's cardiovascular and respiratory system suffers little effect from the application of this medication.

With a MAC rating over 100%, another medication must be used in conjunction with N_2O if general anesthesia is required. Further, the inspiration levels of O_2 drop to 33% when N_2O is administered. This drop in levels can endanger the patient. The patient may suffer from of hypoxia if there is a history of respiratory problems. Further, N_2O is contraindicated in animals with gas-occupying conditions such as gastric dilation, intestinal obstruction, or pneumothorax.

Maintenance of an Anesthesia Machine

The oxygen tanks should be turned off when not in use. This reduces any additional pressure on the oxygen tank regulator. Removable parts of the anesthesia machine can be cleaned with a gentle soapy solution. Any parts that have come into contact with the patient should be cleansed. Removable parts should be placed in a tub of cold disinfectant solution to soak. Following the soak, the parts should be thoroughly rinsed and left to air dry. Cleaning should be performed following each anesthesia induction. Vaporizers should be turned off when not in use. In addition, these appliances should be emptied to prevent any undue buildup of preservatives or residue. A good rule is to check the color of the barium hydroxide or soda lime granules. A color change is a good indication that it is time to change the solution. If the substance becomes rigid and/or brittle, then it should be replaced. It is important to note that rubber does require replacing, as it wears out with use.

Universal F-Circuit and the Bain System

A modified circle system contains a universal F-circuit with the inspiration hose on the inside of the expiration hose. This system requires the following: a CO_2 absorber, rebreathing bag, unidirectional valves, pop-off valve, and a scavenger. The expired gases heat the inward-bound fresh gases. The universal F-circuit is lightweight. It is less cumbersome than the circle system version. It also incorporates safety measures through an end-of-the-inspiration hose and end-of-the-expiration hose pull away connection. This juncture disconnects when the circuit is stretched. The empty space of this system is fashioned like the one found in the circle system. However, the empty space does increase when the hoses stretch.

The Bain system is also known as the Bain coaxial anesthesia circuit. It holds a tube inside another tube. The interior tube allows fresh gas to flow in, and the exterior tube conducts exhaled gasses away.

Use of the Bain System in the Breathing Circuit

The **Bain system** does not incorporate a CO_2 absorber. Instead, it incorporates a rebreathing bag sandwiched between the reservoir bag and scavenger. The following is drawn from the interior tube during the patient's inspiration or inhalation process: fresh gases, either 100% fresh gas or a mixture of fresh and expired gases. A **nonrebreathing system** utilizes the fresh flow rate of 200 to 300 mL/kg/minute in the mechanism. A **partial breathing** system can utilize a flow rate of 130 to 200 mL/kg/minute in the system. The Bain system is compact and light. It has a minimum amount of empty space, which promotes effortless breathing. This is an ideal system for a patient that is under 7 kg or 15 lb. The Bain system is also ideal for treatments that are applied to the head or where there is a need for a great deal of physical manipulation of the patient during a procedure.

A Closed Rebreathing System

Rebreathing or circle systems operate by circulating a combination of expired and fresh gases. The amount of CO_2 in the inhaled gas is regulated by the flow rate of the fresh air and the presence or absence of a CO_2 absorber.

The fresh gas flow rate should not exceed the metabolic oxygen expenditure of the patient. This rate is typically 5 to 10 mL/kg/minute with a closed rebreathing system. The pop-off valve can be in the closed position during operation of the system. Incoming fresh gases are recirculated in combination with expired gases that have gone through a CO_2 extraction process. If the CO_2 absorber is not working effectively, then the patient can be exposed to unhealthy levels of CO_2. It is important to consistently monitor the operation to keep the O_2 flow at the desired metabolic levels. This monitoring will prevent undue pressure from developing in the rebreathing system's operation.

Precision and a Nonprecision Vaporizer

A **precision vaporizer** incorporates an anesthetic vapor concentration that is regulated independently, and based on the time, temperature, and fresh gas flow rate. An anesthetist can compensate for the temperature flow rate manually. This can be accomplished with a vaporizer. The percentage of the anesthetic is fixed according to dials, charts, and/or mathematical calculations. It is impossible for the patient to physically extract gases out of a precision vaporizer. This is due to the internal resistance inherent in the device. The problem is alleviated with an out-of-circle position. The complexity of this device requires particular skill when it is being serviced. **Nonprecision vaporizers** are not appropriate for the administration of a specific, continuous percentage of anesthesia. This is because nonprecision vaporizers are unable to accommodate the following variables: changes in temperature, fresh gas flow rates, ventilation changes, liquid and wick surfaces, and the volume of liquid anesthetic. Thus, these vaporizers do not lend to an accurate calculation and consistent maintenance of the percentage of anesthetic given to the patient. Even so, the low internal resistance allows an in-the-circle application, and this application can include an out-of-circle operation. The nonlinear concentrations given make it hard to regulate the anesthesia depth. However, this simple device does not require as much maintenance as the precision vaporizer requires.

Aseptic Cleaning Method

Aseptic cleaning of the surgical suite must be done before and after each use and at least monthly if the suite is not being used. The aseptic technique prevents contamination to the surgical site from bacteria, viruses, and disease-causing microorganisms. An **effective aseptic technique** involves removing any debris from the area such as blood, feces, or vomit and then cleaning the surfaces with a general cleaner and wiping dry. Next, apply a disinfectant and allow it to sit for the desired amount of time, rinse, and then dry again. To obtain asepsis, the surgical site must be cleaned from top to bottom daily. Start with the walls, which must be wiped down with a disinfectant, as well as all monitoring equipment, lamps, and operating tables. Next, the floors must be swept and mopped using a separate mop and then the mop for the rest of the hospital. Other preventative measures to take to maintain asepsis in the surgical suite are to have a separate area to prep the patient for surgery, as well as a separate area for the surgeon to scrub in for surgery.

Steam Autoclaving

In order to sterilize surgical instruments, **steam autoclaving** is vital for all instruments prior to use to prevent infection. Before being placed into the autoclave, the instruments must be thoroughly cleaned, lubricated, and double wrapped in a pack with a steam indicator strip inside the pack, as well as indicator tape on the outside of the pack. Always leave the hinges of the instruments open so the steam can properly sterilize the entire instrument and to prevent the box locks from cracking. The **autoclave reservoir** must always be filled with distilled water because it will generate pure steam for sterilization unlike tap water, which can leave mineral deposits that can stain instruments and promote buildup in the autoclave itself. The **chamber** will be cleaned with a specific autoclave cleaner and scrubbed with a bristle brush to prevent buildup at least once a week. The **gasket** inside of the autoclave door will need to be wiped down weekly. The steam-line filter will need to be cleaned monthly (or according to the manufacturer's guidelines), by draining the water out and filling it with new distilled water and running a couple of short cycles with a specialized cleaning solution.

Materials Used to Wrap Instruments

Peel pouches come in different sizes, and they are easy to open and close without tearing and dropping the sterile instrument. When packing an instrument in a peel pouch, make sure it is the right size for the instrument because if it is too small the instrument could pierce the pouch. Allow one inch of space between the instrument and all of the sealed edges of the pouch, and place the instrument in with the handle end first because when the pouch is opened the surgeon can grab this end first. **Sterilization drapes** are designed to stop microorganisms from getting to the instruments while also allowing sterilant to pass through to the instruments. **Paper and linen wraps** should be one-time use because they function as a mesh-type filter and after washing and being used, the threads get larger, allowing microorganisms to get through. **SMS polypropylene wraps** are made of dense microfibers and are more reliable for not allowing dust and microorganisms through.

Properly Caring for and Disinfecting an ET

After each use, the **endotracheal tube (ET)** needs to be rinsed and any secretions should be cleaned off right away to prevent the secretions from drying on the tube because this can prevent disinfectants from working properly. The inside of the tracheal tube can be cleaned by using a baby bottle brush or pipe cleaners and then running water and disinfectant through. After being cleaned inside and out, the tracheal tube should be soaked in a disinfectant solution such as dilute chlorhexidine to further reduce the chance of nosocomial infection. After soaking for up to 10 minutes, the tube should be rinsed thoroughly because if there is any chemical residue on the tube it can cause tissue reactions when used again. Let tracheal tubes sit out to air dry completely before the next use.

Finding a Leak in the Anesthetic Machine

Certain areas of the anesthetic machine must be checked to see where the **leak** may be coming from. If the pressure check shows a large leak (500 ml/min), then a few areas must be checked including the pop-off valve, rebreathing bag, soda lime canister, and the breathing circuit. The rebreathing bag should be inspected for holes as well as the breathing tube. The soda lime canister should be removed, and the anesthetic machine should be checked for loose granules that may be preventing the canister from making a proper seal. Thoroughly clean the area of granules and soda lime dust, replace the canister, and pressure check the machine again. A soap solution can be sprayed around common areas on the machine that may leak, and bubbles will rise during the pressure test to show where the leak is coming from.

Setting Up the Surgery Room Prior to a Procedure

To **prepare the surgical suite** for the patient, a checklist would be helpful. First, the surgical suite needs to be inspected to be sure it is clean of all hair and debris. Next, check the anesthetic machine to be sure that the sevoflurane or isoflurane is full and that the oxygen tank is full. Perform a leak test on the anesthetic machine with the correct-sized rebreathing bag and breathing tube for the patient's weight. Gather the necessary supplies needed for the specific procedure to be performed such as a sterile spay pack containing the instruments and gauze, a sterile drape, a sterile scalpel blade of the appropriate size, and the appropriate size suture needed. Place all sterile items on the Mayo stand until they need to be opened. Any patient-warming devices should be warmed up prior to surgery, and all monitoring equipment needs to be turned on to ensure that it is working correctly. An IV fluid stand, pump, appropriate fluids, fluid line, and extension set need to be set up with the fluids run through the line to ensure that there is no air in the line. Overhead lights should be turned on and adjusted accordingly.

Emergency Medicine/Critical Care

Triage

Forms of Trauma and How Begin Treatment of the Trauma Patient

Trauma that commonly causes bleeding in the abdomen, fractures, and ruptured organs is categorized under blunt trauma. Penetrating trauma is specific to the path of the object that penetrated the body such as bite wounds. A patient presenting with any form of trauma should be thoroughly examined for any obvious fractures or hemorrhaging. The veterinarian will listen to the patient's heart for any abnormalities, as well as the lungs to make sure that they sound clear. During the overall exam, the patient should be supported in case of spinal injury or a fractured extremity. The veterinarian will palpate the abdomen to feel for any free fluid or see if the patient is in pain in that area. Close monitoring of the patient is essential because an underlying injury may be present even if the patient presents seemingly normally. The hospital should have a triaging scale created for trauma cases ranging from 0–3 with 0 being no injury noted and a 3 being severe. There should also be categories set for triaging trauma cases, such as cardiac or skeletal.

Cases in Need of Being Triaged

Triage is defined by the assignment of the degree of urgency to the illness or injury to determine the order in which to be treated. Certain cases that require triage are ones that are emergencies such as heat stroke, exposure to any sort of poison, or a patient that has been hit by a car. Certain illnesses that require triaging include seizures, hypoglycemia, or abdominal distension. The first person to communicate information to the client would be the person who answers the phone when they call. If unsure of the severity of the call, the veterinarian must be notified so they can take the call. Once the patient arrives, they must be assessed quickly by the front-desk staff. To quickly but efficiently assess the patient, check the eyes for dullness or if they appear sunken, check the ears for any blue or pale color, and check for respirations to see if the patient is having difficulty. Also check to make sure the patient is alert and responds to you. If the patient exhibits these signs, they must be triaged as STAT or urgent and brought to the veterinarian immediately.

Classifying Patients on a Triage (Priority) Scale

In an emergency hospital, there must be a **triaging** protocol in place along with an overall assessment of the patient to determine how urgent of a case it is. First-priority cases need to be treated within seconds of arriving and include patients having difficulties breathing, excessive bleeding, shock, allergic reactions, ingestion of any form of poison, and a patient hit by a car. Second-priority cases involve patients who are currently stable but need to be monitored closely because their status could change quickly, involving patients with excessive vomiting and diarrhea, seizing patients, and a possible urethral obstruction. Third-priority cases are patients who are stable and not critical that can be treated in a few hours such as patients with a fever, ear hematoma, or small wound. Third-priority cases include patients that are nonurgent or critical and are completely stable.

Triaging a Patient That Has Been Hit by a Car

If an owner calls and says their pet has been **hit by a car,** the triage begins with the receptionist who should tell the owner to bring the pet in right away and alert the veterinarian. If an owner walks in with their pet without calling, this is a level 1 on a scale of 1–5 with 1 being the most urgent on an emergency scale. The veterinary technician will need to immediately bring the pet to the treatment area and obtain a TPR. If the patient has no heart rate, CPR will begin, but if the patient is breathing and alert, then further assessment can begin. The veterinarian may have the technician place an IV catheter and administer IV fluids along with taking radiographs of the dog's chest and abdomen to check for internal bleeding.

Common Eye Injuries in Dogs

Proptosis is when the eye bulges due to an eye injury that disconnects the eyeball from the orbit and the eyelid spasms keeping it from going back into the socket. **Foreign objects** can become lodged in the patient's eye causing irritation, swelling, and tearing. Foreign objects may be dislodged by flushing the eye with saline and obtaining the object with forceps. **Glaucoma** is an increased pressure in the eye, which results in fluid buildup in the eye, bulging, and pain if the pressure gets too high. Lowering the pressure in the eye is the first thing to address when dealing with glaucoma, which can be done with medication or surgery may be needed. **Corneal ulcers** are caused by scratches or other injuries to the eye. Corneal ulcers can cause the eye to bulge if the cornea becomes weak, and surgery may be required. Triaging an eye injury will be done by initial assessment; if it is a case of proptosis, this will need to be addressed immediately, whereas a patient that presents with a possible eye infection or dry eye will be less urgent. Any suspected **eye injuries** should be seen the same day as when the owner calls.

Emergency Nursing Procedures

Four Types of Feeding Tubes

A **flexible PVC catheter** is normally used as an orogastric **feeding tube** and is placed through the mouth, down the esophagus, and into the stomach. **Orogastric feeding tubes** are good for short term use, but they hold a risk of the patient biting the tube as well as possibly causing gastric reflux. **Nasogastric tubes** are passed to the stomach through the patient's nostril, and a nasoesophageal tube is put through the nostril and passed just to the thoracic esophagus. Nasogastric and nasoesophageal feeding tubes run the risk of the patient developing irritation and swelling of the nose (rhinitis) and nosebleed (epistaxis). An **esophagostomy tube** is placed while the patient is under anesthesia, and while the patient is on its right side, a surgical incision is made on the left side of the neck and the tube (red rubber or silicone) is pulled into the esophagus, then into the mouth and turned around to be placed directly down to the distal esophagus and sutured in place on the neck.

Canine Parvovirus

Canine parvovirus causes **acute GI sickness** mainly in dogs younger than 6 months of age and those that are unvaccinated. Canine parvovirus is commonly seen in the intestinal form, which causes vomiting, diarrhea, weight loss, anorexia, and dehydration because this form inhibits the dog's ability to absorb nutrients causing them to become weak from the lack of protein and dehydration. The canine parvovirus can also take on a less common cardiac form and infect the dog's heart muscles, causing death. Canine parvovirus is transmitted mainly through direct oral of nasal contact with infected feces or through personnel that handled an infected dog or contaminated equipment and housing. Parvovirus is shed in the feces of the infected dog after around 5 days from exposure and all the way up until 10 days past recovery.

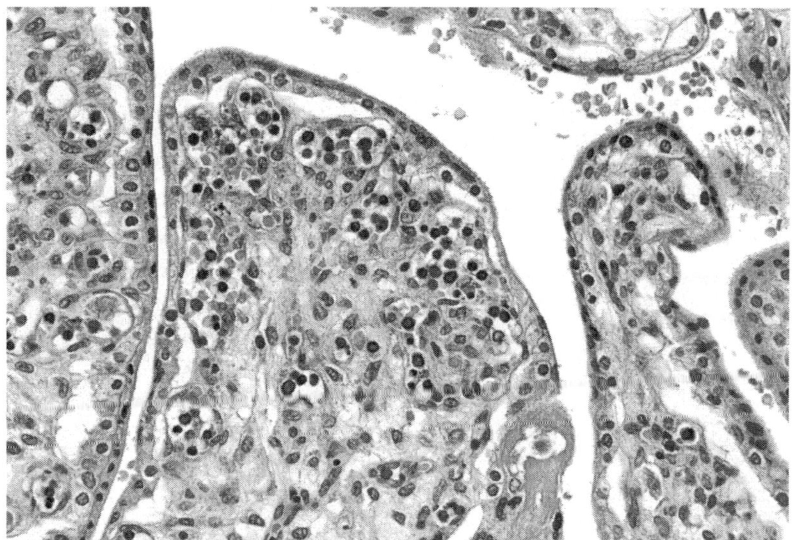

Equine Strangles

Equine strangles refers to the infectious and contagious bacteria, *Streptococcus equi equi* causing abscesses on the lymph nodes under and behind the jaw in the upper respiratory tract. *S. equi equi* organisms can survive more than 4 weeks outside of the host if kept from heat and out of sunlight. Transmission of strangles occurs mainly through direct contact or shared items between horses such as feeding bins or anywhere a draining abscess has touched because they are infective. Strangles can also be transmitted by a handler's clothes or tools that has been exposed to the bacteria. Some horses may be carriers, which means they look otherwise healthy but carry the bacteria and can randomly shed the bacteria for years, therefore always risking infecting other horses.

Function of the Respiratory System

The **respiratory system** starts with oxygen entering the body through the nose or mouth and into the trachea. The oxygen travels down the trachea, which divides into two bronchi and into the lungs. Once it enters the lungs, it ends up in the alveoli where gas exchange occurs, which provides the tissues of the body with oxygen taken in with inspiration and removes carbon dioxide with expiration. The oxygen taken in at inspiration that enters the alveoli will attach to the hemoglobin in the body's RBCs and then is carried to the tissues, then the oxygen molecules detach from the hemoglobin to enter the tissues to provide them with energy. Carbon dioxide is then sent back to the alveoli where it leaves the body via exhalation.

Requirements for Dogs and Cats to be Blood Donors

In order to be able to be a **blood donor,** the dog must be at least 1 year old but not more than 8 years old and weigh at least 55 pounds allowing for around 450 ml of blood to be drawn without causing harm. If the donor is a cat, then it also must be at least 1 year of age and younger than 8 years of age, weighing at least 10 pounds allowing for at least 60 ml of blood to be drawn without causing harm. The PCV of the donor must be checked prior to blood donation to make sure it is within the normal range, which is between 37% and 55% in dogs and 30% and 45% in cats. The donor should have up-to-date vaccines and should not be ill. Cats should be tested for FIV/FeLV to be sure that they are negative, and only indoor cats should be considered to be donors. Dogs and cats can donate blood every 5 weeks if they meet the requirements. Routine blood work, fecal checks, and heartworm tests should be done for regular donors.

Types of Circulatory Shock

Circulatory shock is the result of a decrease in adequate circulation volume in the body. In order for the body to have effective circulating volume, it must have normal blood pressure and blood volume. Circulatory shock is put into three categories: hypovolemic, cardiogenic, and distributive shock. **Hypovolemic shock** occurs when blood volume is low due to a traumatic injury, resulting in excessive blood loss. **Cardiogenic shock** happens when circulating blood volume drops even though there is normal blood volume. Cardiogenic shock happens when the stroke volume decreases and is seen in patients with heart failure. **Distributive shock** is a result of an issue with peripheral blood vessels causing blood to flow away from central circulation, normally due to serious infection of the body. A fast heart rate, pale MM, low blood pressure, and weak pulse are all signs of shock that can progress to a drop in oxygen delivery to the tissues that can lead to organ failure and death.

Ethylene Glycol Toxicity

Ethylene glycol toxicity is caused by the ingestion of ethylene glycol, which is lethal in small doses and is the main component to antifreeze (95%). Ethylene glycol tastes sweet, and in most instances, patients willingly ingest it off of a garage floor or driveway. In smaller doses and less concentrations, ethylene glycol can be found in motor oils, brake fluid, paints, and printer cartridges. The minimum lethal dose of undiluted ethylene glycol in cats is 1.4 ml/kg and 4.4 ml/kg in dogs. Ethylene glycol is absorbed through the GI tract, and within a few hours the concentration of ethylene glycol is at its highest in the blood. Metabolic acidosis and renal tubular epithelial damage result from the toxic metabolites of ethylene glycol. Ethylene glycol produces glycolaldehyde from the enzyme alcohol dehydrogenase, which is metabolized to glycolic acid. Glycolic acid is metabolized to oxalic acid, which forms calcium oxalate crystals when bound to calcium. The buildup of these crystals causes acute kidney failure.

Clinical Signs of Ethylene Glycol Toxicity

The first noticeable **clinical signs** in a patient with ethylene glycol toxicity are that the patient appears intoxicated as well as having vomiting, polyuria, polydipsia, a low body temperature, and seizures. Neurological signs normally appear within the first half hour post ingestion. These symptoms may improve after 24 hours, but then the patient may become very dehydrated and could develop an increased heart rate and respiratory rate. Two to three days after a dog ingests ethylene glycol, acute renal failure develops (24 hours in cats) and the patient may have virtually no urine output. They also will appear lethargic, anorexic, may have seizures, and possibly die. Patients that ingest ethylene glycol must be treated within a few hours of ingestion for the best possible outcome.

Treating Ethylene Glycol Toxicity in Dogs and Cats

To treat a patient with **ethylene glycol toxicity**, absorption must be decreased, as well as preventing it from further metabolizing, attempting to rid the toxin already metabolized, and correcting metabolic acidosis resulting from metabolized ethylene glycol. To induce vomiting will prevent ethylene glycol from being absorbed, but it must be done within 2 hours of ingestion to be effective. IV fluid therapy will help hydrate the patient and increase urine output while aiding in the excretion of metabolized ethylene glycol. The compound 4-Methylpyrazole is used to inactivate alcohol dehydrogenase, which will prevent the metabolism of ethylene glycol. Metabolic acidosis that results from the metabolism of ethylene glycol can be corrected with sodium bicarbonate.

Chocolate Toxicity in Dogs

Theobromine is the toxic chemical found in all **chocolate**, but the darker the chocolate, the more theobromine is found, which dogs are unable to metabolize. Baking chocolate and dark chocolate can contain up to 130–450 mg of theobromine per ounce, whereas milk chocolate only contains up to 58 mg per ounce. Agitation, hyperactivity, diarrhea, and vomiting can be seen at concentrations as low as 20 mg/kg of theobromine. At 40 mg/kg, a racing heart rate, high blood pressure, and arrhythmias can be seen, and at a concentration of greater than 60 mg/kg, neurological signs are seen, including seizures. Fatalities are rare but can occur at concentrations of around 200 mg/kg. Early treatment for chocolate toxicity is vital and can be achieved by administering medications such as Apomorphine to induce vomiting and giving activated charcoal orally to block the theobromine from being absorbed from the body, along with IV fluids to help with the removal of theobromine from the body.

Laryngeal Paralysis

A patient presenting with **laryngeal paralysis** may exhibit stridor on inspiration, noisy respirations, exercise and heat intolerance, dyspnea, and cyanosis. Patients with severe laryngeal paralysis will be hyperthermic and experience coughing, vomiting, and anxiety. Certain activities may cause these symptoms to become worse, such as going on a walk in hotter temperatures. Laryngeal paralysis happens when stimulation of the laryngeal muscles is disrupted, causing the arytenoid cartilage and vocal folds to open at inspiration and close at expiration.

Urethral Obstruction (Blocked Tom) in a Cat

Male cats can develop **stones** and/or **debris** in their urine that can **obstruct their urethra**, which is the pathway from the bladder to the penis, preventing urine from leaving the body. This is an extremely painful condition and a medical emergency that must be treated as soon as possible because it can lead to complete blockage, causing damaged kidneys and even death in a matter of days. Signs and symptoms to look for include the cat frequently going to the litter box to urinate and tiny amounts of urine or even no urine is produced, vocalizing in pain while using the litter box, decreased appetite, and licking at his hind end are all signs that the owner may mention when calling with an issue in need of an exam. Occasionally the owner may think the cat is constipated and trying to have a bowel movement when in actuality the cat is straining to urinate and should be seen immediately to be checked for a **urethral obstruction**.

Performing CPR on Dogs

To perform **CPR**, the animal is laid on its side and 100–120 chest compressions are given per minute for all sizes and species. The person performs chest compressions by placing the hands flat with the palm of one on top of the other, locking elbows, and pushing in a downward motion onto the compression point. Compressions must be forceful enough to compress the chest 1/3–1/2 of its normal width. For deep-chested dogs, compressions will be given over the widest part of the chest, and for narrow-chested dogs, compressions are given over the heart. The patient will be ventilated (if intubated) at 10 breaths per minute. If the patient is not intubated, a veterinary team member must put their mouth around the patient's snout, holding their mouth closed and give 2 breaths per 30 compressions. To maintain the strength of compressions, it is recommended to switch people giving compressions every 2 minutes. Also, vasopressors should be administered every 5 minutes during CPR.

Stabilizing and Placing a Splint in an Emergency Fractured Limb with an Open Wound

If a patient presents with an **emergency fractured limb and an open wound,** the first thing to accomplish is stabilizing the patient and controlling the pain. Once the patient is stable, then the wound will need to be clipped, flushed, and cleaned out with a 0.9% sterile saline solution to remove most of the bacteria. An antimicrobial solution such as chlorhexidine is then used to clean the wound. To apply a splint to the limb, stirrups are formed from nonporous white tape and are placed on the dorsal and palmar sides of the foot and then stuck together off of the paw onto a tongue depressor so the ends don't stick to each other. Cast padding is then applied over the fracture to stabilize the leg; then a second layer of synthetic cast padding is applied around the leg with extra padding over areas that can develop pressure sores from the splint such as the proximal and distal ends of the injured limb. On top of the padding, a type of elastic or roll gauze is placed to create a smooth surface to place the splint on; then secure the splint to the limb with a layer of roll gauze followed by a layer of vet wrap.

Treating a Dog with Heatstroke

If a patient presents with **heatstroke**, the first thing to accomplish is cooling the patient down by use of cool water or towels applied to the patient's body and alcohol on the patient's feet. Cold water and ice are NOT recommended because they can cause vasoconstriction, moving the blood flow toward the body's main organs rather than to the body surface to help cool it down. If the patient is cooled too quickly, the body will not be able to regulate its own temperature due to heatstroke, so it is recommended to cool down to about 102.5 °F over the course of an hour. Cooling methods must be stopped after the patient's body temperature reaches around 102.5 °F to prevent them from shivering because that will increase their muscle activity and can raise their body temperature again. Oxygen supplementation must be administered to the patient via a mask to improve tissue perfusion, and room-temperature IV crystalloid fluids will be administered to help fight dehydration.

Types of Catheters Available for Use

Butterfly catheters have wings on the end with the needle in between so you can hold the wings during placement, and there is a line of tubing with an adaptor end to connect a syringe. Butterfly catheters are not for long-term use, but they are more commonly used to obtain blood samples or administer IV medications in cats and small dogs, ideally using the medial saphenous vein. Over-the-needle catheters are over the needle when placed, and then the needle is pulled out while the catheter is pushed into the vein. Over-the-needle catheters can be placed in any accessible vein, but they are normally placed in the cephalic vein and are used to administer IV fluids and medications and to administer emergency medications. Over-the-needle catheters can be placed and kept patent for up to 72 hours. Through-the-needle catheters are longer catheters used for critically ill patients requiring long-term venous access, and they must be placed using sterile technique in the jugular or lateral saphenous vein.

Catheter Use for Critically Ill Patients

Depending on what the patient is presenting for will help better determine which **catheter** type and vein to use for placement. If the patient will be hospitalized for the next couple of days, then an over-the-needle catheter can be used because it can be maintained for up to 72 hours. If a critically ill patient requires central venous access for parenteral nutritional supplementation, numerous blood draws, and to administer long-term medications for longer than 72 hours, then a through-the-needle catheter must be placed. When trying to determine which vein to use for catheter placement, you should consider if there is any injury to the limb and avoid using that limb.

Intraosseous catheterization (meaning directly into the marrow of the bone) is used in critical situations especially in neonates with limited IV access due to vascular collapse. Intraosseous catheterization can be used to administer fluids as well as emergency medications when a vein is not accessible in critically ill patients.

Oxygen Supplementation Techniques

Any patient experiencing hypoxemia will need oxygen supplementation, and there are a few ways to do it. The blow-by **oxygen supplementation** method is done by holding oxygen up to the patient's nose either by a breathing tube hooked to the oxygen tank or one with a mask attached. The **blow-by technique** will deliver oxygen concentrations of around 35% if given at 5 L/min. An oxygen cage will be able to deliver greater than 50% oxygen concentrations to patients, and the oxygen concentration in the cage can be regulated as well as the temperature and humidity inside the cage. **Intranasal oxygen catheters** can be placed inside the patient's nostril for oxygen delivery. Transtracheal catheters can be done by passing a catheter into the trachea to deliver oxygen, and this method will be able to deliver the highest oxygen concentration to the patient

Blood Transfusions and Administration

Blood transfusions can be given to treat anemia, coagulopathies, and acute blood loss. Packed RBCs, fresh frozen plasma, whole blood, frozen plasma, and synthetic blood substitutes are blood products that are available for use. Blood products are administered intravenously through an IV catheter. Blood products should be administered through an IV set designed solely for blood transfusions because they have fibers that remove blood clots and debris. A blood transfusion should be complete in less than 4 hours at up to 4 ml/kg/hr, and plasma transfusions can be given at up to 6 ml/kg/hr. Bolus amounts may be given if the patient is having severe hemorrhaging, which could result in death. If the patient reacts to the transfusion, they will have vomiting, diarrhea, and respiratory distress. The patient needs to be carefully monitored during the entire process of all vital signs.

Providing the Nutritional Support Needed for a Critically Ill Patient

Nutritional support is a vital part of managing a critically ill patient, and patients without it can have an impaired immune system and the patient will be more prone to infection. A lack of nutritional support can also lead to dehydration, muscle weakness, fatigue, organ failure, and death. With appropriate nutritional support in the hospital, wound healing will be enhanced, organ function will be maintained, and body mass will be maintained for critically ill patients. The enteral route (feeding tubes) for nutritional support is the method of choice if the patient will not tolerate syringe feeding or eating on its own. The type of food will be chosen based on the patient's degree of malnutrition and the calorie and protein requirements.

Performing Evaluations of the Patient's Physical and Mentation Status

The veterinary technician will review the patient's medical history and current status, along with any medications being administered, and nutrition. After reviewing the patient's history, the technician can perform the physical examination. A TPR and the patient's mentation should be noted, along with the patient's hydration status. The patient's **mentation** status will be noted as **bright**, **alert**, and **responsive** (BAR), quiet, alert, and responsive (QAR), dull, or depressed. The veterinary technician should evaluate the patient for any signs of pain. Signs of pain include a fast heart rate, vocalizing, abdominal pain upon palpation, hunched posture, trembling, and depression. The technician will also note how much the patient is eating and drinking or will be administering food via a feeding tube and recording the time and amount. The technician will also note and evaluate any urine and bowel movement output as well. The technician must make sure that the patient is provided comfort with blankets and make sure that they are clean and dry at all times. If the patient is a cat, make sure that the litter box is being cleaned.

Evaluate the Patient's Behavioral Status in Critical Status

When a client brings their pet in for an emergency or critical event, probing questions should be asked about the **patient's behavior**. Asking questions such as if the owner has noticed any sudden behavior changes recently and what the behaviors are can aid in diagnosing the issue. Certain sudden behavior changes, such as hiding, aggression, and anxiety, can indicate pain. Once the owner may realize that their pet has acted aggressively lately, further questions should be asked such as the following: When does the pet show aggression? Does the pet show aggression if you touch a certain area of its body, indicating it is in pain? If the patient is being hospitalized, their behavior must be monitored throughout their stay along with vital signs. Watching for trends in behavior while in the hospital can prove whether supportive care and medications are helping if the animal seems more relaxed and is resting. If the patient is restless and panting, this could also be due to stress, so ongoing behavior evaluation is vital to have a baseline of how the patient has acted since they presented to the hospital.

Pain Management/Analgesia

Pain Types and Severity

Four Components of Pain Transmission

The four components of **pain transmission** include transduction, transmission, modulation, and perception. **Transduction** is the process in which trauma, infection, or inflammation activates the nerve endings (nociceptors). The three categories of damaging stimuli are mechanical, such as pressure or swelling; heat, such as a burn; and chemical, which includes infection or contact with a toxic substance. When a damaging stimulation occurs, it causes chemical mediators to be released from damaged cells, causing the nociceptors to become sensitive. **Transmission** is the process by which the message is carried from the injury site to the brain. When the pain impulses reach the thalamus, they are sent to different areas of the brain where they are processed and the perception of pain takes place. **Perception** of pain includes noticing the pain, expecting it, and the anticipation of it. The **modulation** phase changes or inhibits the transmission of pain impulses in the spinal cord and can develop into an increase or decrease in the transmission of pain impulses.

Five Classifications of Pain

The **five classifications of pain** include clinical pain, peripheral pain, neuropathic pain, idiopathic pain, and physiologic pain. Pain that results when the spinal cord or peripheral nerves are injured and painful impulses are repeatedly picked up by the nociceptors is **clinical pain**. **Visceral pain** or somatic pain that involves the joints and muscles is considered peripheral pain. Visceral pain includes the chest and abdomen and causes cramping, whereas somatic pain is more confined and causes an aching feeling. **Neuropathic pain** causes a random burning sensation after peripheral nerves or spinal cord damage is done. **Idiopathic pain** has no real cause, and pain that is caused by a quick and sharp painful stimulus to the peripheral nerve, such as touching a hot iron, is **peripheral pain**.

Physiology of Pain

Nociceptors, otherwise known as pain receptors, are found all throughout the body and are sensitive to mechanical, thermal, and chemical stimuli. Once the stimulus triggers the nociceptor, a **nerve impulse** is made and transmitted to the dorsal horn of the spinal cord. Once it reaches the spinal cord, it causes a release of excitatory and inhibitory neurotransmitters. **Excitatory neurotransmitters** will continue to send the signal to the brain, and inhibitory neurotransmitters will inhibit the signal from traveling any further. The three nerve fibers include A-delta, A-beta, and C fibers. A **nerve fibers** are more sensitive to thermal or mechanical stimuli, whereas C fibers can be sensitive to all stimuli including mechanical, chemical, and thermal.

Four Most Common Types of Pain Seen in Dogs and Cats

The **four most common types of pain** are acute, chronic, cancer, and neuropathic pain. **Acute pain** is the body's response to a harmful stimulus or injury to the tissues, such as a burn or wound that causes pain described as throbbing, aching, or burning, and it will normally improve within a few days. **Chronic pain** lingers longer than the usual healing time and is a result of a disease such as osteoarthritis, which the patient will need to manage for the duration of their lives. Pain associated with cancer results from the actual tumor or from the cancer if it has metastasized, and it also encompasses painful effects from chemotherapy and radiation. Damage to the CNS causes neuropathic pain, in which damage to the nerves in the body creates chronic pain for the patient and can impair the patient's mobility and bodily functions if it originates in the spinal cord.

Intervertebral disc disease affects the spinal cord and can create pain to other areas of the body and cause the patient to be hypersensitive in that area.

Treatment of Pain

Pain Management for the Patient Undergoing a Dental Procedure

Pain must be managed before, during, and after a **dental procedure**. The benefits of pain management during the dental procedure include the ability to maintain the patient at a lighter anesthesia plane, which significantly reduces that patient's anesthetic risk. Pain management after the procedure includes pain medications that go home with the client to administer, and this helps with the recovery process. If the patient has oral surgery including extractions or removing oral masses and is not treated adequately for pain, then once the pet gets home it will show signs of being in pain such as whining, hiding, not eating well or at all, and excessive drooling. Seeing their pets in pain could encourage the owner to keep up with their pet's dental care in the future.

Osteoarthritis in Small Animals

Osteoarthritis results when the cartilage in the joints degenerates over the course of the patient's lifetime, causing pain and inflammation. The degeneration of joints could be caused by numerous things, such as infection or trauma. Joint and cartilage destruction and inflammation often result from degenerative joint disease, and after enough damage has taken place on the joints, grinding sounds may be heard during movement. Diagnosing osteoarthritis commonly involves the patient's overall disposition, pain upon palpation of the joints, and the owner's evaluation of their pet's movement and painful signs at home. Signs of osteoarthritis are lameness, muscle wasting, the pet can no longer get up and down stairs or jump up onto the bed, and the pet may have trouble getting up after laying down. Radiographs can show soft-tissue swelling around the joint, an increase in joint fluid, and a narrow joint space.

Neuropathic Pain in Dogs

Neuropathic pain in dogs stems from an injury that commonly is from within the spinal cord affecting the body's nerves. Intervertebral disc disease is a specific disease that affects the spinal cord, and depending on which part of the spinal cord is affected, different areas of the patient's body will experience pain. A tumor in the spinal cord may also be a cause of neuropathic pain, as well as limb amputations in which patients may experience phantom pain. When one of these possible causes damages the body tissues and nerves, it creates a chronic pain that has a heightened sensitivity and pain perception for the patient with any contact with the affected area.

Pathophysiology of Pain

Once the patient experiences a painful stimulus, the body releases **catecholamines**. The release of catecholamines will cause high blood pressure, increased heart rate, and it even may lead to left ventricular dysfunction, ischemia, and infarction. The patient can become insulin resistant and hyperglycemic due to the release in cortisol and glucagon resulting from the pain response. If the patient is experiencing abdominal pain, they may have difficulty resting and getting comfortable or they may experience ileus. Patients that experience neck pain may be hypersensitive to slight movements and will exhibit signs of stress and irritability as well as difficulty getting comfortable. Patients that are experiencing chest pain may have difficulty breathing. All forms of pain will present stress to the patient, and when the body is dealing with the stress, the immune system is suppressed and there is a higher chance of infection.

Three Processes That Take Place When a Noxious Stimulus is Experienced

The **three processes** that take place include **transduction**, **transmission**, and **modulation**. The nociceptors change the chemical, thermal, or mechanical energy into electrical impulses at the site of pain during **transduction**. That electrical impulse travels through a three-neuron chain through the **transmission process**. During transmission, the first-order neurons travel to the dorsal horn of the spinal cord, second-order neurons send pain signals to the brain from the spinal cord, and third-order neurons take the pain signals to the cerebral cortex. Finally, the internal analgesic systems inhibit the dorsal horn cells in the spine from processing the pain with natural analgesics in the **modulation phase.**

The Wind-Up Phenomenon

The **wind-up phenomenon** occurs if pain is not adequately treated. The prolonged stimulation of nociceptors causes the CNS to adversely adapt to repetitive pain impulses, causing the nervous system to change the way it is processing the pain. Hyperalgesia results, meaning that there is less stimulation needed to initiate a pain response. Wind-up is also a result of nerve fibers that would normally carry nonpainful information that are now recruited to the pain transmission process resulting in harmless information being interpreted as pain, and this is called allodynia. The presence of hyperalgesia and allodynia together is known as wind-up pain.

Assessing Acute Pain in Dogs

Acute pain refers to pain that is the result of a surgery, sudden trauma, or medical issue that ranges from mild to severe and can last up to a few days but can be managed with analgesia drugs if the pain is assessed regularly. Each dog should have the same pain assessment protocol in place whether they are a hospitalized patient or have just had surgery. The first step would be to watch the dog and assess its posture. If the dog appears hunched over or standing rather than laying down and relaxed, this is an indication of pain that should be addressed right away. The next thing to be done to help assess the dog's pain would be to handle the dog and touch the area where the wound or surgical incision was made to observe the patient's response. If the patient tries to bite, move away, whine, or flinch, this is an indication of pain that would need to be addressed.

Assessing a Cat or Dog's Response to the Treatment of Pain

There must be a protocol in place that is used on every patient to assess pain based on the normal behaviors of cats and dogs compared to how they behave if they are in pain and to what severity. Once the patient arrives at the hospital, there should be an assessment of pain if presenting with an acute trauma or medical issue; therefore, after administering pain control medication, for the duration of the hospital stay, their pain can continue to be assessed compared to the initial exam as to whether it is getting worse, improving, or remaining the same. If the patient appears to still be in pain after pain control medication has been administered, then a different medication may be used or an extra dose may be given. Pain assessment following acute pain such as surgeries should be done every half hour, and then after 8 hours the patient can be assessed every hour depending on the type of surgical procedure.

Preemptive Analgesia for Surgery

Blocking the pain pathway prior to a painful stimulus during surgery is considered **preemptive analgesia.** Blocking the pain pathway decreases **postoperative pain** for the patient. Preemptive analgesia will decrease the amount of induction agent needed as well as maintenance drugs, which lowers the cardiopulmonary effects of general anesthesia on the patient. Using analgesic drugs from more than one analgesic class is a multimodal approach that will increase the success of treating pain because the pain impulse can be blocked at several areas in the pain pathway reaching a synergistic effect in which the drugs will interact and work together for the end result of preventing pain.

Performing Noninteractive and Interactive Assessments of the Patient's Pain

In order to effectively evaluate a patient's level of pain, you must first be familiar with how the patient's normal demeanor is and their normal activity level. Questions to ask the owner are the following: How active is your pet on a normal day? How has their activity level changed recently? You must be able to distinguish between pain and stress. When the pet comes into the hospital, they may hide in the corner and not move because they are scared and not necessarily because they are in pain. To evaluate the patient without being interactive would be to monitor their actions when they think nobody is watching. Watch their movements, if they are eating or drinking, and note if they seem to become more relaxed. Interactive evaluation involves manipulating joints that may be causing pain to elicit a response to pain or palpating different parts of the body suspected to be causing pain for the patient. An ongoing evaluation of pain should continue with documenting any changes in the status of the patient's pain level or any medications administered and how they helped alleviate the pain.

Recognizing a Patient Having Chronic Pain Through Behavioral Changes

The owner is normally the first to recognize if their pet is having **chronic pain** issues because they will notice certain behavior changes. They could also bring their pet in because it will not sleep at night, won't lay down, and is constantly panting, which indicates that the pet could be in pain. Even if the patient is not presenting with an issue, it is important that the veterinary staff asks questions relating to possible behavior issues that could indicate chronic pain. If the pet is becoming aggressive, hiding, or acting lethargic, these can be signs of a chronic pain issue. Also, if the pet is moving around slower than normal, having trouble going up or down the stairs, or even having trouble jumping up and down, these would be possible signs of osteoarthritis. Asking the client probing questions is the key to catching pain issues early so that a therapy plan can be started to help the pet live a long and healthy life with well-managed pain control.

The Tibial Plateau Leveling Esteotomy (TPLO) Procedure

A **tibial plateau leveling osteotomy** (TPLO) surgery is performed on dogs with a torn **anterior cruciate ligament** (ACL). Approximately 90% of all orthopedic injuries in canines are from a torn ACL, and the TPLO surgery has been proven to be an extremely effective solution. A dog's knee is at a constant 110-degree bend; therefore, there is a constant stress put on the ACL, which is inside of the knee joint. Occasionally, this constant stress will cause injury or tearing of the ACL, which then results in the femur rubbing along the back of the tibia causing pain and inflammation. A TPLO surgery will be performed to rotate the tibial plateau where it is rubbing with the femur so that the femur will no longer be able to slide back on it, which creates stabilization for that knee. The first 12 weeks post-surgery are critical, but a full recovery usually takes 6 months. Each dog will recover at its own pace, but home rehabilitation is crucial. The owner should be made aware to avoid infection of the surgical site, and the dog must be kept from licking at the wound by wearing an **Elizabethan collar**. The owner must keep the dog quiet and avoid overactivity for a minimum of 8 weeks because the joint will need to heal.

Client Assessing Their Feline Pet's Pain Level

Educate clients on the fact that **felines hide their pain wel**l and that they must be able to notice the signs and symptoms of pain. The owner should be looking for subtle signs or **behaviors that are outside of the cat's normal behavior** and daily habits. If the cat is normally very active, playful, and interactive, then a sign that something is wrong would be if the cat was sleeping more, hiding, or uninterested in toys. **Inappropriate urination** or **bowel movements** outside of the box could be a sign of pain once a UTI is ruled out. **Aggression** can also be a sign that the cat is in pain as well as fast/shallow breathing patterns and an increased heart rate. **Physical characteristics** of the cat's facial appearance such as dilated pupils, squinting eyes, and ears down or back could indicate pain as well. Educate the client that all of these signs could be pain from a variety of reasons or other serious medical issue and the cat should be evaluated by the veterinarian. If the cat is currently being given long-term medications such as NSAIDs for chronic pain, then the owner will want to be aware of any changes in the pet's pain level to see if medication adjustments are necessary.

Efficacy of NSAID Use in Dogs for Osteoarthritis

NSAIDs are commonly used for **long-term pain management** for dogs with osteoarthritis. NSAIDs are very effective with treating the patient's long-term arthritis pain by **decreasing inflammation and stiffness**. NSAIDs will regulate the body's production of certain enzymes, called prostaglandins, that are responsible for inflammation. Common prescription brands of NSAIDs include Rimadyl, Previcox, and Metacam. While taking long-term NSAIDs, the patient should have annual blood work done to evaluate kidney and liver enzymes because NSAIDs can have a negative effect on these organs. NSAIDs are very effective pain management medications that work to alleviate inflammation and pain so the patient will be more active, allowing for muscle strength to build up so the patient can have more sturdy control over its joints. NSAIDs are much more effective when given daily, so they are getting ahead of the pain rather than given only when the pet shows signs of pain.

Efficacy of Hydrotherapy Used for Dogs and Cats with Osteoarthritis Pain

Hydrotherapy is used for dogs and cats. This effective therapy **strengthens the patient's muscles and allows for joints that are normally painful to move freely**. Hydrotherapy **stimulates the cardiovascular** system as well. While the patient is walking or swimming in water, the therapy is working by making this workout weightless, and it is painless because there are no hard surfaces to step on and there is a reduced effect of gravity. Goals of hydrotherapy, whether it be in underwater treadmills or pools, are to increase the patient's range of motion, improve the strength of the muscles, stimulate circulation of the lymph system, and work out the cardiovascular system. Patients suffering from osteoarthritis benefit greatly from hydrotherapy, as well as patients with hip dysplasia, torn cruciate ligaments, and other musculoskeletal injuries.

Ways the Owner Can Help Manage Osteoarthritis Pain in Dogs at Home

Nonsteroidal anti-inflammatory medications (NSAIDs) are often prescribed to a patient with **osteoarthritis**, and they work by blocking the inflammatory process, which in turn blocks the pain. An **opioid** such as tramadol may be given to the patient as well for added pain relief or if the patient cannot take NSAIDs due to kidney or liver issues. Maintaining a healthy weight, limiting exercise, along with providing cushion and support in the sleeping area will need to be implemented to manage osteoarthritis pain. Weight management is important because any extra weight puts more pressure on the bones and joints, causing further deterioration of the cartilage. Patients with osteoarthritis pain will need to move around and get exercise but cannot overdo it because this can add strain to their joints. Exercises should include short leash walks and physical therapy such as a water treadmill to improve the patient's range of motion, proprioception, and to build muscle mass.

Alternative Therapies for Managing Osteoarthritis

Alternative treatment options such as cold laser therapy, acupuncture, and shockwave therapy are available to use along with other forms of treatment for the management of osteoarthritis pain. Cold therapy lasers work by sending red laser and infrared laser light wavelengths to promote cell metabolism and enhance the health of the cells through increased circulation. Acupuncture is a form of therapy that stimulates areas of the body to release certain neurotransmitters including beta endorphins and serotonin by inserting tiny needles into areas composed of free nerve endings, blood, and lymphatic vessels. If certain points are stimulated at the same time, this creates pain relief and promotes healing. Shockwave therapy uses sound waves to work on specific areas in the body and trigger the repair mechanisms of the body to reduce inflammation, promote the healing and overall health of bones, and to develop new blood vessels.

Prescription Medication and Supplements to Help Relieve Pain

NSAIDs are commonly prescribed for patients experiencing **acute or chronic pain** and work by reducing inflammation to relieve pain. Because NSAIDs are metabolized through the liver and can also affect the kidneys, it is important to perform **annual blood chemistry screenings** on patients who are taking these medications **long term** to monitor kidney and liver function. Opioids work on the CNS to relieve pain and are mainly prescribed for acute pain management. Local anesthetics such as lidocaine are used to numb the area for certain surgical procedures such as debriding and suturing a small wound. Glucosamine and chondroitin supplements can help to rebuild cartilage in the joints. Glucosamine hydrochloride is a part of the cartilage and will stimulate the growth of cells within the cartilage. Chondroitin sulfate is a molecule that works by stopping the enzymes attempting to destroy the cartilage.

Epidural Single-Injection Technique for Administering Analgesia

An **epidural single injection** should be performed once the patient has been induced and is in sternal positioning. The **epidural space**, where the spinal needle is placed, is between the spinal processes of L7 and S1 (the lumbosacral space), and it must be surgically shaved and scrubbed using sterile gloves. The needle with the stylet pierces the skin to almost 1 inch deep, and then the stylet is removed. The hub of the needle is filled with sterile saline and advanced until a "pop" is felt as it advances through the ligament, and the saline is pulled through the needle as it enters the epidural space. If blood enters the hub of the needle, it should be removed and the procedure is tried again. If the needle is passed into the subarachnoid space, then cerebrospinal fluid will flow into the needle and the epidural will need to be redone. The agent to be administered is given slowly, and once it is given, the spinal needle can be slowly pulled out and removed. Morphine is a common analgesic administered via the epidural technique, and it has a slightly slower onset of action (up to 1 hour), so it is best given directly after induction.

Simbadol

Simbadol is an **opioid agonist** and is a controlled substance under Schedule III. Simbadol is a high-concentration buprenorphine (not sustained release) that can be used in cats and has a 24-hour duration of action. Simbadol is routinely administered SQ, but when given IM, its duration of action is reduced to 6 hours. Simbadol is indicated for postoperative pain in cats and is dosed at 0.24 mg/kg. Simbadol should be used with caution in cats with liver disease because it is metabolized through the liver, but it is not excreted in the urine. Simbadol can be administered once daily for up to 3 days for pain control.

Veterinary Technician Code of Ethics

The **veterinary technician code of ethics** states that veterinary technicians should provide excellent care to animals with compassion and competence. Veterinary technicians should commit to lifelong learning through continuing education and educate the public about disease control and zoonotic diseases, as well as assisting with the control of such diseases. Technicians will keep client information confidential unless this information should be disclosed as required by law. Veterinary technicians should act responsibly and uphold the laws and regulations that apply to their position.

Veterinary technicians are held accountable for their actions and must protect the public and the profession against other individuals within the profession who lack competence and ethics.

Image Credits

LICENSED UNDER CC BY 4.0 (CREATIVECOMMONS.ORG/LICENSES/BY/4.0/)

Anatomy of the Tooth: "Tooth Anatomy" by Wikimedia user BruceBlaus (https://commons.wikimedia.org/wiki/File:Tooth_Anatomy_Part_1.png)

Toxocar Cati: "Extremite Anterieure de Toxacar Cati"by Wikimedia user Leodras (https://commons.wikimedia.org/wiki/File:Extr%C3%A9mit%C3%A9_ant%C3%A9rieure_de_Toxocara_cati.jpg)

Strongylus Vulgaris Larva: "Strongylus Vulgaris – Parasite of Horses 01" by Wikimedia user Vitaliy Kharchenko (https://commons.wikimedia.org/wiki/File:Strongylus_vulgaris_-_parasite_of_horses_01.jpg)

Blood Smear: "Blood Smear" by Wikimedia user Анастасія Грущенко (https://commons.wikimedia.org/wiki/File:Blood_Smear.jpg)

Doppler BP Measurement: "Blood Pressure Cat Doppler" by Wikimedia user Kalumet (https://commons.wikimedia.org/wiki/File:Blood_pressure_cat_doppler.JPG)

LICENSED UNDER CC BY-SA 3.0 (CREATIVECOMMONS.ORG/LICENSES/BY-SA/3.0/DEED.EN)

Dirofilaria Immitis: "Dirofilaria-Immitis-Dog-Heart" by Wikimedia user Alan R Walker (https://commons.wikimedia.org/wiki/File:Dirofilaria-immitis-dog-heart.jpg)

Dirofilaria Immitis: Dirofilaria Immitis Lifecycle by Wikimedia user Cú Faoil (https://commons.wikimedia.org/wiki/File:Dirofilaria_immitis_lifecycle.svg)

Ctenocephalides SSP: "Catflea small" by Wikimedia user Evanherk (https://commons.wikimedia.org/wiki/File:Catflea_small.jpg)

Demodectic Mange: "Demodex Milbe Adult" by Wikimedia user Kalumet (https://commons.wikimedia.org/wiki/File:Demodex_Milbe_adult.jpg)

Leukocytes: "1907 Granular Leukocytes" by Openstax user OpenStax (https://cnx.org/contents/FPtK1zmh@6.27:zMTtFGyH@4/Introduction)

Field Stain: "Hodgkin Lymphoma Cytology Small" by Wikimedia user Nephron (https://commons.wikimedia.org/wiki/File:Hodgkin_lymphoma_cytology_small.jpg)

Phagocytic Cell: "TEM Image of Legionella Pneumophila within a Phagocytic Cell" by Wikimedia user Clares Back (https://commons.wikimedia.org/wiki/File:TEM_image_of_Legionella_pneumophila_within_a_phagocytic_cell.tif)

ECG Waveform: "Electrocardiogram of a Healthy Man, 21 Years Old" by Wikimedia user Novic84 (https://commons.wikimedia.org/wiki/File:Electrocardiogram_of_a_healthy_man,_21_years_old.jpg)

Canine Parvovirus: "Parvovirus Infection-wo cond-very high mag" by Wikimedia user Nephron(https://commons.wikimedia.org/wiki/File:Parvovirus_infection_-_wo_cond_-_very_high_mag.jpg)

LICENSED UNDER CC BY-SA 2.0 (HTTPS://CREATIVECOMMONS.ORG/LICENSES/BY/2.0/)

Howell-Jolly Bodies: "Corps de Howell-Jolly-3" by Wikimedia user Guy Waterval (https://commons.wikimedia.org/wiki/File:Corps_de_Howell-Jolly-3.JPG)

VTNE Practice Test

1. Which of the following pieces of information is NOT required on a prescription label?

a. Date of the prescription
b. Age of the patient
c. Name of the prescriber
d. Address of the dispensing pharmacy

2. Fluoroquinolones should not be used in

a. young animals because they cause arthropathy.
b. growing animals because they cause heart conduction disturbance.
c. pregnant animals because they cause abortion.
d. older animals because they cause arthropathy.

3. Which of the following is the most nephrotoxic aminoglycoside?

a. Streptomycin
b. Amikacin
c. Tobramycin
d. Neomycin

4. Which class of drugs is NOT a good choice to treat an infection by a gram-positive anaerobe?

a. Tetracyclines
b. Macrolides
c. Aminoglycosides
d. Beta-lactams

5. When a cat is in compensatory shock the cat should receive isotonic replacement crystalloid fluids intravenously at a rate of

a. 60 mL/kg/h
b. 90 mL/kg/h
c. 30 mL/kg/h
d. 45 mL/kg/h

6. If a patient presented with dry and retracted eyes, dry mucous membranes, weak and rapid pulses, and a significant loss of skin turgor, at what percentage of interstitial dehydration would you estimate the patient to be?

a. More than 11%
b. 8% - 10%
c. 4 - 5%
d. 0 - 3%

7. To create a 5% dextrose solution in a 500 mL bag of 0.45% NaCl, how many mL of a 50% dextrose solution must be added? (Assume that a corresponding amount of NaCl solution will be removed prior to the dextrose being added.)

a. 5 mL
b. 25 mL
c. 50 mL
d. 100 mL

8. Hydromorphone, fentanyl, and pentobarbital are classified by Drug Enforcement Administration regulations as belonging to which of the following groups of controlled substances?

a. Schedule I
b. Schedule II
c. Schedule III
d. Schedule IV

9. Which of the following statements is/are true about the inventory of controlled substances?

a. A new inventory of controlled substances on hand must be taken at least every 2 years.
b. An inventory must include the number of commercial containers of each finished form.
c. An inventory must include the date the inventory was conducted.
d. All of the above are true.

10. What is a reverse distributor?

a. A supplier who resells returned merchandise
b. A supplier who resells returned pharmacy merchandise only
c. A Drug Enforcement Administration registered pharmacist who is authorized to sell items from their inventory to practitioners
d. A Drug Enforcement Administration registrant authorized to receive unusable or unwanted controlled substances

11. Which of the following is an effective surface disinfectant?

a. 1:32 dilution of 5.25% solution of sodium hypochlorite
b. 5.25% solution of sodium hypochlorite
c. 1:5 dilution of 5.25% solution of sodium hypochlorite
d. All of the above

12. Which of the following is NOT true about recombinant human erythropoietin (rh-EPO)?

a. rh-EPO is indicated in canine and feline patients with renal disease and a PCV of 25% or less.
b. There is a high incidence of antibody formation to rh-EPO in dogs and cats.
c. rh-EPO should be given to dogs and cats three times weekly until the target PCV is reached.
d. The maximum dose of rh-EPO that should be given to a dog or cat is 100 U/kg.

13. Which of the following is the best description of strangles?

a. A contagious disease of horses caused by Streptococcus equi var equi
b. An autoimmune disease of dogs causing a skin disorder
c. A bacterial disease of horses that can be prevented with vaccination
d. All of the above.

14. Which of the following is false regarding endotoxins?

a. Endotoxin is a component of the external cell wall of gram-negative bacteria.
b. Endotoxin causes the release of cytokines, vasoactive amines, and proteases.
c. Glucocorticoids are used to treat endotoxic shock.
d. Antibiotics are used to treat endotoxic shock.

15. Which of the following is NOT a statement of the Veterinary Technician Code of Ethics?

a. "Veterinary technicians shall remain competent through commitment to life-long learning."
b. "Veterinary technicians shall safeguard the public and the profession against individuals deficient in professional competence or ethics."
c. "Veterinary technicians shall assume accountability for their professional actions as well as those with whom they work."
d. "Veterinary technicians shall represent their credentials or identify themselves with specialty organizations only if the designation has been awarded or earned."

16. Which of the following groups contains all reportable diseases?

a. Bluetongue, paratuberculosis, Rift Valley fever, lumpy skin disease
b. Anthrax, coronavirus, Marek's disease, ascariasis
c. Rinderpest, sheep pox virus, toxoplasmosis, feline infectious peritonitis
d. Camel pox virus, Q fever, Trichinellosis, feline immunodeficiency virus

17. Which of the following is/are important post-surgical instructions following an ovariohysterectomy?

a. Directions for use of pain relief
b. Limit movement
c. Return for suture removal in 3 days
d. Both A and B

18. What is the proper order of procedures for cleaning the canine or feline ear canal?

1. Ensure the tympanic membrane is intact.
2. Massage the ear.
3. Apply cleaning/flushing fluid to the ear canal.
4. Remove debris from the canal.

a. 1, 2, 3, 4
b. 4, 1, 2, 3
c. 1, 3, 2, 4
d. 3, 2, 4, 1

19. Which of the following is true about heat therapy during cranial cruciate ligament rehabilitation?

a. Damp heat is applied to muscles prior to exercise.
b. Dry heat is applied to the joint and muscles.
c. Heat is applied immediately following surgery.
d. Heat is applied every hour during recovery.

20. When considering the dietary needs of a dog or cat with liver disease, which of the following is true?

a. Protein must be restricted.
b. Normal amounts of protein are fed.
c. A high fat diet is recommended.
d. High amounts of sugar are fed.

21. Calculate a constant rate infusion of lidocaine for a 20-kg dog. The dog must receive lidocaine at 60 mcg/kg/minute. The dog is currently receiving NaCl at a rate of 60 mL/kg/day.

a. 68 mL
b. 72 mL
c. 78 mL
d. 90 mL

22. When a pet dies, its owner often experiences grief. Correctly identify the order and stages of the five stages of grief as identified by Kubler-Ross.

a. Denial, anger, bargaining, depression, and acceptance
b. Anger, depression, denial, bargaining, and acceptance
c. Anger, depression, bargaining, acceptance, and peace
d. Bargaining, anger, depression, peace, acceptance

23. When evaluating a dog or cat for middle ear disease, which radiographic view is best to use?

a. VD or lateral
b. VD, open mouth, or parallel open jaw
c. DV or open mouth
d. DV and lateral

24. "Fill the cat's bladder with contrast and saline. Place the cat in lateral recumbency. Apply gentle pressure to the bladder. Take a radiograph as fluid leaks out." Which of the following is the proper name for this procedure?

a. Bladder study
b. Vesicoureterogram
c. Voiding urethrogram
d. Positive contrast urethrogram

25. A non-rebreathing circuit on an anesthesia machine should only be used

a. for patients weighing 6 kg or less.
b. for patients weighing more than 6 kg.
c. during anesthetic induction.
d. when using isoflurane anesthesia.

26. Which of the following steps is NOT necessary to check an anesthesia machine and circuit prior to use?

a. Fill vaporizers.
b. Confirm waste gas scavenging system is connected.
c. Check the system for leaks by pressurizing a closed circuit to 30 cm H2O.
d. Allow oxygen and gas to flow for five minutes prior to use.

27. Which of the following is not a parameter of perfusion?

a. Capillary refill time
b. Mucous membrane color
c. Heart rate
d. Respiratory rate

28. Food should be withheld for how long prior to surgery in horses?

a. 1 hour
b. 4-8 hours
c. 24 hours
d. Food should not be withheld

29. Which of the following anesthetics is the only one licensed for use in fish?

a. Isoflurane
b. Etomidate
c. Tricaine methanesulfonate (MS-222)
d. Ketamine

30. Surgical anesthesia is attained in rabbits and rodents

a. when the patient has been on anesthetic gas for five minutes.
b. when reflexes have decreased such that ear, toe, and tail pinches do not result in withdrawal.
c. when heart rate decreases to 40 beats per minute.
d. in none of the above situations.

31. Which of the following types of forceps would NOT be included in a standard surgical pack?

a. Kelly hemostatic forceps
b. Adson-Brown tissue forceps
c. Babcock forceps
d. Backhaus towel clamp

32. What is the correct use of Metzenbaum scissors?

a. To cut delicate tissue
b. To cut bandages
c. To cut sutures
d. For routine cutting and dissection

33. Which of the following is true about steam sterilization of surgical packs?

a. Cotton muslin wrap should never be used.
b. A minimum temperature of 160 °F is needed for sterilization.
c. Wrapping material must be permeable to steam.
d. Autoclave paper can be reused.

34. Which of the following is true regarding cytochrome P450?

1. Cytochrome P-450 gene families are named beginning with the letters CYP.
2. Cytochrome P-450 enzymes metabolize toxins and drugs.
3. Cytochrome P-450 enzymes work primarily in the intestines.
4. Cytochrome P-450 enzymes synthesize steroids.
5. Cytochrome P-450 enzymes synthesize bile acids.
6. Drugs can cause cytochrome P-450 enzyme induction.

a. 2, 4, 5, 6
b. 1, 2, 4, 5, 6
c. 1, 2, 5, 6
d. 1, 2, 3, 4, 5, 6

35. Diffusion across the cell membrane with the assistance of carrier proteins is called

a. diffusion.
b. osmosis.
c. facilitated diffusion.
d. filtration.

36. When delivered fluid is more concentrated than intravascular fluid, the delivered fluid is considered

a. hypertonic.
b. isotonic.
c. hypotonic.
d. none of the above.

37. Adipose is what type of tissue?

a. Epithelial tissue
b. Muscle tissue
c. Nervous tissue
d. Connective tissue

38. If something is plantar, it is

a. at the bottom of the rear foot.
b. toward the tail.
c. toward the backbone.
d. farthest from the medial plane.

39. Which of the following is equivalent?

a. 1 tbsp = 5 mL
b. 1 tbsp = 15 mL
c. 1 in = 2.45 cm
d. 1 in = 2.50 cm

40. A dog that weighs 80 pounds weighs

a. 36 kg.
b. 31 kg.
c. 176 kg.
d. 203 kg.

41. The proper name for a neutered male pig is a

a. gelding.
b. wether.
c. gib.
d. barrow.

42. The gestational period of the horse is

a. 285 days.
b. 148 days.
c. 336 days.
d. 365 days.

43. Which of the following is FALSE about canine hookworms?

a. Uncinaria stenocephala is a canine hookworm.
b. Canine hookworms have a worldwide incidence.
c. The prepatent period of canine hookworms is 7 days.
d. Dogs are infected by the ingestion of 3rd stage larvae.

44. Alternaria species, grain mite eggs, and Planarian are all

a. pseudoparasites.
b. spurious parasites.
c. parasites of chicken.
d. parasites of geese.

45. Which of the following life cycles is correctly ordered?

a. Dirofilaria immitis: mature larvae in the pulmonary arteries and right heart; then microfilaria develop in the blood to the L2 stage; then mosquito ingests the L2 larvae and larvae develop to the L3 stage; then mosquito transmits infective L3 by bite.
b. Taenia spp.: adult worms live in an animal's small intestine; then eggs and posterior segments of adult worms are shed in feces; then eggs are released from segments in feces; then intermediate hosts ingest eggs; then intermediate host tissue is eaten by the animal.
c. Toxascaris leonina: larvae mature in the small intestine and adult worms lay eggs; then eggs pass with feces; then eggs embryonate; then eggs undergo three molts; then animals pick up the L5 larvae in the environment.
d. Echinococcus granulosus: adult worms in the small intestine lay eggs; then eggs pass in the feces; then larvae develop to the infective L3 stage; then larvae are eaten and develop to adult worms.

46. When performing a barium study of the upper gastrointestinal tract of a bird, ventrodorsal and lateral radiographs should be taken at

a. 0, 15, 30, 60, and 120 minutes.
b. 0, 15, 30, 45, and 60 minutes.
c. 0, 30, 60, 120, and 240 minutes.
d. 30, 60, 90, and 120 minutes.

47. Which is NOT a radiographic view commonly used to evaluate the navicular bone?

a. Dorsoproximal-palmarodistal view
b. Tangential coronary view
c. Lateral-medial view
d. Flexor tangential view

48. You would expect to see which of the following radiographic changes in a dog with patent ductus arteriosus?

1. Enlarged left ventricle
2. Enlarged right ventricle
3. Segmental enlargement of the descending aortic arch
4. Enlarged left atrium
5. Enhanced pulmonary vascular pattern
6. Pulmonary effusion

a. 1, 2, 4, 6
b. 2, 3, 5, 6
c. 3, 5, 6
d. 1, 3, 4, 5

49. A deficiency in which nutrients is known to cause canine cardiomyopathy?

a. Taurine and carnitine
b. Taurine and glycine
c. Folic acid and carnitine
d. Calcium and folic acid

50. Guinea pigs have an absolute requirement for

a. Vitamin A
b. Vitamin B
c. Vitamin C
d. Vitamin D

51. Topical steroids should never be used on the eye when

a. a corneal ulcer is present.
b. uveitis is present.
c. a cataract is present.
d. systemic steroids are also used.

52. A 40-kg nursing bitch presents with hypocalcemia. She is to be treated with a constant rate infusion of 10% calcium gluconate at a rate of 10 mg/kg/hr. Calculate the amount of calcium gluconate to be delivered per minute.

a. 4 mg/min
b. 6.7 mg/min
c. 67 mg/min
d. 400 mg/min

53. What is true about testing for viral infection?

a. Positive viral serology proves active infection.
b. To prove active infection, viral serology must be performed twice, two weeks apart, and show a rising viral titer.
c. Positive viral serology that shows a viral antigen load of at least 1:128 is consistent with active infection.
d. Negative viral serology proves that the animal has not been exposed to, and is not infected with, the virus.

54. A common test to establish the presence of ringworm infection is

a. Response to antibiotics
b. Fecal flotation
c. Culture on dermatophyte medium
d. Culture on blood agar

55. The feline dental formula - permanent is

a. $2\left(\frac{3\ 1\ 3\ 1}{3\ 1\ 2\ 1}\right)$
b. $2\left(\frac{3\ 1\ 3}{3\ 1\ 2}\right)$
c. $2\left(\frac{3\ 1\ 4\ 2}{3\ 1\ 4\ 3}\right)$
d. $2\left(\frac{3\ 1\ 4\ 3}{3\ 1\ 4\ 3}\right)$

56. The owner of two cats calls to report that she is often finding feces outside the litter box. Which of the following would you recommend?

a. Allowing the cats to go outdoors
b. Medicating the cats for anxiety
c. Confining the cats to the bathroom with the litter pan
d. A second litter pan and more frequent cleaning of the litter pans

57. The frequencies used for veterinary ultrasound range from

a. 10 to 20 MHz
b. 25 to 40 MHz
c. 0.1 to 2.0 MHz
d. 2.25 to 10 MHz

58. Electrical activity that stimulates a heartbeat begins at the

a. bundle of His.
b. Purkinje bundle.
c. sinoatrial node.
d. atrioventricular node.

59. SOAP stands for

a. Standard Operating and Assessment Procedure.
b. Subjective Objective Assessment Plan.
c. Slim Overweight Anorexic Postanorexic.
d. Species Order Animalia Plantae.

60. Which of the following conditions are potential complications of a bovine cesarean section?

1. Retained placenta
2. Dehydration
3. Mastitis
4. Incision complications

a. 1, 4
b. 1, 2, 4
c. 1, 2, 3, 4
d. 4

61. Under OSHA regulations, a practice's written safety and health program for employees involved in hazardous waste operations must include

a. the safety and health training program, names of all employees, and work schedules.
b. names of all employees involved in hazardous waste operations, a medical surveillance program, and contractors who share hazardous waste operations.
c. the safety and health training program, a medical surveillance program, and the practice's standard operating procedures for safety and health.
d. a comprehensive work plan, employee phone list, and work schedules.

62. Personal protective equipment for protection against radiation is made from

a. steel.
b. lead.
c. bonded flexible plastic.
d. rubber.

63. In regard to radiographic personal protective equipment, veterinary technicians should do all of the following EXCEPT

a. fill lead gloves with water to check for leaks that allow radiation through.
b. hang safety equipment.
c. wear their own dosimeter whenever taking or assisting with radiographs.
d. radiograph PPE to evaluate for cracks.

64. Patient files are often color-coded to

a. identify the age of the patient.
b. establish the year a patient came to the practice.
c. prevent visual washout.
d. make filing errors easily visible.

65. Procaine penicillin should NEVER be given in which of the following ways?

a. IV
b. IM
c. SQ
d. None of the above

66. Canine body temperature exceeding 104 °F is common with toxic exposure to

a. lilies.
b. metaldehyde.
c. foxglove.
d. rodenticide.

67. Reconstituted vaccines must be used within

a. 1 hour.
b. 1 day.
c. 12 hours.
d. 2 hours.

68. An animal is prescribed prednisone on the following schedule:

"Take 20 mg every morning for 3 days. Take 10 mg every morning for 7 days. Take 5 mg every morning for 7 days. Take 5 mg every other morning for 2 weeks."

How many tablets should be dispensed?

a. 20 tablets (5mg)
b. 30 tablets (5mg)
c. 20 tablets (10mg)
d. 25 tablets (10mg)

69. A refractometer should be calibrated to 0 every week using

a. control solution.
b. refraction fluid.
c. deionized water.
d. distilled water.

70. "Walking dandruff" is

a. Demodex, diagnosed with a tape preparation.
b. Demodex, diagnosed by skin scraping.
c. Cheyletiella, diagnosed with a tape preparation.
d. Cheyletiella, diagnosed by skin scraping.

71. Use of a 40x objective on a standard light microscope will provide magnification of the studied object of

a. 400x.
b. 40x.
c. 4x.
d. 4000x.

72. The presence of a large number of erythrocytes with a wide variation in size is referred to as

a. microcytosis.
b. poikilocytosis.
c. macrocytosis.
d. anisocytosis.

73. Which are observed artifacts of histological sections?

1. Shrinkage
2. Precipitates
3. Folds
4. Growth distortion

a. 2, 3
b. 1, 2, 3
c. 1, 3, 4
d. All of the above

74. Put the following steps in order for proper Gram staining procedure.

1. Decolorize with ethyl alcohol.
2. Rinse with water.
3. Stain with crystal violet.
4. Stain with Gram's iodine.
5. Stain with safranin.

a. 3, 2, 4, 1, 2, 5, 2
b. 1, 4, 2, 3, 2, 5
c. 1, 3, 2, 5, 2, 4, 2
d. 4, 2, 3, 2, 5, 2, 1

75. A cat with isosthenuric urine will have what measure on the refractometer?

a. Below 1.008
b. 1.008 to 1.012
c. 1.012 to 1.020
d. Above 1.020

76. Neurontin, the proprietary liquid formulation of gabapentin, is contraindicated in dogs because it

a. causes seizures.
b. causes irreversible myelosuppression.
c. contains xylitol.
d. contains glycerin.

77. Dogs treated with bromide as an anticonvulsant that are already past the initiation phase must have blood levels checked every

a. 6 months.
b. 3 months.
c. 1 month.
d. 2 weeks.

78. For a cat at risk, an appropriate vaccination plan against the feline leukemia virus is

a. a two-dose primary series with annual vaccination thereafter.
b. vaccines every two to four weeks until 14 weeks of age and annual vaccination thereafter.
c. annual vaccination.
d. a two-dose primary series.

79. Total parenteral nutrition is administered through a large gauge catheter aseptically placed in the jugular vein or the

a. cranial vena cava.
b. caudal vena cava.
c. saphenous vein.
d. brachial vein.

80. Rabbits are known to have chronic and subclinical infections with which bacteria?

a. Pasteurella multocida
b. Klebsiella
c. Escherichia coli
d. Pseudomonas aeruginosa

81. Compared to the commonly unstained wet preparation for feline or canine urine sediment evaluation, the air-dried, modified-Wright stain is

a. more accurate for determination of crystalluria.
b. less accurate for determination of crystalluria.
c. more accurate for detection of bacteriuria.
d. less accurate for detection of bacteriuria.

82. For feline and canine patients that have not been premedicated, an appropriate dose of propofol for anesthetic induction is

a. 3 mg/kg IV given to effect.
b. 6 mg/kg IV given to effect.
c. 3-4 mg/kg IV.
d. 10 mg/kg.

83. You are advising a client with a new retriever about canine hip dysplasia. Which of the following statements would NOT be appropriate to mention?

a. Retrievers fed a controlled diet have a lower incidence of osteoarthritis than free-fed retrievers.
b. No commercial test ascertains the likelihood of a dog developing significant hip dysplasia.
c. If hip dysplasia develops, signs could include stiffness and lameness in the hind limbs, a hopping gait, and difficulty jumping or walking up stairs.
d. Because it is genetic, nothing can be done to prevent hip dysplasia in a pet.

84. Goals for personal or professional achievement should be SMART. SMART stands for

a. specific, manageable, attainable, realistic, timely.
b. specific, measurable, attainable, reliable, timely.
c. specific, manageable, attainable, reliable, targeted.
d. specific, measurable, attainable, realistic, timely.

85. A 10-kg dog requires a red cell transfusion. Calculate the rate of transfusion.

a. 20 mL/hr
b. 2 mL/hr
c. 0.1 mL/min
d. 1 mL/min

86. What is the most common bacterium associated with urinary tract infections of the dog or cat?

a. Streptococcus
b. Staphylococcus
c. E. coli
d. Klebsiella

87. Based on the oxygenation curve, a measured O2 value should be concerning if it is below what percent?

a. 60%
b. 75%
c. 85%
d. 95%

88. Which is NOT a potential problem identified by a high CO2 level on the end-tidal CO2 monitor during surgery?

a. Hypercapnia
b. Leak in system
c. Elevated inspired CO2
d. Bradycardia

89. What is the drug of choice for a tick-borne pathogen such as Borrelia burgdorferi?

a. Doxycycline
b. Tetracycline
c. Penicillin
d. Fluoroquinolones

90. The bovine fetal bladder attaches to the placental sac by the

a. urachus.
b. umbilical cord.
c. ureter.
d. vesiculosus.

91. Horses with painful colic often have heart rates exceeding

a. 100 bpm.
b. 140 bpm.
c. 120 bpm.
d. 50 bpm.

92. Which of the following is NOT a recognized category of shock?

a. Hypovolemic
b. Proliferative
c. Cardiogenic
d. Obstructive

93. Every time a radiograph is taken, a radiographic exposure log is commonly updated with which of the following information?

a. Date, patient name, measurements, type of cassette, exposure factors
b. Date, patient name, position, thickness of studied region, exposure factors, initials
c. Date, patient name, number of views, measurements
d. Patient name, number of views, exposure factors, cassette size

94. Inoculated agar plates should be evaluated for growth and change every

a. 24 hours.
b. 48 hours.
c. 1 week.
d. 12 hours.

95. MIC stands for

a. medial ileal cancer.
b. medial ileal cartilage.
c. minimum inhibitory concentration.
d. maximum inhibitory concentration.

96. Small intestinal cells absorb fluid droplets by the process of

a. phagocytosis.
b. pinocytosis.
c. membrane binding.
d. exocytosis.

97. A 14.6 kg animal weighs

a. 6.6 pounds.
b. 5 pounds.
c. 25 pounds.
d. 32.1 pounds.

98. A 50-pound dog ingests 8 sticks of gum, each containing 0.17g of xylitol. Has the dog eaten a potentially toxic dose?

a. Yes
b. No
c. Depends on the breed
d. Depends on the dog's age

99. Which position of the anesthetized horse results in the greatest V/Q mismatch?

a. Left lateral recumbency
b. Right lateral recumbency
c. Dorsal recumbency
d. Sternal recumbency

100. Which animal experiences fur slip when roughly handled?

a. Ferret
b. Guinea pig
c. Rabbit
d. Chinchilla

101. A roaster is a

a. 5-pound chicken.
b. 6-month-old chicken.
c. 3-5-month-old chicken weighing about 5-7 pounds.
d. 1-year-old chicken weighing about 7 pounds.

102. Which breed of chicken would not be farmed as a meat breed?

a. Silkie Bantam
b. New Hampshire Red
c. Rhode Island Red
d. Wyandotte

103. The primary survey during triage includes assessment of

a. history and complete physical examination.
b. minimum database.
c. obvious trauma only.
d. airway, breathing, and circulation.

104. A chick egg takes how many days to hatch?

a. 14 days
b. 21 days
c. 28 days
d. 35 days

105. A duck with limber neck has

a. chlamydiosis.
b. tetanus.
c. avian influenza.
d. botulism.

106. A twitch is usually placed on a horse's upper lip. Less commonly, it is placed on

a. both lips.
b. the lower lip and ear.
c. the tail.
d. both ears.

107. Proper general restraint of the ferret is achieved by

a. scruffing the neck and allowing the body to hang freely down.
b. using an arm to hold the length of the ferret against the body.
c. placing one hand under the shoulders with the thumb under the jaw, and using the other hand to support and restrain the hindquarters.
d. holding the ferret forward of the pelvis and allowing the rest of the body to hang freely down.

108. Which breed is an example of a dolichocephalic dog?

a. Collie
b. Westie
c. Pug
d. Saint Bernard

109. Aside from heart rate maintenance, atropine is used as a pre-anesthetic medication to

a. maintain respiration.
b. control secretions.
c. reduce the risk of seizure activity.
d. ease catheterization.

110. Which of these is NOT a sign of dystocia in a dog?

a. 68 days of gestation without signs of labor
b. 4 hours of weak contractions without production of a fetus
c. 30 minutes of strong contractions without production of a fetus
d. Overt disorder interfering with delivery

111. Hyperkalemia may be treated with

a. chloride.
b. sodium.
c. insulin and glucose.
d. insulin and dexamethasone.

112. Complete the sequence of viral replication:

Adsorption, then penetration, then __, then synthesis of viral nucleic acid and protein, then assembly/maturation, then release.

a. Uncoating
b. Destruction of cell
c. Replication of virions
d. Adherence

113. The U.S. Food and Drug Administration prohibits the use of which antibiotic in livestock?

a. Penicillin
b. Cephalosporins
c. Tetracycline
d. Monensin

114. Which common painful lesions of feline teeth are the result of odontoclast activation?

a. Reline caries
b. Feline oral resorptive lesions
c. Feline oral squamous cell carcinoma
d. Feline ulcerative disease

115. Cheyne-Stokes respiration refers to

a. deep, rapid breathing with no end-expiratory pause.
b. an unpredictable breathing pattern.
c. periods of apnea alternating with periods of tachypnea and hyperpnea.
d. a pause at the end of inspiration.

116. Which species has the potential for substantial stress-related hyperglycemia?

a. Horse
b. Pig
c. Cat
d. Rabbit

117. The process of setting a sheep on its hindquarters to work on its hooves or undersides is called

a. straddling.
b. tipping.
c. blocking.
d. cradling.

118. Complete the stages of the estrous cycle: proestrus, then estrus, then __, then diestrus.

a. Biestrus
b. Transestrus
c. Postestrus
d. Metestrus

119. A frantic owner calls to report worms in her dog's feces. You respond:

a. "That's an emergency. Bring your dog right in."
b. "Don't worry. Come in and pick up some medicine, I'll get it ready for you."
c. "Don't worry. Just keep your dog on monthly heartworm preventative."
d. "I'll schedule an appointment for you. Please bring a sample of feces with you for evaluation."

120. Flea larvae are

a. hydrophilic and photophilic.
b. hydrophilic and photophobic.
c. photophilic and kinesophobic.
d. photophobic and kinesophobic.

121. Pentobarbital should be used with great care, or not at all, in what kind of dogs?

a. Scent hounds
b. Sight hounds
c. Brachycephalics
d. Dolichocephalics

122. A pet has been placed on an elimination diet to evaluate response in assessing a food allergy. For what length of time must the pet remain on the elimination diet to ensure there has been NO response?

a. 2 weeks
b. 4 weeks
c. 6 weeks
d. 12 weeks

123. A loud murmur with a palpable thrill is a

a. grade 1 murmur.
b. grade 2 murmur.
c. grade 4 murmur.
d. grade 5 murmur.

124. When a urinalysis will not be run immediately, what test should be performed at the time of storage and at the time of evaluation?

a. Specific gravity
b. pH
c. Protein
d. Bilirubin

125. The veterinarian has asked you to perform a skin scraping and microscopic evaluation of an animal suspected of having a mite infestation. The collected material is placed on a slide. What is the correct method for slide evaluation?

a. 5 randomly chosen spots under high magnification
b. 5 randomly chosen spots under low magnification
c. A Z pattern under high magnification
d. A Z pattern under low magnification

126. The SNAP 4Dx Test tests for all of the following diseases EXCEPT

a. heartworm.
b. bartonellosis.
c. anaplasmosis.
d. ehrlichiosis.

127. Which of the following is NOT a round cell tumor?

a. Transmissible venereal tumor
b. Mast cell tumor
c. Melanoma
d. Cutaneous lymphoma

128. Horses have a blind spot in their visual field directly behind their head at approximately

a. 3°.
b. 20°.
c. 52°.
d. 87°.

129. When bandaging horses' legs, the legs should be wrapped in what direction(s)?

a. Right legs counterclockwise, left legs clockwise
b. Left legs counterclockwise, right legs clockwise
c. Clockwise
d. Counterclockwise

130. On a rebreathing system, the appropriate oxygen flow rate for a 5 kg cat is

a. 500 mL/min
b. 300 mL/min
c. 250 mL/min
d. 150 mL/min

131. The most common arrhythmia in a patient with GDV is

a. asystole.
b. VPCs.
c. sinus arrhythmia.
d. prolonged PR interval.

132. Hyperkalemia leads to what electrocardiographic change?

a. Asystole
b. VPCs
c. Absent PR interval
d. Peaked T waves

133. Between the ages of 4 and 20, a horse should have his or her teeth floated every

a. 3 months.
b. 6 months.
c. 1 year.
d. 2 years.

134. An adult rabbit should NOT be fed what type of hay routinely?

a. Timothy
b. Orchard grass
c. Alfalfa
d. Johnson grass

135. Small breed rabbits will be sexually mature as early as

a. 5 months.
b. 9 months.
c. 1 year.
d. 2 years.

136. Raptors are more easily handled with what placed on them?

a. Hood
b. Muzzle
c. Leash
d. Tape

137. Sweet clover poisoning causes

a. blindness.
b. diarrhea.
c. kidney failure.
d. hemorrhaging.

138. A repetitious behavior with no obvious purpose or function that interferes with normal function is a

a. redirected activity.
b. displaced activity.
c. stereotypic behavior.
d. frustration.

139. Approximately 18% of dogs of what breed are unilaterally or bilaterally deaf?

a. Basenji
b. Dalmatian
c. German Shepherd
d. Dogue de Bordeaux

140. A lesion that develops at pressure points, especially in large dogs, is

a. parakeratosis.
b. ecthyma.
c. acanthosis nigricans.
d. a hygroma.

141. Regarding drug pricing, a higher markup should NOT be charged for drugs that

a. are expensive.
b. have a lower turnover rate.
c. have a short expiration date.
d. require special handling.

142. The reorder point is the

a. time to requisition new stock to maintain predetermined inventory levels.
b. maximum number of a product to be inventoried at any time.
c. point that gives maximum pricing benefit.
d. guarantee of proper stock maintenance.

143. Which of the following is NOT an accepted technique following cruciate ligament rupture?

a. Cruciate ligament graft
b. Tibial tuberosity advancement
c. Tibial plateau leveling osteotomy
d. Extracapsular repair

144. Which of the following items is included in an employee handbook?

1. Disciplinary procedures
2. Dress code
3. Social media policy
4. Job descriptions

a. 1, 2, 3, 4
b. 1, 4
c. 2, 3, 4
d. 1, 2, 3

145. A vicious cat is at the practice for surgery. Where should the staff mark this is an aggressive animal?

a. The pet's record
b. On the cat's cage
c. On the surgery schedule
d. All of the above

146. When should surgical patients be marked with identification?

a. When transferred to the surgical ward
b. Upon arrival
c. Just before surgery
d. At home prior to arrival

147. Cross-training is

a. continuing education through in-house training, online training, and outside seminars.
b. training provided by a superior who is not a technician.
c. learning tasks that are the responsibility of other staff members.
d. training with another species.

148. Pups under what age may not have complete bladder control and cannot reliably avoid house soiling?

a. 12 weeks
b. 16 weeks
c. 20 weeks
d. 26 weeks

149. Eye caps on a snake are directly related to

a. old age.
b. fungal disease.
c. low humidity.
d. cancer.

150. Absorption of plain catgut suture occurs in

a. 30-45 days.
b. 60-70 days.
c. 80-90 days.
d. 100-120 days.

151. Which of these flowers is NOT known to cause acute renal failure in cats?

a. Peace lily
b. Tiger lily
c. Day lily
d. Stargazer lily

152. Shamrock and rhubarb may cause acute renal failure in large animals because they contain

a. insoluble oxalates.
b. soluble oxalates.
c. glycosides.
d. urates.

153. Digibind is an antidote for

a. opioid toxicity.
b. cardiac glycoside toxicity.
c. propylene glycol toxicity.
d. foreign body trauma.

154. Which of the following client behaviors is NOT consistent with an animal hoarder?

a. Reluctance to identify the number of pets in the home
b. Client presenting a large number of pets in inconsistent patterns
c. Client having 5 pets that are consistently seen
d. Client attempting to get medication refills without brining pets in

155. A patient is scheduled for surgery and will be placed on inhalant anesthesia. To calculate the proper size of the breathing bag for the patient,

a. multiply the tidal volume by 2.
b. multiply the patient's weight in kg by 5.
c. multiply the tidal volume by 6.
d. multiply the patient's weight in kg by 10.

156. Neonatal isoerythrolysis is a(n)

a. allergic reaction.
b. delayed hypersensitivity reaction.
c. type II hypersensitivity reaction.
d. type III hypersensitivity reaction.

157. Puppies begin to wean from their mothers at what age?

a. 3 weeks
b. 5 weeks
c. 8 weeks
d. 12 weeks

158. A saddle thromboembolism is generally a sign of

a. liver disease.
b. a low platelet count.
c. heart disease.
d. pelvic injury.

159. An increase in canine distemper may be caused by all the following EXCEPT

a. an increase in insect vectors.
b. a failure of vaccination.
c. an increase in virulence.
d. a reduced rate of vaccination.

160. Chagas disease is contracted by

a. direct contact.
b. mosquito bite.
c. worm infestation.
d. triatomine bite.

161. A hyperbaric oxygen chamber is used to deliver __% oxygen and to __ pressure relative to air pressure.

a. 21%, decrease
b. 21%, increase
c. 100%, decrease
d. 100%, increase

162. What somewhat-controversial program is used to manage feral cat colonies?

a. TNR
b. TAK
c. DNR
d. DTR

163. How much time does the typical horse at pasture spend in grazing behavior?

a. 90%
b. 70%
c. 50%
d. 30%

164. A canine patient is diagnosed with lymphoma. How long will the dog probably survive without treatment?

a. 4-6 weeks
b. 3-4 month
c. 9-12 months
d. 1-2 years

165. Clients may interpret the sound of what activity in their small dog as choking or trouble breathing?

a. Vomiting
b. Reverse sneezing
c. Chattering
d. Snoring

166. The most prevalent metabolic disease of cattle is

a. diabetes.
b. hypothyroidism.
c. hyperinsulinism.
d. ketosis.

167. Universal precautions should be taken when dealing with a patient with a potentially zoonotic or contagious disease. Which is NOT a universal precaution?

a. Minimize the number of staff in contact with the patient.
b. Contain contaminated waste.
c. Use disinfectant procedures for contaminated environmental surfaces.
d. Keep the patient a minimum of 12 feet from other patients at all times.

168. Vaccine-associated feline sarcomas occur in one of every __ vaccinated cats.

a. 1,000
b. 10,000
c. 100,000
d. 1,000,000

169. The incidence of what disease or disorder does not increase with animal obesity?

a. Renal failure
b. Diabetes
c. Musculoskeletal disease
d. Heat intolerance

170. The crystals in a carbon dioxide absorber are changed when what percent of crystals have changed color?

a. 25%
b. 50%
c. 75%
d. 100%

171. Scrubbing of a surgical site is performed in a

a. target pattern.
b. side to side pattern.
c. Z-pattern.
d. random pattern.

172. Which of these agents is NOT an appropriate rinse solution during surgical scrubbing?

a. 70% rubbing alcohol
b. Sterile water
c. 70% propylene glycol
d. Sterile saline

173. What type of knot is used to secure a patient to a surgical table?

a. Square knot
b. Bowline knot
c. Quick-release knot
d. Double knot

174. If the veterinary surgeon is performing a Zepp procedure, what part of the body must be prepared for surgery?

a. Carpus
b. Ear
c. Prepuce
d. Perianal area

175. Lacrimation refers to

a. type of motion.
b. aural discharge.
c. tearing.
d. panting.

176. "Bicipital" refers to

a. the bicuspid valve.
b. a bicuspid tooth.
c. the occipital area.
d. the biceps brachii muscle or tendon.

177. Postoperatively, extubation of the endotracheal tube should occur after

a. the blink reflex is present.
b. the patient is fully awake.
c. the swallowing reflex is present.
d. surgery and before recovery.

178. The receptive nerve cells responsible for colored images in daylight are

a. tapetum.
b. fovea.
c. rods.
d. cones.

179. PCR is a revolutionary laboratory technique that

a. diagnoses lameness.
b. amplifies DNA.
c. separates white blood cells.
d. fast freezes histological samples.

180. Which of these is not a major type of canine aggression?

a. Pack
b. Predation
c. Pain
d. Protectiveness

181. A 950-pound horse is prescribed trimethoprim-sulfadiazine. The dosage of trimethoprim-sulfadiazine is 30 mg/kg every 12-24 hours. Trimethoprim-sulfadiazine is available as 960 mg tablets. How many tablets must the horse be given for each dose?

a. 11
b. 13.5
c. 15
d. 18.5

182. Before recommending or feeding a canine or feline diet, the diet should be checked to ensure it

a. contains a minimum 30% protein content.
b. is supplemented with taurine and carnitine.
c. contains no more than 20% fiber content.
d. meets AAFCO nutritional standards as a complete and balanced food.

183. When walking up stairs, the load is on the

a. right limbs.
b. left limbs.
c. forelimbs.
d. hind limbs.

184. Patients receiving glucocorticoids are prone to developing what metabolic disorder?

a. Hypothyroidism
b. Hyperthyroidism
c. Diabetes mellitus
d. Hyperestrogenemia

185. Prednisone is activated in the liver to

a. cortisol.
b. dexamethasone.
c. prednisolone.
d. deoxycorticosterone acetate.

186. Which of these is the best source of protein for an iguana's diet?

a. Alfalfa
b. Chicken
c. Chick peas
d. Egg

187. Aleutian disease in ferrets is caused by

a. autoimmune disease.
b. streptococcal infection.
c. a migrating parasite.
d. a parvovirus.

188. What percentage of dogs and cats, aged 4 and up, have periodontal disease?

a. 85%
b. 75%
c. 50%
d. 35%

189. Which of the following is an absorbable suture?

a. Prolene
b. Dexon
c. Ethilon
d. Silk

190. On the dental mobility index, a tooth that moves less than the distance of its crown width is classified as a class

a. I.
b. II.
c. III.
d. IV.

191. To assess canine liver function, serum bile acids should be measured fasting and

a. immediately post-prandial.
b. 2 hours post-prandial.
c. 4 hours post-prandial.
d. 8 hours post-prandial.

192. Misdirected canine syndrome is

a. abnormal behavior based on poor and ineffective training.
b. canine aggression where the dog retaliates against a justifiable source by acting aggressively toward an innocent source.
c. a congenital disorder in which the cecum opens in an abnormal location in the bowel.
d. a bite abnormality where a retained deciduous tooth tilts the erupting permanent canine into an abnormal location.

193. A patient has a serum calcium level of 8 mg/dL. The patient's serum albumin level is 3.2 g/dL. What is the patient's corrected calcium level?

a. 7.2
b. 7.6
c. 8.2
d. 8.6

194. A giraffe has how many cervical vertebrae?

a. 7
b. 9
c. 11
d. 12

195. Which of the following does NOT occur with reperfusion injury?

a. Reactive oxygen species
b. Endothelial cell dysfunction
c. Increased erythrocyte production
d. Activation of platelets

196. The most common primary brain tumor of the cat is the

a. glioma.
b. pituitary adenoma.
c. meningioma.
d. adenocarcinoma.

197. What does STT stand for and what does it assess?

a. Sexually Transmitted Test, exposure to sexually transmitted diseases
b. Semitendinosus tracking, presence of bursitis
c. Schirmer Tear Test, corneal ulcers
d. Schirmer Tear Test, tear production

198. When assessing the results of Schiotz tonometry, use the

a. Mackay-Marg calibration.
b. 10-gram weight.
c. plus or minus 2 rule.
d. multiplication factor of 2.

199. The universal birthday for all thoroughbreds born in the Northern hemisphere is

a. January 1.
b. May 1.
c. August 1.
d. November 1.

200. The most practical and efficient method to assessing a mare's readiness to breed is

a. serum estrogen sampling.
b. serum progesterone sampling.
c. teasing.
d. temperature.

201. Rattlesnake envenomation produces this type of poikilocyte:

a. Spherocytes
b. Echinocytes
c. Acanthocytes
d. Schistocytes

202. Over-the-counter nonsteroidal anti-inflammatory drugs (NSAIDs) such as ibuprofen, naproxen, and aspirin represent a leading cause of toxicoses in small animals. What is their common mechanism of action?

a. Bone marrow suppression
b. Smooth muscle contraction
c. Prostaglandin synthesis inhibition
d. Vasodilation of renal vessels

203. Improper handling or restraint of rabbits can result in this common injury:

a. Diaphragmatic hernia
b. Spinal fracture or luxation
c. Splenic rupture
d. Skull fracture

204. Which small mammal has a high risk of dystocia if bred after 6 months of age?

a. Chinchilla
b. Rabbit
c. Guinea pig
d. Ferret

205. Animals poisoned with ethylene glycol (antifreeze) often have large numbers of these crystals in the urine:

a. Struvite
b. Ammonium biurate
c. Cystine
d. Calcium oxalate

206. Which of the following statements regarding dermatophyte test medium (DTM) is TRUE?

a. Sample DTM jars should be closed tightly to prevent the introduction of saprophytic fungi.
b. Dermatophytes rapidly change the color of the DTM agar to red in as little as 3-5 days.
c. Samples should be placed in an incubator for 1-2 weeks.
d. All of the above.

207. In a nonrebreathing system, which of the following has the most influence on the amount of carbon dioxide (CO2) rebreathed?

a. Fresh gas flow rate
b. CO2 absorbent
c. Scavenger system
d. Design of rebreathing system

208. What will happen to a patient if the positive-pressure-relief (pop-off) valve is accidentally left closed during anesthesia?

a. Pressure will build up in the system and the patient will not be able to exhale.
b. The lungs will rupture causing a pneumothorax, a life-threatening emergency.
c. Venous return to the heart will be compromised.
d. All of the above.

209. An increase in heart rate that is accompanied with normal P-QRS-T complexes on electrocardiogram (ECG), and occurs as a result of increased activity of the sinoatrial (SA) node is termed:

a. Ventricular tachycardia
b. Atrial fibrillation
c. Sinus tachycardia
d. Atrial tachycardia

210. What drug is the emetic of choice in canines?

a. Xylazine
b. Apomorphine
c. Hydrogen peroxide
d. Syrup of ipecac

211. A technician is about to administer an intramuscular injection of antibiotic to a box turtle suffering from an aural abscess. Where should the technician administer this injection?

a. Front leg
b. Back leg
c. None of the above
d. a or b

212. Which of the following statements is NOT true regarding jugular intravenous drug administration in horses?

a. The needle should be inserted caudally into the jugular vein in order to match the direction of blood flow.
b. The cranial third of the neck should be used to access the jugular vein to avoid accidental entry into the carotid artery.
c. The medication should be bolused as quickly as possible.
d. Arterial versus venous blood cannot be differentiated by color when drawn into a syringe filled with fluid.

213. Which of the following syndromes will result in a postrenal azotemia?

a. Shock
b. Antifreeze intoxication
c. Feline urologic syndrome (FUS).
d. Dehydration

214. A 75-pound Labrador Retriever requires 8 mg/kg of injectable phenobarbital for initial treatment of status epilepticus. If the concentration of this drug is 30 mg/mL, how many milliliters should this patient receive?

a. 9 mL
b. 20 mL
c. 60 mL
d. 18 mL

215. Which of the following statements regarding grids is incorrect?

a. Grids help reduce the amount of scatter radiation.
b. Grids are used when the area to be radiographed is equal to or exceeds 10 cm in thickness.
c. Grids do not absorb any part of the primary beam.
d. Grids improve the quality of the radiograph by increasing contrast.

216. A client brings in his 5-month-old puppy for vomiting and diarrhea of 2-day duration. He indicates that he himself vaccinated the puppy with injectables purchased at a local feed and grain store. He also states that he followed a vaccine protocol described on the Internet. Despite this owner's good intentions, the puppy tests positive for parvovirus. What is a plausible explanation for this test result?

a. The puppy was immunosuppressed at the time of vaccination and could therefore not mount a sufficient immune response to the vaccines.
b. The owner administered the vaccine incorrectly or at inappropriate intervals.
c. The vaccine was stored at an improper temperature by the retail store or by the owner, thereby rendering the vaccine ineffective.
d. All of the above.

217. Which of the following statements regarding feline transfusion medicine is incorrect?

a. There is no universal feline blood type due to the presence of naturally occurring alloantibodies.
b. Type A cats have weak anti-B alloantibodies.
c. A type AB cat can be safely used as an in-house blood donor.
d. Transfusion of a type B cat with type A blood can produce a potentially fatal acute hemolytic crisis.

218. Alkaline urine does not result from, nor is produced by

a. Diets rich in vegetable products.
b. A urinary tract infection with urease producing bacteria (i.e., Staph or Proteus).
c. Time (>1 hr the voided sample stands at room temperature).
d. Diets consisting of milk or animal products.

219. What type of drug is activated charcoal?

a. Laxative
b. Cathartic
c. Purgative
d. Adsorbent and protectant

220. Which of the following is NOT a function of diazepam?

a. Anxiolytic
b. Anticonvulsant
c. Analgesic
d. Muscle relaxant

221. What is the earliest day of gestation that a small animal pregnancy can be confirmed using ultrasound?

a. Day 5
b. Day 11
c. Day 20
d. Day 45

222. The components of fresh whole blood remain effective for up to:

a. 1 hour
b. 2 hours
c. 8 hours
d. 12 hours

223. What type of injection should be avoided in meat-producing animals?

a. Subcutaneous
b. Intravenous
c. Intramuscular
d. Intraperitoneal

224. What is ultimately responsible for the resolution of an ultrasound image?

a. Size of patient
b. Gain
c. Transducer frequency
d. Power

225. On electrocardiograms (ECGs), ectopic foci that discharge prematurely anywhere within the ventricular walls give rise to:

a. Ventricular tachycardia
b. Ventricular fibrillation
c. Ventricular premature complexes
d. Accelerated idioventricular rhythm

226. What is the most commonly encountered diet-related illness in pet hedgehogs?

a. Rickets
b. Obesity
c. Hepatic lipidosis
d. Periodontal disease

227. In ultrasonography, this artifact is produced when soundwaves are unable to traverse certain types of tissue or anomalies, such as bone or calculi:

a. Distance enhancement
b. Reverberation
c. Acoustic shadowing
d. Mirror image

228. What is the anesthetic of choice in patients with cardiac disease?

a. Ketamine
b. Propofol
c. Fentanyl
d. Etomidate

229. Etomidate should not be administered in repeated boluses because it is a hypertonic solution. What term best describes the changes a red blood cell (RBC) undergoes when introduced into a hypertonic solution?

a. Autoagglutination
b. Hemolysis
c. Crenation
d. Rouleaux formation

230. Which of the following statements regarding equine nasogastric intubation and medication is FALSE?

a. The nasogastric tube should be guided into the dorsal meatus of the horse's nasal passages.
b. When placed properly, the tube can be seen on the left side of the horse's neck as it passes through the esophagus and into the stomach.
c. Force should NEVER be used at any time during nasogastric intubation.
d. A horse could potentially die from gastric rupture when its stomach is overfilled with large volumes of medication or fluid delivered through a nasogastric tube

231. Which of the following statements regarding urine casts is TRUE?

a. Large numbers of casts in urine usually indicate active renal disease.
b. Casts will dissolve in alkaline urine.
c. Casts contain material in their matrix that was present in the renal tubule when the cast was formed.
d. All of the above.

232. Which of the following is the most common oropharyngeal tumor in canines?

a. Fibrosarcoma
b. Squamous cell carcinoma
c. Malignant melanoma
d. Ameloblastoma

233. Cutaneous larval migrans is an important parasitic zoonoses that is caused by:

a. Whipworms
b. Roundworms
c. Tapeworms
d. Hookworms

234. The connective tissue that occupies the space between each tooth and the alveolar bone is called:

a. Cementum
b. Pulp
c. Periodontal ligament
d. Gingiva

235. What is the purpose of polishing in dental prophylaxis?

a. Eliminate calculi
b. Remove sublingual deposits
c. Strengthen the enamel
d. Smooth the enamel

236. Mechanical scalers have the potential to generate excessive heat on the enamel, which can lead to accidental structural damage to the tooth. What step(s) can be taken to avoid this scenario?

a. Use a large amount of water to cool the teeth during scaling.
b. Limit the time spent on each tooth to 5-10 seconds each.
c. Use only at the recommended speed for the particular unit.
d. All of the above.

237. Scissors that are primarily used in intraocular surgery are called:

a. Metzenbaum scissors
b. Iris scissors
c. Mayo scissors
d. Spencer scissors

238. Large hemostatic forceps with longitudinal grooves along the opposing blade surfaces and transverse grooves at the tip are called:

a. Kelly forceps
b. Rochester-Carmalt forceps
c. Mosquito forceps
d. Crile forceps

239. What is the function of surgical milk on instruments?

a. Lubrication
b. Sterilization
c. Anti-corrosive
d. Both a and c

240. In a rebreathing system, how often should the carbon dioxide absorbent be changed?

a. Every 2-4 hours of use
b. Every 6-8 hours of use
c. Every 10-12 hours of use
d. Every 20 hours of use

241. Which knot is recommended to secure a patient's limb to the surgery table?

a. Square knot
b. Sheet bend knot
c. Bowline knot
d. Half hitch

242. Drain placement helps to reduce the occurrence of

a. Seromas.
b. Dead space.
c. Hematomas.
d. All of the above.

243. Which of the following statements regarding hydrogen peroxide (H2O2) is FALSE?

a. Hydrogen peroxide is an effective broad spectrum antimicrobial.
b. Hydrogen peroxide can damage tissue with repeated use.
c. Hydrogen peroxide is a common foaming wound irrigant.
d. Hydrogen is an effective sporicide.

244. Which of the following properties is NOT shared by chlorhexidine AND povidone-iodine scrubs?

a. They are both broad-spectrum antimicrobials.
b. Their residual bactericidal effects are inactivated by blood or alcohol.
c. They have a rapid antimicrobial effect.
d. They both have residual antimicrobial activity that lasts more than 3 hours.

245. Which of the following should never be used to maintain or increase the body temperature of an animal that is undergoing or recovering from surgery?

a. Heated circulating water blanket
b. Electric heating pad
c. Warm water bath
d. Warm air blanket

246. Which of the following pairs of analgesics should NOT be used together?

a. Morphine and lidocaine
b. Butorphanol and fentanyl
c. Dexmedetomidine and buprenorphine
d. Tramadol and nonsteroidal anti-inflammatory drugs

247. Which of the following opioids can be administered transmucosally in the feline?

a. Buprenorphine
b. Hydroxymorphone
c. Fentanyl
d. Butorphanol

248. Which of the following drugs is used to offset the untoward effect of hypersalivation that is commonly seen with barbiturate and dissociative anesthetics?

a. Naloxone hydrochloride
b. Antisedan
c. Glycopyrrolate
d. Thiopental

249. Stay sutures are used to

a. Elevate and stabilize hollow organs.
b. Separate muscle layers.
c. Secure a chest tube to the skin.
d. Prevent recurrence of a rectal prolapse.

250. All of the following drugs are diuretics EXCEPT:

a. Furosemide.
b. Enalapril.
c. Spironolactone.
d. Mannitol.

Answer Key and Explanations

1. B: Age of the patient

- Every prescription label must include:
- Name and address of dispensing pharmacy
- Serial number of the prescription
- Date of the prescription
- Name of the prescriber
- Name of the patient
- Name and strength of the drug
- Directions for use
- Cautionary statements, as appropriate

2. A: Young animals because they cause arthropathy

Fluoroquinolones are toxic to chondrocytes. Damaged chondrocytes form vesicles on articular surfaces. Higher doses of fluoroquinolones are more likely to cause articular damage. Affected animals become lame.

3. D: Neomycin is the most nephrotoxic aminoglycoside.

The significant adverse effects of aminoglycosides include nephrotoxicosis, ototoxicosis, and vestibulotoxicosis. Nephrotoxicosis risk increases with frequent and extended administration of aminoglycosides, particularly when trough concentrations are persistently elevated. Articles in the veterinary literature indicate that neomycin if the most nephrotoxic of the group.

4. C: Aminoglycosides

Beta-lactams and macrolides are reliably useful against gram-positive anaerobes. Tetracyclines are also clinically effective against some gram-positive anaerobes. Aminoglycosides are not clinically useful in fighting gram-positive anaerobes.

5. A: 60 mL/kg/h

In compensatory shock, or early decompensatory shock, cats should be treated with 60 mL/kg/h of isotonic crystalloid replacement fluid. Dogs are treated at a rate of 90 mL/kg/h.

When replacement crystalloids with synthetic colloids are used, the rate to treat a cat in compensatory or decompensatory shock decreases to 24-36 mL/kg/h.

6. B: 8 - 10%

7. C: 50 mL

Each mL of 50% dextrose contains 0.5 g of dextrose. A 5% solution contains of NaCl will contain 50 g of dextrose per liter, or 25 g per half liter. If each mL of 50% dextrose contains 0.5 g, 50 mL of the 50% dextrose will be needed to bring the 500 mL bag of 0.45% NaCl to a 5% dextrose solution. 50 mL of NaCl should be removed from the bag before the corresponding amount of dextrose is added.

8. B: Schedule II

Schedule II substances have a high potential for abuse and include morphine and other narcotics, including hydromorphone, methadone, meperidine, oxycodone, and fentanyl, that may lead to severe psychological or physical dependence. Schedule II controlled substances include stimulants as well as cocaine, amobarbital, glutethimide, and pentobarbital.

Schedule III controlled substances have less potential for abuse. Schedule III also includes some narcotic combination products with a defined, limited dose of narcotic. Schedule IV substances have an even lower potential for abuse that Schedule III substances.

Schedule I controlled substances have a high potential for abuse with no accepted medical use.

9. D: All of the above

According to the Drug Enforcement Administration, an inventory of controlled substances must:

- Be a complete and accurate record of controlled substances on hand
- Include the date the inventory is conducted
- Be in written, typewritten or printed form
- Be conducted at least every two years following an initial inventory
- Be maintained at the registered location for at least two years past the date of the inventory
- Include when the inventory was taken (open or close of business)
- Include names of controlled substances
- Include each finished form of the controlled substances (injectable liquid, powder, tablet and dose or concentration)
- Include the number of dosage units of each finished form in the commercial container (for instance, 50 tablet bottle, 10 mL vial)
- Include the number of commercial containers of each finished form (for example, five 10 mL vials)
- Include the disposition of the controlled substances

10. D: A Drug Enforcement Administration registrant authorized to receive unusable or unwanted controlled substances.

Practitioners dispose of out-of-date, damaged, unusable, and unwanted controlled substances by transferring them to a reverse distributor, a Drug Enforcement Administration registrant authorized to receive them. Local DEA field offices provide a list of authorized reverse distributors. Copies of the records documenting the transfer and disposal must be maintained for 2 years.

11. A: 1:32 dilution of 5.25% solution of sodium hypochlorite

Proper surface disinfection depends on proper cleaning of the surface first. In addition, the surface disinfectant should adequately cover the surface and maintain contact with the surface for a suitable period. Sodium hypochlorite, the active ingredient in bleach, provides optimal disinfection with a 0.16% solution. A 0.16% solution is created by diluting a 5.25% solution to a 1:32 dilution. A dilute bleach or sodium hypochlorite solution is effective against parvovirus as well as other bacteria and viruses.

12. D: The maximum dose of rh-EPO that should be given to a dog or cat is 100 U/kg.

rh-EPO is a therapy for anemia associated with chronic renal disease in people and animals. It is indicated when the PCV drops to 25% or less, and is given at doses of 50-100 U/kg 3 times weekly subcutaneously until the target PCV is reached. Patient PDV should be measured twice weekly to monitor response. When the target PCV is reached, rh-EPO may be given twice weekly. Non-responsive patients may be given a higher dose of rh-EPO. The dose can be increased in 25-50 U/kg increments. No maximum dose has been established but weekly doses up to 1050 U/kg have been reported. Responsive patients have reticulocytosis and a 0.5%-1.0% daily increase in PCV. There is a high incidence of antibody formation in dogs and cats.

13. D: All of the above

Strangles, also known as distemper in horses, is a highly contagious disease caused by S. equi var equi. Vaccines are available and are recommended where strangles is endemic or when horses are expected to be at high risk. Streptococcus equi can be transmitted directly or indirectly, and causes an inflammatory response resulting in fever, dysphagia, anorexia, stridor, nasal discharge, and lymphadenopathy. All symptoms are not necessarily present.

Strangles in dogs is called puppy strangles, juvenile cellulitis, and sterile granulomatous dermatitis and lymphadenitis. It is an uncommon disease related to immune system dysfunction occurring in puppies between 3 weeks and 4 months of age. The face becomes markedly swollen. High doses of corticosteroids are needed to treat the disease. Following resolution, the disease does not recur.

14. D: Antibiotics are used to treat endotoxic shock.

Endotoxin is a lipopolysaccharide and a component of the external cell wall of Gram-negative bacteria. It is released from the bacteria during bacterial growth, and cell lysis and death. When endotoxin binds receptors on host endothelial cells, macrophages or monocytes, or polymorphonuclear leukocytes, biochemical mediators are produced and released. These mediators include cytokines, eicosanoids, nitric oxide, platelet activating factor, proteases, toxic oxygen radicals, and vasoactive amines. The release of these mediators initiates physiologic events resulting in endotoxic shock with cardiopulmonary dysfunction, loss of microvascular integrity, and multiple organ failure.

Glucocorticoids are used in endotoxic shock because they are known to reduce cytokine production, inhibit the inflammatory cascade, and inhibit nitrous oxide. Lazaroids, nonsteroidal anti-inflammatories, pentoxifylline, and nitrous oxide inhibitors are used to treat endotoxic shock, but not antibacterials.

15. C: "Veterinary technicians shall assume accountability for their professional actions as well as those with whom they work."

The full NAVTA Veterinary Technician Code of Ethics covers the obligations, ethical responsibilities, and ideals of veterinary technicians. It was developed by the NAVTA Ethics Committee and contains eleven statements in the Code of Ethics. The line in question correctly reads, "Veterinary technicians shall assume accountability for individual professional actions and judgments."

16. A: Bluetongue, paratuberculosis, Rift Valley fever, lumpy skin disease

Complete lists of reportable diseases for all species can be found on the CDC, USDA, and state websites. Of the disease included, the following are reportable: bluetongue, paratuberculosis, Rift

Valley fever, lumpy skin disease, anthrax, Marek's disease, rinderpest, sheep pox virus, camel pox virus, Q fever, and Trichinellosis.

17. D: Both A and B

Following ovariohysterectomy, patients' movements should be restricted to minimize discomfort as well as pull on the suture line and internal organs. While challenging at times, restriction is important for several days following surgery. Injectable pain relief may be used at the time of surgery with oral pain relievers sent home for use following surgery. Clients must fully understand the dose and administration of pain relievers as well as potential side effects. The surgeon may place intradermal, or subcuticular, sutures, or use skin glue for closure, so that no suture removal is necessary. If skin sutures are placed, they should be removed 7-10 days following surgery. In some cases, sutures may be removed as early as 5 days post-surgery.

18. C: 1, 3, 2, 4

Before applying a cleanser or medication to the ear canal, it is best to determine that the tympanic membrane is intact. When a large amount of debris is present, it may be necessary to first remove some debris to visualize the tympanic membrane. When there is a great deal of inflammation or stenosis, it may not be possible to properly evaluate the tympanic membrane. Ensuring the tympanic membrane is intact is important prior to treatment both to avoid ototoxic cleansers and medications if it is broken and to determine appropriate treatment.

Several drops of cleanser are added to the ear canal and the base of the ear is massaged to move the cleanser through the ear and help break up debris. Debris from the ear canal should be gently, but thoroughly, removed.

19. A: Damp heat is applied to muscles prior to exercise.

Following cranial cruciate ligament injury and/or surgery, the application of heat to the muscles around the stifle joint is helpful to recovery. During the first three postoperative days, only cryotherapy should be used. Beginning day four, heat should be applied three times daily, and should be applied prior to any rehabilitative exercise. Damp heat offers better penetration than dry and is far safer.

20. B: Normal amounts of dietary protein are fed.

Historically, recommended dietary therapy for dogs and cats with liver disease included limits on protein intake. Experts now recommend that normal amounts of protein be fed. Additionally, cats and dogs with liver disease should be fed a high-quality, highly digestible diet in frequent, small amounts. High-fat diets should be avoided; the diet should include normal fat levels.

21. B: 72 mL

The patient is receiving fluids at 1200 mL/day (60mL x 20 kg = 1200 mL) or 50 mL/hour (1200/24 = 50). The 1 L bag of fluids will last this patient 20 hours (1000/50 = 20) or 1200 minutes (20 x 60). The patient must receive 1200 mcg lidocaine per minute. Since the fluids will last 1200 minutes at the current rate of delivery, 1,440,000 mcg (1200 mcg x 1200 minutes) or 1440 mg (1,440,000 mcg/1000 = 1440 mg) of lidocaine must be added to the liter of NaCl. 2% lidocaine contains 20 mg/mL of lidocaine. 1440 mg of 2% lidocaine will be present in 72 mL (1440/20 = 72 mL). 72 mL of NaCl should be discarded from the liter bag, and 72 mL of 2% lidocaine added.

22. A: Denial, anger, bargaining, depression, and acceptance

While grief is an individual process, Elisabeth Kubler-Ross identified five stages people may experience as they come to terms with their loss. Often, people experience the stages of grief as: denial, anger, bargaining, depression, and acceptance. When loss makes life overwhelming, denial helps people survive the loss, slowing the pace of these overwhelming feelings. As a grieving person begins questioning, their denial begins to fade and they often turn to anger.

Anger is a necessary and important step in the healing process. Anger can provide strength and grounding, providing connections, albeit negative. Grieving people may shift between stages, going back and forth between anger and bargaining, for example.

In the bargaining stage, a mourner expresses many "If only" and "What if" statements. People want things returned to their prior state and try to negotiate with a higher power. Post-bargaining, a griever moves his or her attention to the present, feeling grief on a deeper level, and entering the depression stage. This depression is a normal, appropriate response to loss and not mental illness.

Finally, the loss is accepted. Acceptance doesn't mean all is right with the world, it means the mourner has accepted the reality of his or her loss. There is no set time for each stage of grief. Mourners may move through some steps quickly and others for an extended time.

23. B: VD, open mouth, or parallel open jaw

The ventrodorsal view allows a fairly clear view of the bullae as well as comparison of the left and right bulla. Using a block to support the nose and keep the head straight improves the view. An open mouth radiographic view allows visualization of the bulla and surrounding structures with less overlap of other tissues. A parallel open jaw view is equally effective in evaluating middle ear structures. The head is angled up and the radiograph shot with the beam parallel to the lower jaw.

Greater overlap of tissues and interference occurs with a dorsoventral view and shouldn't be used. Lateral views are not useful in the evaluation of the middle ear due to overlapping structures.

24. C: Voiding Urethrogram

This procedure is designed to evaluate the urethra, not the bladder, and will show contrast as it actively moves through the urethra. A positive contrast urethrogram, by contrast, is performed by placing a catheter about 2 cm into the urethra and injecting positive contrast. The catheter is withdrawn and a radiograph is taken. This study shows a passive view of urethral status.

25. A: For patients weighing 6 kg or less

With a non-rebreathing circuit, anesthetic gases flow from the anesthetic machine to the patient to the atmosphere without flowing back to the patient. Adequate gas flow is needed to properly eliminate CO_2. Due to delivery of precise anesthetic concentration with a non-rebreathing system, a change in vaporizer setting effects rapid change in inspired gas concentration and patient anesthesia.

Examples of non-rebreathing circuits are the Bain circuit, Ayre's T piece, Magill system, and Lack system. The amount of dead space in an apparatus and the resistance in the apparatus are limits to the size of the patient.

26. D: Allow oxygen and gas to flow for five minutes prior to use

All anesthetic machines should be checked prior to use by:

1. Restock by filling vaporizers, and filling the CO_2 canister with absorbent.
2. Check to confirm function of unidirectional valves, verify the oxygen supply, check the pressure of the oxygen cylinder and the N_2O cylinder, and check for free movement of the float in flow meters.
3. Check the integrity of the breathing circuit and ensure tight connections. Close the pop-off or pressure relief valve, block the Y-piece, bring the circuit to a pressure of 30 cm H_2O, and check for leaks.
4. Check the gas scavenging system is properly connected and turned on.
5. Check that the ventilator is properly attached to the breathing circuit and is free of leaks.

27. D: Respiratory rate

A patient's perfusion can be assessed by evaluating the patient's heart rate, capillary refill time, mucous membrane color, and arterial blood pressure.

28. B: 4-8 hours

Whenever possible, food should be withheld for 4-8 hours prior to surgery in equine patients. Water should not be withheld. By comparison, food is withheld for 12-18 hours prior to surgery in large ruminants, and 8-12 hours in small ruminants. Cats and dogs should be fasted 6 hours prior to surgery.

29. C: Tricaine methanesulfonate (MS-222)

MS-222, etomidate, clove oil, and isoflurane are effective anesthetic agents in fish. Only MS-222, tricaine methanesulfonate, is licensed for use in fish. MS-222 is used as an immersion bath with 20-50 mg/L causing sedation and 75-125 mg/L causing anesthesia. Anesthesia is maintained at 50-75 mg/L though dose is species-dependent. To achieve proper depth of anesthesia, fish are moved from an anesthetic water bath to a non-medicated water bath. MS-222 has a wide margin of safety and induces anesthesia rapidly, in less than five minutes.

30. B: Reflexes have decreased such that ear, toe, and tail pinches do not result in withdrawal.

Rabbits and rodents have reached a surgical plan of anesthesia when they no longer withdraw to a pinch on the ear, toe, and tail. Corneal reflexes are highly variable under anesthesia. Loss of corneal reflex is not an indicator of reaching a surgical plane of anesthesia, but loss of corneal reflex in a patient that previously had a reflex indicates that anesthesia is too deep. Anesthesia is also too deep if heart rate or respiratory rate is dropping.

31. C: Babcock forceps

Babcock forceps have looped blades designed to hold a short length of intestine without causing tissue compression. They are not part of a standard surgical pack, but would be used for intestinal surgeries. Kelly hemostatic forceps are used to occlude blood vessels or clamp tissue. Adson-Brown forceps, or Brown-Adson forceps, are common grasping forceps. Backhaus towel clamps are commonly used to hold towels and drapes in place.

32. A: To cut delicate tissue

Metzenbaum scissors are a smaller, slightly curved surgical scissor designed to cut delicate tissues. Mayo scissors are used for routine cutting and dissection. Some other scissors are practically named, bandage scissors for cutting bandages, and suture scissors for cutting sutures.

33. C: Wrapping material must be permeable to steam.

Steam autoclaves are used to sterilize surgical packs. Successful sterilization depends upon the steam thoroughly penetrating the pack wrap and the contents. Wrapping should be permeable to steam, but not to microbes. Cotton muslin is a good choice for its durability and flexibility, but offers less storage time than other wraps. When used, muslin should be double layered and double wrapped around the pack. Autoclave paper, such as crepe paper, can be used, but not reused. Paper can be used in single or double layers and offers a superior pack storage time to fabric.

Instruments must be unhinged when they are sterilized for proper effect. Pans should be packed with the open end facing down or horizontally. Linens must be laundered and ironed prior to sterilization. Drapes should be packaged separately and individually to allow proper steam penetration of the compact material.

Instrument packs should be positioned in the direction of steam flow and vertically with empty space between packs. A minimum of 13 minutes saturated steam at 120 °F is the minimum requirement for sterilization. Higher temperatures may be used for highly resistant spores.

34. B: All but 3

Cytochrome P-450 enzymes metabolize toxins and drugs, the process of biotransformation, primarily in the liver. P-450 enzymes also synthesize steroids, fatty acids, and bile acids. These enzymes are also found in the intestines, lungs, and other organs.

Cytochrome P-450 gene families are classified by sequence similarities, not function. A gene family is labeled by the letters "CYP." CYP1, CYP2, and CYP3 gene families metabolize drugs. Individual enzymes in this system are named "CYP" followed by a number, a letter, and a number. CYP2D6, for example, is responsible for metabolizing psychotherapy drugs.

Drug interactions result from cytochrome P-450 enzyme inhibition or enzyme induction. Enzyme inhibition often occurs when drugs compete for the enzyme binding site. Enzyme induction occurs when the body produces additional enzyme protein in response to a drug.

35. C: Facilitated diffusion

Diffusion is a passive process of molecular movement from a high concentration to a low concentration. Osmosis is the movement of water through a semipermeable membrane from an area of low solute to high solute. Facilitated diffusion is diffusion with the assistance of carrier proteins across the cell membrane. Filtration is a process of forcing substances across a cell membrane using hydrostatic pressure.

36. A: Hypertonic

Isotonic fluid is equally as concentrated as the comparison fluid. Hypotonic fluid is less concentrated than the comparison fluid. Hypertonic fluid is more concentrated than the comparison fluid.

37. D: Connective tissue

Areolar, adipose, and reticular tissues are all proper connective tissues. Hyaline, elastic, fibrocartilage, spongy blood, and bone are all specialized connective tissues.

38. A: At the bottom of the rear foot

By definition, plantar refers to the bottom of the rear foot; palmar to the bottom of the front foot. Caudal and posterior refer to toward the tail. Dorsal is towards the backbone. Lateral is farthest from the medial plane.

39. B: 1tbsp = 15 mL

One teaspoon is equivalent to 5 milliliters. One tablespoon is equivalent to 15 milliliters. One inch is equivalent to 2.54 centimeters.

40. A: 36 kg

One kilogram is equivalent to 2.2 pounds.

41. D: Barrow

A neutered male pig is a barrow. A neutered male ferret is a gib. A neutered male horse or llama is a gelding. A neutered male sheep is a wether.

42. C: 336 days

Normal gestational periods, in days, of different species:

Horse	336 days
Cow	285 days
Sheep	148 days
Goat	149 days
Pig	114 days
Dog	63-65 days
Cat	63-65 days

43. C: The prepatent period of canine hookworms is 7 days.

Ancylostoma caninum, uncinaria stenocephala, and ancylostoma braziliense are canine hookworms. Dogs are infected by ingestion of 3rd stage larvae, larval penetration of the skin, ingestion of a vertebrate with infected tissue, and transmammary transmission. The prepatent period ranges from 13 to 27 days, though nursing puppies can shed eggs in just 10 to 12 days. Canine hookworms are present worldwide. A. caninum is highly pathogenic, and A. braziliense causes cutaneous larva migrans.

44. A: Pseudoparasites

Pseudoparasites are mistaken for parasites when found in feces or blood, but are not parasites. Fecal pseudoparasites include Alternaria species, free-living nematodes, grain mite eggs, Planarian, and pollen granules. A spurious parasite is a true parasite in one or more species, but not in the one in which it is found. Spurious parasites are found when an animal ingests invertebrates with larval stages of the parasite or the feces of infected animals.

45. B: Taenia spp.

Adult worms live in an animal's small intestine; then eggs and posterior segments of adult worms are shed in feces; then eggs are released from segments in feces; then intermediate hosts ingest eggs; then intermediate host tissue is eaten by the animal.

The correct order of the life cycle of Dirofilaria immitis is: larvae mature on the heart and pulmonary arteries and release microfilaria; then mosquito takes a blood meal and ingests microfilaria; then microfilaria develop to the L3 stage within the mosquito; then mosquito transmits the infective L3 larvae with a bite.

The correct order of the life cycle of Toxocaris leonina: larvae mature in the small intestines and adult worms lay eggs; then eggs pass with feces; then eggs embryonate; then larvae molts twice within the egg; then embryonated egg is ingested by a transport host; then transport host or embryonated eggs are eaten.

The correct order of the life cycle of Echinococcus granulosus is: adult worms are in the small intestine; then worm segments pass in the feces; then eggs are released from the segments; then eggs in the feces are ingested by an intermediate host; then hydatids form in the intermediate host in the liver or lungs; then intermediate host is ingested.

46. C: 0, 30, 60, 120, and 240 minutes

An upper gastrointestinal tract barium study may be used to evaluate the cause of regurgitation, vomiting, diarrhea, and abnormal palpation in a bird. Positive-contrast medium such as barium may also be used to determine organ location.

Barium is administered to the bird by stomach tube and radiographs are taken at 0 m, 30 m, 60 m, 2 h, and 4 h. In a normal gastrointestinal tract, the crop fills immediately. The proventriculus and gizzard fill after 30 minutes; the small intestine after 1 hour. By 4 hours, the crop should be empty.

47. B: Tangential coronary view

The navicular bone of the horse has an articular surface and a flexor surface. The articular surface is the palmar or plantar part of the distal interphalangeal joint. Radiographs of the navicular bone are used for prepurchase examinations, to evaluate navicular disease, evaluate trauma, and determine the extent of foot abscesses and wounds.

Before radiographs are taken, the horse's show should be removed, when possible, and the sole cleaned and pared. Three views are commonly taken for comprehensive evaluation of the navicular bone. The dorsoproximal-palmarodistal view can be taken by the high coronary route with the foot flat, or the upright pedal route with an angled foot against a vertical plate.

With the lateral-medial view, the horse's foot lies on a wooden block so the x-ray beam can be centered on the lateral axis of the bone. For the flexor tangential view, the horse's foot is positioned caudally while the horse stands on a reinforced cassette or cassette tunnel. The x-ray beam is centered between the bulbs of the heel and tangential to the flexor cortex plane.

48. D: 1, 3, 4, 5

Patent ductus arteriosus is a condition in which a blood vessel, the ductus arteriosus, allows embryonic blood to bypass the lungs and does not close at or immediately following birth. Consequently, the abnormal blood flow and pressure causes some pathologic changes in the heart and cardiopulmonary vasculature. Specifically, the descending aortic arch is segmentally enlarged, the left atrium and left ventricle are enlarged, and the pulmonary vascular pattern is enhanced.

49. A: Taurine and carnitine

Canine dilated cardiomyopathy is an acquired cardiovascular disease more likely to occur in breeds such as the Cocker Spaniel, and in large and giant breeds. Research has identified low taurine and carnitine levels in the blood of a considerable portion of dogs with dilated cardiomyopathy. Taurine is an amino acid. Carnitine is a derivative of the amino acid lysine. Even in dogs with dilated cardiomyopathy without measurable deficits in carnitine and taurine, patients have improved when given these nutritional supplements.

50. C: Vitamin C

Humans, monkeys, apes, guinea pigs, capybaras, and some bats, birds, and fish cannot manufacture their own vitamin C, and, therefore, have an absolute requirement for it.

51. A: A corneal ulcer is present

A corneal ulcer is an erosion through the corneal epithelium. Corneal ulcers may be caused by trauma, chemical burn, infection, and disease. For example, keratoconjunctivitis sicca dries the cornea and predisposes it to ulceration. Corneal ulcers are treated with antibiotic drops or ointment to prevent infection, atropine drops or ointment to relieve spasm, and, often, surgery to close and protect the eye. Steroids are contraindicated during the initial healing phase of corneal ulceration because steroids inhibit healing of the epithelium and the response to infection.

52. B: 6.7 mg/min

The female must receive 10 mg/kg/hr. She weighs 40 kg. Thus she needs 400 mg calcium gluconate per hour (10 mg x 40 kg = 400 mg/hour) or 6.7 mg per minute (400 mg/hour / 60 min/hour = 6.67 mg/min).

53. B: To prove active infection, viral serology must be performed twice, two weeks apart, and show a rising viral titer.

Viral serology tests for the presence of antibodies specific to a given virus. A positive value, the presence of serum antibody to a virus, indicates an animal's exposure to a virus. A single positive value, no matter the quantity of antibody, does not necessarily indicate active infection. To prove active infection, current and convalescent blood samples must be taken and viral serology performed on both. A rising titer of viral antibody confirms active infection. Generally, samples are taken two weeks apart. Negative viral serology does not prove an animal has not been exposed to a virus or is not infected with a virus. The test will be negative in the days prior to the body mounting an antibody response, when the animal is unable to generate a response (usually because of significant immune disease or immunosuppressive medications), or when the animal was exposed to the virus a considerable time ago and no measurable antibodies remain in the serum.

54. C: Culture on dermatophyte medium

Ringworm is a contagious fungal skin infection. The type of fungi that cause ringworm are dermatophytic, specifically Microsporum, Trichophyton, and Epidermophyton, with Microsporum canis particularly common. Affected animals experience pruritus and alopecia. Crusting, scaling, redness, and hyperpigmentation may exist. A Wood's lamp may be used to check for fluorescence of suspected infected hairs. Fluorescence suggests ringworm infection, but neither the presence nor absence of fluorescence is diagnostic. Definitive diagnosis of ringworm depends on culturing the fungus from plucked hairs. Hairs are placed on dermatophyte test medium and gently pressed into the medium. Results are often seen within days, but up to two weeks are allowed for growth and color change of the medium.

55. A: $2\left(\frac{3\,1\,3\,1}{3\,1\,2\,1}\right)$

Response B is the feline deciduous dental formula. Response C is the canine permanent dental formula. Response D is the porcine permanent dental formula.

56. D: A second litter pan and more frequent cleaning of the litter pans

When two or more cats are present in a household, the litter pan must be cleaned at least once a day as fastidious, and even less fastidious cats, may find the shared litter pan too dirty to use. In this case, one or more of the cats may defecate outside the litter pan, often in close proximity. More frequent cleaning of the litter pan, sometimes more than once a day, or offering multiple litter pans—at least one per cat—should solve the problem.

If the scenario had included evidence of a new addition to the family, pain, or another stressful event, anxiety might be a consideration. In the case of anxiety, however, both urine and feces would typically be found outside the litter pan. Similarly, territorial marking generally includes inappropriate urination.

57. D: 2.25 to 10 MHz

Veterinary ultrasound frequencies of 2.25 to 10 MHz do not penetrate bone or air, which reflect waves in this frequency range. Lower frequency sound waves penetrate farther than higher frequency sound waves and are used for deeper structures. Different frequencies are also used for different animals; for example, dogs are usually evaluated with 5.0 or 7.5 MHZ. Horse tendons are likely to be evaluated at 7.5 MHz.

58. C: Sinoatrial node

The sinoatrial node or S-A node is the natural pacemaker of the heart with cells that initiate the electrical activity that will spread through the heart. From the S-A node, the electrical impulse spreads across the atria to the atrioventricular or A-V node. From the atrioventricular node, the electrical signal passes to the His bundle, through the right and left bundle branches, to the Purkinje fibers.

59. B: Subjective Objective Assessment Plan

Soap is an organization plan for patient record keeping. Notes under (S) Subjective include history and observations. (O) Objective includes factual information including vital statistics, examination notes, and laboratory and radiographic data. (A) Assessment includes conclusions based on the subjective and objective information as well as differential diagnoses. The (P) Plan includes client education, proposed and planned diagnostic procedures and surgery, and therapies.

60. C: 1, 2, 3, 4

A large incision must be made for a bovine cesarean section. Complications at the incision site are not uncommon. Cows should deliver their placenta within 24 hours. A retained placenta will not pass in that time frame. Bacterial infection of the skin, uterus, and mammaries (mastitis) are risks. Dehydration may occur secondary to fluid loss or inadequate intake.

61. C: the safety and health training program, medical surveillance program, and the practice's standard operating procedures for safety and health.

According to OSHA Standard 29 CFR Part 1920, "Employers shall develop and implement a written safety and health program for their employees involved in hazardous waste operations. The program shall be designed to identify, evaluate, and control safety and health hazards, and provide for emergency response for hazardous waste operations." This written safety and health program must include: organizational structure, comprehensive work plan, site-specific safety and health plan, safety and health training program, medical surveillance program, employer's standard operating procedures for safety and health, and necessary interface between general program and site-specific activities.

62. B: Lead

Lead effectively blocks the passage of x-rays and is used to shield bodies during radiographic exposure. Personal protective equipment for taking radiographs includes lead gloves, lead apron, lead thyroid shield, lead gonad shield, and lead glasses.

63. A: Fill lead gloves with water to check for leaks that allow radiation through

Personal protective equipment used to ward against radiographic exposure must be properly cared for to maintain its protective value. Lead-containing safety equipment should never be folded. Aprons and shields should be hung up; gloves should be placed on a glove rack. Equipment should be examined for damage and periodically radiographed to look for cracks or breaks. One of the most important pieces of protective equipment is not a shield, but a measurement devise—the dosimeter that measures radiation exposure. A personal dosimeter must be worn whenever taking, or assisting with, radiographs. Whenever possible, only the radiographic subject should be in the radiology room.

64. D: Make filing errors easily visible.

Patient files are often marked with two or three colored letter labels identifying the first letters of the last name of the client. The colored labels are placed on the outside edge of the file so they are visible when the file is filed away. In this manner, record keepers can visually scan all files and see any file out of place. In some practices, names are replaced with numbers generated by the practice and color-coded numbers are placed on the files. Color can be used in other ways in files to provide easily detected visual information. For example, a blue or pink patient information sheet may be used to identify the sex of the patient or a red sticker may be clearly placed on the file to indicate an aggressive animal.

65. A: IV

Procaine penicillin is a long-acting formulation. Like benzathine-penicillin it may be used IM or SQ, but never IV.

66. B: Metaldehyde

Slug and snail control products, and rat control products, may contain metaldehyde. When ingested, metaldehyde is absorbed in the stomach and intestines and decreases serotonin, norepinephrine, and GABA. Neurological signs appear including muscle tremors and ataxia. After ingesting metaldehyde, a dog likely also experiences hyperthermia and tachycardia. Symptoms progress to convulsions. Diazepam may be used to reduce excitement and convulsions.

67. A: 1 hour

A vaccine that requires no mixing or reconstitution may be sterilely placed in a syringe and capped. So long as it was handled properly and refrigerated, the vaccine remains stable and safe. Reconstituted vaccines, however, even when handled properly, must be used within an hour of reconstitution. Any exceptions will be noted on the product label.

Vaccine should only be mixed with its own designated diluent. The diluent must be sterilely removed from its vial and injected into the vaccine vial. The dry vaccine and diluent are then gently mixed. After full mixing, the reconstituted vaccine is sterilely removed with a syringe. Biologics, such as vaccines, are kept refrigerated in a designated refrigerator free of food.

68. C: 20 tablets (10 mg)

The patient takes 20 mg every morning for 3 days. 20 x 3 = 60

The patient then takes 10 mg every morning for 7 days. 10 x 7 = 70

The patient next takes 5 mg every morning for 7 days. 5 x 7 = 35

The patient finishes with 5 mg every other morning for 14 days. 5 x 7 = 35

60 + 70 + 35 + 35 = 200 mg

The only choice that contains exactly 200 mg is 20 tablets (10mg)

69. D: Distilled water

A refractometer measures the specific gravity of fluid. A drop of fluid is placed on the glass, the top closed and the specific gravity read by looking through the eyepiece and observing the line against the measures. In between each use, the refractometer is cleaned to the manufacturer's instruction, generally by wiping the glass dry with a non-scratching, lint-free cloth. Once a week, the refractometer is calibrated by placing a drop of distilled water on the glass. Distilled water gives a reading of a specific gravity of 1.000. If the refractometer reads differently, it must be adjusted. As with all device control testing and recalibrations, a record should be kept of the date of recalibration, signed by the person who conducted the recalibration.

70. C: Cheyletiella, diagnosed with a tape preparation

Cheyletiella is a mite commonly referred to as walking dandruff. Cheyletiella is best diagnosed by placing a piece of cellophane tape against the patient's skin and hair then placing the tape on a slide. Microscopic viewing should show any Cheyletiella or other pathologic mites, including Demodex, Sarcoptes, and Notoedres, are diagnosed from a skin scraping. Scraped calls are swiped onto a clean slide. The slide is evaluated microscopically for the presence of mites.

71. A: 400x

A standard light microscope has an ocular projection lens with a magnification of x10. Combined with the magnification power of an objective lens, the total magnification will be the power of the ocular lens times the power of the objective lens, in this case 10 x 40, or 400. The object studied using the microscope is magnified 400 times.

72. D: Anisocytosis

All of these words are descriptors in abnormal variability of red cell size or shape. Anisocytosis describes a substantial percentage of red blood cells with sizes varying from the norm. Microcytosis describes red cells smaller than 6 µm in diameter; macrocytosis larger than normal. Poikilocytes are red cells with distorted shapes.

73. B: 1, 2, 3

Artifacts in histological sections result from manipulation of the samples and must be minimized for best interpretation. The following 6 types of artifacts are known to occur: shrinkage, precipitates, folds and wrinkles, cut defects, mutilation from rough handling, and postmortem degeneration.

Shrinkage results from fixatives or heat and may be uneven. Inadequately buffered fixative may crystallize and precipitate. Folds and wrinkles occur when thin tissue samples are cut or attached to slides.

Any defects in the cutting knife edge may cause straight line defects in the tissue sample. Rough handling from pinching or crushing the tissue may mutilate the tissue. If tissues aren't fixed promptly and properly, tissues will undergo autolysis or degeneration.

74. A: 3, 2, 4, 1, 2, 5, 2

The proper steps to gram-stain a sample on a slide are:

1. Stain with crystal violet, the primary stain.
2. Rinse with water.
3. Stain with Gram's iodine, the mordant.
4. Run 95% ethyl alcohol down the slide as a decolorizing agent.
5. Rinse with water.
6. Stain with safranin, the counter stain.
7. Rinse with water

75. B: 1.008 to 1.012

Isosthenuric urine is neither concentrated nor dilute. It is produced when there is neither excess water the body must get rid of, nor a need to conserve water by the body. Isosthenuric urine may also be a sign of kidney disease, as it may be a sign that the kidney tubules are no longer capable of concentrating or diluting urine. Three-fourths of kidney function must be lost before the kidneys are unable to concentrate or dilute urine.

76. C: It contains xylitol.

Xylitol is a sugar substitute often used in gums and mints. Xylitol is rapidly and completely absorbed by dogs with blood levels peaking 30 minutes post-ingestion. Dogs exposed to xylitol may vomit. A dog's blood sugar may drop within 30 minutes or after several hours. Developing hypoglycemia may secondarily cause lethargy, ataxia, seizure, and collapse. Acute liver failure is also possible following xylitol ingestion. Responsive treatment with IV fluids containing dextrose is necessary.

77. A: 6 months

Dogs treated with bromide as an anticonvulsant initially have their blood levels checked at one and three months. Thereafter, tests occur every 6 months to ensure therapeutic serum bromide concentrations.

Phenobarbital and bromide are commonly used anticonvulsants in dogs. Alternative anticonvulsants include felbamate, gabapentin, levetiracetam, pregabalin, topiramate, and zonisamide.

It is important to maintain a therapeutic level of bromide to reduce the incidence of convulsions. It is equally important to limit the concentration to reduce the incidence of adverse effects including sedation and rear limb lameness.

78. A: A 2-dose primary series with annual vaccination thereafter

Vaccines against the feline leukemia vaccine are known to have considerable effectiveness beyond that expected from natural resistance. The vaccine is often given to kittens after they test negative for the feline leukemia virus. No matter the age at initial vaccination, two doses administered two to three weeks apart are given for the initial series. Thereafter, annual doses of vaccine are given so long as the cat remains at risk for exposure.

79. B: Caudal vena cava

Total parenteral nutrition (TPN) is nutrition delivered intravenously to meet the complete nutritional and caloric needs of a patient. TPN must be administered aseptically and through placement of a large gauge catheter. Either the jugular vein or caudal vena cava is used. Patients are sedated for catheter placement. The TPN mixture is individually formulated.

80. A: Pasteurella multocida

Pasteurella infection is so prevalent in rabbit populations that only severe efforts to eliminate it could be effective. Pasteurella is a highly contagious bacteria transmitted through direct contact, and sometimes through aerosolization. 30 to 90% of healthy rabbits carry the bacteria. Mothers often pass it to their kits.

Rabbits may remain carriers of Pasteurella or develop disease caused by the bacteria. Rabbits may develop snuffles (rhinitis), pneumonia, otitis interna and media, conjunctivitis, genital infections, and abscesses—all from Pasteurella.

While antibiotics may be effectively used for active infection, Pasteurella may not be eradicated.

81. C: More accurate for detection of bacteriuria

Urine sediment examination can yield different results than urine culture, often because of misinterpreted pseudobacteria, small particles that resemble bacteria in size, shape, and movement. An air-dried urine preparation stained with a modified-Wright (Diff-Quik) stain reduces misidentification.

82. B: 6 mg/kg IV given to effect

Propofol can be used for anesthetic induction and anesthetic maintenance. Premedication reduces the amount of propofol needed for induction. The recommended dose of propofol for anesthetic administration in cats and dogs is 6 mg/kg given intravenously and to effect. With pre-administration with an opioid or sedative, propofol doses in the 3-4 mg/kg range are given intravenously for induction. Anesthesia can be maintained with additional boluses of propofol of 0.5 - 1 mg/kg given to effect intravenously or with a constant rate infusion of propofol at 0.1 - 0.4 mg/kg/min.

83. D: Because it is genetic, nothing can be done to prevent hip dysplasia in her pet.

Canine hip dysplasia (CHD) is a significant disease with an increasing incidence. CHD is multifactorial with polygenetic and environmental contributing factors. Limiting food intake and pet body weight reduces radiographic and clinical signs of osteoarthritis in predisposed dogs. Radiographs and examination can be used to evaluate laxity, abnormal bone structure, and osteoarthritic changes, but no available test can determine which dogs will develop significant CHD.

84. D: Specific, measurable, attainable, realistic, timely.

SMART goals make achievement planned and monitored for success. A goal should be specifically defined and detailed. The goal should be measurable to know when it has been reached. Goals must be attainable to be true goals and not wishes. Goals should be aspiring, but also realistic goal with a certainty that achievement is possible. Goals should have a set time frame to focus achievement. A large goal may be broken down into smaller parts for timely and realistic attainment.

85. A: 20 mL/hr

Transfusions are given at a rate of 2 mL/kg/hr. A 10kg dog should receive 20mL of red cells per hour or 0.3 mL per minute.

86. C: E. coli

Staphylococcus, Streptococcus, Enterococcus, Klebsiella, and Proteus all contribute to urinary tract infections in the dog and cat, but Escherichia coli is the most common. E. coli is isolated from 67% of urinary tract infections in cats and 44% in dogs.

87. D: 95%

Due to the sigmoidal shape of the oxygen saturation curve, once hemoglobin saturation drops below 95%, the PaO_2 falls precipitously. Patients monitored with pulse oximetry may be at the edge of a dangerous drop in oxygen concentration when their values fall to 95%.

88. D: Bradycardia

A patient's end-tidal CO_2 is monitored during surgery to assess ventilation. The CO_2 monitor measures the CO_2 level of expired breath as well as waveform shape and baseline. Should the patient breathe in a relatively high level of CO_2 or be hypercapnic, the end-tidal CO_2 will be high. A leak in the breathing system can also result in a high value.

89. A: Doxycycline

90. A: Urachus

91. D: 50 bpm

A horse's at rest heart rate is 28-40 beats per minute. Any painful situation can raise the resting heart rate. Colic ranges from non-painful to severely painful. With a mild obstruction, horses commonly have a resting heart rate elevated in the 50 to 60 beats per minute range. A strangulated bowel causing substantial distress may cause an elevation in heart rate to 80 to 90 beats per minute.

92. B: Proliferative

Traditional categories of shock include hypovolemic or hemorrhagic shock, septic shock, cardiogenic shock, traumatic shock, and anaphylactic shock. Functional categories of shock include hypovolemic, cardiogenic, vasogenic or distributive, and obstructive shock.

Cardiogenic shock results from heart failure. Bleeding or substantial loss of intravascular volume leads to hypovolemic or hemorrhagic shock. Septic shock (from bacterial infection) and traumatic shock (from fluid movement as a result of trauma) interfere with proper distribution of blood throughout the body.

93. B: Date, patient name, position, thickness of studied region, exposure factors, initials

A radiographic exposure log serves a number of functions. It is used to track the number of radiographs taken and assess when calibration and cleaning are needed. Data in the log can be used to determine the efficiency of work, track a patient's radiographs, and monitor the effectiveness of settings for a particular body part and thickness.

The radiographic log commonly tracks:

- Date of radiograph
- Name of patient
- Position
- Thickness of studied region
- Exposure factors
- Initials of person taking radiograph(s)

94. A: 24 hours

Agar plates are inoculated with a concerted effort to avoid contamination, and with the infected or potentially infected material spread evenly across the surface of the agar plate. The agar plate should be stored upside-down with the lid taped plate. The plate should be placed in an incubator and checked every 24 hours to evaluate growth and color change.

95. C: Minimum inhibitory concentration

Following bacterial culture, bacteria are assessed for their sensitivity to different antibiotics and the amount of antibiotic required to inhibit bacterial growth. The minimum concentration of antibiotic that inhibits bacterial growth is the MIC, or minimum inhibitory concentration.

A broth dilution test is one method of evaluating MIC. In a broth dilution test, the bacteria under evaluation are incubated in several tubes of broth with varying amounts of the antibiotic being tested. The tubes are evaluated to determine which allowed bacterial growth and which did not.

The lowest antibiotic concentration that inhibited growth of the bacteria is the MIC. Other methods of evaluating MIC are agar dilution and the Etest.

96. B: Pinocytosis

Endocytosis is an active cell process by which materials are taken into a cell. In pinocytosis, the cell membrane extends around fluid membranes. With phagocytosis, the cell membrane extends around solid particles. Specific substances, including hormones, iron, and cholesterol, enter the cell through a receptor-mediated process. Contrarily, exocytosis is a process of expelling materials from a cell.

97. D: 32.1 pounds

Each kilogram is equivalent to 2.2 pounds. 14.6 x 2.2 = 32.1 pounds.

98. B: No

Xylitol is a sugar substitute found in gum and other foods. A toxic dose results in hypoglycemia and, in high quantities, liver failure. The toxic dose for dogs is 75-100 mg/kg. To determine whether this dog received a potentially toxic dose, calculate the quantity of xylitol ingested and the weight of the dog in kg. A 50-pound dog weighs 22.7 kg (50/2.2 = 22.7). The toxic dose for a dog starts at 75 mg/kg. The minimum toxic dose for this 22.7 kg dog is 1,704 mg xylitol or 1.7 g xylitol (22.7 x 75 = 1704). The dog ate 8 sticks of gum, each containing 0.17 g of xylitol for a total of 1.36 g xylitol (0.17 x 8 = 1.36). As 1.36 is below the threshold of 1.7, this dog is not considered to have eaten a toxic dose.

99. C: Dorsal recumbency

Alveolar ventilation and pulmonary perfusion are optimal in awake, standing horses. A ventilation/perfusion mismatch, or V/Q mismatch, occurs in anesthetized horses. Ventilation/perfusion is most dramatically affected when an anesthetized horse is in dorsal recumbency, and often results in low arterial oxygen tension.

100. D: Chinchilla

Chinchillas will lose large patches of hair when roughly handled, a condition called fur slip.

101. C: 3-5-month-old chicken weighing approximately 5-7 pounds

A roaster is a 3- to 5-month-old chicken that weighs approximately 5 to 7 pounds. A roaster has a higher density of meat than a broiler or a fryer. A broiler is 6 to 8 weeks old.

102. A: Silkie Bantam

While some chickens are farmed for both meat and eggs, the Silkie Bantam is an ornamental breed raised for eggs, but not meat.

103. D: Airway, breathing, circulation

Triage assigns priority to emergency patients and their medical issues. Certain severe problems including excessive bleeding and open fractures warrant immediate treatment without full assessment. For patients surveyed during triage, the primary survey involves assessment of airway, breathing, and circulation. The secondary survey includes history taking, complete physical examination, and a minimum database.

104. B: 21 days

Chicken eggs are commonly incubated to hatch them. An egg takes 21 days to hatch. A still-air incubator is heated to 101.5 °F. Incubator humidity should be 60-65 percent for the first 18 days of incubation, and 80-85 percent for the last 3 days.

105. D: Botulism

Clostridium botulinum, once ingested by a duck, releases a toxin that causes paralysis. They are said to have limber neck. With early supportive treatment, the duck may survive through the toxin wearing off.

106. B: The lower lip and ear

The twitch, properly applied, is an effective means of restraint, distracting the horse from other tasks. A twitch is applied to the lower lip by holding the lip and pulling it into the loop of the twitch. The handle is then rotated to tighten the twitch on the lip. Uncommonly, the lower lip and ear will be twitched.

107. C: Placing one hand under the shoulders with the thumb under the jaw, and using the other hand to support and restrain the hindquarters

Ferrets can be difficult to restrain, but must be safely restrained at both their shoulders and hips to prevent injury.

108. A: Collie

Dolichocephaly indicates a long head, often recognized as an elongated nose in dogs. Brachycephalic breeds, by contrast, have broad heads and short muzzles.

109. B: Control secretions

Anticholinergics atropine and glycopyrrolate control salivary and respiratory tract secretions.

110. A: 68 days of gestation without signs of labor

Canine gestation may last 57-72 days, with an average of 65 days. Dystocia, problems with delivery of one or more pups are caused by fetal factors including oversize and malpresentations, anatomic disorder of the mother, and uterine inertia. Signs of dystocia include gestation past 70 days with no sign of labor, pelvic anatomical disorders, pup lodged in the birth canal, strong contractions without delivery of a pup in 30 minutes, weal contractions without delivery of a pup in 4 hours, severe pain, temperature drop below 100 °F with return to normal but no labor after 24 hours.

111. C: Insulin and glucose

Hyperkalemia, high serum potassium content, is a serious condition requiring prompt treatment. Potassium can be driven into cells by activating the sodium-potassium pump with administration of insulin. Because excess insulin will also drive glucose into cells, supplemental glucose must be given to prevent hypoglycemia while treating hyperkalemia.

112. A: Uncoating

The first step of viral replication is adsorption, when the virus attaches to the cell surface. Second, the virus penetrates the cell by fusing with the plasma membrane, entering through endosomes at the cell surface, or crossing the membrane directly. Next, the virus uncoats so that virus replication can begin.

During the fourth step, the virus synthesizes viral nucleic acid and protein. New virus particles are then assembled, and, in the sixth and final step, the newly assembled virus particles are released due to cell lysis or budding from the cell.

113. B: Cephalosporins

Antibiotics are used in food animals to treat active infections and control infections that may limit growth. Some medications may not be used within a defined time period prior to slaughter to limit the risk of human exposure to medication through food. The Food and Drug Administration expressly prohibits the use of some antibiotics, including fluoroquinolones and cephalosporins, in livestock.

114. B: Feline oral resorptive lesions

Feline oral resorptive lesions have been observed with increasing frequency since the 1970s. The lesions are caused by activation of odontoclasts, though the cause of activation remains under study. With this disease, odontoclasts abnormally remodel tooth structure, causing excess, and potentially extensive, tooth resorption. Lesions tend to occur at the gumline and are very painful.

115. C: Periods of apnea alternating with periods of tachypnea and hyperpnea

Cheyne-Stokes respiration is an abnormal breathing pattern characterized by periods of apnea alternating with periods of tachypnea and hyperpnea. This breathing pattern can have negative cardiopulmonary effects including oxygen desaturation and arrhythmias. Treatment depends on the underlying cause, which may be advanced cardiac disease.

116. C: Cat

While other animals can experience an elevated serum glucose concentration secondary to stress, cats may have such substantial elevation as to confuse stress hyperglycemia with diabetes. When in doubt, serum fructosamine levels can be evaluated to differentiate chronic elevation in glucose from a limited episode.

117. B: Tipping

A sheep is tipped to trim hooves or work on its underside. Tipping can be performed humanely and without injury to the sheep. The handler should hold the sheep's head and position his or her body aside the sheep. By swinging the head outward while rotating the body down and inward, the sheep can be moved into a position of resting on its hindquarters or rump.

118. D: Metestrus

Progesterone levels decline and estradiol increases as the corpus luteum regresses in the proestrus stage. The follicle grows during proestrus and estrus. Ovulation occurs during estrus in most species. Metestrus is the first part of the luteal phase when the corpus luteum develops. Ovulation occurs during metestrus in the cow. Diestrus completes the luteal phase.

119. D: "I'll schedule an appointment for you. Please bring a sample of feces with you for evaluation."

While worms in the feces are not an emergency, they are of great concern and must be addressed. Dogs may be infected with multiple intestinal parasites, and should not be diagnosed or treated solely on the basis of visible worms. Medication should not be dispensed without a valid doctor-client-patient relationship and a doctor's prescription. The dog should be evaluated for signs of disease. The dog's feces should be evaluated for other parasites. The client should be educated on treatment and limiting the likelihood of further infection.

120. D: Photophobic and kinesophobic

Understanding the flea life cycle and characteristics is useful to avoid fleas and treat infestations. Flea eggs can be picked up by vacuums. Flea larvae eat flea feces. Vacuuming removes flea feces and reduces the food supply for larvae. Because larvae are photophobic and kinesophobic, they will more likely be found in dark, poorly trafficked areas. Treatment should focus on these areas.

121. B: Sight hounds

122. D: 12 weeks

To properly assess the presence of a food allergy and define the one or more causative patients, cats and dogs are placed on novel protein-limited ingredient elimination diets. Because it takes time to build an allergic response, the animal will not have an allergic reaction to ingredients to which the animal has not been previously exposed. A positive response is a reduction or elimination of allergic symptoms while on the elimination diet. A diagnosis depends on confirmation with return of allergic symptoms when reintroduced to the offending protein. A positive response, a reduction in allergy symptoms, can be detected early in the course of assessment. Contrarily, a negative response takes 12 weeks to confirm. A lack of response to the novel diet over the first few weeks is not diagnostic. Some animals take up to three weeks to resolve their inflammatory response.

123. D: Grade 5 murmur

Heart murmurs are graded based on their loudness and intensity. A grade 1 heart murmur will be difficult to detect even under ideal conditions. A grade 3 murmur is moderately loud or intense and can be heard in more than one location. Grade 4 and grade 5 murmurs are loud. They are differentiated by the presence of a palpable thrill. A loud murmur with a palpable thrill is categorized as grade 5.

124. B: pH

Refrigeration of urine leads to degeneration of casts and, in some cases, ex vivo crystal formation. To assess the likelihood of changes in sediment, pH can be monitored. A change in pH indicates a likelihood of cast and crystal changes.

125. D: A Z pattern under low magnification

Mites are relatively large and easily spotted under microscopic examination. Low power magnification, either 4x or 10x, is most appropriate for visualizing mites. For thorough evaluation, the slide is moved in a Z pattern to ensure all fields are viewed and evaluated. Using the Z pattern, viewing begins at one corner of the slide and viewing continues in a straight line. When the edge of the sample or edge of slide is reached, the slide is moved to the next line, with slight overlap of the first line. Evaluation of the entire slide continues in this manner.

126. B: Bartonellosis

The SNAP 4Dx Test by IDEXX Laboratories is a commonly used rapid screening test for heartworm, Lyme disease, Anaplasma phagocytophila, and Ehrlichia canis.

127. C: Melanoma

Round cell tumors are named for their shape under microscopic examination. The cells are discrete cells, round to oval in shape, that exfoliate from the tumor mass well. Generally speaking, they are easily identified with fine needle aspiration and microscopic evaluation. Canine round cell tumors include mast cell tumor, histiocytoma, plasmacytomas, transmissible venereal tumors, and cutaneous lymphoma.

Llamas and alpacas have malignant round cell tumors that include lymphoma, neuroblastoma, Ewing's sarcoma, rhabdomyosarcoma, and primitive neuroectodermal tumor.

128. A: 3°

Horses have large eyes, positioned laterally. The horizontal field of vision for each eye is 190°, with an overlapping binocular field of 65°. The vertical field of vision of each eye is 180°. Horses have two very narrow blind spots. One is below the nose. The other is behind the head, extending over the spine of the horse. The rear blind spot is only 3° wide.

129. B: Left legs counterclockwise, right legs clockwise

Proper bandaging technique of horse limbs requires wrapping in a spiral pattern beginning at the inside of the cannon bone above the fetlock. Each leg should be wrapped from front to back and from outside to inside. This pattern equates to counterclockwise wrapping of left legs, and clockwise wrapping of right legs. Bandages should not begin or end over a joint. Each layer should overlap the prior layer by 50%.

130. D: 150 mL/min

On a rebreathing system, the appropriate flow rate for oxygen is 30 mL/kg/min. A 5-kg cat receives 150 mL/min (5 kg x 30mL = 150 mL). Alterations in flow rate would be made to accommodate disease states and inhibited ventilation.

131. B: VPCs

When a patient has gastric dilatation and volvulus (GDV), the distended stomach may compress the abdominal caudal vena cava, thereby decreasing venous return to the heart and decreasing cardiac output. The cascade of deleterious effects continues as systolic blood pressure drops and peripheral vasoconstriction follows. The decreasing circulation of oxygen-rich blood and venous return increases the risk of myocardial damage.

As the heart experiences injury, the electrical rhythm changes as demonstrated in an ECG: P waves disappear as ventricles spontaneously fire and the QRS complex becomes wide and irregular as electrical communication is disrupted. These VPCs (ventricular premature contractions) develop 12+ hours following dilatation and volvulus.

132. D: Peaked T waves

Serum potassium concentrations above 5.5 mEq/L accelerate depolarization of the heart. Electrically, the result will be seen in the ECG as the T waves become tall and tented or peaked. If serum potassium concentrations continue to rise above 6.5 mEq/L, cardiac conduction slows and intervals are prolonged. Serum potassium levels above 7 mEq/L further affect the heart's conduction, flattening the P wave, inducing ventricular fibrillation, and, in the most severe cases, causing cardiac arrest.

133. C: 1 year

A horse's chewing motion causes sharp points to develop on the molars over time. If left alone, the points will interfere with the ability to chew food properly. The horse may also have difficulty with a bit. Consequently, the points are filed down, known as floating teeth.

Floating is generally first needed at three to four years of age, and then every year on an ongoing basis. Some horses may be able to go as long as a year and a half in between floatings.

134. C: Alfalfa

Rabbits should have hay offered ad libitum. Young, growing rabbits should have alfalfa hay that is higher in protein and calcium levels. Adult rabbits should not have legume hays like alfalfa, peanut, clover, vetch, or pea. Instead the maintenance diet of adult rabbits should include grass hay. Timothy hay is most often fed, but orchard, Timothy, oat, brome, Bermuda, and Johnson grass are acceptable options.

135. A: 5 months

While different breeds of rabbit become sexually mature at different ages, all rabbit breeds are able to reproduce by one year of age. Smaller rabbits mature sexually sooner than larger rabbits. The smallest breeds, those under 4 kg, mature at four to five months of age. Breeds in the 2-4 kg range tend to become sexually mature at five to six months of age. Larger breeds become sexually mature at six to eight months of age, though some mature slightly after that.

136. A: Hood

When handling raptors, long leather gloves should be worn and the bird permitted to perch atop the glove. A hood can be used to cover the eyes, and calm the bird.

137. D: Hemorrhaging

The natural coumarins in sweet clover change into toxic dicumarol when the sweet clover spoils or gets moldy. Dicumarol is an anticoagulant, interfering with production of coagulation factor VII. Poisoning, therefore, causes hemorrhaging, massive bleeding. Blood transfusions, vitamin K1, and removal of spoiled sweet clover are necessary for treatment.

138. C: Stereotypic behavior

Stereotypic behaviors are repetitious movements with no obvious purpose. They are usually derived from normal maintenance behaviors, but now interfere with normal function. Stereotypic behaviors are a description, not a diagnosis.

Redirected activity is focused away from the actual target and on to another target. Displaced activity has similarities to redirected behavior, but involves an activity performed out-of-context or with a different behavior because the animal cannot perform the original activity.

139. B: Dalmatian

Although the precise number varies slightly among different studies, 18-20% of Dalmatians have congenital deafness. The incidence of unilaterally deaf Dalmatians is almost three times the number of bilaterally deaf Dalmatians. Hearing is evaluated with the BAER test. Evaluation has shown an inherited pattern. Unilaterally deaf Dalmatians with blue eyes should not be bred.

140. D: A hygroma

The repeated trauma to pressure points from lying on a hard surface induces an inflammatory response, and, secondarily, a fluid-filled, painless false bursae. This lesion is called a hygroma.

141. A: Are expensive

Good inventory management and pricing strategies are highly important to the financial success of veterinary practices. Prices are set based not only on the direct cost of the drug but the additional costs of inventorying and handling each drug. Costs increase when drugs have a low turnover rate resulting in higher storage costs, have a short expiration date—increasing the chance of waste—or require special handling.

142. A: Time to requisition new stock to maintain predetermined inventory levels

Each practice establishes its own inventory reorder point. A point is set for every item in inventory to minimize the cost of carrying product as well as any disruption in supply. Reorder point formulas are available, but the point may be set by a fairly simple interpretation of minimum tolerable stock, the length of time required to restock, and turnover rate.

143. A: Cruciate ligament graft

The cranial cruciate ligament is injured fairly frequently, and is the most common knee injury of the dog. Veterinarians will often be able to elicit a drawer sign when the ligament is ruptured. Rupture of the ligament destabilizes the knee joint and establishes an environment for arthritis.

Surgical repair stabilizes the knee joint, and may limit the progression of osteoarthritis. Different surgical approaches are used: TPLO (tibial plateau leveling osteotomy), TTA (tibial tuberosity advancement), and extracapsular repair. Intracapsular repair, or the "over the top" method, is no longer commonly used.

144. D: 1, 2, 3

Employee handbooks can be extensive summaries of a practices rules and policies. An employee handbook includes information on the practice and the type of employment, general employment information including ADA and EEO information, attendance policies, work safety issues, reimbursement policies, compensation and benefits information, time off work, performance evaluation procedures, complaint procedures, and workplace monitoring. It does not include job descriptions.

145. D: All of the above

Safety is a priority. The safest solution is to mark the cat's aggressive status in every location staff may look for information about the cat. Marking the cage is important for any staff members who may have responsibility for cages, but are less likely to check records prior to basic care.

146. B: Upon arrival

To minimize the possibility of confusion and misidentification, patients arriving for surgery should be marked with identification upon arrival at the practice.

147. C: Learning tasks that are the responsibility of other staff members

Practices with a team philosophy and efficient work habits cross-train staff. Each staff member learns the responsibilities of his or her own position as well as responsibilities of staff members in other roles. A kennel worker, for example, is trained to restrain animals and set up laboratory samples. A technician learns receptionist duties including handling payment at discharge.

148. A: 12 weeks

Puppies may be too young to be fully house-trained. The ability to reliably avoid soiling the house depends upon good bladder control. Under twelve weeks of age, bladder control is incomplete and unreliable.

149. C: Low humidity

Snakes normally shed every few weeks to once or twice per year. The skin normally sheds in one piece. Poor shedding may be indirectly related to poor health. It is directly related to low humidity and mite infestation. When a snake does not shed properly and fully, old skin may be retained over the eyes, called eye caps. Substantial retention requires removal so the snake can see clearly and eat properly.

150. B: 60-70 days

151. A: Peace lily

True lilies are highly toxic to cats, and known to cause acute renal failure in that species. True lilies include the Easter lily, tiger lily, stargazer lily, day lily, and all Asiatic lilies. Other flowers have lily in their name, but are not true lilies and do not cause acute renal failure. These flowers include the calla lily, peace lily, lily of the valley, and Peruvian lily.

152. B: Soluble oxalates

Rhubarb leaves, star fruit, and shamrock contain soluble oxalates. When eaten, these oxalates are absorbed through the gastrointestinal tract and bind with serum calcium and cause acute hypocalcemia. Additionally, calcium oxalate crystals accumulate in the kidneys and cause damage.

153. B: Cardiac glycoside toxicity

Digibind is a human product and antidote to cardiac glycoside toxicity. Toxicity can occur with administration of digitalis or ingestion of foxglove, oleander, or other plants containing cardiac glycosides.

154. C: Client has 5 pets that are consistently seen

True animal hoarding is a type of mental illness. Hoarders attempt to maintain far more animals than they can adequately care for. Hoarders are often experienced at hiding signs of this behavior. Some tip-offs that a patient lives with a hoarder or that a client is a hoarder are:

- Inconsistent or unidentified number of pets in the home
- Interest in further animal acquisition
- Inconsistent care of individual patients, but many visits with different patients
- Attempting to obtain medications for unseen animals
- Bringing in one or more poorly conditioned animals claiming stray status

Not every client with multiple pets, or a higher than average number of pets is a hoarder. An owner taking proper care of all pets is not likely to be a hoarder.

155. C: Multiply the tidal volume by 6

Tidal volume, the air inhales and exhaled with each breath, is 10-20 mL/kg. The volume of the breathing bag should be 6 times the tidal volume. The result will be in mL and should be translated to L to match bag sizing.

156. C: Type II hypersensitivity reaction

In this condition, animals are born healthy, but develop a serious hemolytic anemia after drinking their mother's colostrum. The anemia develops within days, or even hours. A mother exposed to red cell antigens of the father or neonate develops a sensitivity to the antigens and produces alloantibody. Antibodies are released in colostrums, causing the newborn to be exposed to antibodies to the antigens on its red cells. Red cell lysis follows. This is a type II hypersensitivity.

157. A: 3 weeks

Puppies begin to wean from their mother at 3 weeks of age. Formula is offered, first. Later, thin cereal is mixed into the formula. Canned food is next offered. At around 5 weeks, puppies can be offered dry puppy food.

158. C: Heart disease

Turbulent blood flow in the heart precipitated blood clots forming. This happens at a substantially higher rate in the presence of heart disease, and is often associated with hypertrophic cardiomyopathy. Often, a large clot forms in the left atrium and attaches to the wall. A piece of thrombus may break free and enter the circulation. The clot may then catch in the narrowed blood vessel, the aortic trifurcation. A clot in this location blocks blood flow to the hind limbs and is called a saddle thrombus or thromboembolism.

A cat with a saddle thrombus presents with partial or complete paralysis of the hind limbs and is often in substantial pain. Pain relief, treatment for hypertrophic cardiomyopathy, anticoagulants, and fluid therapy are given.

159. A: An increase in insect vectors

Canine distemper is a viral disease caused by contact with infected animals and environments. Canine distemper is not carried by insect vectors. A vaccine is routinely used to prevent infection. The incidence of canine distemper increases if the distemper virus mutates to a more virulent form, if fewer patients are vaccinated so that more are susceptible, and if the vaccine against canine distemper is flawed so that it does not provide as much immunity and protection.

160. D: Triatomine bite

Chagas disease, caused by the organism Trypanosoma cruzi, is passed to animals by triatomines, blood-feeding insects. Trypanosoma cruzi is actually in the insect feces, often rubbed into the wounds left by the insect bites by the animals themselves. Once the organism is rubbed into the wound, eyes, or mouth, the animal is infected. When animals in the home are exposed, the risk of human exposure increases.

161. D: 100%, increased

A hyperbaric oxygen chamber provides 100% oxygen under increased pressure, relative to room air, resulting in an up to fifteen time increase in dissolved oxygen. Increasing oxygen concentration in the blood increases the amount of oxygen in tissues as well as the depth of diffusion into tissues. Treatment is useful with compromised circulation, smoke inhalation, anaerobic infection, and some injuries. Barotrauma and oxygen toxicity can occur, but are minimized by proper treatment procedures.

162. A: TNR

TNR or "trap, neuter, release" programs are often run by charitable organizations hoping to minimize feral cat populations without killing colonies. Groups identify a feral colony, develop a plan to trap the cats, have them neutered, and release them back to their colony once safely awake. Groups may also have volunteers bring in feral cats or stray cats not identified as part of a colony. Opponents argue the method is ineffective as the colony will be healthier and live longer. New cats may be added more easily, and any intact females in the group will have larger litters. Supporters argue that they not only improve the quality of life for these cats, but anecdotal and numerical evidence show the success of TNR.

163. B: 70%

A typical horse at pasture spends 17 hours per day, or 70% of its time, in grazing behavior. The other 30% of time is distributed between sleep, play, socialization, and herd behaviors. A typical horse sleeps 1 to 4 hours per day.

164. A: 4-6 weeks

Canine lymphoma is an aggressive and common white blood cell cancer. Without treatment, lymphoma is fatal within 6 weeks. Aggressive treatment with today's best protocols results in an 85-90% likelihood of complete remission, though less than 5% of dogs are ever cured. 50% of treated patients live 1 year after diagnosis with a good quality of life, 25% live 2 years with a good quality of life.

165. B: Reverse sneezing

Reverse sneezing is a paroxysmal sound from the laryngeal region. The episode varies in length. The dog returns to normal immediately following. Reverse sneezing may be related to hypersensitivities or allergies. Antihistamines may help minimize episodes in patients that frequently exhibit this action.

166. D: Ketosis

Ketosis is estimated to occur in 30% of dairy cattle, though some herds have an incidence over 50%. Onset of ketosis often begins within 5 DIM, days in milk. While most cases resolve in seven days, some cows remain ketotic at 16 DIM. Ketotic cows produce less milk, have more reproductive difficulty, and are at increased risk of displaced abomasums. Preventing ketosis, therefore, is important, and involves reducing cow stress and preventing negative energy balance.

167. D: Keep the patient a minimum of 12 feet from other patients at all times

Universal precautions are taken when patients present with any potential zoonotic or contagious disease and include minimizing the number of staff in contact with the patients; wearing protective equipment, often a gown and gloves as a physical barrier; using effective, approved cleaning and disinfecting procedures for staff as well as contaminated environmental surfaces; and containing and disposing of contaminated waste. Waste is bagged in the patient's room, then placed within another bag outside the area and sealed for disposal.

Specific precautions are added depending on diagnosis or suspected diagnosis. A patient contagious only to its own species can freely stay with other species. A patient capable of infecting other patients and staff requires strict quarantine.

168. B: 10,000

Vaccine-associated feline sarcomas are rapidly growing, highly invasive tumors requiring aggressive treatment. They occur at injection sites in approximately one of every 10,000 vaccinated cats.

169. A: Renal failure

Obesity primarily or secondarily affects body systems substantially. Obesity is related to an increased incidence of musculoskeletal disease, cardiovascular disease, heat intolerance, exercise intolerance, diabetes, and liver disease.

170. B: 50%

Carbon dioxide absorbers connect to an anesthetic machine system to capture exhaled carbon dioxide. Carbon dioxide is absorbed by the barium hydroxide lime or sodium hydroxide lime crystals, producing, heat, water, and a color change, and depleting the crystals. Crystals are changed when 50% of the crystals in the absorber have changed color. Hours of use can be tracked to better define the best time to change the canister.

171. A: Target pattern

Surgical sites are always cleaned from the primary incision area out to edge of the field. Movements are circular. Scrubbing begins at the anticipated incision site with circular motions of the localized area. New scrub and gauze are used to scrub a clean ring around the first ring, and so on until the edge of the field is reached. At no time does the hand scrub from the edge of the surgical field toward the center of the surgical field.

172. C: 70% propylene glycol

A rinsing agent is used, in alternating fashion, to remove the scrubbing agent when cleaning a surgical field. 70% isopropyl alcohol, or rubbing alcohol, is commonly used. Sterile water and sterile saline may also be used. Care must be taken not to overly cool the patient using alcohol.

173. C: Quick-release knot

Quick release knots are used to secure surgical patients to the surgery table in correct position for the anticipated procedure. Patients must be secure, yet easy to free for an emergency or when recovery is rapid.

174. B: Ear

The Zepp procedure is also known as a lateral ear resection. This surgery is often performed to mitigate chronic and painful ear infections, but may be used to treat cancer and ear trauma.

175. C: Tearing

176. D: The biceps brachii muscle or tendon

177. C: The swallowing reflex is present

Endotracheal tubes are placed to maintain respiratory access and reduce the risk of aspiration. They are removed before the patient is awake enough, postoperatively, to bite or chew the tube. A good practice is to remove the endotracheal tube after the patient has recovered its swallowing reflex. The cuff on the tube must be deflated prior to extubation.

178. D: Cones

Modified dendrites of nerve cells form photoreceptor cells in the inner layer of the eye. Those receptive to a variety of colors allowing the formation of a colored image in daylight are cones.

179. B: Amplifies DNA

Using PCR, or polymerase chain reaction, scientists can amplify the DNA present in a sample. DNA amplification of a selective piece of DNA is possible. In veterinary practice, this technique is used to maximize the opportunity to identify pathogens present in samples.

180. A: Pack

Borchelt identified 8 major types of canine aggression. Fear aggression relates to a dog's aggressive behavior secondary to a fear response. Dominance aggression is aggression directed at establishing the dog's dominance against another animal. The possessiveness type of dominance is seen when a dog exhibits aggressive behavior to maintain an item as his or hers. Protectiveness of people and territory aggression is exhibited when a dog experiences a perceived threat to protected people or territory—the threat needn't seem substantial or real to humans to be protective aggression. Predation aggression is the aggression used to hunt. Punishment aggression is retaliatory for a real or perceived insult. Pain aggression is seen when a dog exhibits aggressive behavior directly related to an incident in which the dog is in pain. The eighth major type of aggression is intraspecific aggression.

181. B: 13.5

A 950-pound horse is 950/2.2 = 432 kg. A 432-kg horse needs 432 x 30 = 12,960 mg of combined product. If each tablet is 960 mg, 12960/960 = 13.5 tablets are needed.

182. D: Meets AAFCO nutritional standards as a complete and balanced food

AAFCO, the Association of American Feed Control Officials, offers model regulations for pet foods, a checklist for labels, and develops nutritional standards. Nutritional standards are based on substantiated nutrient content and feeding trials. Pets should be fed foods that have undergone feeding trials to prove they are balanced and complete.

183. D: Hind limbs

Ground reaction force patterns can be used to evaluate gait and assess the pressures on each limb through a gait pattern. When an animal climbs stairs, force shifts from a standing distribution, 60% of force on forelimbs and 40% on hind limbs, to being primarily on the hind limbs.

184. C: Diabetes mellitus

Glucocorticoids, particularly when administered at high doses or for extended periods of time, have a substantial incidence of adverse effects. Adverse effects include thromboembolism, infection, stomach ulcers, Cushing's disease, hepatic changes, and diabetes mellitus. Glucocorticoids increase insulin resistance and increase the incidence of hyperglycemia. When persistent hyperglycemia and glucosuria develop, insulin therapy is started, and glucocorticoids are weaned as possible. Remission may occur following cessation of glucocorticoid treatment.

185. C: Prednisolone

Glucocorticoid therapy is available as prednisone and prednisolone. When prednisone is administered, it is activated in the liver into prednisolone. Some cats have difficulty converting prednisone to prednisolone. Prednisolone is, therefore, the preferred form for administration in cats.

186. A: Alfalfa

Iguanas are herbivores and are not fed animal protein. Mature alfalfa contains 15% protein by volume and is an excellent and appropriate source of protein for the iguana.

187. D: A parvovirus

Aleutian disease is caused by a parvovirus, and was first reported in mink in 1940. Mutant strains of the mink Aleutian disease virus affect ferrets. Different strains vary in their virulence. Aleutian disease is primarily transmitted with direct contact of infected body fluids and feces, but can be transmitted through the air or contact with contaminated people and objects. The incubation and shedding periods are unknown. Ferrets can be healthy carriers of the disease.

188. A: 85%

85% of dogs and cats, aged 4 or older, have periodontal disease. Periodontal disease begins when plaque forms. If left alone, mineral salts in food precipitate and form dental calculus irritating gingival tissues. Irritated gingival alters the pH of the mouth and allows subgingival bacteria to survive. As those bacteria thrive, deep periodontal pockets form, and then bone is destroyed.

Daily tooth brushing, a hard diet, and dental cleanings prevent plaque formation and resolve early periodontitis.

189. B: Dexon

Dexon is an example of a synthetic absorbable suture with the generic name of polyglycolic acid.

Prolene, ethilon, and silk are all examples of nonabsorbable suture materials that are used primarily in the skin and removed after an incision is healed.

190. B: Class II

The dental mobility index is a formal way of grading the looseness of a tooth. Classifications are as follows:

- Class I: tooth moves slightly
- Class II: tooth moves less than the distance of its crown width
- Class III: tooth moves more than the distance of its crown width

191. B: 2 hours post-prandial

When symptoms and blood chemistries suggest liver disease, serum bile acids should be tested. Serum bile acids are a highly sensitive and specific test of hepatic function. Serum bile acids are the best available method of assessing liver function, but do not determine the cause or severity of the underlying liver disease.

The first blood draw for serum bile acids takes place when the patient is fasted. The patient is then fed. Two hours later, a post-prandial sample is taken for evaluation of bile acids. Abnormal results suggest the need for a liver biopsy to specifically evaluate the cause of the liver dysfunction.

192. D: A bite abnormality where a retained deciduous tooth tilts the erupting permanent canine into an abnormal location

When a canine tooth has been misdirected in this fashion, opposing canines may not occlude properly. Secondary abnormal wear and periodontal disease can result. Puppies must have their dentition evaluated at every visit to evaluate retained deciduous teeth and abnormal eruption, and allow for early intervention.

193. D: 8.6

Because calcium is protein-bound, when the serum albumin level is elevated, so is the serum calcium level. When the patient has hypoalbuminemia, the patient will not be able to bind as much calcium, and the serum calcium level will appear low even as normal calcium levels exist. To assess the true body calcium level, the serum albumin levels must be assessed, and the calcium levels properly adjusted. The formula to correct measured calcium levels for assessment is:

Corrected Ca = [0.8 x (normal albumin - patient's albumin)] + serum Ca

In this instance the corrected Ca = [0.8 x (4 - 3.2)] + 8 = 8.6 mg/dL

194. A: 7

Mammals have 7 cervical vertebrae no matter the length of neck. Mammals also have 13 thoracic vertebrae, 7 lumbar vertebrae, and 3 sacral vertebrae. The number of caudal vertebrae varies.

195. C: Increased erythrocyte production

Reperfusion injury occurs when tissues previously deprived of oxygen receive an influx of oxygen. While the tissues need oxygen, the rapid alteration results in cellular damage, including the production of reactive oxygen species that interfere with cellular metabolism. Additionally, reperfusion can cause intracellular calcium handling changes and intracellular calcium overload, microvascular and endothelial cell dysfunction, and activation of neutrophils, platelets, and complement.

196. C: Meningioma

The most common primary brain tumor of the cat and dog is the meningioma, a brain tumor that originates in the arachnoid mater of the meninges, or membranes lining the brain. Meningiomas, fortunately, are rather slow-growing tumors and are relatively easily resected. Symptoms result from compression of brain tissue resulting in neurologic deficits.

197. D: Schirmer tear test, tear production

The Schirmer tear test is an easy, rapid test to assess tear production. The test strip is placed between the conjunctiva and the cornea. Tear movement up the strip is monitored and measured using either markings on the test strip or comparison against markings on the container. 15 mm or more of tear production over 1 minute is deemed sufficient for a dog. Some testers will end the test at 30 seconds so long as tear production is at or above 15mm.

The Schirmer tear test measures only the middle aqueous layer of tear production, not the inner mucin layer or outer lipid layer. Deficiency in tear production will leave the eye dry and predispose it to damage.

198. C: Plus or minus 2 rule

Schiotz tonometry is used to measure intraocular pressure. A topical anesthetic should be used on the cornea prior to tonometry. The tonometer should be zeroed and the foot plate rested evenly on the patient's cornea. The results are interpreted using the plus or minus 2 rule. If the 5-gram weight is used, a normal intraocular pressure is between 3 and 7 (5 minus 2 to 5 plus 2). A normal pressure falls between 5.5 and 9.5 when the 7.5-gram weight is used.

199. A: January 1

No matter the actual date of birth of a thoroughbred, all horses born in the same year are given a January 1 birthday. This birthday is set so that all horses born in a given year are all considered yearlings, two-year olds, or three-year olds. Horse owners attempt to manage thoroughbred reproduction so that foals are born as close to January 1 as possible, making them older, and likely larger, than foals born later in the year.

200. C: Teasing

A mare or group of mares under evaluation is exposed to a stallion. One on one, a mare is presented head to head to a stallion followed by his head to her tail. If the mare is estrual, or in heat, the stallion will exhibit a flehmen response. Teasing should take place every day or every other day to assess a mare's readiness to breed.

201. B: Echinocytes

Echinocytes are small, crenated (shrunken) erythrocytes characterized by the presence of 10-30 spikes or spicules on their outer membrane. Normally they are most numerous within the first 24 hours of envenomation, before the development of clinical signs, and will affect almost 100% of the red blood cells. After 2-3 days, the echinocytes steadily decrease in number and eventually become absent on a blood smear. It is important to note, however, that in some animals echinocytes do not appear at all following envenomation and that appropriate medical therapy will still need to be implemented.

202. C: Prostaglandin synthesis inhibition

Prostaglandins are chemicals that mediate an array of normal physiologic functions such as platelet aggregation, renal blood flow, and gastric acid production. In addition, they protect the cells lining the gastrointestinal (GI) tract from noxious chemicals. When over-the-counter NSAIDs are mistakenly given or accidentally ingested in large quantities, they work to inhibit prostaglandin synthesis, which can potentially lead to a myriad of life-threatening problems such as GI ulceration, clotting abnormalities, and kidney failure.

It is important to note that the toxic dose of any NSAID can vary between animals depending on individual sensitivities, and actual manifestation of clinical signs (melena, vomiting, etc.) can be delayed by up to 4 days following ingestion. This being said, many owners do not seek out veterinary care unless clinical signs are present and only after the damage has already been done. Thus, it is important to recommend to clients who may have administered or suspect that their animals have ingested any NSAID that their animal be seen immediately for a consultation.

203. B: Spinal fracture or luxation

Rabbits that are allowed to frantically kick, whether confined in a cage or while being restrained, or rabbits that are dropped can fracture or dislocate their lumbar vertebrae. The result is hind limb paresis or paralysis that only rarely responds to emergency medical therapy.

When handled or restrained, rabbits need to have their hind end fully supported. This can be accomplished with a "football" hold, whereby the rabbit's head is tucked into the handler's arm with one hand, and the other hand supports its hind end. If rabbits are kept at the clinic and become too excited in a cage, then they will need to be moved to a small carrier to prevent excessive movement.

204. C: Guinea pig

The pubic symphysis of guinea pigs fuses together between 7 and 8 months of age and is normally not an issue with nonbreeding females. Guinea pigs that are acquired for breeding purposes, however, and are bred after 6 months of age will experience difficult labor and possibly dystocia if they are unable to separate the symphysis during parturition.

205. D: Calcium oxalate

Calcium oxalate monohydrate urolithiasis is a common occurrence in animals that have ingested antifreeze (ethylene glycol). It occurs as a result of ethylene glycol metabolism in the liver, the end products of which are several potentially lethal toxic metabolites, one of which is oxalate. These metabolites direct their toxic effects on the kidneys by destroying renal epithelial cells as well as by obstructing the renal tubules, which ultimately results in acute renal failure.

206. B: Dermatophytes rapidly change the color of the DTM agar to red in as little as 3-5 days.

Dermatophytes can quickly change the color of the DTM agar to red in as few as 3-5 days, and before growth can be visualized by the naked eye. The caps on these samples need to be secured loosely to permit the flow of air into the sample, thus allowing growth of the dermatophyte. The sample should be kept at room temperature in a place where it can be easily seen and evaluated each day.

207. A: Fresh gas flow rate

In a nonrebreathing system, there is no CO_2 absorption, so the clearance of CO_2 is dependent on the use of high fresh gas flow rates (200-300 mL/kg/min). These rates are required to prevent buildup of CO_2, which can lead to the rebreathing of exhaled air. Flow rates below 200 mL/kg/min will result in the accumulation and rebreathing of exhaled gases, and the potential for the development of hypoxemia and hypercarbemia.

208. D: All of the above

A pop-off valve that is accidentally left closed during anesthesia can have catastrophic repercussions. Pressure will build up in the system, and as a result, the patient will not be able to exhale. If pressure continues to build in the thorax, there will be inadequate venous return to the heart. Ultimately, a patient could suffer a ruptured lung and subsequent pneumothorax. Thus, it is EXTREMELY important to remember to open a pop-off valve that has been closed, and always put the anesthetic machine away with the valve in the open position.

209. C: Sinus tachycardia

Sinus tachycardia is an increase in heart rate that can occur due to a variety of physiologic (i.e., exercise, pain, fear), pharmacologic (drugs such as atropine, epinephrine, acepromazine) or pathologic influences (i.e., anemia, heart failure, shock). The heart remains under the control of a normal SA node and the P-QRS-T complexes appear normal.

210. B: Apomorphine

Apomorphine is the most reliable and effective drug for the induction of emesis in canines. When administered intravenously or intramuscularly, apomorphine can produce emesis in a matter of minutes. It is also available in a tablet form that can be crushed and a small amount placed in the conjunctival sac.

Xylazine is an effective and fast-acting (1-2 minutes) emetic in cats. Hydrogen peroxide can induce vomiting in dogs by irritating the gastric mucosa. Results, however, are often not immediate and may not occur at all. Syrup of ipecac can also induce vomiting in dogs, but only after 15-30 minutes following administration. It must reach the intestine before it exerts is effects.

211. A: Front leg

The technician should administer the injection in a front leg in order to avoid the renal portal system in the caudal half of the body. The renal portal system is a complex of blood vessels associated with the kidneys. Injections given in the caudal half of the body could potentially be carried to the kidneys before entering the systemic circulation. As a result, the drug may not reach therapeutic levels because a portion may be excreted prematurely. Renal damage could also occur since the drug has not had an opportunity to be metabolized by the body.

212. C: The medication should be bolused as quickly as possible.

Caution must always be exercised when performing an intravenous (IV) injection in the jugular vein of horses because the carotid artery lies in close proximity to the jugular vein, and can therefore be mistakenly accessed even by the most experienced technicians. Steps to help minimize this error include utilizing the cranial third of the neck for venipuncture. This is because the artery does not lie in such close proximity to the vein as it does in the more caudal aspect of the neck.

Another tactic would be to insert a large bore needle first and watch the blood as it exits the hub. If it is a gentle drip, then the needle is in the vein. If it is a steady, pulsating stream, the needle is in the artery and needs to be readjusted. Once the needle is in the vein, the drug should be administered slowly in order to give the technician or veterinarian ample time to stop the injection in the event of an adverse reaction. For example, sometimes horses move during an injection and cause the needle to be redirected into the carotid artery. If medication is injected into the carotid artery, it travels straight to the brain where it can cause potentially lethal consequences. Thus, it is extremely important not to be overconfident with these injections, and always use good judgment and safe techniques.

213. C: Feline urologic syndrome (FUS).

Postrenal azotemia results from either an obstruction (i.e., foreign body, FUS, neoplasia) in the urinary outflow tract or interruption (i.e., rupture, laceration) of the urinary outflow tract leading to the escape of urine into the peritoneal cavity. Early in the course of the disease, lab findings usually demonstrate an increase in both the blood urea nitrogen (BUN) and creatinine values. Urine specific gravity is usually normal. Postrenal azotemia, however, can progress to intrinsic renal disease due to increased pressure in the urinary system or due to a sustained decrease in renal blood flow. The prognosis of postrenal azotemia is good if the underlying cause can be treated or corrected early in the course of disease.

214. A: 9 mL

First, convert pounds to kilograms: 75 lbs * 1 kg/2.2 lbs = 34 kg. Second, calculate how many milligrams of drug the patient requires: 34 kg * 8 mg/kg = 272 mg. Third, calculate the volume that will yield 272 mg of drug: 272 mg * 1 mL/30 mg = 9 mL.

215. C: Grids do not absorb any part of the primary beam.

In radiology, grids are used to help reduce the amount of scatter radiation when radiographing large areas (≥10 cm thick). They are needed because larger subjects require more kVp for penetration, and more kVp produces more scatter radiation, which ultimately results in a poor quality radiograph.

An important fact about grids is that they do indeed absorb some of the primary beam thereby necessitating an increase in exposure. This is accomplished by increasing the mAs before taking the radiograph.

216. D: All of the above.

The efficacy of any one vaccine is dependent on several variables. First and foremost, it must be stored in the proper conditions once it leaves the manufacturer. As a consumer, it is impossible to know if the store immediately refrigerated the vaccines after they arrived. Also, the consumer must transport the vaccine back home and may do so in less than optimal conditions. Perhaps this individual forgets that the vaccine is in the car, or runs errands on a hot day, thereby further endangering the vaccine's potency.

If the vaccine does happen to make it home without insult, there are still other variables that could produce a less than optimal immune response once it is injected. For example, the owner could inadvertently inject all the way through the skin, in which case the puppy receives no vaccine at all. If the owner starts the vaccine series too early (before 6 weeks), maternal antibodies will destroy the vaccine. Also, if the puppy is sick or is born with a weak immune system, it may not be able to mount a sufficient antibody response to the vaccine. In all these instances, vaccines will lose their efficacy, which is why it is important to educate the public about the dangers of store-bought vaccines and why exams are recommended before any vaccine is administered.

217. C: A type AB cat can be safely used as an in-house blood donor.

There are 3 described blood types in cats: A, B, and AB. Blood type A is the most prevalent and is seen in most domestic longhairs and shorthairs. Blood type B is not as common and is seen mostly in purebred cats, but not exclusively. Type AB is very rare and can be present in any cat. All cats have naturally occurring alloantibodies to blood types that are not their own. These antibodies can be very strong, as in the case of type B cats, or weak as with the type A cats. As a result, type B cats will undergo a severe reaction if transfused with type A blood. However, type A cats may not react at all with a transfusion of type B blood, but the transfused blood will only last a few days. Because of the presence of these alloantibodies, there can be no universal feline donor. A type AB cat is no exception.

218. D: Diets consisting of animal products and/or milk are acid producing and therefore, lower the pH of urine.

Diets rich in vegetable products will produce an alkaline urine sample. A urine sample that is allowed to stand at room temperature for an hour or more will become alkaline, so these must be checked within 20-30 minutes of collection or at least refrigerated to help prevent the sample from degrading. A urinary tract infection with urease producing bacteria will cause an alkaline urine sample because the enzyme urease converts urea to ammonia, which raises pH.

219. D: Adsorbent and protectant

Activated charcoal adsorbs to its surface many chemicals, toxins, and drugs in the upper gastrointestinal tract that would otherwise be absorbed systemically.

220. C: Analgesic

Diazepam is a benzodiazepine drug that has several clinical indications. In prescribed doses, it can function as an anxiolytic, a short-duration anticonvulsant, a muscle relaxant, and an appetite stimulant. Diazepam does not, however, provide any analgesia when administered by itself and therefore must be used in conjunction with specific pain-relieving drugs, such as opioids, when used for anesthetic purposes.

221. C: Day 20

Ultrasonography provides the earliest detection of pregnancy on day 20 of gestation in small animals. At this time the gestational sac should be readily visible.

222. C: 8 hours

It is always recommended to transfuse fresh whole blood immediately after collection so that the patient reaps the benefits of all the active components (coagulation factors, platelets, etc.). If this is not possible, however, the blood may be transfused within the next 6-8 hours and still retain is effectiveness. After 8 hours, the blood will need to be refrigerated to preserve the blood components that are still useful (proteins, cells, Vitamin K dependent clotting factors). Platelets and other more "delicate" coagulation factors in the blood become ineffective over time and with refrigeration.

223. C: Intramuscular

Bruising is a common sequela of intramuscular injections. Any bruised meat that is found at the time of slaughter will be either trimmed away, if possible, or thrown out altogether, which results in a financial loss for the cattle rancher.

224. C: Transducer frequency

The transducer frequency is ultimately responsible for the resolution of the ultrasound image. As frequency increases, the wavelength decreases and shorter wavelengths produce better resolution and overall quality of the image.

225. C: Ventricular premature complexes

Ventricular premature complexes (VPCs) occur as a result of an ectopic foci that discharge anywhere in the myocardial wall of the ventricle. The impulse is conducted cell-to-cell through the myocardium at a slow rate, versus more quickly through the intended Purkinje system, thereby producing an abnormally wide and bizarre QRS-T complex on ECG. VPCs are commonly seen with primary cardiac disease, secondary to trauma or systemic disease, or secondary to drug therapy.

It is important to understand that they rarely cause any hemodynamic impairment unless they occur frequently, in which case they should be treated to prevent progression to more serious and potentially fatal arrhythmias such as ventricular tachycardia or ventricular fibrillation.

226. B: Obesity

Obesity is the most common diet-related illness in pet hedgehogs and may occur as a result of overfeeding, lack of exercise, or high-fat diets. Obesity may lead to poor skin condition, hepatic lipidosis, respiratory and/or immune related disease, as well as skin fold dermatitis. It is therefore important to monitor the animal's weight frequently and to adjust the amount or type of food fed to the animal accordingly. Rickets and periodontal disease are other types of diet-related illness in hedgehogs that occur in unbalanced diets or diets that lack a hard consistency.

227. C: Acoustic shadowing

Acoustic shadowing is produced when soundwaves fail to travel through certain tissue like bone, or anomalies like bladder or gall stones. Since these soundwaves are completely attenuated, there is a shadow present directly posterior to these types of structures due to an absence of echoes.

228. D: Etomidate

Etomidate is a fast acting and short-lived induction agent that produces minimal cardiopulmonary effects, and is therefore the anesthetic of choice in patients with heart disease. Heart rate and rhythm, blood pressure, as well as respiratory rate are all maintained throughout anesthesia. Due to its short duration of action, etomidate is ideal to conduct brief studies such as examination and diagnostics on patients in extreme distress from cardiopulmonary disease that could easily die with any manipulation.

229. C: Crenation

Crenation occurs when RBCs lose water through osmosis because the extracellular fluid is more concentrated (hypertonic) than the intracellular fluid (isotonic). Hemolysis occurs when RBCs gain water through osmosis because the extracellular fluid is less concentrated (hypotonic) than the intracellular fluid. Clumping of RBCs is termed autoagglutination and is usually indicative of immune-mediated hemolytic anemia. RBCs that are clumped or stacked into a linear arrangement create a rouleaux formation (a normal finding in horses).

230. A: The nasogastric tube should be guided into the dorsal meatus of the horse's nasal passages.

A nasogastric tube placed properly into the ventral meatus will feed easily into the esophagus and meet little resistance along the way, providing there are no obstructions such as tumors or foreign objects.

Excessive force during nasogastric intubation can damage the ethmoturbinates of the equine nasal passages, which will result in an exorbitant amount of bleeding. Force can also rupture the esophagus if there is a foreign body present.

An equine stomach should always be checked for gastric reflux before introducing any water or medication. If an abnormally large amount of ingesta is present in the stomach (this is usually indicated when ingesta flows freely out of the nasogastric tube), then the delivery of medication or water should be postponed until the stomach empties. This will reduce the risk of gastric overfilling and potential rupture.

231. D: All of the above.

Casts are formed by the slow movement of material in the renal tubules and are molded by the tubular lumen. Casts are comprised predominantly of a protein matrix that also contains substances that were present in the tubule when the cast was formed, such as hyaline, white or red blood cells, or epithelial cells. When present in large numbers, they indicate active renal disease. Few casts, however, may not be significant, especially if not found on repeat sediment exams.

Casts readily dissolve in alkaline urine, so it is imperative that urine samples be evaluated immediately before the urine chemistry changes.

232. C: Malignant melanoma

Malignant melanoma is the most common oropharyngeal tumor in dogs and is usually located on the gingiva or on the buccal or labial mucosa. It may or may not be pigmented. Metastasis is very common with malignant melanoma (50% or more of cases), as is bone invasion (66% of cases), so preliminary diagnostics to determine stage of disease is recommended. Treatment usually involves a combination of surgical excision, radiation, immunotherapy, and/or chemotherapy. These treatments, however, still only afford a guarded prognosis.

233. D: Hookworms

Cutaneous larval migrans is a zoonotic disease in humans that is caused by the burrowing and migration of hookworm larvae intracutaneously, resulting in an intense dermatitis. Children who play in the dirt as well as people who are exposed to infected soil (gardeners, utility workers) are at risk of hookworm infection. These larvae migrate for long periods of time, and may penetrate into deeper tissues.

The zoonotic potential of many parasites necessitates the adoption of a comprehensive deworming program in any clinic. Technicians play a vital role in providing clients with vital information regarding these parasites so they can make informed decisions regarding the health of their pets and their families.

234. C: Periodontal ligament

The periodontal ligament is composed of connective fibers that serve to anchor the tooth root to the alveolar bone. In addition to this function, the periodontal ligament also provides nutrients to the alveolar bone and cementum through a network of arterioles, and also serves as a "shock absorber" during mastication.

235. D: Smooth the enamel

Dental polishing represents an integral part of the dental prophylaxis. Polishing decreases total tooth surface area by smoothing the enamel that was roughened and made irregular by the scaling process. By decreasing this surface area, polishing decreases the rate of plaque and calculus reattachment.

236. D: All of the above.

Mechanical scalers are an indispensable instrument during any prophylaxis and must be used properly to avoid accidental heat damage to the tooth surface. The amount of heat generated by the scaler can be reduced by using large amounts of water during the scaling process to cool the teeth, limiting the time spent on each tooth to only 5-10 seconds a piece, and only using the scaler at the speed that is recommended for the particular unit. In addition, it also helps not to use excessive force with the scaler, which can also create heat and further damage the enamel, possibly exposing the pulp.

237. B: Iris scissors

Iris scissors are small, fine, delicate scissors that are reserved for precise surgeries, usually involving the eye. Spencer scissors are used to remove sutures. Mayo scissors are common in surgery for cutting dense, thick tissue. Metzenbaum scissors are also used in surgery for delicate tissue dissection.

238. B: Rochester-Carmalt forceps

Rochester-Carmalt forceps are large, crushing, hemostatic forceps that are used to secure tissue bundles containing blood vessels such as uterine stumps or ovarian pedicles.

239. D: Both a and c

Instruments are placed in surgical milk following ultrasonic cleaning to keep the instruments lubricated as well as to help prevent the formation of rust. It has no cleaning or sterilizing properties.

240. B: Every 6-8 hours of use

The carbon dioxide absorbent needs to be changed after 6-8 hours of use, or every 30 days regardless of how little it has been used. The absorbent serves to "capture" exhaled CO_2 and convert it to carbonate. If all the absorbent has been consumed, the patient will start to accumulate CO_2 in the bloodstream (hypercapnia), which leads to respiratory acidosis.

241. D: Half hitch

A half hitch knot is recommended because it not only allows for easy release in case of an emergency, but also alleviates direct pressure on the skin when it is applied over 2 areas of contact.

242. D: All of the above.

When a surgeon requests a drain during a surgical procedure, he/she is anticipating an accumulation of air (dead space) or fluid (i.e., pus, serum, blood) in and/or around the surgical site. Procedures or conditions that warrant drain placement include abscesses, removal of large tumors that leave large gaps in muscle or tissue, limb amputation, or wounds that are difficult to clean completely. If drains are not utilized for these types of situations, the surgical site could swell or leak fluid, or continue to be infected, all of which can lead to suture dehiscence and the need for more surgery.

243. A: Hydrogen peroxide is an effective broad-spectrum antimicrobial.

Hydrogen peroxide is a common foaming wound irrigant that should only be used once for the initial cleansing of a contaminated wound. If used repeatedly, hydrogen peroxide can damage the surrounding healthy tissue, which results in delayed wound healing.

Hydrogen peroxide does not possess any significant antimicrobial properties and thus should not be used solely for this purpose. It does, however, have a certain amount of effectiveness against spores.

244. B: Their residual bactericidal effects are inactivated by blood or alcohol.

Chlorhexidine and povidone-iodine scrubs share many properties, however only povidone-iodine scrub is inactivated by alcohol and organic matter such as blood or body fluids.

245. B: Electric heating pad

Electric heating pads are extremely dangerous when used to warm an animal and should never be used. They provide intense, focal areas of heat to which an unconscious animal cannot react, resulting in very painful and necrosing thermal burns.

246. B: Butorphanol and fentanyl

Butorphanol should not be used in conjunction with fentanyl or any pure opioid agonist because it blocks the receptor (mu) in the brain to which the opioids bind to produce analgesia. Butorphanol is a mixed opioid agonist/antagonist meaning it stimulates certain receptors of the brain (kappa) to produce mild analgesia and moderate sedation, however it blocks the mu receptors, which are responsible for profound analgesia and mild sedation. So, when used together, a patient only receives the fleeting (45 minutes) analgesic effects of butorphanol versus the longer analgesic duration of the other pure opioid agonists, and is therefore experiencing pain most of the time.

247. A: Buprenorphine

Buprenorphine is an opioid analgesic in small animals that is used to control mild to moderate pain. Due to the unusual chemistry of the feline oral cavity, buprenorphine can be administered orally and still retain the same efficacy as an intramuscular or intravenous injection.

248. C: Glycopyrrolate

Glycopyrrolate is a preanesthetic anticholinergic that prevents or remedies the adverse effects (bradycardia, hypersalivation) of opioids, barbiturates, and dissociative anesthetics such as morphine, thiopental, and ketamine, respectively. As a parasympatholytic drug, glycopyrrolate also functions as a mydriatic, a bronchodilator as well as in inhibitor of intestinal motility. Because glycopyrrolate does not cross significantly through the blood-brain barrier, its effects on the central nervous system are less pronounced. It also should be noted that glycopyrrolate does not cross the placental barrier, which makes it an excellent preanesthetic drug for pregnant animals.

249. A: Elevate and stabilize hollow organs.

Stay sutures are an invaluable tool for isolating and elevating hollow organs that need to be incised, such as the bladder, intestine, or stomach. They are placed in the serosal surface of these organs on either side of the incision linearly and then secured with mosquito forceps. The organ is then gently elevated out of the abdominal cavity and placed over laparotomy pads, which will catch or reduce any spillage of urine or intestinal material that would otherwise contaminate the surgical area. They allow for better visualization and control over the surgical site.

250. B: Enalapril is an angiotensin-converting enzyme inhibitor and functions to reduce the workload on a diseased heart by promoting vasodilation.

Diuretics are substances that promote urine secretion, usually through a mechanism that enhances the excretion of sodium and water in the renal tubules. They are most commonly used to treat edema that occurs as a result of congestive heart failure, liver failure, or neuronal edema from head trauma. For example, mannitol is an osmotic diuretic that has a low molecular weight and is freely filtered by the kidneys. Its presence in the kidney will draw water and sodium into the tubules, thereby increasing urine flow. It is used primary in cases of cerebral edema. Furosemide is a drug that inhibits sodium chloride reabsorption in the ascending loop of Henle, again serving to increase urine flow. This drug is commonly used for congestive heart failure. Spironolactone is a drug that blocks the effects of the hormone aldosterone, a hormone that would ordinarily allow for sodium reabsorption in the renal tubules.

How to Overcome Test Anxiety

Just the thought of taking a test is enough to make most people a little nervous. A test is an important event that can have a long-term impact on your future, so it's important to take it seriously and it's natural to feel anxious about performing well. But just because anxiety is normal, that doesn't mean that it's helpful in test taking, or that you should simply accept it as part of your life. Anxiety can have a variety of effects. These effects can be mild, like making you feel slightly nervous, or severe, like blocking your ability to focus or remember even a simple detail.

If you experience test anxiety—whether severe or mild—it's important to know how to beat it. To discover this, first you need to understand what causes test anxiety.

Causes of Test Anxiety

While we often think of anxiety as an uncontrollable emotional state, it can actually be caused by simple, practical things. One of the most common causes of test anxiety is that a person does not feel adequately prepared for their test. This feeling can be the result of many different issues such as poor study habits or lack of organization, but the most common culprit is time management. Starting to study too late, failing to organize your study time to cover all of the material, or being distracted while you study will mean that you're not well prepared for the test. This may lead to cramming the night before, which will cause you to be physically and mentally exhausted for the test. Poor time management also contributes to feelings of stress, fear, and hopelessness as you realize you are not well prepared but don't know what to do about it.

Other times, test anxiety is not related to your preparation for the test but comes from unresolved fear. This may be a past failure on a test, or poor performance on tests in general. It may come from comparing yourself to others who seem to be performing better or from the stress of living up to expectations. Anxiety may be driven by fears of the future—how failure on this test would affect your educational and career goals. These fears are often completely irrational, but they can still negatively impact your test performance.

Review Video: 3 Reasons You Have Test Anxiety
Visit mometrix.com/academy and enter code: 428468

Elements of Test Anxiety

As mentioned earlier, test anxiety is considered to be an emotional state, but it has physical and mental components as well. Sometimes you may not even realize that you are suffering from test anxiety until you notice the physical symptoms. These can include trembling hands, rapid heartbeat, sweating, nausea, and tense muscles. Extreme anxiety may lead to fainting or vomiting. Obviously, any of these symptoms can have a negative impact on testing. It is important to recognize them as soon as they begin to occur so that you can address the problem before it damages your performance.

Review Video: 3 Ways to Tell You Have Test Anxiety
Visit mometrix.com/academy and enter code: 927847

The mental components of test anxiety include trouble focusing and inability to remember learned information. During a test, your mind is on high alert, which can help you recall information and stay focused for an extended period of time. However, anxiety interferes with your mind's natural processes, causing you to blank out, even on the questions you know well. The strain of testing during anxiety makes it difficult to stay focused, especially on a test that may take several hours. Extreme anxiety can take a huge mental toll, making it difficult not only to recall test information but even to understand the test questions or pull your thoughts together.

Review Video: How Test Anxiety Affects Memory
Visit mometrix.com/academy and enter code: 609003

Effects of Test Anxiety

Test anxiety is like a disease—if left untreated, it will get progressively worse. Anxiety leads to poor performance, and this reinforces the feelings of fear and failure, which in turn lead to poor performances on subsequent tests. It can grow from a mild nervousness to a crippling condition. If allowed to progress, test anxiety can have a big impact on your schooling, and consequently on your future.

Test anxiety can spread to other parts of your life. Anxiety on tests can become anxiety in any stressful situation, and blanking on a test can turn into panicking in a job situation. But fortunately, you don't have to let anxiety rule your testing and determine your grades. There are a number of relatively simple steps you can take to move past anxiety and function normally on a test and in the rest of life.

Review Video: How Test Anxiety Impacts Your Grades
Visit mometrix.com/academy and enter code: 939819

Physical Steps for Beating Test Anxiety

While test anxiety is a serious problem, the good news is that it can be overcome. It doesn't have to control your ability to think and remember information. While it may take time, you can begin taking steps today to beat anxiety.

Just as your first hint that you may be struggling with anxiety comes from the physical symptoms, the first step to treating it is also physical. Rest is crucial for having a clear, strong mind. If you are tired, it is much easier to give in to anxiety. But if you establish good sleep habits, your body and mind will be ready to perform optimally, without the strain of exhaustion. Additionally, sleeping well helps you to retain information better, so you're more likely to recall the answers when you see the test questions.

Getting good sleep means more than going to bed on time. It's important to allow your brain time to relax. Take study breaks from time to time so it doesn't get overworked, and don't study right before bed. Take time to rest your mind before trying to rest your body, or you may find it difficult to fall asleep.

Review Video: The Importance of Sleep for Your Brain
Visit mometrix.com/academy and enter code: 319338

Along with sleep, other aspects of physical health are important in preparing for a test. Good nutrition is vital for good brain function. Sugary foods and drinks may give a burst of energy but this burst is followed by a crash, both physically and emotionally. Instead, fuel your body with protein and vitamin-rich foods.

Also, drink plenty of water. Dehydration can lead to headaches and exhaustion, especially if your brain is already under stress from the rigors of the test. Particularly if your test is a long one, drink water during the breaks. And if possible, take an energy-boosting snack to eat between sections.

Review Video: How Diet Can Affect your Mood
Visit mometrix.com/academy and enter code: 624317

Along with sleep and diet, a third important part of physical health is exercise. Maintaining a steady workout schedule is helpful, but even taking 5-minute study breaks to walk can help get your blood pumping faster and clear your head. Exercise also releases endorphins, which contribute to a positive feeling and can help combat test anxiety.

When you nurture your physical health, you are also contributing to your mental health. If your body is healthy, your mind is much more likely to be healthy as well. So take time to rest, nourish your body with healthy food and water, and get moving as much as possible. Taking these physical steps will make you stronger and more able to take the mental steps necessary to overcome test anxiety.

Review Video: How to Stay Healthy and Prevent Test Anxiety
Visit mometrix.com/academy and enter code: 877894

Mental Steps for Beating Test Anxiety

Working on the mental side of test anxiety can be more challenging, but as with the physical side, there are clear steps you can take to overcome it. As mentioned earlier, test anxiety often stems from lack of preparation, so the obvious solution is to prepare for the test. Effective studying may be the most important weapon you have for beating test anxiety, but you can and should employ several other mental tools to combat fear.

First, boost your confidence by reminding yourself of past success—tests or projects that you aced. If you're putting as much effort into preparing for this test as you did for those, there's no reason you should expect to fail here. Work hard to prepare; then trust your preparation.

Second, surround yourself with encouraging people. It can be helpful to find a study group, but be sure that the people you're around will encourage a positive attitude. If you spend time with others who are anxious or cynical, this will only contribute to your own anxiety. Look for others who are motivated to study hard from a desire to succeed, not from a fear of failure.

Third, reward yourself. A test is physically and mentally tiring, even without anxiety, and it can be helpful to have something to look forward to. Plan an activity following the test, regardless of the outcome, such as going to a movie or getting ice cream.

When you are taking the test, if you find yourself beginning to feel anxious, remind yourself that you know the material. Visualize successfully completing the test. Then take a few deep, relaxing breaths and return to it. Work through the questions carefully but with confidence, knowing that you are capable of succeeding.

Developing a healthy mental approach to test taking will also aid in other areas of life. Test anxiety affects more than just the actual test—it can be damaging to your mental health and even contribute to depression. It's important to beat test anxiety before it becomes a problem for more than testing.

Review Video: Test Anxiety and Depression
Visit mometrix.com/academy and enter code: 904704

Study Strategy

Being prepared for the test is necessary to combat anxiety, but what does being prepared look like? You may study for hours on end and still not feel prepared. What you need is a strategy for test prep. The next few pages outline our recommended steps to help you plan out and conquer the challenge of preparation.

Step 1: Scope Out the Test

Learn everything you can about the format (multiple choice, essay, etc.) and what will be on the test. Gather any study materials, course outlines, or sample exams that may be available. Not only will this help you to prepare, but knowing what to expect can help to alleviate test anxiety.

Step 2: Map Out the Material

Look through the textbook or study guide and make note of how many chapters or sections it has. Then divide these over the time you have. For example, if a book has 15 chapters and you have five days to study, you need to cover three chapters each day. Even better, if you have the time, leave an extra day at the end for overall review after you have gone through the material in depth.

If time is limited, you may need to prioritize the material. Look through it and make note of which sections you think you already have a good grasp on, and which need review. While you are studying, skim quickly through the familiar sections and take more time on the challenging parts. Write out your plan so you don't get lost as you go. Having a written plan also helps you feel more in control of the study, so anxiety is less likely to arise from feeling overwhelmed at the amount to cover. A sample plan may look like this:

- Day 1: Skim chapters 1–4, study chapter 5 (especially pages 31–33)
- Day 2: Study chapters 6–7, skim chapters 8–9
- Day 3: Skim chapter 10, study chapters 11–12 (especially pages 87–90)
- Day 4: Study chapters 13–15
- Day 5: Overall review (focus most on chapters 5, 6, and 12), take practice test

Step 3: Gather Your Tools

Decide what study method works best for you. Do you prefer to highlight in the book as you study and then go back over the highlighted portions? Or do you type out notes of the important information? Or is it helpful to make flashcards that you can carry with you? Assemble the pens, index cards, highlighters, post-it notes, and any other materials you may need so you won't be distracted by getting up to find things while you study.

If you're having a hard time retaining the information or organizing your notes, experiment with different methods. For example, try color-coding by subject with colored pens, highlighters, or post-it notes. If you learn better by hearing, try recording yourself reading your notes so you can listen while in the car, working out, or simply sitting at your desk. Ask a friend to quiz you from your flashcards, or try teaching someone the material to solidify it in your mind.

Step 4: Create Your Environment

It's important to avoid distractions while you study. This includes both the obvious distractions like visitors and the subtle distractions like an uncomfortable chair (or a too-comfortable couch that makes you want to fall asleep). Set up the best study environment possible: good lighting and a comfortable work area. If background music helps you focus, you may want to turn it on, but otherwise keep the room quiet. If you are using a computer to take notes, be sure you don't have any other windows open, especially applications like social media, games, or anything else that could distract you. Silence your phone and turn off notifications. Be sure to keep water close by so you stay hydrated while you study (but avoid unhealthy drinks and snacks).

Also, take into account the best time of day to study. Are you freshest first thing in the morning? Try to set aside some time then to work through the material. Is your mind clearer in the afternoon or evening? Schedule your study session then. Another method is to study at the same time of day that you will take the test, so that your brain gets used to working on the material at that time and will be ready to focus at test time.

Step 5: Study!

Once you have done all the study preparation, it's time to settle into the actual studying. Sit down, take a few moments to settle your mind so you can focus, and begin to follow your study plan. Don't give in to distractions or let yourself procrastinate. This is your time to prepare so you'll be ready to fearlessly approach the test. Make the most of the time and stay focused.

Of course, you don't want to burn out. If you study too long you may find that you're not retaining the information very well. Take regular study breaks. For example, taking five minutes out of every hour to walk briskly, breathing deeply and swinging your arms, can help your mind stay fresh.

As you get to the end of each chapter or section, it's a good idea to do a quick review. Remind yourself of what you learned and work on any difficult parts. When you feel that you've mastered the material, move on to the next part. At the end of your study session, briefly skim through your notes again.

But while review is helpful, cramming last minute is NOT. If at all possible, work ahead so that you won't need to fit all your study into the last day. Cramming overloads your brain with more information than it can process and retain, and your tired mind may struggle to recall even previously learned information when it is overwhelmed with last-minute study. Also, the urgent nature of cramming and the stress placed on your brain contribute to anxiety. You'll be more likely to go to the test feeling unprepared and having trouble thinking clearly.

So don't cram, and don't stay up late before the test, even just to review your notes at a leisurely pace. Your brain needs rest more than it needs to go over the information again. In fact, plan to finish your studies by noon or early afternoon the day before the test. Give your brain the rest of the day to relax or focus on other things, and get a good night's sleep. Then you will be fresh for the test and better able to recall what you've studied.

Step 6: Take a practice test

Many courses offer sample tests, either online or in the study materials. This is an excellent resource to check whether you have mastered the material, as well as to prepare for the test format and environment.

Check the test format ahead of time: the number of questions, the type (multiple choice, free response, etc.), and the time limit. Then create a plan for working through them. For example, if you have 30 minutes to take a 60-question test, your limit is 30 seconds per question. Spend less time on the questions you know well so that you can take more time on the difficult ones.

If you have time to take several practice tests, take the first one open book, with no time limit. Work through the questions at your own pace and make sure you fully understand them. Gradually work up to taking a test under test conditions: sit at a desk with all study materials put away and set a timer. Pace yourself to make sure you finish the test with time to spare and go back to check your answers if you have time.

After each test, check your answers. On the questions you missed, be sure you understand why you missed them. Did you misread the question (tests can use tricky wording)? Did you forget the information? Or was it something you hadn't learned? Go back and study any shaky areas that the practice tests reveal.

Taking these tests not only helps with your grade, but also aids in combating test anxiety. If you're already used to the test conditions, you're less likely to worry about it, and working through tests until you're scoring well gives you a confidence boost. Go through the practice tests until you feel comfortable, and then you can go into the test knowing that you're ready for it.

Test Tips

On test day, you should be confident, knowing that you've prepared well and are ready to answer the questions. But aside from preparation, there are several test day strategies you can employ to maximize your performance.

First, as stated before, get a good night's sleep the night before the test (and for several nights before that, if possible). Go into the test with a fresh, alert mind rather than staying up late to study.

Try not to change too much about your normal routine on the day of the test. It's important to eat a nutritious breakfast, but if you normally don't eat breakfast at all, consider eating just a protein bar. If you're a coffee drinker, go ahead and have your normal coffee. Just make sure you time it so that the caffeine doesn't wear off right in the middle of your test. Avoid sugary beverages, and drink enough water to stay hydrated but not so much that you need a restroom break 10 minutes into the test. If your test isn't first thing in the morning, consider going for a walk or doing a light workout before the test to get your blood flowing.

Allow yourself enough time to get ready, and leave for the test with plenty of time to spare so you won't have the anxiety of scrambling to arrive in time. Another reason to be early is to select a good seat. It's helpful to sit away from doors and windows, which can be distracting. Find a good seat, get out your supplies, and settle your mind before the test begins.

When the test begins, start by going over the instructions carefully, even if you already know what to expect. Make sure you avoid any careless mistakes by following the directions.

Then begin working through the questions, pacing yourself as you've practiced. If you're not sure on an answer, don't spend too much time on it, and don't let it shake your confidence. Either skip it and come back later, or eliminate as many wrong answers as possible and guess among the remaining ones. Don't dwell on these questions as you continue—put them out of your mind and focus on what lies ahead.

Be sure to read all of the answer choices, even if you're sure the first one is the right answer. Sometimes you'll find a better one if you keep reading. But don't second-guess yourself if you do immediately know the answer. Your gut instinct is usually right. Don't let test anxiety rob you of the information you know.

If you have time at the end of the test (and if the test format allows), go back and review your answers. Be cautious about changing any, since your first instinct tends to be correct, but make sure you didn't misread any of the questions or accidentally mark the wrong answer choice. Look over any you skipped and make an educated guess.

At the end, leave the test feeling confident. You've done your best, so don't waste time worrying about your performance or wishing you could change anything. Instead, celebrate the successful completion of this test. And finally, use this test to learn how to deal with anxiety even better next time.

Review Video: 5 Tips to Beat Test Anxiety
Visit mometrix.com/academy and enter code: 570656

Important Qualification

Not all anxiety is created equal. If your test anxiety is causing major issues in your life beyond the classroom or testing center, or if you are experiencing troubling physical symptoms related to your anxiety, it may be a sign of a serious physiological or psychological condition. If this sounds like your situation, we strongly encourage you to seek professional help.

How to Overcome Your Fear of Math

The word *math* is enough to strike fear into most hearts. How many of us have memories of sitting through confusing lectures, wrestling over mind-numbing homework, or taking tests that still seem incomprehensible even after hours of study? Years after graduation, many still shudder at these memories.

The fact is, math is not just a classroom subject. It has real-world implications that you face every day, whether you realize it or not. This may be balancing your monthly budget, deciding how many supplies to buy for a project, or simply splitting a meal check with friends. The idea of daily confrontations with math can be so paralyzing that some develop a condition known as *math anxiety*.

But you do NOT need to be paralyzed by this anxiety! In fact, while you may have thought all your life that you're not good at math, or that your brain isn't wired to understand it, the truth is that you may have been conditioned to think this way. From your earliest school days, the way you were taught affected the way you viewed different subjects. And the way math has been taught has changed.

Several decades ago, there was a shift in American math classrooms. The focus changed from traditional problem-solving to a conceptual view of topics, de-emphasizing the importance of learning the basics and building on them. The solid foundation necessary for math progression and confidence was undermined. Math became more of a vague concept than a concrete idea. Today, it is common to think of math, not as a straightforward system, but as a mysterious, complicated method that can't be fully understood unless you're a genius.

This is why you may still have nightmares about being called on to answer a difficult problem in front of the class. Math anxiety is a very real, though unnecessary, fear.

Math anxiety may begin with a single class period. Let's say you missed a day in 6th grade math and never quite understood the concept that was taught while you were gone. Since math is cumulative, with each new concept building on past ones, this could very well affect the rest of your math career. Without that one day's knowledge, it will be difficult to understand any other concepts that link to it. Rather than realizing that you're just missing one key piece, you may begin to believe that you're simply not capable of understanding math.

This belief can change the way you approach other classes, career options, and everyday life experiences, if you become anxious at the thought that math might be required. A student who loves science may choose a different path of study upon realizing that multiple math classes will be required for a degree. An aspiring medical student may hesitate at the thought of going through the necessary math classes. For some this anxiety escalates into a more extreme state known as *math phobia*.

Math anxiety is challenging to address because it is rooted deeply and may come from a variety of causes: an embarrassing moment in class, a teacher who did not explain concepts well and contributed to a shaky foundation, or a failed test that contributed to the belief of math failure.

These causes add up over time, encouraged by society's popular view that math is hard and unpleasant. Eventually a person comes to firmly believe that he or she is simply bad at math. This belief makes it difficult to grasp new concepts or even remember old ones. Homework and test grades begin to slip, which only confirms the belief. The poor performance is not due to lack of ability but is caused by math anxiety.

Math anxiety is an emotional issue, not a lack of intelligence. But when it becomes deeply rooted, it can become more than just an emotional problem. Physical symptoms appear. Blood pressure may rise and heartbeat may quicken at the sight of a math problem – or even the thought of math! This fear leads to a mental block. When someone with math anxiety is asked to perform a calculation, even a basic problem can seem overwhelming and impossible. The emotional and physical response to the thought of math prevents the brain from working through it logically.

The more this happens, the more a person's confidence drops, and the more math anxiety is generated. This vicious cycle must be broken!

The first step in breaking the cycle is to go back to very beginning and make sure you really understand the basics of how math works and why it works. It is not enough to memorize rules for multiplication and division. If you don't know WHY these rules work, your foundation will be shaky and you will be at risk of developing a phobia. Understanding mathematical concepts not only promotes confidence and security, but allows you to build on this understanding for new concepts. Additionally, you can solve unfamiliar problems using familiar concepts and processes.

Why is it that students in other countries regularly outperform American students in math? The answer likely boils down to a couple of things: the foundation of mathematical conceptual understanding and societal perception. While students in the US are not expected to *like* or *get* math, in many other nations, students are expected not only to understand math but also to excel at it.

Changing the American view of math that leads to math anxiety is a monumental task. It requires changing the training of teachers nationwide, from kindergarten through high school, so that they learn to teach the *why* behind math and to combat the wrong math views that students may develop. It also involves changing the stigma associated with math, so that it is no longer viewed as unpleasant and incomprehensible. While these are necessary changes, they are challenging and will take time. But in the meantime, math anxiety is not irreversible—it can be faced and defeated, one person at a time.

False Beliefs

One reason math anxiety has taken such hold is that several false beliefs have been created and shared until they became widely accepted. Some of these unhelpful beliefs include the following:

There is only one way to solve a math problem. In the same way that you can choose from different driving routes and still arrive at the same house, you can solve a math problem using different methods and still find the correct answer. A person who understands the reasoning behind math calculations may be able to look at an unfamiliar concept and find the right answer, just by applying logic to the knowledge they already have. This approach may be different than what is taught in the classroom, but it is still valid. Unfortunately, even many teachers view math as a subject where the best course of action is to memorize the rule or process for each problem rather than as a place for students to exercise logic and creativity in finding a solution.

Many people don't have a mind for math. A person who has struggled due to poor teaching or math anxiety may falsely believe that he or she doesn't have the mental capacity to grasp mathematical concepts. Most of the time, this is false. Many people find that when they are relieved of their math anxiety, they have more than enough brainpower to understand math.

Men are naturally better at math than women. Even though research has shown this to be false, many young women still avoid math careers and classes because of their belief that their math abilities are inferior. Many girls have come to believe that math is a male skill and have given up trying to understand or enjoy it.

Counting aids are bad. Something like counting on your fingers or drawing out a problem to visualize it may be frowned on as childish or a crutch, but these devices can help you get a tangible understanding of a problem or a concept.

Sadly, many students buy into these ideologies at an early age. A young girl who enjoys math class may be conditioned to think that she doesn't actually have the brain for it because math is for boys, and may turn her energies to other pursuits, permanently closing the door on a wide range of opportunities. A child who finds the right answer but doesn't follow the teacher's method may believe that he is doing it wrong and isn't good at math. A student who never had a problem with math before may have a poor teacher and become confused, yet believe that the problem is because she doesn't have a mathematical mind.

Students who have bought into these erroneous beliefs quickly begin to add their own anxieties, adapting them to their own personal situations:

I'll never use this in real life. A huge number of people wrongly believe that math is irrelevant outside the classroom. By adopting this mindset, they are handicapping themselves for a life in a mathematical world, as well as limiting their career choices. When they are inevitably faced with real-world math, they are conditioning themselves to respond with anxiety.

I'm not quick enough. While timed tests and quizzes, or even simply comparing yourself with other students in the class, can lead to this belief, speed is not an indicator of skill level. A person can work very slowly yet understand at a deep level.

If I can understand it, it's too easy. People with a low view of their own abilities tend to think that if they are able to grasp a concept, it must be simple. They cannot accept the idea that they are capable of understanding math. This belief will make it harder to learn, no matter how intelligent they are.

I just can't learn this. An overwhelming number of people think this, from young children to adults, and much of the time it is simply not true. But this mindset can turn into a self-fulfilling prophecy that keeps you from exercising and growing your math ability.

The good news is, each of these myths can be debunked. For most people, they are based on emotion and psychology, NOT on actual ability! It will take time, effort, and the desire to change, but change is possible. Even if you have spent years thinking that you don't have the capability to understand math, it is not too late to uncover your true ability and find relief from the anxiety that surrounds math.

Math Strategies

It is important to have a plan of attack to combat math anxiety. There are many useful strategies for pinpointing the fears or myths and eradicating them:

Go back to the basics. For most people, math anxiety stems from a poor foundation. You may think that you have a complete understanding of addition and subtraction, or even decimals and percentages, but make absolutely sure. Learning math is different from learning other subjects. For example, when you learn history, you study various time periods and places and events. It may be important to memorize dates or find out about the lives of famous people. When you move from US history to world history, there will be some overlap, but a large amount of the information will be new. Mathematical concepts, on the other hand, are very closely linked and highly dependent on each other. It's like climbing a ladder – if a rung is missing from your understanding, it may be difficult or impossible for you to climb any higher, no matter how hard you try. So go back and make sure your math foundation is strong. This may mean taking a remedial math course, going to a tutor to work through the shaky concepts, or just going through your old homework to make sure you really understand it.

Speak the language. Math has a large vocabulary of terms and phrases unique to working problems. Sometimes these are completely new terms, and sometimes they are common words, but are used differently in a math setting. If you can't speak the language, it will be very difficult to get a thorough understanding of the concepts. It's common for students to think that they don't understand math when they simply don't understand the vocabulary. The good news is that this is fairly easy to fix. Brushing up on any terms you aren't quite sure of can help bring the rest of the concepts into focus.

Check your anxiety level. When you think about math, do you feel nervous or uncomfortable? Do you struggle with feelings of inadequacy, even on concepts that you know you've already learned? It's important to understand your specific math anxieties, and what triggers them. When you catch yourself falling back on a false belief, mentally replace it with the truth. Don't let yourself believe that you can't learn, or that struggling with a concept means you'll never understand it. Instead, remind yourself of how much you've already learned and dwell on that past success. Visualize grasping the new concept, linking it to your old knowledge, and moving on to the next challenge. Also, learn how to manage anxiety when it arises. There are many techniques for coping with the irrational fears that rise to the surface when you enter the math classroom. This may include controlled breathing, replacing negative thoughts with positive ones, or visualizing success. Anxiety interferes with your ability to concentrate and absorb information, which in turn contributes to greater anxiety. If you can learn how to regain control of your thinking, you will be better able to pay attention, make progress, and succeed!

Don't go it alone. Like any deeply ingrained belief, math anxiety is not easy to eradicate. And there is no need for you to wrestle through it on your own. It will take time, and many people find that speaking with a counselor or psychiatrist helps. They can help you develop strategies for responding to anxiety and overcoming old ideas. Additionally, it can be very helpful to take a short course or seek out a math tutor to help you find and fix the missing rungs on your ladder and make sure that you're ready to progress to the next level. You can also find a number of math aids online: courses that will teach you mental devices for figuring out problems, how to get the most out of your math classes, etc.

Check your math attitude. No matter how much you want to learn and overcome your anxiety, you'll have trouble if you still have a negative attitude toward math. If you think it's too hard, or just have general feelings of dread about math, it will be hard to learn and to break through the anxiety. Work on cultivating a positive math attitude. Remind yourself that math is not just a hurdle to be cleared, but a valuable asset. When you view math with a positive attitude, you'll be much more likely to understand and even enjoy it. This is something you must do for yourself. You may find it helpful to visit with a counselor. Your tutor, friends, and family may cheer you on in your endeavors. But your greatest asset is yourself. You are inside your own mind – tell yourself what you need to hear. Relive past victories. Remind yourself that you are capable of understanding math. Root out any false beliefs that linger and replace them with positive truths. Even if it doesn't feel true at first, it will begin to affect your thinking and pave the way for a positive, anxiety-free mindset.

Aside from these general strategies, there are a number of specific practical things you can do to begin your journey toward overcoming math anxiety. Something as simple as learning a new note-taking strategy can change the way you approach math and give you more confidence and understanding. New study techniques can also make a huge difference.

Math anxiety leads to bad habits. If it causes you to be afraid of answering a question in class, you may gravitate toward the back row. You may be embarrassed to ask for help. And you may procrastinate on assignments, which leads to rushing through them at the last moment when it's too late to get a better understanding. It's important to identify your negative behaviors and replace them with positive ones:

Prepare ahead of time. Read the lesson before you go to class. Being exposed to the topics that will be covered in class ahead of time, even if you don't understand them perfectly, is extremely helpful in increasing what you retain from the lecture. Do your homework and, if you're still shaky, go over some extra problems. The key to a solid understanding of math is practice.

Sit front and center. When you can easily see and hear, you'll understand more, and you'll avoid the distractions of other students if no one is in front of you. Plus, you're more likely to be sitting with students who are positive and engaged, rather than others with math anxiety. Let their positive math attitude rub off on you.

Ask questions in class and out. If you don't understand something, just ask. If you need a more in-depth explanation, the teacher may need to work with you outside of class, but often it's a simple concept you don't quite understand, and a single question may clear it up. If you wait, you may not be able to follow the rest of the day's lesson. For extra help, most professors have office hours outside of class when you can go over concepts one-on-one to clear up any uncertainties. Additionally, there may be a *math lab* or study session you can attend for homework help. Take advantage of this.

Review. Even if you feel that you've fully mastered a concept, review it periodically to reinforce it. Going over an old lesson has several benefits: solidifying your understanding, giving you a confidence boost, and even giving some new insights into material that you're currently learning! Don't let yourself get rusty. That can lead to problems with learning later concepts.

Teaching Tips

While the math student's mindset is the most crucial to overcoming math anxiety, it is also important for others to adjust their math attitudes. Teachers and parents have an enormous influence on how students relate to math. They can either contribute to math confidence or math anxiety.

As a parent or teacher, it is very important to convey a positive math attitude. Retelling horror stories of your own bad experience with math will contribute to a new generation of math anxiety. Even if you don't share your experiences, others will be able to sense your fears and may begin to believe them.

Even a careless comment can have a big impact, so watch for phrases like *He's not good at math* or *I never liked math*. You are a crucial role model, and your children or students will unconsciously adopt your mindset. Give them a positive example to follow. Rather than teaching them to fear the math world before they even know it, teach them about all its potential and excitement.

Work to present math as an integral, beautiful, and understandable part of life. Encourage creativity in solving problems. Watch for false beliefs and dispel them. Cross the lines between subjects: integrate history, English, and music with math. Show students how math is used every day, and how the entire world is based on mathematical principles, from the pull of gravity to the shape of seashells. Instead of letting students see math as a necessary evil, direct them to view it as an imaginative, beautiful art form – an art form that they are capable of mastering and using.

Don't give too narrow a view of math. It is more than just numbers. Yes, working problems and learning formulas is a large part of classroom math. But don't let the teaching stop there. Teach students about the everyday implications of math. Show them how nature works according to the laws of mathematics, and take them outside to make discoveries of their own. Expose them to math-related careers by inviting visiting speakers, asking students to do research and presentations, and learning students' interests and aptitudes on a personal level.

Demonstrate the importance of math. Many people see math as nothing more than a required stepping stone to their degree, a nuisance with no real usefulness. Teach students that algebra is used every day in managing their bank accounts, in following recipes, and in scheduling the day's events. Show them how learning to do geometric proofs helps them to develop logical thinking, an invaluable life skill. Let them see that math surrounds them and is integrally linked to their daily lives: that weather predictions are based on math, that math was used to design cars and other machines, etc. Most of all, give them the tools to use math to enrich their lives.

Make math as tangible as possible. Use visual aids and objects that can be touched. It is much easier to grasp a concept when you can hold it in your hands and manipulate it, rather than just listening to the lecture. Encourage math outside of the classroom. The real world is full of measuring, counting, and calculating, so let students participate in this. Keep your eyes open for numbers and patterns to discuss. Talk about how scores are calculated in sports games and how far apart plants are placed in a garden row for maximum growth. Build the mindset that math is a normal and interesting part of daily life.

Finally, find math resources that help to build a positive math attitude. There are a number of books that show math as fascinating and exciting while teaching important concepts, for example: *The Math Curse; A Wrinkle in Time; The Phantom Tollbooth;* and *Fractals, Googols and Other Mathematical Tales*. You can also find a number of online resources: math puzzles and games, videos that show math in nature, and communities of math enthusiasts. On a local level, students can compete in a variety of math competitions with other schools or join a math club.

The student who experiences math as exciting and interesting is unlikely to suffer from math anxiety. Going through life without this handicap is an immense advantage and opens many doors that others have closed through their fear.

Self-Check

Whether you suffer from math anxiety or not, chances are that you have been exposed to some of the false beliefs mentioned above. Now is the time to check yourself for any errors you may have accepted. Do you think you're not wired for math? Or that you don't need to understand it since you're not planning on a math career? Do you think math is just too difficult for the average person?

Find the errors you've taken to heart and replace them with positive thinking. Are you capable of learning math? Yes! Can you control your anxiety? Yes! These errors will resurface from time to time, so be watchful. Don't let others with math anxiety influence you or sway your confidence. If you're having trouble with a concept, find help. Don't let it discourage you!

Create a plan of attack for defeating math anxiety and sharpening your skills. Do some research and decide if it would help you to take a class, get a tutor, or find some online resources to fine-tune your knowledge. Make the effort to get good nutrition, hydration, and sleep so that you are operating at full capacity. Remind yourself daily that you are skilled and that anxiety does not control you. Your mind is capable of so much more than you know. Give it the tools it needs to grow and thrive.

Thank You

We at Mometrix would like to extend our heartfelt thanks to you, our friend and patron, for allowing us to play a part in your journey. It is a privilege to serve people from all walks of life who are unified in their commitment to building the best future they can for themselves.

The preparation you devote to these important testing milestones may be the most valuable educational opportunity you have for making a real difference in your life. We encourage you to put your heart into it—that feeling of succeeding, overcoming, and yes, conquering will be well worth the hours you've invested.

We want to hear your story, your struggles and your successes, and if you see any opportunities for us to improve our materials so we can help others even more effectively in the future, please share that with us as well. **The team at Mometrix would be absolutely thrilled to hear from you!** So please, send us an email (support@mometrix.com) and let's stay in touch.

If you'd like some additional help, check out these other resources we offer for your exam:
http://MometrixFlashcards.com/VTNE

Additional Bonus Material

Due to our efforts to try to keep this book to a manageable length, we've created a link that will give you access to all of your additional bonus material.

Please visit https://www.mometrix.com/bonus948/vtne to access the information.